Diseases of the Parathyroid Glands

Angelo A. Licata • Edgar V. Lerma
Editors

Diseases of the Parathyroid Glands

Springer

Editors
Angelo A. Licata, MD, PhD
Departments of Biomedical Engineering
and Endocrinology-Metabolism
Cleveland Clinic
Cleveland, OH, USA

Edgar V. Lerma, MD
Department of Medicine
Section of Nephrology
University of Illinois at Chicago
College of Medicine
Associates in Nephrology, SC
Chicago, IL, USA

ISBN 978-1-4419-5549-4 e-ISBN 978-1-4419-5550-0
DOI 10.1007/978-1-4419-5550-0
Springer New York Dordrecht Heidelberg London

Library of Congress Control Number: 2012933755

Printed on acid-free paper

Springer is part of Springer Science+Business Media (www.springer.com)

To my mentors, colleagues, and friends, at the University of Santo Tomas Faculty of Medicine and Surgery in Manila, Philippines, and Northwestern University Feinberg School of Medicine, who have guided me to where I am right now …

To all the medical students, interns, and residents at Advocate Christ Medical Center whom I have taught or learned from,

To my parents and my brothers, without whose unremitting love and caring, and support through thick and thin, I would not have persevered and reached my goals in life …

Most especially, to my two lovely daughters Anastasia Zofia and Isabella Ann, whose smiles and laughter constantly provide me joy and happiness; and my very loving and understanding wife Michelle, who has always been supportive of my endeavors, and who sacrificed a lot of time and exhibited unparalleled patience as I devoted a significant amount of time and effort to this project. Truly, they are my inspiration.

– Edgar V. Lerma

To Cookie,

For her smiles, laughter, happiness, and patience

– Angelo A. Licata

Preface

Parathyroid disease is one of the most common endocrine disorders in general medical practice. It is generally manifested by hyperparathyroidism and less often by hypoparathyroidism. Hyperparathyroid disease is seen more often than previously. It is usually present as solitary disease but can rarely be associated with multiple endocrine neoplastic disorders. It is generally sporadic in nature but a genetic component is now appreciated in many families. Due to automated chemical testing procedures run in general medical practice, hypercalcemia, the telltale sign of the disorder, is found very frequently in the early stage of the disease when it is generally asymptomatic in most patients. Although kidney stones, osteoporosis, fractures, gastrointestinal disease, and psychological problems are the classic textbook findings once considered pathognomonic of the disorder, these problems are now relatively rare. The presence of hypercalcemia and increased parathyroid hormone levels is generally considered diagnostic for the disease. Nowadays, however, normal levels of calcium in the blood along with elevated, or inappropriate levels of parathyroid hormone with respect to the ambient serum calcium, may be characteristic of the entity called eucalcemic or normocalcemic hyperparathyroidism. This is an especially challenging entity to diagnose because of the sporadic fluctuations in serum calcium levels seen in patients from day-to-day. Coupling this with the commonly seen Vitamin D deficiency wherein a high serum PTH level and normal serum calcium is very frequently seen, makes this eucalcemic entity harder to diagnose.

Another entity that involves hyperfunctioning of the parathyroid gland is secondary hyperparathyroidism (also traditionally referred to as renal osteodystrophy), and its relation to chronic kidney disease. It has been recognized that as kidney function deteriorates, there is a progressive alteration in normal mineral homeostasis, with a disruption of serum and tissue concentrations of phosphorus and calcium, and changes in circulating levels of hormones which include parathyroid hormone (PTH), 25-hydroxyvitamin D (25(OH)D), 1,25-dihydroxyvitamin D (1,25(OH)$_2$D), and other Vitamin D metabolites, fibroblast growth factor-23 (FGF-23), and growth hormone. Even in moderately advanced kidney disease (Stage 3 CKD), the ability of the kidneys to appropriately excrete a phosphate load is compromised, thereby leading to hyperphosphatemia, elevated PTH, and decreased 1,25(OH)$_2$D with associated elevations in the levels of FGF-23. The conversion of 25(OH)D to

$1,25(OH)_2D$ is also impaired, leading to decreased intestinal calcium absorption and increased PTH. The kidney fails to respond (resistance) adequately to PTH, which normally promotes phosphaturia and calcium reabsorption, or to FGF-23, which also enhances phosphate excretion. At the tissue level, there is also downregulation of Vitamin D receptor and of resistance to the actions of PTH. In fact, therapy is generally centered on correcting these biochemical and hormonal abnormalities in an effort to limit the complications that arise there from.

The mineral and endocrine functions disrupted in CKD are critically important in the regulation of both initial bone formation during growth (bone modeling) and bone structure and function during adulthood (bone remodeling). As a result, bone abnormalities are found almost universally in patients with advanced stages of CKD (stage 5 CKD; or those requiring dialysis), and in the majority of patients with CKD stages 3–5. More recently, there has been an increasing concern of extraskeletal calcification, i.e. calciphylaxis, that may result from the deranged mineral and bone metabolism of CKD and from the therapies used to correct these abnormalities.

Hypoparathyroidism, on the other hand, tends to be a more symptomatic problem in most cases because it is associated with hypocalcemia and its resulting muscular and neurological problems. Most of these cases follow from postoperative sequellae of neck surgery and resulting parathyroid gland(s) injury; congenital problems are seen, but rarely so. Hypocalcemia, the hallmark of this particular disorder, is not generally missed on routine laboratory testing. Corroboration of its existence by adjusting for serum albumin is well appreciated by all practitioners. Failure to find increased parathyroid hormone levels in this scenario is the hallmark of hypoparathyroidism. Rare problems such as pseudo-hypoparathyroidism can clinically mimic true hypoparathyroidism. Attention to clinical history and symptoms usually aides clinicians in recognizing the distinction. But with the advent of the new assays for parathyroid hormone, these particular problems have become easier to diagnose. The assay for intact parathyroid hormone has made it possible to accurately discern excess of the hormone in the pseudo-state and deficiency of the hormone in real hypoparathyroid state.

For practitioners of all stages of experience, diseases of the parathyroid glands are not as easily deciphered as most textbooks would indicate. There are many subtleties to its pathology and diagnosis. The wealth of new information from molecular medicine makes it very challenging for the individual practitioner to have a total picture of these entities. To help clinicians, this book was developed. It is a small user-friendly text. It provides a present day background on mineral physiology and its regulation and couples this with a variety of clinical topics on parathyroid gland pathology.

Introductory chapters cover calcium regulation and parathyroid gland physiology, drawing upon many of the new aspects of glandular control mechanisms beyond the classical ones associated with calcium alone. The majority of the text covers clinical problems. Although most chapters address problems in adult medicine, three separate chapters are devoted to pediatric problems of hyper- and hypoparathyroidsm and parathormone resistance states. The clinical material for adults is introduced with a general chapter about the patient with calcium problems. The following chapters cover a broad spectrum of topics, such as diseases of the calcium receptor, new aspects of primary and secondary parathyroid disease, the hypoparathyroid and pseudohypoparathyroid patient, pathophysiology of PTH-related protein and its diseases, multiple endocrine neoplasia, and familial hypocalcuric hypercalcemia. There are several chapters on less common but equally challenging problems, such as parathyroid cancer, calciphylaxis, cystic lesions of the glands, and ectopic glandular disease. The final chapters of the text detail the techniques of parathyroid gland imaging and surgical treatment.

From personal experience, we know that very few people read a textbook from cover to cover. For a variety of reasons, the majority would read only one or a few chapters at any given time. Therefore, we tried to ensure that each chapter would be complete in itself. As a consequence, there is unavoidable overlap among some of the information provided in some chapters; we, however, feel that this was truly necessary, at least from an information-retrieval standpoint, and in this way it will not be necessary for readers to read bits of information between one or more chapters just to get complete information regarding a particular subject.

We trust our readers will refer to this text often in the course of their clinical experiences. As it is with any text of this type, the flow of new material outpaces publishing deadlines. New information accumulates even as the book goes to press. As a result, we welcome useful comments from our audience about what directions future editions should take.

Cleveland, OH, USA — Angelo A. Licata
Chicago, IL, USA — Edgar V. Lerma

Contents

1 **Molecular Mechanisms of Parathyroid Hormone Synthesis** 1
Tally Naveh-Many and Morris Nechama

2 **Regulation of Calcium and Phosphate Metabolism** 13
Arthur D. Conigrave

3 **Diagnosis and Treatment of the Patient with Abnormal Calcium** 53
Elizabeth H. Holt

4 **The Calcium-Sensing Receptor: Physiology and Pathophysiology** 69
Friedhelm Raue and Christine Haag

5 **New Concepts for Primary and Secondary Hyperparathyroidism** 91
Joachim Beige and Peter Lamesch

6 **Calcific Uremic Arteriolopathy (Calciphylaxis)** 113
Earl H. Rudolph and Edgar V. Lerma

7 **Cystic Parathyroid Lesions** 147
Jean-François Henry and Maurizio Iacobone

8 **Parathyroid Cancer** 157
Maurizio Iacobone and Jean-François Henry

9 **Biochemistry, Physiology, and Pathophysiology of Parathyroid Hormone-Related Peptide** 179
Bandana Chakravarti, Shailendra K. Dhar Dwivedi, Ambrish Mithal, and Naibedya Chattopadhyay

10 **Ectopic Parathyroid Glands** 203
Jean-François Henry and Maurizio Iacobone

11 **Hyperparathyroidism in Multiple Endocrine Neoplasia** 219
Syeda S. Zaidi, Vipul T. Lakhani, and James T. Broome

12 **Familial Hypocalciuric Hypercalcemia** 237
Ogo I. Egbuna and Edward M. Brown

13 **Hyperparathyroidism–Jaw Tumor Syndrome** 253
Andrew C. Calabria and Michael A. Levine

14 **Hypoparathyroidism and Pseudohypoparathyroidism** 273
Rajesh V. Thakker

15 **Primary Hyperparathyroidism in Neonates and Children** 289
Eric Mallet and Mireille Castanet

16 **Hypoparathyroidism in Children** 299
Anne Lienhardt-Roussie and Agnès Linglart

17 **Parathormone Resistance in Children** 311
Agnès Linglart and Eric Mallet

18 **The Use of Ultrasonography in the Management of Parathyroid Diseases** 323
Zvonimir L. Milas and Mira Milas

19 **Imaging in Parathyroid Diseases** 343
Donald R. Neumann and Joyce J. Shin

20 **Parathyroid Surgery** 363
Zvonimir L. Milas and Mira Milas

Index 379

Contributors

Joachim Beige, MD, PhD Department of Nephrology and KfH Renal Unit, Hospital St. Georg, Leipzig, Saxony, Germany

James T. Broome, MD Division of Surgical Oncology/Endocrine Surgery, Department of Surgical Sciences, Vanderbilt University, Nashville, TN, USA

Edward M. Brown, MD Division of Endocrinology, Diabetes and Hypertension, Brigham and Women's Hospital, Boston, MA, USA

Andrew C. Calabria, MD Division of Endocrinology and Diabetes, The Children's Hospital of Philadelphia, Philadelphia, PA, USA

Mireille Castanet, MD, PhD Department of Pediatric, Rouen University Hospital, Rouen, France

Bandana Chakravarti, MSc Department of Endocrinology, Central Drug Research Institute, Lucknow, Uttar Pradesh, India

Naibedya Chattopadhyay, PhD Department of Endocrinology, Central Drug Research Institute, Lucknow, Uttar Pradesh, India

Arthur D. Conigrave, MD, PhD, FRACP School of Molecular Bioscience, University of Sydney, NSW, Australia

Shailendra K. Dhar Dwivedi, MSc Department of Endocrinology, Central Drug Research Institute, Lucknow, Uttar Pradesh, India

Ogo I. Egbuna, MD, MSc, FASN Amgen Inc, Bone Therapeutic Area, Thousand Oaks, CA, USA

Christine Haag, PhD Endocrine Practice, Laboratory of Molecular Genetics, Heidelberg, Germany

Jean-François Henry, MD, FRCS Department of Endocrine Surgery, University Hospital La Timone, Marseilles, France

Elizabeth H. Holt, MD, PhD Section of Endocrinology and Metabolism, Department of Internal Medicine, Yale University of Medicine, New Haven, CT, USA

Maurizio Iacobone, MD, FEBS (Endocrine Surgery) Endocrine Surgery Unit, Department of Surgical, Oncological and Gastroenterological Sciences, University of Padua, Padua, Italy

Vipul T. Lakhani, MD Division of Endocrinology, Department of Medicine, Vanderbilt University School of Medicine, Nashville, TN, USA

Peter Lamesch, MD, FACS Department of Endocrinological Surgery, Hospital St. Georg, Leipzig, Saxony, Germany

Edgar V. Lerma, MD Department of Medicine, Section of Nephrology, University of Illinois at Chicago College of Medicine, Chicago, IL, USA

Michael A. Levine, MD Department of Pediatrics, University of Pennsylvania School of Medicine, Children's Hospital of Philadelphia, Philadelphia, PA, USA

Angelo A. Licata, MD, PhD Endocrine Calcium Clinic & Center Space Medicine, Cleveland Clinic, Cleveland, OH, USA

Anne Lienhardt-Roussie, MD, PhD Department of Pediatric, National Reference Center for Calcium/Phosphorus metabolic diseases, Limoges, France

Agnes Linglart, MD, PhD Department of Pediatric Endocrinology, Bicêtre-Paris-Sud hospital, French Center of Reference for rare disorders of calcium and phosphate metabolism and INSERM unit U986, le Kremlin-Bicêtre, France

Eric Mallet, MD, PhD Department of Pediatrics and CIC INSERM 204, Rouen University Hospital, Rouen, France

Mira Milas, MD The Thyroid Center, Department of Endocrine Surgery, Cleveland Clinic, Cleveland, OH, USA

Zvonimir L. Milas, MD Head and Neck Surgical Oncology, MD Anderson Cancer Center, Orlando, FL, USA

Ambrish Mithal, MD, DM Department of Endocrinology and Diabetes, Medanta, The Medicity, Gurgaon, Haryana, India

Tally Naveh-Many, PhD Department of Nephrology, Hadassah Hebrew University Medical Center, Jerusalem, Israel

Morris Nechama, PhD Department of Nephrology, Hadassah Hebrew University Medical Center, Jerusalem, Israel

Donald R. Neumann, MD, PhD Department of Nuclear Medicine, Cleveland Clinic Imaging Institute, Cleveland, OH, USA

Friedhelm Raue, MD Endocrine Practice, Heidelberg, Germany

Earl H. Rudolph, DO Department of Nephrology and Hypertension, Georgetown University Medical Center, Washington, DC, USA

Joyce J. Shin, MD Department of Endocrine Surgery, Endocrinology & Metabolism Institute, Cleveland, OH, USA

Rajesh V. Thakker, MD, ScD, FRCP, FRCPath, FMedSci Nuffield Department of Medicine, University of Oxford, OCDEM, Churchill Hospital, Oxford, UK

Syeda S. Zaidi, MD Department of Endocrinology and Metabolism, Vanderbilt University Hospital, Nashville, TN, USA

Molecular Mechanisms of Parathyroid Hormone Synthesis

1

Tally Naveh-Many and Morris Nechama

Abstract

Parathyroid hormone (PTH) is central for the hormonal and cellular responses that determine mineral metabolism and bone strength. Small changes in serum calcium are sensed by the parathyroid G-protein coupled calcium-sensing receptor (CaR) and alter PTH secretion, gene expression, and if prolonged parathyroid cell proliferation. The major trigger for PTH secretion is a low extracellular calcium. PTH then binds to its receptor on its target tissues, the bone, and kidney to correct serum calcium. The parathyroid also responds to changes in serum phosphate (Pi), 1,25(OH)2 vitamin D (1,25D), and fibroblast growth factor-23 (FGF23). The regulation of PTH gene expression by dietary-induced changes in serum calcium, phosphate, and in chronic kidney failure is post-transcriptional and is mediated by the regulated binding of *trans*-acting proteins to a defined *cis* element in the PTH mRNA 3′-untranslated region (UTR). These protein–PTH mRNA interactions are orchestrated by the peptidylprolyl isomerase Pin1. In contrast, 1,25D decreases PTH gene transcription. This chapter discusses the molecular mechanisms of regulation of PTH gene expression that determine serum PTH levels and mineral metabolism.

Keywords

Parathyroid hormone • G-protein • Calcium-sensing receptor • Serum phosphate • 1,25 (OH)2 vitamin D • Fibroblastic growth factor • FGF23 • PTH gene • Gene expression • Chronic kidney failure • CKD • *Trans*-acting proteins • *Cis* element • Messenger RNA • mRNA • Peptidylprolyl isomerase P • Secretory granules • Phosphaturic hormone • Klotho • Transmembrane • MAP kinase pathway • Feedback loop • PTH mRNA • VDR • DNA sequence • 5′Flanking region • Oligonucleotide • Osteocalcin • Osteosarcoma • VDRE • Upregulatory 1,25D response element • Retinoid

T. Naveh-Many, PhD • M. Nechama, PhD (✉)
Department of Nephrology, Hadassah Hebrew University Medical Center, Ein Karem, Jerusalem 91120, Israel
e-mail: tally@cc.huji.ac.il; Moris.Nehama@umassmed.edu

A.A. Licata and E.V. Lerma (eds.), *Diseases of the Parathyroid Glands*,
DOI 10.1007/978-1-4419-5550-0_1, © Springer Science+Business Media, LLC 2012

X receptor • Heterodimer • Chloramphenicol acetyltransferase • Histone deacetylase • Transrepression • Hypocalcemia • Calreticulin • Post-transcriptional regulation • Hypophosphatemia • Lanthanum carbonate • Calcimimetic • AU-rich elements • ARE • Pentanucleotide • Exoribonuclease • Exosome • Proto-oncogenes • Exon • Eukaryotic • In vitro degradation assay • mRNA *cis*-acting protein binding element • mRNA *trans*-acting stabilizing protein • Isoforms • Chimeric • KSRP decay promoting protein • RNA immunoprecipitation • RIP • TGFβ • GM-CSF • Dephosphorylation • AUF1 • AU rich binding protein-1 • PMR1 • un-translated region • UTR • 5′-UTR • 3′-UTR • chronic kidney disease

Introduction

Parathyroid hormone (PTH) regulates serum calcium and phosphate levels and bone strength. The parathyroid is unique in that the trigger for PTH secretion is a low extracellular calcium rather than high calcium as for other hormones. Small decreases in serum calcium and more prolonged increases in serum phosphate (Pi) stimulate the parathyroid to secrete PTH which then acts on its target organs, the kidney and bone, to correct serum calcium and Pi levels [1]. Parathyroid cells have few secretory granules as compared to other endocrine cells and, therefore, PTH production is regulated largely at the levels of PTH gene expression and parathyroid cell proliferation [2]. The regulation of PTH gene expression by changes in calcium, Pi levels, and chronic kidney disease (CKD) is post-transcriptional involving regulated protein–PTH mRNA interactions [3]. The parathyroid also responds to changes in serum 1,25(OH)$_2$ vitamin D (1,25D) which decreases PTH levels. In contrast to the post-transcriptional regulation of PTH gene expression by changes in serum calcium and Pi levels, 1,25D decreases PTH gene transcription [4]. Fibroblast growth factor-23 (FGF23) is a bone-derived phosphaturic hormone that acts on the kidney to increase Pi excretion and suppress biosynthesis of 1,25D. FGF23 signals through fibroblast growth factor receptors (FGFRs) bound by the transmembrane protein Klotho [5]. We have identified the parathyroid as a new target organ for FGF23 [6]. Recombinant FGF23 decreases PTH gene expression and secretion in vivo and in vitro by activation of the MAP kinase pathway. In this chapter, we discuss the molecular mechanisms of regulation of PTH gene expression by 1,25D, calcium, Pi, and FGF23.

Regulation of PTH Gene Transcription by 1,25(OH)$_2$ Vitamin D

1,25(OH)$_2$ vitamin D (1,25D) has independent effects on calcium and Pi levels and also participates in a well-defined feedback loop with PTH. PTH increases the renal synthesis of 1,25D. 1,25D then increases blood calcium largely by increasing the efficiency of intestinal calcium absorption. The increased serum calcium would shut down PTH secretion by activating the parathyroid cell 7 *trans* membrane G-protein coupled calcium-sensing receptor (CaR) [7]. 1,25D also potently decreases PTH gene transcription. This action was first demonstrated in vitro in bovine parathyroid cells in primary culture, where 1,25D led to a marked decrease in PTH mRNA levels and a consequent decrease in PTH secretion [8]. The physiological relevance of these findings was established by in vivo studies in rats [4]. Rats injected with 1,25D at concentrations that did not increase serum calcium showed a marked decrease in PTH mRNA levels, reaching <4% of control at 48 h. This effect was shown to be transcriptional both in vivo in rats [4] and in vitro in primary cultures of bovine parathyroid cells [9]. In situ hybridization first showed the expression of the

1,25D receptor (VDR) mRNA in the rat parathyroid, confirming that the parathyroid is indeed a target organ for vitamin D [10].

Several groups have identified DNA sequences in the 5′-flanking region of the PTH gene that may mediate the negative regulation of PTH gene transcription by 1,25D. Demay et al. [11] identified DNA sequences in the human PTH gene that bind the 1,25D receptor (VDR). A 25-bp oligonucleotide containing sequences from −125 to −101 relative to the transcription start site bound nuclear proteins that were recognized by monoclonal antibodies against the VDR. The sequence contained a single copy of a motif (AGGTTCA) that is homologous to the motifs repeated in the upregulatory 1,25D response element (VDRE) of the osteocalcin gene. This 25-bp oligonucleotide mediated transcriptional repression in response to 1,25D in GH4C1 cells but not in a rat osteosarcoma cell line ROS 17/2.8 [11]. Russell et al. [12] have shown that there are two negative VDREs in the rat PTH gene. One is situated at −793 to −779 and bound a VDR/RXR (retinoid X receptor) heterodimer with high affinity and the other at −760 to −746 bound the heterodimer with a lower affinity. Transfection studies with a VDRE-CAT (chloramphenicol acetyltransferase) constructs showed that they had an additive effect. Liu et al. [13] have identified such sequences in the chicken PTH gene and demonstrated their functionality after transfection into the opossum kidney (OK) cell line. They showed that there was a p160 protein that specifically interacted with a heterodimer complex bound to the wild-type VDRE, but was absent from complexes bound to response elements associated with positive transcriptional activity. Thus, the sequence of the individual VDRE appears to play an active role in dictating transcriptional responses that may be mediated by altering the ability of a VDR/RXR heterodimer to interact with accessory factor proteins. Further work is needed to demonstrate that any of these differing negative VDREs function in this fashion in parathyroid cells. The *trans*-repression by 1,25D has also been shown to be dependent upon another promoter element. Kato et al. have identified an E-box (CANNTG)-like motif as another class of negative VDRE (nVDRE) in the human 1α(OH) ase promoter [14, 15]. In sharp contrast to the previously reported motif in the hPTH gene promoter, a basic helix–loop–helix factor, designated VDR interacting repressor (VDIR), transactivates through direct binding to this E-box-type element (1αnVDRE). The functions of VDIR and E-box motifs in the human (h) PTH and PTH related protein hPTHrP gene promoters have been characterized [16] in a mouse renal tubule cell line. The hPTH nVDRE alone was enough to direct ligand-induced *trans* repression mediated through VDR/RXR and VDIR. It was concluded that negative regulation of the hPTH gene by liganded VDR is mediated by VDIR directly binding to the E-box-type nVDRE at the promoter, together with recruitment of a histone deacetylase (HDAC) co-repressor for ligand-induced transrepression [16]. These studies were specific to a mouse proximal tubule cell line and await the development of a parathyroid cell line to confirm them in a homologous cell system.

A further level at which 1,25D may regulate the PTH gene would be at the level of the VDR. 1,25D in physiologically relevant doses led to an increase in VDR mRNA levels in the parathyroid glands in contrast to the decrease in PTH mRNA levels [10]. 1,25D may also amplify its effect on the parathyroid by increasing the CaR protein levels. Functional VDREs have been identified in the CaR gene promoter and probably provide the mechanism, whereby 1,25D upregulates parathyroid CaR expression [17].

Weanling rats fed a diet deficient in calcium were markedly hypocalcemic at 3 weeks and had very high serum 1,25D levels. Despite the chronically high serum 1,25D levels, serum PTH and PTH mRNA levels did not fall and were increased markedly [18]. Calreticulin is a calcium-binding protein present in the cell endoplasmic reticulum that may also have a nuclear function to regulate gene transcription. Calreticulin has been shown to bind a protein motif in the DNA-binding domain of nuclear hormone receptors of sterol hormones. Calreticulin prevents vitamin D's binding and action on the osteocalcin gene in vitro [19]. Sela-Brown et al. [20] showed that calreticulin may inhibit the action of vitamin D on the PTH gene in hypocalcemic rats. These rats had increased levels of calreticulin protein in their parathyroid nuclear fraction. It was postulated that the high calreticulin levels would prevent the effect of 1,25D to suppress the PTH gene. The lack of suppression of PTH synthesis in the setting of hypocalcemia and increased serum 1,25D is relevant physiologically because it allows an increase in both PTH and 1,25D at a time of chronic hypocalcemic stress. Extracellular calcium increases parathyroid VDR mRNA in vitro suggesting that the activation of the CaR upregulates the parathyroid VDR mRNA [21].

The action of 1,25D to decrease serum PTH is used therapeutically in the management of patients with chronic kidney disease (CKD). They are given 1,25D or its prodrug 1α(OH)-vitamin D_3 to treat or prevent the secondary hyperparathyroidism (2HPT) of CKD. The poor response to this treatment in some patients may well result from poor control of serum Pi, decreased VDR concentration in the patients' parathyroids [22], an inhibitory effect of a uremic toxin(s) on VDR-VDRE binding [23], or tertiary hyperparathyroidism with monoclonal parathyroid tumors [24].

Post-Transcriptional Regulation of PTH Gene Expression by Calcium, Phosphate, and CKD

In contrast to the transcriptional effect of 1,25D on PTH gene expression described above, the regulation of PTH gene expression by hypocalcemia, hypophosphatemia, and CKD is post-transcriptional. Dietary-induced hypocalcemia and experimental CKD markedly increases PTH secretion, mRNA levels, and after prolonged stimulation, parathyroid cell proliferation [25, 26]. In the rat, hypocalcemia leads to a >tenfold increase in PTH mRNA levels and this increase in mRNA levels is post-transcriptional affecting mRNA stability [25]. Serum Pi also has a direct effect on PTH secretion, PTH mRNA levels, and parathyroid cell proliferation [26, 27]. Careful in vivo studies showed that the regulation of PTH gene expression by dietary-induced hypophosphatemia is independent of changes in serum calcium and 1,25D [27]. In vitro studies, when tissue architecture was maintained, confirmed the direct effect of Pi on the parathyroid. This was shown in whole glands or tissue slices of parathyroids from different species, but not in isolated cells [28–32]. In vivo studies showed that Pi depletion leads to a dramatic decrease in rat PTH mRNA levels and that this effect is post-transcriptional as is the effect of hypocalcemia to increase PTH mRNA levels [25, 27]. There is a ~60-fold difference in PTH mRNA levels between hypocalcemic and hypophosphatemic rats and these dietary models were used as tools to define the mechanism of the post-transcriptional regulation of PTH gene expression [25, 33].

2HPT is a common disorder in patients with CKD [34]. Experimental kidney failure induces an increase in PTH gene expression, secretion, and parathyroid hyperplasia which are primarily attributed to the retention of Pi and the decreased renal capacity to produce 1,25D. Low serum 1,25D reduces intestinal calcium transport, and high serum Pi further decreases the levels of serum calcium. The resulting hypocalcemia as itself is a strong stimulus to increase PTH gene expression and secretion [18]. However, as mentioned, the parathyroid glands also respond directly to changes in serum Pi. The high Pi levels can increase PTH synthesis directly, enhance PTH mRNA levels, and stimulate parathyroid cell proliferation [26].

In CKD patients with 2HPT, calcimimetics and oral Pi binders are effective drugs used to control the high serum PTH levels [35–38]. In a rat model of CKD induced by an adenine high phosphate diet, PTH mRNA levels were increased already after 3 days of the diet and more so at 7 and 21 days [39]. The addition of the calcimimetic R568 or an oral Pi binder, lanthanum carbonate (La), decreased PTH mRNA and serum PTH levels in the CKD rats at both 7 and 21 days [40]. The effects of the adenine diet and the calcimimetic or La, as the effects of calcium or Pi depletion, on PTH gene expression are all post-transcriptional [25, 41, 42]. This regulation of PTH mRNA stability is mediated by protein–PTH mRNA interactions that determine the susceptibility of PTH mRNA to the degradation machinery. The balanced interaction of stabilizing and destabilizing proteins with the PTH mRNA determines PTH mRNA stability and levels, serum PTH and the resultant response of the parathyroid to hypocalcemia, hypophosphatemia, and CKD [33, 42].

The PTH mRNA *Cis*-Acting Protein Binding Element

For many mRNAs, post-transcriptional regulation involves critical *cis*-acting elements, mostly in the untranslated regions (UTRs) that are targets for *trans*-acting proteins regulating mRNA stability and translation [43]. AU-rich elements (AREs) are a well-defined family of *cis*-acting elements critical for the expression of many unstable mRNAs that code for cytokines, transcription factors, proto-oncogenes, and other mRNAs [44]. Three classes of AREs have been identified, two of which contain several scattered or overlapping copies of the pentanucleotide AUUUA, while the class III AREs lack this motif but contain A and U rich sequences and possibly other unknown determinants. A number of ARE binding proteins have been identified. KH-type splicing regulatory protein (KSRP) is an example for decay promoting factors [43, 45]. KSRP interacts with the large multiprotein 3′–5′ exoribonuclease complex, the exosome and recruits it to target ARE containing mRNAs thereby promoting their rapid degradation [46, 47]. Other ARE binding proteins, such as the ELAV protein family members (mainly HuR), are stabilizing factors and AU-rich binding factor 1 (AUF-1) promotes either decay or stabilization, depending on the mRNA and cell type [48].

PTH mRNAs are typical eukaryotic mRNAs that contain a 7-methylguanosine cap at the 5′ terminus and a poly adenylic nucleic acid (poly A) stretch at the 3′ terminus. PTH mRNA consists of three exons coding for the 5′-UTR (exon I), the prepro region (exon II), and the structural PTH hormone together with the 3′-UTR (exon III) (Fig. 1.1). The PTH mRNA 3′-UTR in all species is rich in A and U nucleotides [49]. A specific sequence at the 3′ end of the rat PTH mRNA 3′-UTR was identified as a *cis*-acting type III ARE that determines PTH mRNA stability and its regulation [50].

Protein–PTH mRNA binding experiments demonstrated specific interaction of rat and human parathyroid extracts with transcripts for the rat and human PTH mRNA 3′-UTR terminal region. This binding was regulated by calcium or phosphate depletion and correlated with PTH mRNA levels and stability in vivo [25]. A 26-nucleotide sequence at the 3′ end of the PTH mRNA 3′-UTR is the minimal protein binding region and is highly conserved in the PTH mRNA 3′-UTRs of rat, mouse, man, dog, and cat (Fig. 1.1). The conservation of sequences within a region that does not code for protein (UTR) suggests that the binding element is a functional unit that has been evolutionarily conserved [50, 51]. This PTH mRNA 3′-UTR element is a *cis*-acting sequence that determines PTH mRNA stability and its regulation by changes in serum calcium, Pi, and CKD (see below) [33, 50].

There is no parathyroid cell line; therefore, a cell-free mRNA in vitro degradation assay (IVDA) was utilized to identify the factors involved in PTH mRNA decay. The IVDA has been shown to reproduce differences in mRNA stability that occur in vivo and, specifically, the differences in PTH mRNA stability induced by calcium, Pi, and CKD [25, 42, 52]. Parathyroid extracts from hypocalcemic and CKD rats stabilized and extracts from hypophosphatemic rats destabilized transcripts for the PTH mRNA compared to parathyroid extracts from control rat, correlating with steady-state PTH mRNA levels in vivo. These effects were dependent upon the terminal 60 nucleotides of the PTH mRNA 3′-UTR [25, 41, 42]. A 63-nucleotide transcript containing the conserved 26 nucleotide ARE and flanking regions was both necessary and sufficient to regulate PTH mRNA stability and to confer responsiveness of reporter mRNAs to changes in calcium and Pi [50]. Structural analysis showed that the PTH mRNA 3′-UTR and, in particular, the ARE is dominated by significant open regions with little folded base pairing [53].

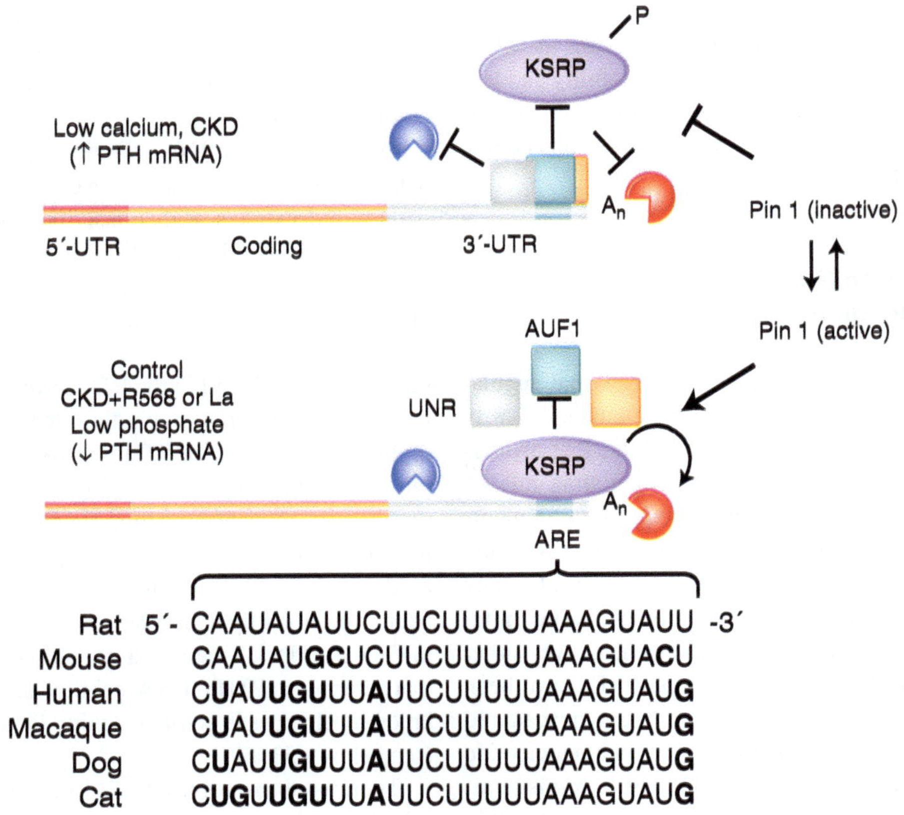

Fig. 1.1 Model for the regulation of parathyroid hormone mRNA stability by changes in calcium and Pi levels and CKD. Schematic representation of the PTH mRNA and binding proteins. The nucleotide sequence of the 26-nucleotide *cis* element in different species is shown. Nucleotides that differ from the rat sequence are in *bold*. AUF1 and Unr stabilize and KSRP destabilizes PTH mRNA. The peptidylprolyl *cis/trans* isomerase Pin1 is upstream of KSRP and leads to KSRP dephosphorylation and activation. In hypocalcemic and experimental CKD rats, the enzymatic activity of Pin1 is reduced. As a result, KSRP is phosphorylated and hence less active. The stabilizing proteins AUF1 and Unr then bind the PTH mRNA 3′-UTR ARE with a greater affinity leading to increased PTH mRNA stability and levels. In control and more so in phosphate depleted rats or in CKD rats treated with a calcimimetic (R568) or an oral Pi binder (La), there is increased association of PTH mRNA with KSRP and decreased association with AUF1 and Unr. KSRP then recruits the exosome leading to PTH mRNA decay. Adapted with permission from Naveh-Many T. Minireview: the play of proteins on the parathyroid hormone messenger ribonucleic acid regulates its expression. Endocrinol 2009 [3]. Copyright 2010, The Endocrine Society

The PTH mRNA *Trans*-Acting Stabilizing Proteins

Two PTH mRNA binding and stabilizing proteins have been identified by PTH RNA affinity chromatography. These *trans*-acting proteins are AUF1 and Up-stream of N-*ras* (Unr) [54, 55]. AUF1 consists of four isoforms (p37, p40, p42, and p45) that are generated by alternative pre-mRNA splicing of the AUF1 mRNA [56]. These proteins bind the PTH mRNA 3′-UTR and are part of the PTH mRNA–parathyroid protein binding complex. Addition of recombinant AUF1 isoforms to parathyroid extracts from Pi-depleted rats prevented the rapid degradation of PTH transcripts in IVDAs [54]. AUF1 is modified post-translationally in the parathyroids of rats fed a calcium or a phosphate-depleted diet or CKD rats [39, 57]. These modifications could lead to differences in AUF1–PTH mRNA binding affinity and PTH mRNA stability. Overexpression of AUF1 or Unr in human embryonic kidney (HEK) 293 cells co-transfected with expression plasmids for the PTH gene or a chimeric GH gene containing the PTH mRNA 3′-UTR 63 nucleotide *cis*-acting element, stabilized the PTH mRNA and chimeric reporter mRNA, but not a PTH mRNA lacking the *cis* element nor a reporter mRNA containing a truncated PTH element [51, 55]. Knock-down of all four AUF1 isoforms or Unr by siRNA led to the opposite effect, decreasing PTH mRNA levels [55, 57]. AUF1 also stabilized a reporter mRNA containing the bovine PTH mRNA protein-binding element that is different from the one characterized in rat [51]. These results identified AUF1 and Unr as PTH mRNA stabilizing proteins (Fig. 1.1). However, the half-life of mRNAs is determined by the coordinate association of both stabilizing and destabilizing factors with the specific mRNA in the cytoplasm. We therefore studied the relationship between the PTH mRNA stabilizing proteins and other ARE-binding proteins that would affect mRNA decay.

KSRP Is a PTH mRNA *Trans*-Acting Destabilizing Protein

We demonstrated that the decay promoting protein KSRP binds the PTH mRNA 3′-UTR ARE both in vivo in the parathyroid and in vitro. In HEK293 cells, KSRP overexpression and knock down experiments showed that KSRP decreases co-transfected PTH mRNA steady-state levels through the PTH mRNA ARE. Overexpression of the PTH mRNA stabilizing protein AUF1 isoform p45 blocked KSRP–PTH mRNA binding and partially prevented the KSRP mediated decrease in PTH mRNA levels [33]. KSRP and AUF1 protein–PTH mRNA interactions in the parathyroid were studied using a RNA immunoprecipitation (RIP) assay which provides a measure of protein–mRNA interactions at a specific time point in vivo. In this assay, the parathyroid glands were cross-linked, AUF1 or KSRP-containing complexes immunoprecipitated, and the amount of PTH mRNA associated with each of the proteins determined by qRT-PCR analysis. KSRP-PTH mRNA interaction was decreased in glands from calcium depleted or CKD rats, where PTH mRNA is more stable, and increased in parathyroids from phosphate depleted rats, where PTH mRNA is less stable. In contrast, AUF1–PTH mRNA interactions were increased by hypocalcemia and CKD and decreased in the phosphate depleted rat parathyroids [33]. This differential interaction of KSRP and AUF1 suggests that these proteins compete for their interaction with the same PTH mRNA 3′-UTR *cis* element, having antagonistic effects on PTH mRNA stability (Fig. 1.1) [58].

KSRP–PTH mRNA interaction was increased by both the calcimimetic R568 and the oral Pi binder La which decrease PTH mRNA levels in CKD rats. IVDAs showed that PTH mRNA is destabilized by parathyroid extracts from CKD rats treated with R568 or La compared to parathyroid extracts from untreated CKD rats. This destabilizing effect of R568 and La was dependent upon KSRP and the PTH mRNA 3′-UTR. Therefore, the calcimimetic R568 and correction of serum phosphorus by La determine PTH mRNA stability through KSRP-mediated PTH mRNA decay, thereby decreasing PTH expression [42]. The changes in binding of the *trans*-acting factors to the PTH mRNA, therefore, determine PTH gene expression in CKD and after management of the 2HPT by both calcimimetics or oral phosphorus binders as well as in dietary-induced hypocalcaemia or hypophosphatemia (Fig. 1.1).

Of interest, recent studies have shown that KSRP also interacts with the endoribonuclease polysomal ribonuclease 1 (PMR1) that facilitates PTH mRNA degradation. PMR1 mediated decrease in PTH mRNA levels involves the PTH mRNA 3′-UTR ARE, KSRP and the exosome. These findings suggest that KSRP recruits a degradation complex, comprising both exo- and endo-ribonucleases to PTH mRNA, thus controlling its mRNA half-life [59].

The Peptidylprolyl Isomerase Pin1 Determines PTH mRNA Levels and Stability in Secondary Hyperparathyroidism

The above results indicate that KSRP and AUF1 directly or indirectly respond to changes in serum calcium and Pi concentrations and CKD by altering their association with PTH mRNA leading to differences in PTH mRNA stability and levels [33, 42]. These changes could be a result of post-translational modifications of these ARE-binding proteins, affecting their binding affinity to the PTH mRNA. Indeed, AUF1 is post-translationally modified in the parathyroids of 2HPT rats and this is at least in part due to differences in protein phosphorylation [39, 57]. KSRP is also a phospho-protein with two identified phosphorylation sites at serine 193 (S193) and threonine residue 692 (T692). Phosphorylation at these sites prevents KSRP association with the ribonuclease degradation complex exosome (S193) or compromises KSRP binding to ARE-containing target mRNAs and hence their decay (T692) [60, 61]. Therefore, the differential interaction of KSRP and AUF1 with PTH mRNA after changes in serum calcium and Pi may involve KSRP and AUF1 post-translational modifications.

The peptidylprolyl *cis/trans* isomerase Pin1 specifically binds phosphorylated serine/threonine–proline protein motifs and catalyzes the *cis/trans* isomerization of the peptide bonds thereby changing the biological activity, phosphorylation, and turn-over of its target proteins [62, 63]. Pin1-catalyzed conformational regulation has a profound impact on many key proteins involved in various cell functions [64, 65]. Pin1 was shown to regulate the turnover of ARE-containing mRNAs, mainly cytokine mRNAs, through the interaction and isomerization of ARE-binding proteins. Pin1 interacts with AUF1 and thereby stabilizes both GM-CSF and TGFβ mRNAs [66, 67]. These observations led us to speculate that Pin1 may be involved in PTH gene expression through AUF1 and/or KSRP interaction and isomerization. Indeed, we have recently identified Pin1 as a PTH mRNA destabilizing protein in rat parathyroids and in transfected cells [68]. The regulation of PTH mRNA stability by Pin1 was mediated by the PTH mRNA 3′-UTR ARE and by the mRNA destabilizing protein KSRP. We show for the first time that KSRP is a Pin1 target protein. Pin1 interacts with phosphorylated KSRP at S181, leading to KSRP dephosphorylation and activation. Importantly, Pin1 enzymatic activity was decreased in parathyroid extracts from rats with 2HPT due to either a calcium depleted diet or CKD. Pharmacological inhibition of Pin1 increased PTH mRNA levels and stability and decreased KSRP–PTH mRNA interaction in the parathyroid. This decreased interaction would contribute to the increased PTH gene expression after Pin1 inhibition. Furthermore, *Pin1*$^{-/-}$ mice display increased serum PTH and PTH mRNA levels. Therefore, Pin1 determines basal PTH expression in vivo and in vitro and decreased Pin1 activity correlates with increased PTH mRNA levels in rats with 2HPT. These results demonstrate that Pin1 is a key mediator of PTH mRNA stability and indicate a role for Pin1 in the pathogenesis of the 2HPT of CKD [68]. Our data suggest that phosphorylated KSRP at S181 is inactive. Upon interaction with Pin1, *cis–trans* isomerization of the proline bond in KSRP leads to conformational change, exposing the phosphorylated S181 residue and possibly additional phosphorylation sites. This leads to KSRP dephosphorylation by a still unidentified phosphatase thus activating KSRP, which then interacts with PTH mRNA and enhances its decay. A low calcium diet and CKD lead to decreased Pin1 isomerase activity in the parathyroids of these rats. This decreased Pin1 activity would prevent KSRP dephosphorylation, resulting in decreased KSRP–PTH mRNA interaction, inhibition of PTH mRNA degradation, and increased PTH mRNA levels (Fig. 1.1). The trigger for the reduced Pin1 activity in the parathyroid glands of 2HPT rats is not known. It is possible that post-translational modifications of Pin1 protein play a role in this regulation. It was recently shown that Pin1 is post-translationally modified by phosphorylation that affects its ability to interact with target proteins and its activity. PKA mediated phosphorylation at Ser residue 16 affects Pin1 ability to interact with its target proteins while phosphorylation at Ser residue 71 by the protein kinase DAPK1, inhibits Pin1 isomerization activity [69, 70]. Future studies may identify the factors that decrease Pin1 activity in the hyper-functioning parathyroid glands of 2HPT. Another main challenge will be to unravel the cell-signaling cascade and the particular kinases responsible for KSRP phosphorylation at S181 that determine PTH mRNA–KSRP interactions and PTH mRNA decay. Understanding these mechanisms will hopefully enhance the development of parathyroid-specific modulators of ARE-binding proteins which may result in drugs effective for the control of the high PTH mRNA stability and serum PTH levels of 2HPT.

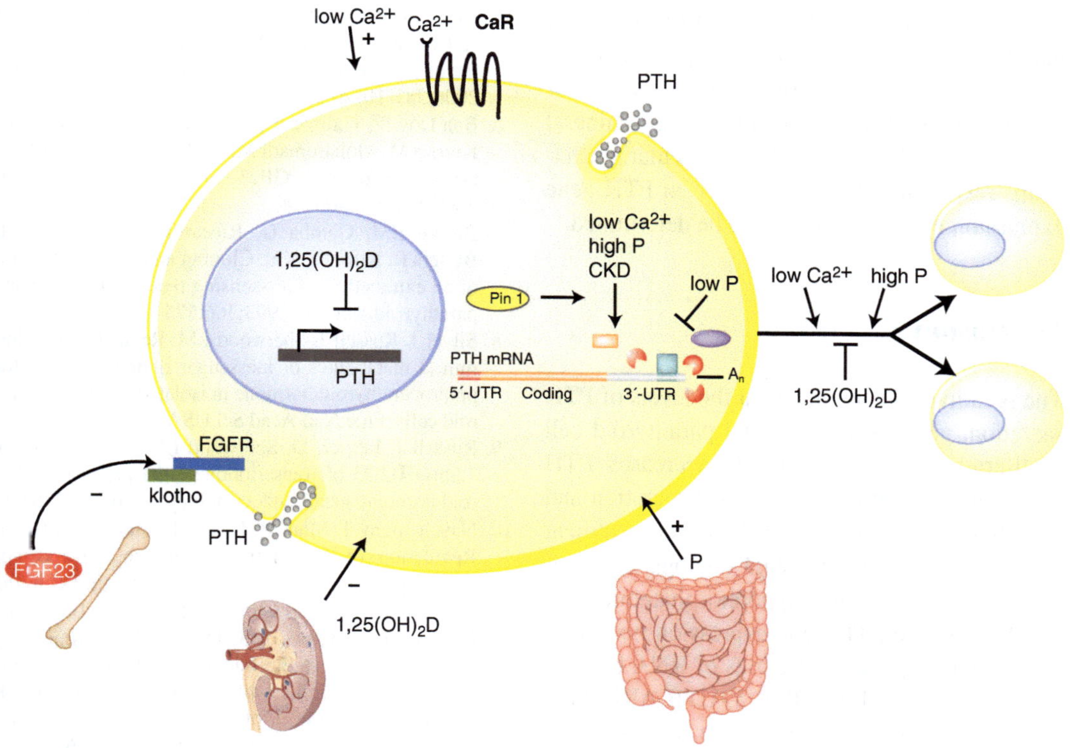

Fig. 1.2 Regulation of parathyroid hormone gene expression, secretion, and parathyroid cell proliferation. Parathyroid synthesizes and secretes PTH unless it is restrained by the parathyroid calcium receptor (CaR) which senses serum [Ca^{2+}] levels. A low serum calcium leads to decreased activation of the CaR and thus increased PTH mRNA stability and levels, PTH secretion, and parathyroid cell proliferation. A high serum Pi and chronic kidney disease (CKD) lead to similar changes in all these parameters. PTH mRNA stability is regulated by the balanced interactions of the protective parathyroid *trans*-acting factors AUF1 and Unr and the decay promoting protein KSRP, that bind to a defined *cis* element in the PTH mRNA 3′-UTR. These interactions are regulated by the peptidylprolyl *cis/trans* isomerase Pin1. 1,25D decreases PTH gene transcription and parathyroid cell proliferation. Fibroblast growth factor 23 (FGF23) is a bone-derived hormone that decreases PTH gene expression and secretion. Adapted with permission from Naveh-Many T. Minireview: the play of proteins on the parathyroid hormone messenger ribonucleic acid regulates its expression. Endocrinol 2009 [3]. Copyright 2010, The Endocrine Society

Fibroblast Growth Factor-23 and PTH Gene Expression

Pi homeostasis is maintained by a counterbalance between efflux from the kidney and influx from intestine and bone. FGF23 is a bone-derived phosphaturic hormone that acts on the kidney to increase Pi excretion and suppress biosynthesis of 1,25D. FGF23 signals through FGFR bound by the transmembrane protein Klotho [5]. Since most tissues express FGFRs, expression of Klotho virtually determines FGF23 target organs. Klotho protein is expressed not only in the kidney but also in the parathyroid brain, pituitary, and sino-atrial node [6, 71]. We have identified the parathyroid as a new target organ for FGF23. We showed that the rat parathyroid gland expresses Klotho and that the administration of recombinant FGF23 leads to an increase in parathyroid Klotho levels. In addition, FGF23 activates the MAP kinase pathway in the parathyroid through ERK1/2 phosphorylation and increased Egr-1 mRNA levels. Importantly, FGF23 suppresses PTH gene expression and secretion in vivo and in vitro. The FGF23-induced decrease in PTH secretion was prevented by a MAPK inhibitor. These data indicate that FGF23 acts directly on the parathyroid through the MAPK pathway to decrease serum PTH. FGF23 also leads to a decrease in PTH secretion in bovine parathyroid primary cultures [72]. This novel bone–parathyroid endocrine axis adds a new dimension to the understanding of mineral homeostasis [6] (Fig. 1.2). The molecular mechanisms responsible for the decrease in PTH gene expression by FGF23 remain to be determined.

Conclusion

The parathyroid is regulated at the levels of PTH secretion, gene expression, and parathyroid cell proliferation (Fig. 1.2). 1,25D decreases PTH gene transcription and hence PTH secretion and this effect is the scientific basis for the treatment of CKD patients with 1,25D analogs. Dietary-induced hypocalcemia, hypophosphatemia, and CKD determine PTH gene expression post-transcriptionally by the interactions of RNA binding protein with the PTH mRNA 3′-UTR ARE. Pin1 enzymatic activity affects these protein–PTH mRNA interactions and consequently PTH mRNA decay (Fig. 1.1). The data suggest that it is possible to modulate PTH mRNA stability and levels by altering the activity of Pin1 thus changing KSRP phosphorylation status and KSRP–AUF1–PTH mRNA interactions in the parathyroid cell. FGF23 decreases PTH expression through the MAPK pathway. The stimulus to PTH expression is a low serum calcium and high serum Pi as in CKD. 1,25D and FGF23 act together to suppress PTH levels (Fig. 1.2).

References

1. Silver J, Naveh-Many T. Phosphate and the parathyroid. Kidney Int. 2009;75(9):898–905.
2. Habener JF, Rosenblatt M, Potts JTJ. Parathyroid hormone: biochemical aspects of biosynthesis, secretion, action, and metabolism. Physiol Rev. 1984;64:985–1053.
3. Naveh-Many T. Minireview: the play of proteins on the parathyroid hormone messenger ribonucleic acid regulates its expression. Endocrinology. 2010;151(4):1398–402.
4. Silver J, Naveh-Many T, Mayer H, Schmelzer HJ, Popovtzer MM. Regulation by vitamin D metabolites of parathyroid hormone gene transcription in vivo in the rat. J Clin Invest. 1986;78:1296–301.
5. Kurosu H, Ogawa Y, Miyoshi M, Yamamoto M, Nandi A, Rosenblatt KP, et al. Regulation of fibroblast growth factor-23 signaling by klotho. J Biol Chem. 2006;281(10):6120–3.
6. Ben Dov IZ, Galitzer H, Lavi-Moshayoff V, Goetz R, Kuro-o M, Mohammadi M, et al. The parathyroid is a target organ for FGF23 in rats. J Clin Invest. 2007;117(12):4003–8.
7. Brown EM, Gamba G, Riccardi D, Lombardi M, Butters R, Kifor O, et al. Cloning and characterization of an extracellular Ca^{2+}-sensing receptor from bovine parathyroid. Nature. 1993;366:575–80.
8. Silver J, Russell J, Sherwood LM. Regulation by vitamin D metabolites of messenger ribonucleic acid for preproparathyroid hormone in isolated bovine parathyroid cells. Proc Natl Acad Sci USA. 1985;82:4270–3.
9. Russell J, Lettieri D, Sherwood LM. Suppression by 1,25(OH)2D3 of transcription of the pre-proparathyroid hormone gene. Endocrinology. 1986;119:2864–6.
10. Naveh-Many T, Marx R, Keshet E, Pike JW, Silver J. Regulation of 1,25-dihydroxyvitamin D3 receptor gene expression by 1,25-dihydroxyvitamin D3 in the parathyroid in vivo. J Clin Invest. 1990;86:1968–75.
11. Demay MB, Kiernan MS, DeLuca HF, Kronenberg HM. Sequences in the human parathyroid hormone gene that bind the 1,25-dihydroxyvitamin D-3 receptor and mediate transcriptional repression in response to 1,25-dihydroxyvitamin D-3. Proc Natl Acad Sci USA. 1992;89:8097–101.
12. Russell J, Ashok S, Koszewski NJ. Vitamin D receptor interactions with the rat parathyroid hormone gene: synergistic effects between two negative vitamin D response elements. J Bone Miner Res. 1999;14(11):1828–37.
13. Liu SM, Koszewski N, Lupez M, Malluche HH, Olivera A, Russell J. Characterization of a response element in the 5′-flanking region of the avian (chicken) parathyroid hormone gene that mediates negative regulation of gene transcription by 1,25-dihydroxyvitamin D_3 and binds the vitamin D_3 receptor. Mol Endocrinol. 1996;10:206–15.
14. Murayama A, Kim MS, Yanagisawa J, Takeyama K, Kato S. Transrepression by a liganded nuclear receptor via a bHLH activator through co-regulator switching. EMBO J. 2004;23(7):1598–608.
15. Fujiki R, Kim MS, Sasaki Y, Yoshimura K, Kitagawa H, Kato S. Ligand-induced transrepression by VDR through association of WSTF with acetylated histones. EMBO J. 2005;24(22):3881–94.
16. Kim MS, Fujiki R, Murayama A, Kitagawa H, Yamaoka K, Yamamoto Y, et al. 1Alpha,25(OH)2D3-induced transrepression by vitamin D receptor through E-box-type elements in the human parathyroid hormone gene promoter. Mol Endocrinol. 2007;21(2): 334–42.
17. Canaff L, Hendy GN. Human calcium-sensing receptor gene. Vitamin D response elements in promoters P1 and P2 confer transcriptional responsiveness to 1,25-dihydroxyvitamin D. J Biol Chem. 2002;277(33):30337–50.

18. Naveh-Many T, Silver J. Regulation of parathyroid hormone gene expression by hypocalcemia, hypercalcemia, and vitamin D in the rat. J Clin Invest. 1990;86:1313–9.
19. Wheeler DG, Horsford J, Michalak M, White JH, Hendy GN. Calreticulin inhibits vitamin D3 signal transduction. Nucleic Acids Res. 1995;23:3268–74.
20. Sela-Brown A, Russell J, Koszewski NJ, Michalak M, Naveh-Many T, Silver J. Calreticulin inhibits vitamin D's action on the PTH gene *in vitro* and may prevent vitamin D's effect *in vivo* in hypocalcemic rats. Mol Endocrinol. 1998;12:1193–200.
21. Garfia B, Canadillas S, Canalejo A, Luque F, Siendones E, Quesada M, et al. Regulation of parathyroid vitamin D receptor expression by extracellular calcium. J Am Soc Nephrol. 2002;13(12):2945–52.
22. Fukuda N, Tanaka H, Tominaga Y, Fukagawa M, Kurokawa K, Seino Y. Decreased 1,25-dihydroxyvitamin D3 receptor density is associated with a more severe form of parathyroid hyperplasia in chronic uremic patients. J Clin Invest. 1993;92:1436–43.
23. Patel S, Simpson RU, Hsu CH. Effect of vitamin D metabolites on calcitriol metabolism in experimental renal failure. Kidney Int. 1989;36:234–9.
24 Arnold A, Brown MF, Urena P, Gaz RD, Sarfati E, Drueke TB. Monoclonality of parathyroid tumors in chronic renal failure and in primary parathyroid hyperplasia. J Clin Invest. 1995;95:2047–53.
25. Moallem E, Silver J, Kilav R, Naveh-Many T. RNA protein binding and post-transcriptional regulation of PTH gene expression by calcium and phosphate. J Biol Chem. 1998;273:5253–9.
26. Naveh-Many T, Rahamimov R, Livni N, Silver J. Parathyroid cell proliferation in normal and chronic renal failure rats: the effects of calcium, phosphate and vitamin D. J Clin Invest. 1995;96:1786–93.
27. Kilav R, Silver J, Naveh-Many T. Parathyroid hormone gene expression in hypophosphatemic rats. J Clin Invest. 1995;96:327–33.
28. Almaden Y, Canalejo A, Hernandez A, Ballesteros E, Garcia-Navarro S, Torres A, et al. Direct effect of phosphorus on parathyroid hormone secretion from whole rat parathyroid glands in vitro. J Bone Miner Res. 1996;11:970–6.
29. Almaden Y, Hernandez A, Torregrosa V, Canalejo A, Sabate L, Fernandez CL, et al. High phosphate level directly stimulates parathyroid hormone secretion and synthesis by human parathyroid tissue in vitro. J Am Soc Nephrol. 1998;9(10):1845–52.
30. Nielsen PK, Feldt-Rasmusen U, Olgaard K. A direct effect of phosphate on PTH release from bovine parathyroid tissue slices but not from dispersed parathyroid cells. Nephrol Dial Transplant. 1996;11:1762–8.
31. Slatopolsky E, Finch J, Denda M, Ritter C, Zhong A, Dusso A, et al. Phosphate restriction prevents parathyroid cell growth in uremic rats. High phosphate directly stimulates PTH secretion in vitro. J Clin Invest. 1996;97:2534–40.
32. Rodriguez M, Almaden Y, Hernandez A, Torres A. Effect of phosphate on the parathyroid gland: direct and indirect? Curr Opin Nephrol Hypertens. 1996; 5(4):321–8.
33. Nechama M, Ben Dov IZ, Briata P, Gherzi R, Naveh-Many T. The mRNA decay promoting factor K-homology splicing regulator protein post-transcriptionally determines parathyroid hormone mRNA levels. FASEB J. 2008;22:3458–68.
34. Silver J, Kilav R, Naveh-Many T. Mechanisms of secondary hyperparathyroidism. Am J Physiol Renal Physiol. 2002;283(3):F367–76.
35. Joy MS, Finn WF. Randomized, double-blind, placebo-controlled, dose-titration, phase III study assessing the efficacy and tolerability of lanthanum carbonate: a new phosphate binder for the treatment of hyperphosphatemia. Am J Kidney Dis. 2003; 42(1):96–107.
36. D'Haese PC, Spasovski GB, Sikole A, Hutchison A, Freemont TJ, Sulkova S, et al. A multicenter study on the effects of lanthanum carbonate (Fosrenol) and calcium carbonate on renal bone disease in dialysis patients. Kidney Int Suppl. 2003;85:S73–8.
37. Block GA, Martin KJ, de Francisco AL, Turner SA, Avram MM, Suranyi MG, et al. Cinacalcet for secondary hyperparathyroidism in patients receiving hemodialysis. N Engl J Med. 2004;350(15):1516–25.
38. Moe SM, Cunningham J, Bommer J, Adler S, Rosansky SJ, Urena-Torres P, et al. Long-term treatment of secondary hyperparathyroidism with the calcimimetic cinacalcet HCl. Nephrol Dial Transplant. 2005;20(10):2186–93.
39. Levi R, Ben Dov IZ, Lavi-Moshayoff V, Dinur M, Martin D, Naveh-Many T, et al. Increased parathyroid hormone gene expression in secondary hyperparathyroidism of experimental uremia is reversed by calcimimetics: correlation with posttranslational modification of the trans acting factor AUF1. J Am Soc Nephrol. 2006;17(1):107–12.
40. Ben Dov IZ, Pappo O, Sklair-Levy M, Galitzer H, Ilan Y, Naveh-Many T, et al. Lanthanum carbonate decreases PTH gene expression with no hepatotoxicity in uraemic rats. Nephrol Dial Transplant. 2007;22(2):362–8.
41. Yalcindag C, Silver J, Naveh-Many T. Mechanism of increased parathyroid hormone mRNA in experimental uremia: roles of protein RNA binding and RNA degradation. J Am Soc Nephrol. 1999;10(12): 2562–8.
42. Nechama M, Ben Dov IZ, Silver J, Naveh-Many T. Regulation of PTH mRNA stability by the calcimimetic R568 and the phosphorus binder lanthanum carbonate in CKD. Am J Physiol Renal Physiol. 2009;296(4):F795–800.
43. Barreau C, Paillard L, Osborne HB. AU-rich elements and associated factors: are there unifying principles? Nucleic Acids Res. 2006;33(22):7138–50.
44. Brewer G. Messenger RNA decay during aging and development. Ageing Res Rev. 2002;1(4):607–25.
45. Gherzi R, Lee KY, Briata P, Wegmuller D, Moroni C, Karin M, et al. A KH domain RNA binding protein, KSRP, promotes ARE-directed mRNA turnover by

recruiting the degradation machinery. Mol Cell. 2004;14(5):571–83.
46. Linker K, Pautz A, Fechir M, Hubrich T, Greeve J, Kleinert H. Involvement of KSRP in the post-transcriptional regulation of human iNOS expression-complex interplay of KSRP with TTP and HuR. Nucleic Acids Res. 2005;33(15):4813–27.
47. Chou CF, Mulky A, Maitra S, Lin WJ, Gherzi R, Kappes J, et al. Tethering KSRP, a decay-promoting AU-rich element-binding protein, to mRNAs elicits mRNA decay. Mol Cell Biol. 2006;26(10):3695–706.
48. Wilusz CJ, Wilusz J. Bringing the role of mRNA decay in the control of gene expression into focus. Trends Genet. 2004;20(10):491–7.
49. Bell O, Silver J, Naveh-Many T. Parathyroid hormone, from gene to protein. In: Naveh-Many T, editor. Molecular biology of the parathyroid. New York: Landes Bioscience and Kluwer Academic; 2005. p. 8–28.
50. Kilav R, Silver J, Naveh-Many T. A conserved cis-acting element in the parathyroid hormone 3′-untranslated region is sufficient for regulation of RNA stability by calcium and phosphate. J Biol Chem. 2001;276:8727–33.
51. Bell O, Silver J, Naveh-Many T. Identification and characterization of *cis*-acting elements in the human and bovine parathyroid hormone mRNA 3′-untranslated region. J Bone Miner Res. 2005;20:858–66.
52. Fritz DT, Ford LP, Wilusz J. An in vitro assay to study regulated mRNA stability. Sci STKE. 2000; 2000(61):L1.
53. Kilav R, Bell O, Le SY, Silver J, Naveh-Many T. The parathyroid hormone mRNA 3′-untranslated region AU-rich element is an unstructured functional element. J Biol Chem. 2004;279(3):2109–16.
54. Sela-Brown A, Silver J, Brewer G, Naveh-Many T. Identification of AUF1 as a parathyroid hormone mRNA 3′-untranslated region binding protein that determines parathyroid hormone mRNA stability. J Biol Chem. 2000;275(10):7424–9.
55. Dinur M, Kilav R, Sela-Brown A, Jacquemin-Sablon H, Naveh-Many T. In vitro evidence that upstream of N-ras participates in the regulation of parathyroid hormone messenger ribonucleic acid stability. Mol Endocrinol. 2006;20(7):1652–60.
56. Wagner BJ, DeMaria CT, Sun Y, Wilson GM, Brewer G. Structure and genomic organization of the human AUF1 gene: alternative pre-mRNA splicing generates four protein isoforms. Genomics. 1998;48(2): 195–202.
57. Bell O, Gaberman E, Kilav R, Levi R, Cox KB, Molkentin JD, et al. The protein phosphatase calcineurin determines basal parathyroid hormone gene expression. Mol Endocrinol. 2005;19:516–26.
58. Naveh-Many T, Nechama M. Regulation of parathyroid hormone mRNA stability by calcium, phosphate and uremia. Curr Opin Nephrol Hypertens. 2007; 16(4):305–10.
59. Nechama M, Peng Y, Bell O, Briata P, Gherzi R, Schoenberg DR, Naveh-Many T. KSRP-PMR1-exosome association determines parathyroid hormone mRNA levels and stability in transfected cells. BMC Cell Biol. 2009;10:70.
60. Gherzi R, Trabucchi M, Ponassi M, Ruggiero T, Corte G, Moroni C, et al. The RNA-binding protein KSRP promotes decay of beta-catenin mRNA and is inactivated by PI3K-AKT signaling. PLoS Biol. 2006; 5(1):e5.
61. Ruggiero T, Trabucchi M, Ponassi M, Corte G, Chen CY, al Haj L, et al. Identification of a set of KSRP target transcripts upregulated by PI3K-AKT signaling. BMC Mol Biol. 2007;8:28.
62. Wulf GM, Liou YC, Ryo A, Lee SW, Lu KP. Role of Pin1 in the regulation of p53 stability and p21 transactivation, and cell cycle checkpoints in response to DNA damage. J Biol Chem. 2002;277(50):47976–9.
63. Zhou XZ, Kops O, Werner A, Lu PJ, Shen M, Stoller G, et al. Pin1-dependent prolyl isomerization regulates dephosphorylation of Cdc25C and tau proteins. Mol Cell. 2000;6(4):873–83.
64. Winkler KE, Swenson KI, Kornbluth S, Means AR. Requirement of the prolyl isomerase Pin1 for the replication checkpoint. Science. 2000;287(5458):1644–7.
65. Lu PJ, Wulf G, Zhou XZ, Davies P, Lu KP. The prolyl isomerase Pin1 restores the function of Alzheimer-associated phosphorylated tau protein. Nature. 1999;399(6738):784–8.
66. Shen ZJ, Esnault S, Malter JS. The peptidyl-prolyl isomerase Pin1 regulates the stability of granulocyte-macrophage colony-stimulating factor mRNA in activated eosinophils. Nat Immunol. 2005;6(12):1280–7.
67. Shen ZJ, Esnault S, Rosenthal LA, Szakaly RJ, Sorkness RL, Westmark PR, et al. Pin1 regulates TGF-beta1 production by activated human and murine eosinophils and contributes to allergic lung fibrosis. J Clin Invest. 2008;118(2):479–90.
68. Nechama M, Uchida T, Yosef-Levi IM, Silver J, Naveh-Many T. The peptidyl-prolyl isomerase Pin1 determines parathyroid hormone mRNA levels and stability in rat models of secondary hyperparathyroidism. J Clin Invest. 2009;119(10):3102–14.
69. Lu PJ, Zhou XZ, Liou YC, Noel JP, Lu KP. Critical role of WW domain phosphorylation in regulating phosphoserine binding activity and Pin1 function. J Biol Chem. 2002;277:2381–4.
70. Lee TH, Chen CH, Suizu F, Huang P, Schiene-Fischer C, Daum S, Zhang YJ, Goate A, Chen RH, Zhou XZ Lu KP. Death-associated protein kinase 1 phosphorylates Pin1 and inhibits its prolyl isomerase activity and cellular function. Mol Cell. 22 2011;42(2):147–59.
71. Takeshita K, Fujimori T, Kurotaki Y, Honjo H, Tsujikawa H, Yasui K, et al. Sinoatrial node dysfunction and early unexpected death of mice with a defect of klotho gene expression. Circulation. 2004; 109(14):1776–82.
72. Krajisnik T, Bjorklund P, Marsell R, Ljunggren O, Akerstrom G, Jonsson KB, et al. Fibroblast growth factor-23 regulates parathyroid hormone and 1alpha-hydroxylase expression in cultured bovine parathyroid cells. J Endocrinol. 2007;195(1):125–31.

Regulation of Calcium and Phosphate Metabolism

2

Arthur D. Conigrave

Abstract

This is an up-to-date discussion of calcium and phosphorus metabolism and the many regulators both old and new involved in the control of these minerals. The author provides a discussion of dietary sources of these minerals, their intestinal and renal handling. He focuses on the well-established regulators such as parathyroid hormone and vitamin D and also provides new insights into this regulation by the new compounds FGF-23 and Klotho. The author also highlights the molecular sensors for calcium and phosphorus, membrane receptors, and their importance in controlling mineral metabolism at the intestine, kidney, and bone. He ends the chapter with discussions of how macronutrients such as carbohydrates and proteins influence the overall regulation of these minerals.

Keywords

Metabolism • Regulation • Hydroxyapatite • Calcium • Phosphorus • Parathyroid hormone • PTHrP • CYP27B1 gene • Calbindin • CYP24A1 gene • Calcitriol • 1,25(OH)$_2$ vitamin D$_3$ • 24,25(OH)$_2$ vitamin D$_3$ • FGF-23 • Klotho • Calcium-sensing receptor • Synthesis • Secretion • GALNT3 gene • TRPV5,6 channels • Depolarization • Intestinal transport • Ionized calcium • Phosphoric acid • Phosphate carrier • Renal handling calcium and phosphorus • Intracellular calcium function • Extracellular calcium function • Bone mineral • Hypocalcemia • Hypercalcemia • Secretion • Osteoblasts • Osteoclasts • Kidney reabsorption • Intestinal absorption • 25-Hydroxyvitamin D$_3$ • 1α-Hydroxylase • IGF-1 • Vitamin D binding protein • Osteomalacia • Phosphatonin • Mutations calcium-sensing receptor • Phosphate-sensing mechanisms • Calcium transport mechanisms • Intestinal calcium transport • Macronutrients • Intestinal phosphate absorption • Renal control mechanism of calcium and phosphate transport

A.D. Conigrave, MD, PhD, FRACP (✉)
School of Molecular Bioscience, University of Sydney, NSW 2006, Australia
e-mail: arthur.conigrave@sydney.edu.au

A.A. Licata and E.V. Lerma (eds.), *Diseases of the Parathyroid Glands*,
DOI 10.1007/978-1-4419-5550-0_2, © Springer Science+Business Media, LLC 2012

• Hormonal regulation of calcium renal transport • Calcitonin • Renal tubular phosphate transport • Renal proximal tubule • Cartilage and bone and mineral regulation • Bone resorption • Remodeling • Modulators bone resorption • Calcitonin • Estrogen • Leptin • β-adrenergic signaling • Bone formation • Mineralization • SIBLING • Rickets • Hypophosphatemic rickets • ADHR • XLH • ARHR • Bone calcium-sensing receptor • Thick ascending limb • Phosphate transporters (Npt2a and Npt2c and PiT-2) • Secreted frizzled-related protein-4 • Na/H exchanger regulatory factors • Null mice • Apoptosis • Cathepsin proteases • Sclerostin • Hypocalciuric hypercalcemia • Cytokine TNF-α • RANK ligand • Tissue nonspecific alkaline phosphatase • Dentin matrix protein-1 • Matrix extracellular phosphoglycoprotein • PHEX • Phosphatonin • Ossification

Introduction

The metabolisms of calcium and inorganic phosphate are intimately connected as, respectively, the cationic and anionic components of crystalline hydroxyapatite, which confers rigidity on the bone matrix (Fig. 2.1). In this chapter, the author considers the biological processes that underlie the balances of Ca^{2+} and phosphate as well as the key points of exchange in the gut, kidney, and bone, together with their regulation. These balances depend on dietary composition and the effectiveness with which calcium and phosphate are released from ingested food. They also depend on the efficiencies of intestinal absorption, glomerular filtration, and renal tubular reabsorption along with rates of transfer between the blood and the bone mineral store as well as the magnitudes of unavoidable losses associated, for example, with small and large intestinal secretions. Regulation of calcium and phosphate metabolism depends on several important hormones, chiefly parathyroid hormone (PTH), $1,25(OH)_2$ vitamin D_3 (calcitriol), and fibroblast growth factor-23

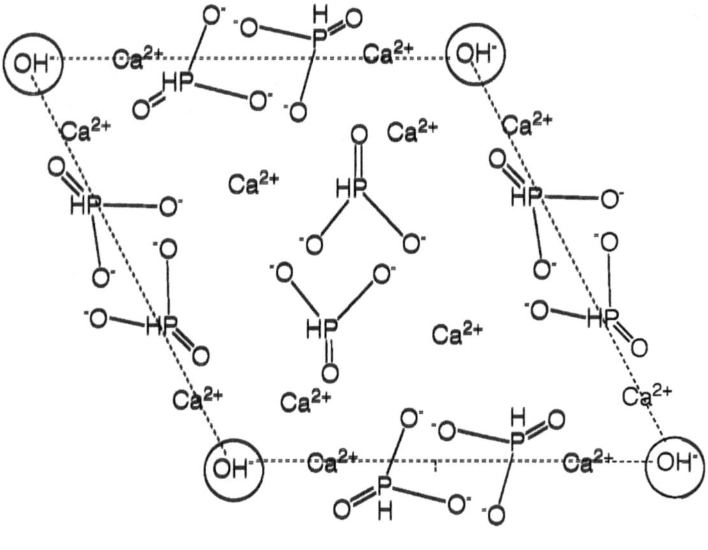

Fig. 2.1 Partial structure of the bone mineral hydroxyapatite. A view of the repeating structural unit of hydroxyapatite based on the analysis in [269]. The corners of the repeating unit are occupied by hydroxyl ions. The hydroxyl groups are typically carboxylated by reaction with carbon dioxide. Note the presence of two distinct Ca^{2+} binding sites

(FGF-23) as well as molecular sensors for Ca^{2+}, including the so-called calcium-sensing receptor (CaSR), and phosphate. In some cases, these sensors coordinate the synthesis and release of hormones with actions on both Ca^{2+} and phosphate transfers in targets including intestine, kidney, and bone. In other cases, they directly modulate Ca^{2+} and/or phosphate transport in key target cells. In addition, macronutrients including carbohydrates and protein are important modulators of calcium and phosphate metabolism with notable positive effects on intestinal absorption.

Introduction to Calcium and Phosphate

In serum, calcium is present in three main forms: ionized, complexed with small anions such as citrate, and bound to serum proteins, chiefly albumin. After ingestion, calcium is released from foods, in part by the action of gastric acid as well as digestive enzymes in the stomach and small intestine. Calcium absorption is mediated by transport mechanisms in all segments of the small intestine. Even so it is inherently inefficient. Typically, significantly less than 50% of ingested calcium is absorbed (Fig. 2.2).

Phosphoric acid is a strong acid with three pH titratable hydroxyl (OH) groups. For this reason, inorganic phosphate exists in three forms: $H_2PO_4^-$, HPO_4^{2-}, and PO_4^{3-}. Under standard conditions at 25°C, the p*K*as that govern the equilibria between the species are (1) 2.13; (2) 7.20; and (3) 12.36 [1]. At physiological ionic strength and temperature, these p*K*a values shift so that pKa_2, for example, falls from 7.2 to around 6.8. Thus, in blood plasma at pH 7.4 with a total inorganic phosphate concentration of around 1.0 mM, the HPO_4^{2-} concentration is approximately 0.8 mM and the $H_2PO_4^-$ concentration is around 0.2 mM; the concentrations of other species are negligible. In the acid environment of the distal nephron, where pH values frequently drop below 5.5 as a result of proton secretion [2], $H_2PO_4^-$ becomes the predominant species. In general, the negative

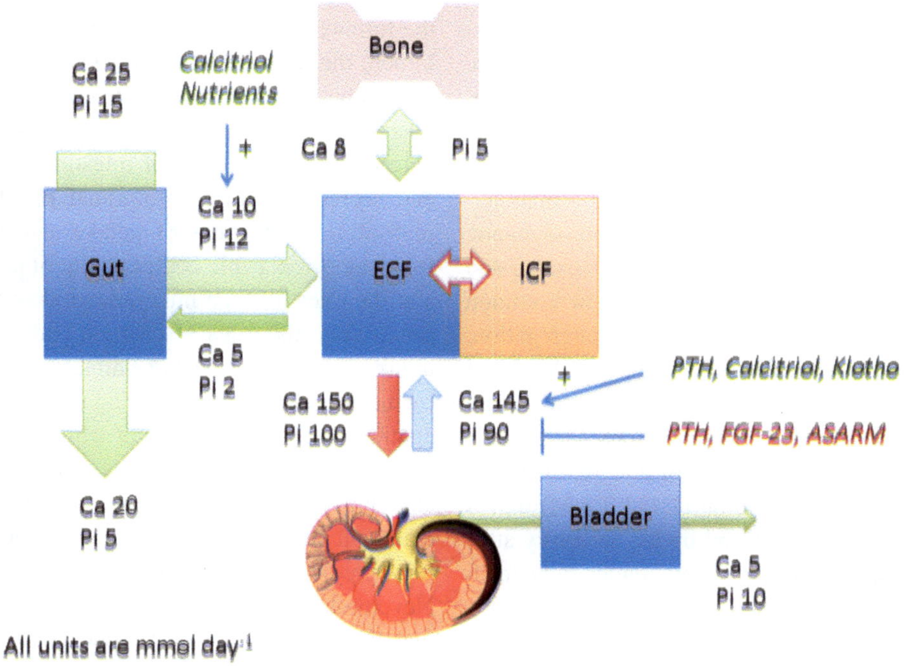

Fig. 2.2 Whole body calcium and phosphate fluxes in adult humans. Representative fluxes are shown for calcium and phosphate transfers between the extracellular fluid and the gut, kidney, and bone and have been based on previous analyses [208, 270]. The ratio of the fluxes for calcium and phosphate between bone and the extracellular fluid reflects the composition of hydroxyapatite. The fluxes shown between the ECF and kidney refer to glomerular filtration and tubular reabsorption. ECF, extracellular fluid; ICF, intracellular fluid

charge on phosphate is balanced in body fluids by the monovalent cations Na^{+} or K^{+} with no implications for its water solubility. However, HPO_4^{2-} forms insoluble precipitates with Ca^{2+} ions in the presence of water with a solubility product of around 5×10^{-7} $(mol/L)^2$. At the normal ionized concentrations for Ca^{2+} of 1.2 mM and HPO_4^{2-} of 0.8 mM in human plasma, this product is exceeded. Nevertheless, precipitation and bone mineral formation do not proceed spontaneously in body fluids or in the interstitium due, in part, to the presence of Mg^{2+}, which competes with Ca^{2+} [3], and forms phosphate complexes of greater solubility [4], as well as inhibitory polyphosphates and proteins (see below).

Intracellular and Extracellular Roles of Calcium and Phosphate

Ca^{2+} and inorganic phosphate play multiple physiological roles, many of which are independent of their roles in mineralization. *Intracellularly*, Ca^{2+} acts as a pluripotent regulator of biochemical pathways via high affinity interactions with rate-limiting enzymes or protein modulators. Phosphate, on the other hand, acts as a substrate for the synthesis of organic phosphates in biochemical interconversions, molecular recognition, energy storage (e.g., in ATP and creatine phosphate) or as a regulator of protein conformation.

Extracellularly, Ca^{2+} also supports synaptic transmission, the contractile state of vascular and nonvascular smooth muscle, the final common pathway of coagulation, and platelet aggregation; it also acts as a reservoir for the replenishment of intracellular Ca^{2+} pools. The requirements of all these processes have led to the establishment of a tight physiological range for the extracellular ionized Ca^{2+} concentration (1.1–1.3 mM) that is defended at the lower end by the secretory state of the four parathyroid glands under tight feedback control mediated by extracellular Ca^{2+}-sensing receptors (review: [5]) and at the higher end by renal Ca^{2+}-sensing receptors coupled to stimulated calcium excretion [6]. Calcitriol and FGF-23 modulate the parathyroid response: calcitriol by enhancing Ca^{2+}-sensing receptor expression [7] and suppressing PTH expression [8, 9]; FGF-23 by suppressing PTH gene expression [10]. Interestingly, the immediate precursor of calcitriol, 25-hydroxyvitamin D significantly suppresses PTH secretion and mRNA levels at physiologically relevant concentrations [11], suggesting either that 25-hydroxyvitamin D directly activates the parathyroid vitamin D receptor or acts as the substrate for the local generation of calcitriol.

Like Ca^{2+}, the extracellular inorganic phosphate concentration is tightly regulated. However, there is greater variation in its normal range from around 0.7 to 1.4 mM, providing variation in the Ca^{2+}-phosphate solubility product and, thus, in the potential rates of hydroxyapatite formation. Hypophosphatemia is a recognized cause of rickets and osteomalacia (review: [12]) as considered below.

An Overview of Calcium and Phosphate Metabolism

Calcium and phosphate exchange between the blood plasma and extracellular fluid as well as the following major compartments: the intestinal lumen, the intracellular fluid, bone mineral, and renal tubular fluid (Fig. 2.2). In consequence, the overall balances for calcium and phosphate are determined by the rates of intestinal absorption and secretion, the rates of renal filtration and reabsorption, the rates of uptake and extrusion from the cytoplasmic compartment of all tissues, and the rates of bone mineralization and resorption. While the rates of calcium and phosphate uptake and release from bone mineral are matched by the structure of the repeating unit of hydroxyapatite, $(Ca_{10}(PO_4)_6(OH)_2)$, in which the relative proportion of Ca:phosphate is 5:3, the rates of calcium and phosphate transfers between the extracellular fluid and other compartments are less predictable and regulated independently. Nevertheless, key hormonal regulators of calcium metabolism also impact on phosphate metabolism. Notable examples are PTH and, calcitriol. Major relationships between calcium, phosphate, PTH, calcitriol, and FGF-23, the key phosphate regulating hormone, as well as calcitonin are presented in Fig. 2.3 and discussed below.

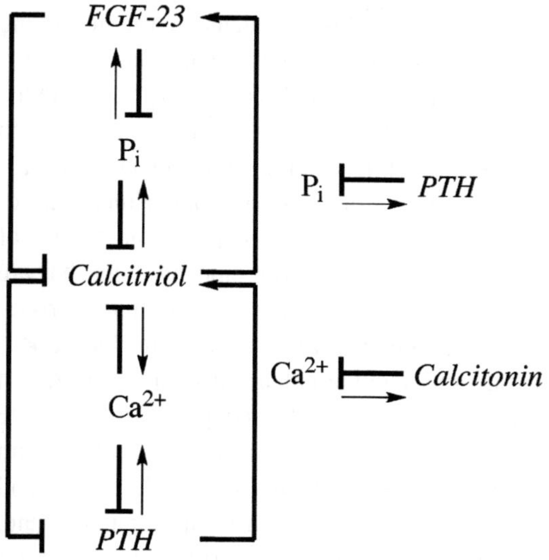

Fig. 2.3 Relationships between calcium and phosphate with key mineral-regulating hormones. The *left-hand panel* shows the relationships between calcium and phosphate with calcitriol, the key positive modulator of their intestinal absorption. In addition, the feedback relationships between calcium and PTH (*bottom*) as well as the phosphate and FGF-23 (*top*) are shown. Elevated calcium suppresses PTH secretion within minutes; hypocalcemia acutely stimulates PTH secretion. Elevated phosphate, on the other hand, promotes the production of FGF-23 only after a delay of several hours. Also shown in the *left-hand panel* are the major reciprocal relationships between PTH and calcitriol, and calcitriol and FGF-23. PTH stimulates calcitriol synthesis; calcitriol promotes the production of FGF-23, thereby reducing the risk of hyperphosphatemia following enhanced intestinal phosphate absorption. On the other hand, FGF-23 suppresses calcitriol synthesis and calcitriol suppresses PTH synthesis. These relationships may contribute to a reported positive effect of PTH on FGF-23 synthesis and a reported negative effect of FGF-23 on PTH synthesis. The *right-hand panels* show the feedback relationships between phosphate and PTH as well as calcium and calcitonin. PTH lowers the serum phosphate concentration by suppressing its reabsorption in the proximal tubule and calcitonin suppresses the serum calcium concentration by suppressing osteoclastic resorption of bone

Parathyroid Hormone

PTH secretion is under the tight inhibitory control of the serum ionized calcium (Ca^{2+}) concentration acting via the CaSR (review: [5]). Thus, PTH secretion is markedly stimulated by hypocalcemia. In addition, PTH secretion is negatively modulated by various factors including L-amino acids [13], which enhance the extracellular Ca^{2+} sensitivity of the CaSR (reviews: [14, 15]), as well as calcitriol, which upregulates CaSR expression [7] and suppresses PTH expression (review: [16]), 25-hydroxyvitamin D [11], and FGF-23 [10]. Inorganic phosphate promotes parathyroid hyperplasia and PTH secretion and these effects appear to contribute to secondary hyperparathyroidism in chronic kidney disease [17]. Endogenous expression of the single-pass integral membrane protein, α-klotho, in the parathyroid has been reported to facilitate PTH secretion [18].

Consistent with the stimulatory impact of hypocalcemia on its secretion, key actions of PTH are directed to elevating the serum Ca^{2+} concentration and restraining or suppressing the inorganic phosphate concentration to prevent inappropriate crystallization. Thus, PTH promotes osteoclastic bone resorption via type-I PTH/PTHrP receptors (PTH1Rs) on cells of the osteoblast–osteocyte lineage as well as T lymphocytes [19]. It also modulates renal tubular transport via independent effects to stimulate Ca^{2+} reabsorption and inhibit phosphate reabsorption. Finally, it promotes 1α-hydroxylase activity in the renal proximal tubule to boost serum calcitriol levels [20] and, thus, stimulate intestinal calcium absorption. In consequence, endogenous PTH is best viewed as a surveillance and emergency-response hormone directed to the prevention and reversal of hypocalcemia ([6]; review: [21]).

PTH stimulates calcium reabsorption in the distal nephron [22]; thereby, enhancing total renal calcium reabsorption from around 95% to 98.5% and thus suppressing renal calcium excretion from around 5% to 1.5% of a largely fixed, filtered load [23]. On the other hand, PTH suppresses phosphate reabsorption in the proximal tubules [24], markedly elevating renal phosphate excretion from around 15–20% to greater than 50% of the filtered load. Correspondingly, parathyroidectomy suppresses fractional phosphate excretion to around 10% [25]. PTH-induced renal phosphate wasting would appear to be an appropriate compensatory response to calcitriol-stimulated small intestinal phosphate uptake and osteoclastic release of phosphate from resorbed hydroxyapatite in bone. Evidence that PTH [26] and, indeed, calcitriol [27] promote the production of the phosphatonin FGF-23 in bone provides additional mechanisms for the activation of renal phosphate wasting under conditions of PTH-stimulated bone resorption and calcitriol synthesis.

Although prolonged elevations in PTH induce osteoclastic bone resorption, acute administration of PTH, in pharmacological doses and in the context of normal serum calcium levels, promotes bone formation (review: [28]), possibly simulating some of the effects of bone cell-derived PTHrP (review: [29]). Thus, acute repetitive stimulation of PTH1Rs on osteoblasts and/or osteocytes for 1–2 h promotes bone formation and mineralization. Perhaps consistent with this, the immediate response to acute administration of PTH is a *fall* rather than a rise in serum Ca^{2+} concentration associated with calcium uptake by bone [30, 31].

The outcome of PTH action is, thus, dependent upon context. The duration of exposure, the serum level of calcitriol and its precursor 25-hydroxyvitamin D, the dietary intakes and serum levels of calcium and phosphate, together with the relative levels of the responses in bone and kidney all contribute to the outcome. In the context of prolonged elevation of PTH, the serum calcium concentration rises because the effects of PTH, whether direct or indirect, on all key targets promote Ca^{2+} accumulation in the extracellular fluid whether from bone, kidney, or gut. However, the impact of prolonged elevation of PTH on phosphate is less predictable and depends on whether the primary effect is on the kidney, in which case serum phosphate levels may drop or the gut, via calcitriol, or on bone in which case serum phosphate levels are more likely to be normal. In the setting of chronic kidney disease, in which there is resistance to PTH actions, serum phosphate levels are typically elevated and serum calcium levels are normal or suppressed (review: [32]).

Calcitriol and 25-Hydroxyvitamin D

Calcitriol is synthesized from 25-hydroxyvitamin D by the action of 1α-hydroxylase, the product of the *CYP27B1* gene (review: [33]). In serum, calcitriol is a tightly regulated hormone arising from the actions of multiple nutrient and hormonal inputs on 1α-hydroxylase expression in the renal proximal tubules. Its primary actions are to promote intestinal calcium and phosphate absorption via effects on duodenal and jejunal enterocytes, respectively (review: [33]) and failure of these effects can be overcome by diets that are rich in calcium, phosphate, and certain macronutrients including lactose and protein. Its secondary actions include enhanced renal reabsorption of calcium (review: [33]) and, possibly, phosphate [34]. Together, enhanced absorptions of calcium and phosphate ions are detected by local Ca^{2+} and phosphate sensors in the gastrointestinal tract and, if sufficient to elevate the serum calcium and/or phosphate levels, by sensors strategically positioned in endocrine, bone, and kidney cells. In this way, enhanced calcium absorption, whether arising from calcitriol-stimulated vitamin D receptors (VDRs) in the duodenum or via an alternative small intestinal absorption pathway can shut down PTH secretion via extracellular Ca^{2+}-sensing receptors on parathyroid cells (review: [5]). Together with the elevated serum calcium and phosphate levels, suppressed PTH levels remove an important stimulatory drive for renal calcitriol synthesis (review: [33]).

In company with adequate levels of serum calcium, calcitriol also suppresses the growth of parathyroid glands in 1α-hydroxylase null mice (review: [35]). Nevertheless, the normal physiological significance of these effects is unclear. In part, this uncertainty arises from observations of a lack of correlation between the serum calcitriol and PTH levels in human subjects, and from the primacy of the serum Ca^{2+} concentration in determining serum PTH levels.

25-Hydroxyvitamin D is both the substrate for the synthesis of calcitriol and a nutritional modulator in its own right. With respect to mineral metabolism, its primary target appears to be the parathyroid where, in concert with the serum Ca^{2+} concentration, it suppresses PTH synthesis. This explains highly reproducible negative correlations between serum 25-hydroxyvitamin D and PTH levels (review: [36]) and is supported by evidence that 25-hydroxyvitamin D suppresses

PTH gene expression and secretion from cultured parathyroid cells in both the absence and presence of a 1α-hydroxylase inhibitor [11]. Furthermore, in *CYP27B1* null mice, vitamin D3 supplements sufficient to raise the serum 25-hydroxyvitamin D level to 400 nmol/L prevented hypocalcemia and markedly increased the expressions of the VDR-sensitive targets, intestinal calbindin-D_{9K}, and renal 24-hydroxylase on a standard diet [37]. Whether these effects operate at more commonly observed concentrations in humans (around 30–80 nmol/L) is currently unclear.

The significance of serum calcitriol levels and calcitriol-dependent activation of small intestinal VDRs for whole body mineral metabolism depends on dietary context. It is critical under conditions of low calcium and/or phosphate intake and in the absence of dietary lactose upon weaning in mice (review: [33]). Under these circumstances, 1α-hydroxylase null or VDR null mice develop hypocalcemia, hypophosphatemia, and secondary hyperparathyroidism taking the form of massively elevated serum PTH levels [38, 39]. However, calcium and phosphate absorption is restored, as reported by serum calcium, phosphate, and PTH levels, upon the introduction of a diet containing 2% calcium, 1-2% phosphate, and 20% lactose [40]. These findings are consistent with the notion of a calcitriol-independent absorption pathway linked to macronutrient digestion and absorption (see below). Under conditions in which dietary calcium and phosphate intake is high and intestinal absorption is supported by adequate levels of key macronutrients, as may frequently occur in humans, the impact of serum calcitriol on mineral metabolism may be limited, as extracellular Ca^{2+}-dependent suppression of PTH removes a key drive for renal calcitriol synthesis. Under these conditions, there is no correlation between serum PTH and calcitriol levels and the negative impact of exogenously administered calcitriol on PTH synthesis and secretion (review: [41]) may be primarily of pharmacological significance. Nevertheless, under these conditions, serum 25-hydroxyvitamin D retains significance as a nutritional modulator with the ability to suppress PTH whether alone or in concert with calcium [42].

As bodily vitamin D stores fall in humans whether due to inadequate diet or intestinal absorption, poor sunlight exposure or skin biosynthesis, or a combination of these factors, as frequently occurs in the elderly (review: [43]), serum 25-hydroxyvitamin D levels fall with attendant increases in serum PTH levels. The serum calcium concentration typically remains in the normal range. Whether elevated serum PTH levels act to maintain or boost serum calcitriol levels under these circumstances is unclear—typically, serum calcitriol levels also remain within the normal reference range. However, there is a cost: accelerated consumption of 25-hydroxyvitamin D. Oral calcium supplements can facilitate calcium absorption in the context of vitamin D deficiency and thereby boost serum ionized Ca^{2+} levels, typically, still within the normal range. This provides Ca^{2+}-dependent feedback inhibition of renal calcitriol synthesis as well as PTH secretion, further relieving the drive for calcitriol synthesis [44]. Conversely, repletion of vitamin D stores is reflected first in elevated 25-hydroxyvitamin D levels with corresponding falls in serum PTH [45].

25-Hydroxyvitamin D is converted to the key calcium and phosphate-elevating hormone, calcitriol via the action of 1α-hydroxylase. Although the gene *CYP27B1* appears to universally encode 1α-hydroxylase in tissues including the kidney, testis, brain, placenta, bone, and skin, thereby catalyzing the local production of calcitriol (review: [46]), only the renal enzyme controls the synthesis of calcitriol for release into the circulation under physiological conditions and is selectively controlled by key micronutrient and hormonal regulators of mineral metabolism (review: [33]). These regulators include elevations in the serum levels of calcium or phosphate (negative), as well as the hormones FGF-23 and calcitriol (also negative), and PTH and IGF-1 (both positive). Downregulation of renal 1α-hydroxylase by calcium, phosphate, FGF-23 (as a delayed reporter of ingested phosphate), and calcitriol itself may all be viewed as physiologically appropriate forms of negative feedback. On the other hand, upregulation of 1α-hydroxylase by PTH and IGF-1 would appear to arise in quite different physiological contexts with distinct implications. Thus, upregulation of 1α-hydroxylase by PTH may be viewed as a component of an "emergency response to hypocalcemia," whose goal is the restoration of normal serum calcium levels. Upregulation of 1α-hydroxylase by IGF-1, on the other hand, would appear to provide a mechanism by which intestinal calcium and phosphate absorption can be enhanced together with their renal retention in the context of growth and an associated stimulation of bone formation [47–49].

Together, 25-hydroxyvitamin D and calcitriol are carried in the circulation by a 52-kDa vitamin D binding protein (DBP) and both are deactivated by a widely expressed 24-hydroxylase, encoded by the CYP24A1 gene, whose expression is powerfully upregulated by calcitriol [50, 51] and possibly 25-hydroxyvitamin D [52] leading to the generation of 24,25(OH)$_2$ vitamin D or 1α-hydroxy-23-carboxy-24, 25, 26, 27-tetranorvitamin D$_3$ (calcitroic acid). Based on findings in CYP24a1 null mice, 24-hydroxylase prevents inappropriate elevation of serum calcitriol levels as well as attendant hypercalcemia and hypoparathyroidism [53].

In the renal synthesis of calcitriol, the DBP–25-hydroxyvitamin D complex enters the proximal tubular cytoplasm following glomerular filtration and uptake via apical megalin/cubulin-mediated endocytosis [54–56]. DBP null mice exhibit markedly suppressed levels of circulating calcitriol and 25-hydroxyvitamin D, and a demineralizing phenotype [57]. Surprisingly, serum calcium, phosphate, and PTH levels were normal in DBP null mice on control chow but administration of a vitamin D-deficient diet for 4 weeks induced a significant decrease in serum phosphate and a significant increase in serum PTH without a change in serum calcium [57] indicating that the elevated PTH had normalized serum calcium in the context of vitamin D deficiency while suppressing the serum phosphate level. Whether serum FGF-23 levels changed under the conditions of these experiments is unknown. The results indicate that DBP provides a store of circulating vitamin D metabolites and prolongs their serum half-lives but is not necessary for their actions (review: [58]).

The significance of calcitriol for normal mineral homeostasis has been assessed in 1α-hydroxylase (*CYP27B1*) null mice and VDR null mice. Although the phenotypes of these mice are not identical suggesting the existence of calcitriol-independent actions of VDR in the skin and hair follicles, and VDR-independent actions of calcitriol in the epiphyseal growth plates (review: [33]), they both exhibit severe rickets and osteomalacia after weaning, arising from markedly impaired intestinal calcium and phosphate absorption. The findings indicate that, postweaning, adequate circulating levels of calcitriol together with the expression of its cognate VDRs in the small intestine are required for normal mineral metabolism (review: [33]). Thus, intestinal calcium and phosphate transport was restored in *CYP27B1* null mice following administration of exogenous calcitriol [59], and in global VDR null mice by intestine-specific transgenic expression of the VDR [60]. Furthermore, the hypo-mineralizing bone phenotype was clearly dependent upon impaired intestinal calcium and phosphate absorption because it could be overcome by rescue diets containing enhanced contents of calcium and phosphate as well as lactose (review: [33]). The expression of the phenotype only after weaning and the striking impact of lactose in the rescue diet suggests the existence of a calcitriol-independent, macronutrient-associated absorption pathway (see below).

FGF-23 and Klotho

FGF-23 is a "phosphatonin," i.e., a circulating factor that promotes renal proximal tubular phosphate wasting and thereby lowers serum phosphate levels (reviews: [61, 62]). Although its impact on phosphate metabolism in certain pathological contexts seems clear, its role in the normal surveillance of bodily phosphate metabolism and the time-scale over which it operates are uncertain.

The significance of FGF-23 for the control of renal phosphate excretion and serum phosphate levels was first established in human studies of inherited forms of rickets and/or osteomalacia including autosomal dominant hypophosphatemic rickets (ADHR) [63] and X-linked hypophosphatemia (XLH) [64] as well as tumor-induced osteomalacia [64] in all of which serum FGF-23 levels are elevated in association with renal phosphate wasting, hypophosphatemia, and inappropriately suppressed serum calcitriol levels (review: [41]). Correspondingly, tumoral calcinosis in humans in the context of hyperphosphatemia and elevated serum calcitriol levels typically arises from impaired FGF-23 secretion whether associated with specific FGF-23 mutations [65] or mutations of UDP-GalNAc transferase 3 (GALNT3) that impair FGF-23 processing (review: [66]).

The significance of FGF-23 in the control of phosphate metabolism is supported by transgenic mouse studies, most notably *fgf-23* null mice, which exhibit hyperphosphatemia, elevated serum calcitriol levels, hypercalcemia, and widespread calcification [67]. Elevated serum calcitriol levels appear to be critical for the development of both hyperphosphatemia and hypercalcemia in these mice. Consistent with this notion, the double mutant $fgf23^{-/-}/1\alpha\text{-}OHase^{-/-}$ mouse exhibits normal or near-normal serum calcium and phosphate levels as well as normal growth and markedly improved lifespan [68].

FGF-23 is a key negative regulator of serum calcitriol levels. Thus, an acute bolus intravenous injection of FGF-23 in mice suppressed 1α-OHase expression and promoted 24-hydroxylase expression, resulting in markedly suppressed serum calcitriol levels [69]. The effect of FGF-23 on serum calcitriol levels was detected between 3 and 24 h (trough around 9 h) indicating that its effects are likely to be dependent on changes in gene expression. Interestingly, the effect of FGF-23 on the serum calcitriol level in these studies occurred several hours earlier, and was substantially greater, than its effect on the serum phosphate level [69]. Thus, although FGF-23 promotes phosphaturia by downregulating the expressions of Npt2a and Npt2c in the renal proximal tubular luminal membrane [70], and suppresses serum phosphate levels, it is not yet clear whether its effects are mediated directly by FGF receptors in the renal proximal tubule or indirectly via other hormonal factors, e.g., arising from the processing of small integrin-binding ligand N-linked glycoproteins (SIBLINGs) to acidic serine and aspartate-rich motif (ASARM) peptides in bone or via paracrine factors, e.g., from the distal tubule (review: [71]). Complicating these considerations is an observation that FGF-23 suppresses intestinal Npt2b expression in wild-type but not Npt2a or Npt2c null mice [72] independent of serum calcitriol levels, which were markedly suppressed in all three cases. The results point to the existence of, as yet unrecognized, phosphate regulatory signals that operate between the kidney and small intestine and are mediated by Npt2a and 2c and/or one of their partner proteins.

The pronounced negative effect of serum FGF-23 on serum calcitriol levels raised the possibility of a novel feedback loop involving the two hormones. Consistent with this idea, calcitriol activates FGF-23 expression [27, 73, 74]. In addition, prolonged elevations of calcitriol upregulate the expression of FGF-23 and prolonged elevations of FGF-23 coordinately downregulate renal 1α-hydroxylase and upregulate renal 24-hydroxylase (review: [41]). The feedback loop between calcitriol and FGF-23 may contribute to the support of a natural diurnal rhythm in whole body calcium and phosphate metabolism, which in part takes the form of a coordinated trough in the serum levels of calcium (–2%), phosphate (–10%), calcitriol (–10%), and PTH (–20%) at around 0800 [75]. In a recent study, no diurnal rhythm was observed in serum FGF-23 levels, however, there was a pronounced trough in the level of the soluble form of its co-receptor α-klotho (–40%) at around 0000 [76]. The significance of these findings is currently unclear.

FGF-23 is synthesized in osteocytes and osteoblasts and its secretion depends, in part, on the enzyme GALNT3 which O-glycosylates the peptide (review: [41]). Its expression and serum levels are increased by elevated dietary phosphate intake [77–79] and elevated serum calcitriol levels [27] and these effects have been demonstrated in both mouse and human studies. However, serum FGF-23 levels do not appear to be regulated by acute changes in serum phosphate concentration. Data obtained in acute human studies, for example, suggest that serum FGF-23 levels do not normally respond within 6 h of exposure to a substantial increase in either dietary phosphate intake or the serum phosphate level [79, 80] and possibly not before 12 h [81].

PTH has been reported to promote FGF-23 expression and elevate its serum levels. Thus, PTH administered subcutaneously in mice for 3 days by osmotic mini-pump induced an elevation in serum FGF-23 levels in the context of elevated serum calcium and suppressed serum phosphate levels [26] and in a study in healthy men who received 18-h intravenous infusions of PTH 1–34, serum FGF-23 levels were elevated from 6 to 18 h in association with elevated serum levels of calcitriol and calcium [82]. Whether reported reciprocal interactions between PTH and FGF-23 [10, 26] constitute an additional regulatory loop or are dependent upon the intermediary actions of calcitriol and/or phosphate is currently uncertain.

α-Klotho

α-Klotho is an important partner of FGF-23 and exists in both circulating and integral membrane forms. It contributes to the formation of high affinity FGF-23 receptors by forming ternary complexes with FGF receptors [83] including FGFR1c in the proximal tubule [70]. Consistent with the notion that the actions of α-klotho and FGF-23 are interdependent, the phenotypes of α-klotho null mice and FGF-23 null mice are similar and both include marked elevations of serum phosphate and increased serum levels of calcitriol [84]. In addition, FGF-23 levels are markedly elevated in α-klotho null mice [85] suggesting the existence of a resistance state with dysregulated FGF23 secretion arising from elevated serum calcitriol and/or serum phosphate levels.

More recent work suggests that α-klotho may have additional actions on mineral metabolism that arise, at least in part, from its β-glucuronidase activity. Thus, α-klotho promotes the surface expression of distal nephron TRPV5 [86] by cleaving terminal sialic acid residues to expose an underlying galactose-*N*-acetylglucosamine, which binds to the plasma membrane lectin, galectin-1 [87]. The outcome is enhanced renal Ca^{2+} reabsorption (review: [88]). Consistent with these findings the α-klotho null mouse exhibits impaired distal convoluted tubule (DCT) and connecting tubule Ca^{2+} reabsorption and resistance to the stimulatory action of PTH on Ca^{2+} reabsorption [89]. In addition, as noted above, α-klotho expression in the parathyroid has also been linked to PTH secretion [18].

Calcium-Sensing Mechanisms: Calcium-Sensing Receptors

Although a number of cellular calcium-sensing mechanisms have been defined based on the activities of ion channels and transporters, one of the best understood calcium-sensing mechanism in human biology is dependent upon the expression of a class C G-protein-coupled receptor known as the CaSR. The CaSR was first cloned from the parathyroid [90], where it mediates feedback control of PTH secretion and thus provides a key defense against hypocalcemia (review: [5]) and subsequently the kidney [91], where it regulates renal calcium excretion, providing an important defense against hypercalcemia [6]. The CaSR also modulates renal phosphate, salt, and water transport (review: [92]). It is expressed in various bodily compartments and organs including the gastro-intestinal tract, kidney, thyroid C-cells, and bone in which it is expressed on cells of both the osteoblast and osteoclast lineages [93]. The roles of the CaSR in the control of renal calcium and phosphate transport as well as bone biology are considered below. In gut biology it has multiple roles that include the promotion of interactions between macronutrient and micronutrient metabolism (review: [94]).

Heterozygous inactivating mutations of the CaSR underlie the uncommon, typically benign, hypercalcemic disorder known as familial hypocalciuric hypercalcemia (FHH) [95] in which there is impaired inhibition of calcium reabsorption in the renal cortical thick ascending limb (TAL) [96]. The primary problem is impaired inhibitory control of renal calcium reabsorption but, in addition, the serum PTH level is typically inappropriately normal [97]. The rare, typically homozygous, form of the disorder presents as a neonatal form of severe hyperparathyroidism with markedly elevated serum calcium levels and pathological fractures within the first weeks of life [98]. The problem arises from extreme resistance to the serum Ca^{2+} concentration in both the parathyroid and kidney.

In addition to sensing the extracellular Ca^{2+} concentration, the CaSR is a multimodal chemosensor that responds to L-amino acids and is, thus, sensitive to changes in protein nutrition (review: [99]), as well as ionic strength, pH, Mg^{2+}, neuromodulators including spermine, and glutathione analogs (reviews: [15, 100]). Thus, the CaSR has roles not only in the regulation and modulation of calcium and phosphate metabolism and bone biology but also in various other physiological processes. In the gastro-intestinal tract, these include the modulation of gastrin release and acid secretion (review: [99]) as well as the regulation of cholecystokinin secretion [101–103]. The CaSR may also contribute to well-recognized positive interactions between protein nutrition and calcium and bone metabolism [104].

Phosphate-Sensing Mechanisms

Phosphate-sensing mechanisms have been identified in the intestine, kidney, bone, and growth plate and act to regulate renal phosphate excretion and skeletal development as well as bone mass and mineralization (see below). Biological effects coupled to phosphate-sensing mechanisms include enhanced production of phosphatonins including FGF-23, and MEPE, and suppressed production of calcitriol, both of which are appropriate responses to hyperphosphatemia, as well as apoptosis of hypertrophic chondrocytes in the process of normal growth plate development and osteoblast maturation (review: [105]). In addition, a number of putative phosphate sensors, e.g., based on one or more phosphate transporters, and even elements of potential signaling pathways, e.g., ERK1/2, have been proposed [106]. However, the full significance of these pathways awaits the identification of the molecular sensors and their signaling partners.

Calcium Transport Mechanisms

Epithelial Calcium Transporters in Support of Transcellular Ca^{2+} Transport

Expression cloning of key epithelial Ca^{2+} transporters of the small intestine [107] and kidney [108], permitted the identification and detailed analyses of active transport mechanisms in the duodenum and distal nephron (review: [109]). These transporters are now recognized as members of the TRPV family of ion channels, i.e., TRPV6 and TRPV5, respectively (review: [110]). In support of these transport mechanisms are the cytoplasmic Ca^{2+}-binding proteins calbindin-D_{9k} (intestine and kidney) and calbindin-D_{28k} (kidney), which promote calcium uptake and transport by buffering the intracellular Ca^{2+} concentration, as well as two energy-expending basolateral Ca^{2+} pump mechanisms: the Ca^{2+}-ATPase isoform Ib and the Na^+/Ca^{2+}-exchanger NCX1 coupled to Na^+–K^+-ATPase activity (review: [109, 110]). The Na^+–K^+-ATPase maintains a steep electrochemical gradient for Na^+ ions across the basolateral membrane favoring Na^+ influx from the extracellular fluid to the cytoplasm. The Na^+ gradient is used by NCX1 to drive Ca^{2+} efflux in exchange for Na^+ influx (Fig. 2.4; upper cell). These mechanisms support calcitriol-induced Ca^{2+} absorption in the duodenum (review: [110]) and PTH and calcitriol-induced Ca^{2+} reabsorption in the distal nephron (review: [22]).

In addition, less well-defined transcellular Ca^{2+} transport mechanisms provide a link between calcium absorption and the absorption of key macronutrients (see below).

Paracellular Ca^{2+} Transport Across Epithelia

In addition to transcellular mechanisms of calcium transport, paracellular Ca^{2+} transport mechanisms support Ca^{2+} transport in both the intestine and renal tubules. The key elements of these transport mechanisms are a transepithelial electrochemical gradient and a paracellular pathway (Fig. 2.5). A favorable transepithelial

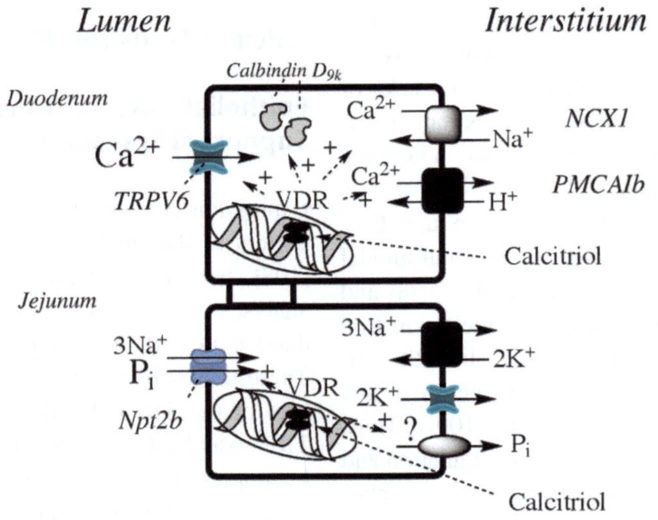

Fig. 2.4 Calcitriol stimulated intestinal absorption pathways for calcium and phosphate. The *upper cell* presents components of a key duodenal calcium absorptive pathway including the luminal membrane Ca^{2+} channel, TRPV6, the intracellular Ca^{2+} binding protein, calbindin D_{9k}, which buffers the cytoplasmic Ca^{2+} concentration, as well as exit pathways via the Na^+/Ca^{2+} exchanger, NCX1 and the Ca^{2+}-ATPase, PMCAIb (review: [110]). The basolateral Na^+/K^+-ATPase, which maintains the Na^+ gradient across the interstitium–facing membrane is not shown. The *lower cell* presents components of a key jejunal phosphate absorptive pathway (review: [114]), including the luminal membrane Na^+-phosphate co-transporter, Npt2b, basolateral Na^+/K^+-ATPase, and a basolateral membrane phosphate channel (or transporter). Calcitriol acts via nuclear vitamin D receptors to upregulate the synthesis of molecular components in both pathways. Additional pathways for the small intestinal absorption of calcium, and possibly phosphate, are linked to macronutrient uptake (not shown)

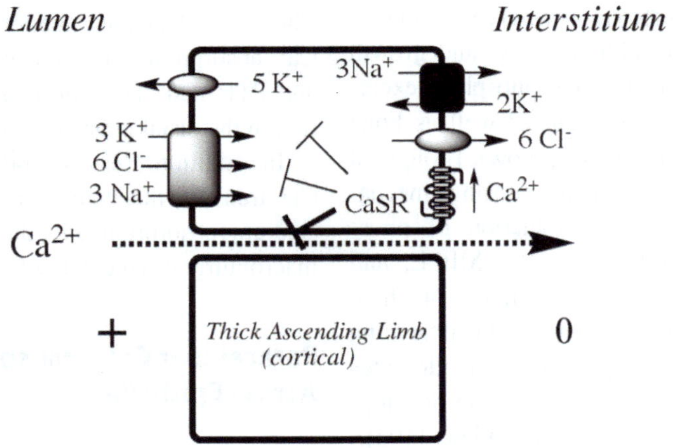

Fig. 2.5 Inhibitory control of paracellular calcium reabsorption in the cortical thick ascending limb by calcium-sensing receptors. Basolateral calcium-sensing receptors are activated by elevated extracellular fluid Ca^{2+} concentration, e.g., in the context of systemic hypercalcemia or in response to transient local hyper-reabsorption (review: [96]). A signaling pathway linked, in part, to the production of arachidonic acid metabolites suppresses either the transepithelial driving force for reabsorption or Ca^{2+} permeation via the intercellular junctions

electrochemical gradient may arise from either a lumen positive potential difference (expressed with respect to a reference electrode in the interstitium) and/or a transepithelial Ca^{2+} concentration gradient that favors transport. In addition, paracellular transport requires the presence of a cation-selective intercellular pathway via the junctional complexes. The cloning and identification of claudins, cation-selective proteins that are expressed in tight junctional complexes (review: [111]) have greatly enhanced understandings of these mechanisms and the nature of their regulation. Key sites for paracellular calcium transport include the renal proximal tubule and TAL of Henle's loop (see below).

Inorganic Phosphate Transport Mechanisms

Inorganic Phosphate Transporters

Three families of inorganic phosphate transporters have been identified: so-called type-I transporters of the SLC17 family, which are now recognized as nonselective organic anion transporters (review: [112]); type-II transporters of the SLC34 family, including NaPi-IIa, -IIb, and -IIc, also known as Npt2a, 2b, and 2c, respectively, which are Na^+-dependent, selective for the divalent HPO_4^{2-} species and expressed in the brush border (luminal) membranes of the renal proximal tubules (2a and 2c) and small intestine (2b); and type-III transporters of the SLC20 family, which are widely expressed, Na^+-dependent, selective for the monovalent $H_2PO_4^-$ species and include PiT-1 and PiT-2 (reviews: [113, 114]).

Despite the identification of transporters on the luminal brush border membranes of transporting epithelia such as small intestine and renal proximal tubule, the identities of phosphate transporters on the basolateral membranes, which are required to deliver inorganic phosphate to the blood, are unclear. Based on energetic considerations, which include a cell-negative membrane potential with respect to the extracellular fluid, and an intracellular inorganic phosphate concentration that is likely to be elevated with respect to the extracellular fluid, phosphate transport across epithelial basolateral membranes is likely to be passive and, thus, mediated by (1) phosphate-permeant anion channels, (2) an electroneutral transporter such as the Band-3 anion exchanger of erythrocytes [115], or (3) a phosphate carrier analogous to mitochondrial SLC25A3 [116].

Intestinal Calcium Absorption

Intestinal calcium absorption is largely confined to the small intestine and is notably inefficient. Thus, despite the existence of various mechanisms to promote absorption, absorption rates are typically less than 50% of ingested loads (Fig. 2.2). Macronutrients including protein [117, 118] and carbohydrates such as glucose [119] and lactose [40, 120] promote calcium absorption. In addition, calcium absorption is powerfully stimulated by calcitriol, which together with the vitamin D receptor is required to prevent hypocalcemia and secondary hyperparathyroidism in mice after, but not prior to, weaning (review: [33]). Intestinal calcium absorption is positively modulated by estrogens [121–123], as well as prolactin [124, 125] and placental lactogen [126]. Consistent with these effects, intestinal calcium absorption is impaired in vitamin D deficiency (review: [127]), reduced in postmenopausal women (review: [128]), and enhanced in pregnancy [129]. The molecular bases for the effects of calcitriol, estrogens, and prolactin/ placental lactogen are not yet clear. Nevertheless, calcitriol and estrogens (reviews: [109, 110]) as well as prolactin [130] upregulate several recognized molecular components of Ca^{2+} transport.

Ca^{2+} ions are absorbed from all three major segments of the small intestine: the duodenum; the jejunum; and the ileum. However, the mechanisms of calcium absorption differ between these segments. In particular, active calcium absorption localizes to the duodenum [131] where it is stimulated by calcitriol [132] and calcium absorption that is coupled to the absorption of glucose or lactose is primarily located in the jejunum and ileum [133, 134]. The location and molecular basis of protein-linked Ca^{2+} absorption are currently unknown.

Several distinct transepithelial transport pathways support calcium absorption. One of the better recognized pathways operates in the duodenum and comprises: *TRPV6 Ca^{2+} channels*, which mediate Ca^{2+} uptake from the intestinal lumen across the enterocyte luminal brush border membrane [107]; *calbindin-D_{9k}*, an intracellular Ca^{2+}-binding protein, which buffers the cytoplasmic ionized Ca^{2+} concentration and promotes transcellular Ca^{2+} transport; and ATP-dependent Ca^{2+} efflux into the extracellular fluid, including (1) the Na^+/Ca^{2+} exchanger NCX1, coupled to Na^+/K^+-ATPase activity, or (2) the plasma membrane Ca^{2+}-ATPase, PMCA1b (reviews: [109, 110]).

Calcitriol-Dependent Activation of Calcium Absorption

As noted above, the primary action of calcitriol is to stimulate duodenal calcium absorption. The significance of the pathway is underscored by the phenotypes of *CYP27B1* null mice, which lack 1α-hydroxylase required for calcitriol synthesis, as well as VDR null mice, which together exhibit very similar phenotypes including impaired intestinal calcium absorption, hypocalcemia, and rickets (review: [33]). Furthermore, in global VDR null mice intestine-specific expression of VDR normalized intestinal calcium absorption, serum calcium levels, and the bone phenotype [60]. Calcitriol promotes the intestinal expression of key components of duodenal Ca^{2+} transport including TRPV6, its isoform TRPV5, which is normally expressed at high levels in the kidney, calbindin-D_{9k}, and PMCAIb inviting the conclusion that calcitriol action is wholly dependent upon the upregulation of a duodenal transport "system" based on these components (reviews: [109, 110]). The key components of this transport pathway are presented in Fig. 2.4 (upper cell). Surprisingly, however, recent studies in transgenic mice indicate that the molecular basis of calcitriol action is more complicated. In particular, calcitriol-stimulated intestinal calcium absorption was intact in calbindin-D_{9k} null mice [135] and, indeed, TRPV6 null mice [136]. Furthermore, active calcium absorption was only partially impaired in TRPV6/calbindin-9k double null mice [137]. These results suggest the existence of redundancy in the actions of calcitriol on intestinal calcium transport, e.g., via upregulation of TRPV5 in compensation for TRPV6, or the existence of an alternative pathway. Consistent with the latter notion, recent evidence suggests that calcitriol promotes paracellular calcium transport in the small intestine by modifying the expression of epithelial junction proteins including upregulation of claudins 2 and 12, which support the formation of a divalent cation-permeable pathway [138].

Macronutrient-Dependent Stimulation of Intestinal Calcium Absorption: Carbohydrates

Although vitamin D deficiency or defective VDR status promotes the development of hypocalcemia and secondary hyperparathyroidism, as well as rickets or osteomalacia (review: [33]), rescue diets with increased contents of calcium and phosphate and containing lactose [120] or glucose [119, 134] can prevent and/or restore normal calcium metabolism and the bone phenotype. In addition, the duodenal (i.e., vitamin D-dependent) contribution to Ca^{2+} absorption appears to be minor, perhaps as low as 15% of the total, when there are plentiful supplies of calcium, phosphate, and macronutrients [134].

Recent work suggests a distinct segmental pattern for macronutrient-dependent calcium absorption based on the jejunum and ileum, and an alternative molecular basis for macronutrient-linked calcium absorption. According to one hypothesis, calcium absorption in the rat jejunum and ileum is dependent upon the expression of $Ca_{v1.3}$ voltage-operated Ca^{2+} channels in the enterocyte brush-border membrane together with SGLT1 Na^+-dependent glucose transporters [119]. SGLT1 mediates membrane depolarization secondary to Na^+ influx as well as glucose transport. Depolarization activates $Ca_{v1.3}$ channels to provide a pathway for Ca^{2+} influx [119]. Thus, the proposed mechanism couples the transports of glucose and Ca^{2+}.

Macronutrient-Dependent Stimulation of Intestinal Calcium Absorption: Protein

The intake of dietary protein, like that of carbohydrates, promotes intestinal calcium absorption [117, 118, 139] and may contribute to the recognized positive impact of dietary protein on bone health (review: [104]). The effect occurs independent of gastric acid production and attendant solubilization of Ca^{2+} salts, at least in healthy young adults [140]. Whether the effect of dietary protein localizes to a particular intestinal segment and depends on a transcellular or paracellular mechanism is not yet clear. Gaffney-Stomberg et al. demonstrated enhanced Ca^{2+} uptake into duodenal brush-border membrane vesicles prepared from female rats fed a high (40%) protein diet when compared with vesicles prepared from rats fed a low (5%) protein diet, suggesting changes in the expression of key Ca^{2+} transport proteins [139]. These results suggest the existence of a dietary protein-modulated transcellular pathway for Ca^{2+} absorption in the small intestine.

Intestinal Phosphate Absorption

The small intestine is also the primary site of inorganic phosphate absorption. Since organic as well as inorganic phosphate is ingested in the diet, the stomach provides an important site for the nonenzymatic hydrolysis of organic phosphates such as nucleotides and sugar phosphates including phytates as well as inorganic polyphosphates including pyrophosphate, octa-calcium phosphate, and hydroxyapatite. Studies in humans and rats indicate that inorganic phosphate absorption occurs throughout the small intestine, primarily localizes to the duodenum (pH 6–7) and jejunum (pH 7–8) and is mediated by the Na^{+}-dependent type-IIb (Npt2b) and PiT-1 or PiT-2 transporters (review: [114]); on the other hand, inorganic phosphate transport in the mouse primarily localizes to the ileum.

Like intestinal calcium absorption, intestinal phosphate absorption is mediated by all three segments of the small intestine. However, as noted above, important species-related differences have been identified between humans and rats on the one hand, in which phosphate transport is highest in the duodenum, and mice on the other, in which it is highest in the ileum [141]. Like intestinal calcium absorption, intestinal phosphate absorption is stimulated by calcitriol ([142]; review: [143]). Surprisingly, however, at variance with the situation for calcium absorption, the jejunum rather than the duodenum is the primary site of calcitriol-dependent phosphate transport in all three species [141]. In addition, intestinal phosphate transport is markedly enhanced by low dietary phosphate (review: [144]). Whether macronutrients promote inorganic phosphate absorption as observed for calcium absorption is unknown.

Intestinal phosphate transport is mediated by Na^{+}-dependent transcellular as well as Na^{+}-independent, possibly paracellular, mechanisms [145]. However, the Na^{+}-dependent mechanisms are better understood and appear to mediate the effect of calcitriol. Na^{+}-dependent transport is mediated primarily by Npt2b transporters and, to a lesser extent, type-III transporters including PiT-1 and PiT-2 expressed in luminal brush-border membranes (review: [114]). Interestingly, calcitriol upregulates small intestinal expression of Npt2b [141] and PiT-2 [146]. In addition, low dietary phosphate upregulates Npt2b expression [147] independent of calcitriol synthesis or the VDR [148]. Key components of the calcitriol-stimulated Npt2b pathway of intestinal phosphate transport are presented in Fig. 2.4 (lower cell).

Other Modulators of Phosphate Transport

Phosphate transport is also positively modulated by estrogens, which upregulate Npt2b expression [149] consistent with the notion that postmenopausal bone loss may arise from reduced absorption of phosphate as well as calcium (review: [150]). Other hormonal influences on dietary phosphate absorption include epidermal growth factor (EGF), which promotes Npt2b expression [151] as well as glucocorticoids [152, 153] and TNF-α [154], which suppress Npt2b expression and phosphate absorption, suggesting potential explanations of the low bone mass phenotypes associated with prolonged high-dose steroids and inflammatory bowel disease. Other negative influences on intestinal phosphate transport include advancing age as well as matrix extracellular phosphoglycoprotein (MEPE) and FGF-23 (review: [114]).

Renal Mechanisms in the Control of Calcium and Phosphate Transport

Renal Tubular Calcium Transport

Renal Ca^{2+} reabsorption occurs in the proximal tubule, medullary and cortical TAL, the DCT and connecting tubules (reviews: [96, 155, 156]). As a result, renal calcium excretion in adults typically varies from 2 to 8 mmol/day (around 1.5–5% of the filtered load). The mechanisms that support renal Ca^{2+} reabsorption differ between tubular segments and include both transcellular and paracellular mechanisms. In addition, they are differentially regulated by hormonal and nutrient-dependent control mechanisms. The primary hormonal regulator of renal Ca^{2+} reabsorption is PTH, which promotes Ca^{2+} reabsorption in the distal nephron (i.e., distinct from its proximal tubule site of action on phosphate transport). Other hormonal modulators include calcitriol (review: [157]) and calcitonin [158], both of which promote Ca^{2+} reabsorption.

Ca^{2+} Reabsorption Mechanisms in the Proximal Tubule and Thick Ascending Limb

The cellular basis of Ca^{2+} reabsorption in the proximal tubule and TAL is predominantly paracellular, i.e., via the tight junctions between neighboring cells (review: [155]). It is, thus, governed by the transepithelial electrochemical gradient as well as the ion selectivity and conductance of the intercellular corridor formed by the tight junctional complex (review [159]).

Proximal Tubule

In the proximal tubule, paracellular reabsorption of Ca^{2+} is favored by both the transepithelial electrical potential difference, which is lumen positive under control conditions [160], as well as the transepithelial concentration gradient in which the luminal Ca^{2+} concentration is elevated by isosmotic coupling of water transport to NaCl reabsorption. As a result of the high level of water reabsorption, which approximates 75%, the luminal Ca^{2+} concentration appears to be held above the interstitial Ca^{2+} concentration throughout the length of the proximal tubule.

Thick Ascending Limb

In the TAL, which is an important site of regulated Ca^{2+} transport, NaCl reabsorption occurs independent of water reabsorption and is more tightly coupled to the generation of a lumen positive transepithelial potential difference (Fig. 2.5). The luminal membrane components of the TAL mechanism include $Na^+/K^+/2Cl^-$ (NKCC2) cotransporters and inwardly rectifying "ROMK" K^+ channels (review: [96]). The basolateral (blood-facing) components include the Na^+/K^+-ATPase, which provides the driving force for transcellular Na^+ reabsorption, and the CLC-KB Cl^- channel, which mediates Cl^- efflux from the cell to the interstitium in response to a cell-negative membrane potential difference (review: [96]). Control of Ca^{2+} transport in the TAL arises from regulated expression and transport rates of NKCC2, ROMK, and CLC-KB and is primarily modulated by (1) PTH1Rs, which promote Ca^{2+} reabsorption in response to elevated serum PTH levels and (2) CaSRs, which suppress Ca^{2+} reabsorption (review: [96]).

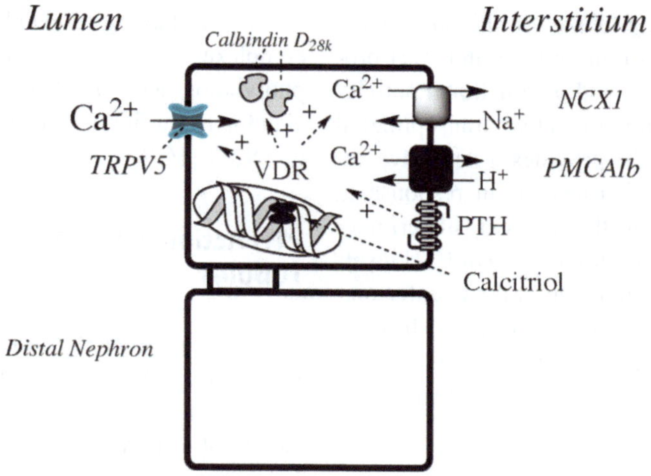

Fig. 2.6 Positive modulation of transcellular calcium reabsorption in the distal nephron by PTH and calcitriol. The mechanism shown in the cell diagram operates in both distal convoluted tubules and connecting tubules (review: [171]). Ca^{2+}-influx across the luminal membrane is mediated by the Ca^{2+}-selective ion channel, TRPV5. Calbindin-D_{28k} and calbindin-D_{9k} (not shown) buffer the cytoplasmic Ca^{2+} concentration and thereby promote continuing Ca^{2+} influx without activating intracellular signaling pathways. Ca^{2+} exits the cell at the basolateral membrane via PMCA1b and NCX1. PTH and calcitriol both upregulate the expressions of TRPV5, the calbindins, and NCX1 [163, 165]. In addition, PTH activates TRPV5-mediated calcium transport [173]. Although a similar calcium transport mechanism operates in the duodenum, there are key differences between the molecular components (e.g., TRPV6 in the duodenum rather than TRPV5 as here in the distal nephron) and regulation. Thus, although calcitriol promotes calcium transport at both sites, PTH has no direct effect on calcium transport in the duodenum

Distal Convoluted Tubules and Connecting Tubules

Unlike the proximal tubule and TAL, Ca^{2+} reabsorption in the DCTs and connecting tubules, amounting to as much as 15% of the total, is primarily transcellular and dependent on the expression of the TRPV5 Ca^{2+}-selective channel in the luminal membrane, which provides a pathway for Ca^{2+} influx into the cell, together with PMCA1b or NCX1 on the basolateral membrane, which provide a pathway for Ca^{2+} efflux to the interstitium (Fig. 2.6; review: [109]). Ca^{2+} transport is facilitated by expression of the Ca^{2+} chelators, calbindin-D_{28k} (review: [161]), and calbindin-D_{9k} in the cytoplasm of DCT cells. The chelator properties of these proteins appear to prevent the cytoplasmic ionized Ca^{2+} concentration from rising to levels ($\geq$200 nM) that might otherwise trigger intracellular signaling events and, by maintaining the steep electrochemical gradient for Ca^{2+} across the apical membrane, facilitate the continuing uptake of Ca^{2+} ions across the luminal membrane [162]. Interestingly, the cellular uptake of nonprotein Ca^{2+} chelators such as the EGTA-analog, BAPTA-AM mimics the effect of calbindins on calcium transport [162]. The expression of both Ca^{2+}-binding proteins is promoted by calcitriol [163] and, based on studies in cultured kidney cells, the effect of calcitriol on calbindin-D_{9k} appears to be enhanced by PTH [164].

Hormonal Regulation of Renal Ca^{2+} Transport

Parathyroid Hormone

PTH regulates renal calcium excretion by promoting Ca^{2+} reabsorption in the cTAL as well as the DCT and connecting tubule segments of the distal nephron (reviews: [96, 165]). In the cTAL, Ca^{2+} reabsorption is primarily paracellular, accompanied by Mg^{2+}, and antagonized by the CaSR located on the basolateral membrane. In the

DCT and connecting tubule, on the other hand, Ca^{2+} reabsorption is transcellular and PTH promotes the expression and/or functional activity of proteins that support active transepithelial transport. While PTH provides a key drive for stimulated renal Ca^{2+} transport in response to hypocalcemia or in the context of primary hyperparathyroidism, suppression of PTH levels plays a relatively minor role in the counter-regulatory response to hypercalcemia. Instead, CaSR-dependent suppression of TAL Ca^{2+} reabsorption provides a key defense against hypercalcemia [6].

PTH Action in the cTAL

Key determinants of paracellular transport include the concentration gradient between the lumen and interstitium, the transepithelial potential, and the ion permeability of the junctional complex. Although the impact of PTH on NaCl transport in the cTAL is mediated, at least in part, by cAMP-dependent trafficking of NKCC2 to the luminal membrane (review: [96]), PTH is reported to have little or no effect on the transepithelial potential [166] and, thus, on the driving force for transport. Given that *TRPV5* and other key components of the DCT transcellular Ca^{2+} reabsorption mechanism are not expressed in the cTAL (reviews: [96, 155]), it seems reasonable to consider whether PTH stimulation of Ca^{2+} reabsorption in the cTAL arises instead from enhanced Ca^{2+} permeability of the junctional complex, e.g., due to increased expression of claudins.

Claudins are a family of four-transmembrane domain, integral membrane proteins that co-localize with occludins in junctional complexes and are widely expressed in epithelial tissues (review: [111]). They are organized so that both their N- and C termini are intracellular, and form homo- and hetero-oligomers with characteristic isoform-specific expression patterns in renal tubular segments (reviews: [111, 167]). Mutations of claudin-16 or -19 have been linked to a rare human disorder of Ca^{2+} and Mg^{2+} reabsorption in the TAL known as familial hypercalciuric hypomagnesemia with nephrocalcinosis [168] (review: [167]). Trafficking of claudins to the junctional complexes is regulated, at least in part, by phosphorylation and a PKA site that is required for claudin-16 trafficking has been identified at residue S217 [169].

PTH Action in the DCT and Connecting Tubules

The cloning of *TRPV5* (originally identified as *ECaC-1*) led to its identification as a key component of a transcellular Ca^{2+} transport apparatus in the distal nephron ([108, 170]; reviews: [156, 171]). The cloning of *TRPV6* (originally identified as *CaT1*) represented a similar advance for understanding transcellular Ca^{2+} transport in the duodenum [107]. PTH was previously observed to activate Ca^{2+} uptake across the luminal membrane of distal tubular cells [172], however, the molecular basis for the effect was unknown. It is now clear that PTH promotes both the expression [165] and functional activity [173] of TRPV5. In addition, PTH promotes the expression of calbindin-D_{28k} [165], calbindin-D_{9k} [164], and NCX1 but not PMCA1b [165]. Thus, PTH is a powerful modulator of the expression of key components required for all rate-limiting steps of transcellular transport in the DCT and connecting tubules (see Fig. 2.6).

Calcitriol

The nature of the effect of calcitriol on renal calcium reabsorption was previously confusing due to its elevation of serum calcium levels and, thus, the filtered load. More recently, the availability of mice that are null either for 1α-hydroxylase or the VDR has permitted a more rigorous assessment of the role of calcitriol in renal calcium handling, leading to the conclusion that it promotes calcium conservation. Thus, VDR null mice exhibit inappropriately high renal Ca^{2+} losses in the context of hypocalcemia, despite the presence of secondary hyperparathyroidism [174]. In addition, 1α-hydroxylase null mice exhibit pronounced decreases in the expressions of key transport proteins of the distal nephron including TRPV5, calbindin D_{28k}, and the basolateral Na^{+}/

Ca^{2+} exchanger, NCX1, which were corrected upon administration of exogenous calcitriol ([163]; see Fig. 2.6).

Calcitonin

Taken together with its well-recognized action in lowering serum Ca^{2+} concentration [175], the apparently paradoxical positive effect of calcitonin on renal calcium reabsorption suggests a primary role in redirecting calcium to bone and retaining it in established hydroxyapatite stores. Consistent with this notion, osteoclast-specific ablation of the calcitonin receptor in mice attenuated their resistance to hypercalcemia [176].

α-Klotho

α-klotho contributes to the control of the renal transport of both calcium and phosphate and is expressed at highest levels in the DCT [177] and at much lower levels in the proximal tubule [178]. It supports renal calcium transport via direct and indirect mechanisms. Thus, it directly stabilizes TRPV5 expression in the plasma membrane via its endogenous β-glucuronidase activity [86, 87]. Indirect roles, dependent in part on the modulation of serum calcitriol levels, are suggested by analyses of the α-klotho null mouse, which in addition to enhanced intestinal calcium absorption exhibits enhanced renal calcium excretion and renal tubular calcium-phosphate precipitation associated with down-regulated expression of calbindin-D_{9k} and NCX1 [179].

Modulation of Renal Ca^{2+} Transport by the CaSR

Elevated extracellular Ca^{2+} concentration promotes renal calcium excretion independent of its action to suppress PTH levels [6]. Consistent with the notion that the kidney senses and responds to changes in the serum ionized Ca^{2+} concentration, the CaSR is widely expressed in the renal tubules. Expression in the proximal tubule provides a mechanism for modulating the effects of PTH and dietary phosphate intake on phosphate reabsorption (see below; [180, 181]). Expression in the mTAL provides a mechanism for suppressing NaCl reabsorption that takes the form of reduced expression of NKCC2 and ROMK, thereby disrupting uptake of Na^+ and Cl^- ions, and K^+ recycling across the luminal membrane as well as reduced expression of CLC-KB in the basolateral membrane, thereby disrupting Cl^- efflux into the extracellular fluid. Consistent with this notion, activating mutations of the CaSR induce a form of Bartter syndrome (type V) typified by salt wasting and hypokalemia (review: [96]).

Robust expression of the CaSR in the basolateral membrane of the cTAL [182] provides a mechanism for suppressing Ca^{2+} reabsorption and an important defense against hypercalcemia even in the PTH-null mouse [6]. Although its molecular basis is unclear, the CaSR appears to suppress the activities of NKCC2, ROMK, and Na^+/K^+-ATPase via the production of arachidonic acid and 20-HETE [183], thereby suppressing the electrical driving force. Alternatively, the CaSR may negatively modulate the insertion of the divalent cation-selective protein, claudin-16 into the junctional complexes thereby reducing the permeability of the paracellular route [184]. CaSR-dependent suppression of PTH-stimulated Ca^{2+} reabsorption in the cTAL arises, in part, from suppression of cAMP levels [185] either by activation of the heterotrimeric G-protein G_i or intracellular Ca^{2+}-dependent inhibition of type-6 adenylyl cyclase or intracellular Ca^{2+}-dependent activation of type-1 PDE (review: [96]).

Renal Tubular Phosphate Transport

Renal phosphate reabsorption localizes to the proximal tubule and is mediated primarily by the type-II transporters Npt2a and Npt2c, and to a lesser extent, by the type-III transporter, PiT-2 (review: [112]). The significance of Npt2a is underscored by the phenotype of Npt2a null mice, which includes frank renal phosphate wasting, hypophosphatemia, impaired trabecular bone development, elevated serum calcitriol levels, attendant hypercalcemia and hypercalciuria, as well as secondary hypoparathyroidism [186]. By comparison, Npt2c null mice failed to exhibit significant phosphate wasting, hypophosphatemia or a bone phenotype but instead prior to, but not after, weaning exhibited hypercalcemia and hypercalciuria associated with elevated serum calcitriol levels and reduced renal 24-hydroxylase mRNA expression [187]. Consistent with these findings, Npt2a mediates around 70% of Na/Pi co-transport in murine isolated brush border vesicles (review: [112]) and Npt2c mediates around 30% of renal Na/Pi cotransport in mice fed a low phosphate diet. The supporting role of Npt2c in murine proximal tubular phosphate reabsorption is underscored by the phenotype of double null Npt2a/Npt2c mice, which in comparison to either of the single null mice exhibit aggravated hypophosphatemia, exaggerated metabolic disturbances including an elevated calcitriol level, hypercalcemia, suppressed PTH and FGF23 levels, as well as a severe bone phenotype that includes rickets [188].

Initial analyses of human kindreds with the autosomal recessive disorder, hereditary hypophosphatemic rickets with hypercalciuria, indicated that Npt2c plays the primary role in renal phosphate transport in humans [189, 190]. However, a recent report indicates that an inactivating mutation of Npt2a that interferes with its surface expression can also induce a severe phosphate-wasting phenotype [191].

Regulation of Proximal Tubular Phosphate Transport

Proximal tubular phosphate reabsorption is regulated by both dietary and hormonal factors. Thus, low dietary phosphate promotes and high dietary phosphate suppresses the expression of proximal tubular phosphate transporters including Npt2a, Npt2c, and PiT-2 in the luminal brush border membrane (reviews: [112, 192]). Various hormonal factors modulate proximal tubule phosphate transport including the phosphaturic factors: PTH, FGF-23, secreted frizzled-related protein-4 (sFRP-4), and FGF-7 (reviews: [41, 112]). Calcitriol does not appear to modulate proximal tubule phosphate transport (review: [112]).

Regulation of Proximal Tubular Phosphate Transport by PTH

PTH acutely suppresses the surface expression of Npt2a in the luminal brush-border membranes of proximal tubule cells within minutes (see Fig. 2.7) and has more delayed effects on the surface expression of Npt2c and PiT-2 [24, 193]. PTH acts on type-I PTH receptors (PTH1Rs) expressed on both luminal and basolateral membranes of proximal tubule cells and stimulation of both PI-PLC, arising from the activation of luminal receptors, and adenylyl cyclase, arising from the activation of basolateral receptors, appear to contribute to the response (review: [112]). Signaling mechanisms downstream of PTH1R in the proximal tubule are dependent upon Na^+/H^+-exchanger regulatory factors (NHERFs), which interact via tandem PDZ domains with ion transporters including Npt2a as well as various GPCRs, including PTH1Rs (review: [112]). Consistent with a key role of NHERF-1 in proximal tubular phosphate transport, NHERF-1-null mice exhibit defective expression of Npt2a transporters along with phosphate wasting, hypophosphatemia, hypercalciuria, and osteomalacia [194], a phenotype that closely resembles that of Npt2a null mice [186]. NHERF1 stabilizes luminal membrane expression of Npt2a and modulates PTH action by promoting PTH1R-dependent activation of PI-PLC [195]. Recent work suggests that PTH triggers PKC-dependent phosphorylation of NHERF1, disabling its interaction with Npt2a thereby inducing Npt2a internalization. A recent report indicates that NHERFs may also contribute to the regulation of Npt2c and/or PiT-2 [196]. PTH has indirect as well as direct effects on renal phosphate transport, e.g., by promoting the expression of FGF-23 [26].

Regulation of Proximal Tubular Phosphate Transport by FGF-23 and α-Klotho

FGF-23 induces phosphaturia and impairs the renal synthesis of calcitriol [69, 70] via actions on the proximal tubules. The phosphaturic action of FGF-23 is dependent on FGF1c receptors [70] in the presence of the co-receptor, α-klotho

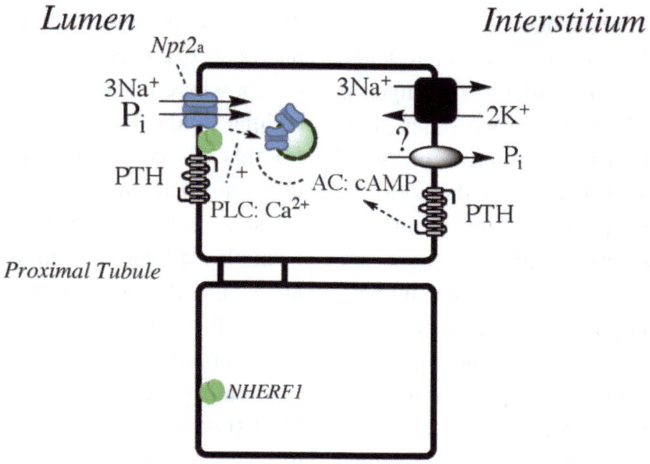

Fig. 2.7 PTH suppresses phosphate reabsorption in the proximal tubule via receptors on both the luminal and basolateral membranes. Transcellular phosphate transport is mediated by Npt2a channels as well as Npt2c and PiT-2 channels (neither of the latter are shown) on the luminal membrane coupled to, an as yet, unidentified phosphate channel or transporter on the basolateral membrane. PTH acutely suppresses phosphate transport by disrupting the interaction between Npt2a and NHERF1 at the plasma membrane. In consequence, Npt2a is rapidly internalized and transcellular transport is markedly inhibited (review: [112]). Npt2c and PiT-2 are inhibited by alternative mechanisms with a much slower time-course. Other modulatory influences on phosphate transport are FGF-23, which like PTH markedly inhibits phosphate transport [70] and luminal calcium-sensing receptors, which dampen the inhibitory effect of PTH [181]

[83, 85] and, like that of PTH, is dependent upon the internalization of Npt2a and Npt2c transporters [70, 72]. However, the actions of FGF-23 on renal phosphate excretion and serum phosphate are delayed in acute studies in humans, i.e., only after 6 h or more [69]. Due to the low level of α-klotho expression in the proximal tubule [177, 178], there has been speculation that the phosphaturic effect of FGF-23 arises indirectly via receptor-dependent expression of paracrine factors from the closely related DCTs ([197]; review: [71]).

Modulation of Proximal Tubular Phosphate Transport by the CaSR

As noted above, the CaSR plays an important role in the inhibitory control of renal calcium reabsorption, which is largely dependent upon its expression in the basolateral membrane of cTAL cells (review: [96]). This mechanism provides a key defense against hypercalcemia [6]. In addition, the CaSR is expressed in the luminal membrane of proximal tubule cells where it reduces the negative impact of PTH on phosphate reabsorption [181]. These results appear to indicate that elevated extracellular Ca^{2+} levels restrain the phosphaturic response to PTH, thereby limiting the magnitude of phosphate losses and the risk of hypophosphatemia. Interestingly, the introduction of a high phosphate diet or acute exposure to high dose PTH by intraperitoneal injection, both of which induce marked phosphaturia, appear to overcome this restraining mechanism by suppressing proximal tubular expression of the CaSR as well as Npt2a in rats ([180]; review: [92]). The findings suggest that a maximal phosphaturic response requires deactivation of CaSR-dependent inhibition of PTH-dependent signaling as well as decreased surface expression of Npt2a and/or Npt2c.

Novel Hormonal Link: Small Intestinal Phosphate Sensing Drives Renal Phosphate Excretion

Recent work indicates the presence of hitherto unrecognized endocrine interactions between the small intestine and the kidney in the control of phosphate metabolism. In one line of enquiry, instillation of phosphate into the rat small intestinal lumen induced prompt phosphaturia in the absence of an elevation in the serum phosphate level [198]. The phosphaturic effect was unaffected by parathyroidectomy or renal denervation, and occurred independent of changes in the serum levels of FGF-23 or two other phosphatonins, secreted frizzled-related protein-4 (sFRP4) or FGF-7. Consistent with the notion of phosphate-dependent, small intestinal production of a hormonal regulator of renal phosphate transport, infusion of a duodenal extract induced prompt phosphaturia [198]. In a second line of enquiry, homozygous null Npt2b mice, in which small intestinal phosphate absorption was markedly impaired, exhibited only a modest fall in the serum phosphate level in association with upregulated expression of renal proximal tubular Npt2a transporters and reduced serum FGF-23 levels [199]. The results indicate that renal phosphate reabsorption can compensate for impaired intestinal phosphate absorption. Finally, overexpression of a stable mutant of FGF-23, R179Q that retains full biological activity, was recently reported to suppress the expression of small intestinal Npt2b in wild-type mice but not in mice that were null for either of the proximal tubular transporters Npt2a or -2c, despite comparable suppression of serum calcitriol levels by FGF-23 (R179Q) in all three models [72]. The findings suggest dynamic coupling of phosphate transport in the kidney and small intestine, via currently unrecognized phosphate-sensing and associated effector mechanisms.

Roles of Bone and Cartilage in Calcium and Phosphate Metabolism

In addition to conferring mechanical rigidity on bone and cartilage, hydroxyapatite acts as the major bodily reservoir of calcium that is released in response to systemic calcium deficiency. It is also a major site of phosphate storage but, as described below, has lesser significance for the maintenance of serum phosphate levels. This section focuses on systemic factors that either control mineralization at the hydroxyapatite surface, and/or promote bone resorption. Clearly bone formation and mineralization are dependent upon the number, activity, and locations of osteoblasts and osteocytes. However, the burgeoning field of the molecular and cellular biology of bone formation has been excluded from the current discussion, except where it is of direct significance for extracellular fluid calcium and phosphate metabolism. For this reason, the author has omitted discussions of the mechanisms that support the anabolic effect of intermittent PTH including key modulators of osteoblastic bone formation. This extends to negative modulators including serotonin (review: [200]), β-adrenergic agonists (review: [201]), and glucocorticoids (review: [202]) as well as positive modulators including PTHrP (review: [203]), PTH (review: [204]), and IGF-1 (review: [205]) together with their interactions [206]. Thus, the sections that follow focus on the mechanisms that control bone resorption, thereby controlling the release of calcium and phosphate, and mineralization, thereby controlling the transfer of calcium and phosphate to bone.

Significance of the Hydroxyapatite Store in Mineral Metabolism

Although hydroxyapatite is a crystalline phosphate salt of calcium, there is no evidence that it buffers the serum phosphate concentration or corrects hypophosphatemia in the same way that it buffers the extracellular Ca^{2+} concentration or corrects hypocalcemia [207]. Thus, enhanced bone resorption is a key physiological response to hypocalcemia but there is no comparable resorptive response to hypophosphatemia. Instead, hypophosphatemia markedly impairs growth plate maturation and bone mineralization thereby restricting inorganic phosphate transfer from the extracellular fluid to bone (review: [105]). In addition, soft tissue phosphate stores in liver and muscle, contribute to the buffering of serum phosphate levels via mechanisms that are not well understood (review: [208]).

Significance of the Hydroxyapatite Store in the Context of Calcium Deficiency

The significance of the hydroxyapatite store for calcium metabolism is underscored by the development of acute hypocalcemia in subgroups

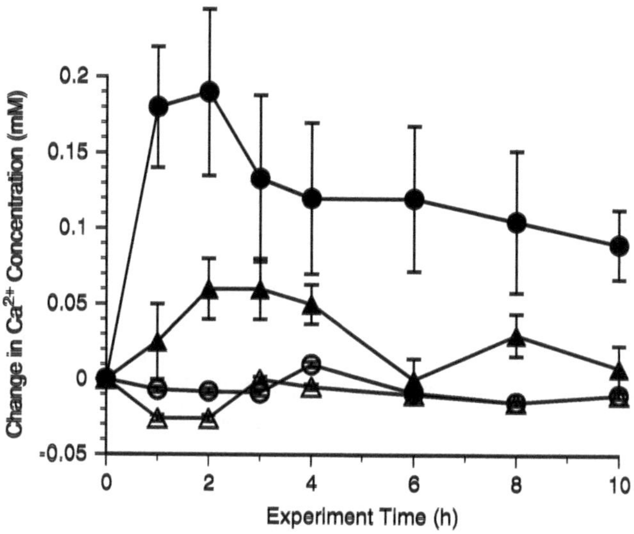

Fig. 2.8 Impaired PTH-induced hypercalcemia in transgenic mice expressing collagenase-resistant type-I collagen. Transgenic *rr* mice that expressed collagenase-resistant type-I collagen exhibited markedly impaired bone resorption and calcium release in response to intraperitoneal injections of PTH. The data have been redrawn from [211]. *Circles*, wild-type mice; *triangles*, transgenic *rr* mice; *open symbols*, vehicle controls; *closed symbols*, PTH-treated. A greater than 50% reduction in PTH-induced hypercalcemia was observed in *rr* mice. (From [211]. Reprinted with permission)

of patients treated with agents that selectively disable bone resorption including bisphosphonates (review: [209]) or denosumab, a RANK-ligand neutralizing monoclonal antibody [210]. In addition, transgenic mice expressing collagenase-resistant type-I collagen, which disables bone resorption, exhibit a markedly impaired calcemic response to PTH (Fig. 2.8; [211]) indicating that bone resorption is a key element of the PTH-dependent defense against hypocalcemia. Furthermore, persistently elevated PTH in primary hyperparathyroidism promotes bone resorption and elevates the serum Ca^{2+} concentration in the context of renal Ca^{2+} retention. Due to its promotion of renal phosphate wasting, however, PTH tends to suppress the serum phosphate concentration in the context of bone resorption. In support of this outcome, PTH also stimulates the production of the phosphatonin FGF-23 [26, 82].

Significance of the Hydroxyapatite Store in the Context of Phosphate Deficiency

Although the primary, bone-based, hormone response to systemic phosphate deficiency is impaired bone mineral formation [105, 212], hypophosphatemia also stimulates calcitriol synthesis and calcitriol, in turn, stimulates intestinal phosphate absorption. Thus, hypophosphatemia arising in Npt2a null, Npt2c null, and double null mice is associated with rickets and osteomalacia together with suppressed serum FGF-23 and PTH levels, an elevated serum calcitriol level and secondary hypercalciuria [188].

Molecular and Cellular Basis of Bone Resorption and its Regulation

Initial activation of the resorbing compartment at the bone surface requires the action of osteoblast lining cell-derived collagenase on type-I collagen (reviews: [213, 214]). Consistent with this conclusion, collagenase-resistant transgenic mice exhibit markedly impaired bone resorption under both basal and PTH-stimulated conditions [211, 215]. Subsequently, exposed extracellular matrix proteins including fibronectin and osteopontin promote β1-integrin-dependent activation of osteoblasts to express key activators of osteoclast maturation including intercellular adhesion molecule-1 (ICAM-1) and receptor activator of NF-κB ligand (RANK-L) [216]. Osteoblast lining cells also express macrophage colony-stimulating factor (M-CSF; [214]). Bone resorption is completed by the actions of mature osteoclasts, which establish membrane-limited resorption pits into which are released HCl and proteases including cathepsin K and, later, neutral matrix metalloproteinases (review: [217]). The action of acid on hydroxyapatite releases calcium and phosphate in ionized form into the extracellular fluid.

Two main bone resorption scenarios need to be considered. The first relates to the maintenance of bone mass and architecture. In this scenario, resorption is a necessary component of remodeling and is targeted to the repair of areas of microdamage or to provide mechanical adaptation to altered strain. The outcomes include revised bone architecture together with enhanced bone quality and strength (reviews: [213, 214]). In one proposed mechanism, apoptotic osteocytes signal to osteoclasts via surface osteoblasts [218], e.g., by the withdrawal of tonic, sclerostin-mediated inhibition of osteoblast expression of the osteoclast activators M-CSF and RANK-ligand.

The second scenario is of particular interest to the present discussion and relates to the role of bone as a calcium store. This store is accessed upon a drop in the serum Ca^{2+} concentration via the release of CaSR-mediated tonic inhibition of PTH secretion leading to elevated serum PTH levels (review: [5]). A similar situation arises in the context of dysregulated PTH secretion, e.g., in primary hyperparathyroidism or FHH (review: [5]). Although hypocalcemia also promotes the synthesis of calcitriol, this effect is generally considered to be of primary significance for intestinal Ca^{2+} absorption rather than bone resorption (review: [33]). Nevertheless, calcitriol may enhance the responsiveness of osteoblasts and/or osteoclasts to persistent elevation of PTH [35].

PTH-Induced Remodeling

Elevated serum PTH levels induce a general activation of remodeling, which is particularly pronounced on the endocortical surface of cortical bone leading to increased porosity [219] but also affects trabecular bone [220]. Enhanced expression of RANK-L and decreased expression of its soluble receptor osteoprotegerin (OPG) are key elements of the response that include osteoclastogenesis and attendant bone resorption [221].

PTH1Rs, which respond to elevated serum PTH levels as well as locally synthesized PTHrP, are expressed on cells of the osteoblast lineage including marrow stromal cells, osteoblast lining cells, mature osteoblasts, and osteocytes [222]. In addition, PTH1Rs are expressed on T lymphocytes and recent work demonstrates that T-cell-specific deletion of PTH1Rs in mice protects against bone loss via impaired production of the cytokine TNF-α [19]. TNF-α promotes osteoclastogenesis, at least in part, by enhanced stromal cell expression of RANK-L and reduced expression of OPG [19].

Modulation of Bone Remodeling by Calcitriol

Calcitriol has multiple actions on bone mass and mineralization. As noted above, the most important of these actions appear to derive from the promotion of intestinal calcium and phosphate absorption since many of the phenotypic features of 1α-hydroxylase null mice and VDR null mice are corrected by rescue diets rich in calcium, phosphate, and macronutrients (review: [33]). Nevertheless, VDRs are expressed in cells of both the osteoblast and monocyte–macrophage–osteoclast lineages and promote bone formation, at least in part, by enhancing the proliferation of osteoblast progenitors [223], as well as bone resorption, by facilitating the expression of RANK-L [224]. These effects appear to be more pronounced with aging [223] and suggest a role for calcitriol in promoting bone remodeling and turnover (review: [35]). Interestingly, the outcomes of vitamin D receptor function appear to be critically dependent upon the differentiation state of the cells in which it is expressed. Thus, transgenic overexpression of the VDR in mature osteoblasts under the osteocalcin promoter enhanced bone mass and impaired bone resorption [225], suggesting a role for VDRs in the local downregulation of osteoclasts once mature osteoblasts have been established in the remodeling zone.

Bone Remodeling by Osteocytes

A role for osteocyte PTH1Rs in PTH-induced bone-resorption is suggested by the impact of over-expressing a constitutively active PTH1R under the control of the osteocyte-specific dentin matrix protein-1 (DMP-1) promoter [226]. Although such a mechanism might involve enhanced osteoclastogenesis and bone remodeling at the bone surface, recent work suggests that osteocytes may directly participate in a wider remodeling process that includes the perilacunar matrix and canalicular network dependent upon the upregulation of key bone resorption genes in osteocytes themselves (reviews: [227, 228]). Consistent with this concept, the volume of the perilacunar space appears to expand during lactation [228]. Thus, although the mechanisms are not well-defined, hormonal control of "osteocytic osteolysis" and osteocytic bone formation may also contribute to the control of whole body calcium and phosphate.

Other Modulators of Bone Resorption

Calcitonin

Calcitonin receptors are class B G-protein coupled receptors [229] expressed by mature osteoclasts [230]. They provide a mechanism by which hypercalcemia-induced calcitonin production impairs bone resorption. Consistent with this concept, both global [175] and osteoclast-specific [176] calcitonin receptor null mice exhibit loss of resistance to induced hypercalcemia. Thus, one key defense against hypercalcemia is based on the activation of the CaSR in thyroid C-cells [231], which promotes calcitonin secretion and, in turn, activates calcitonin receptors in osteoclasts to suppress bone resorption.

Estrogens

Postmenopausal bone loss is responsive to therapy with selective estrogen receptor modulators (SERMs) with a tissue selectivity profile that reduces the risk of major estrogen-related side effects including malignant transformation of mammary epithelial cells (review: [232]). Consistent with this behavior, estrogens negatively modulate bone resorption and bone turnover via effects on osteoclast survival and function, and analyses of transgenic mice indicate that both nuclear receptor subclasses, ER-α and ER-β contribute to the effects (review: [233]). However, the identities of the cell types that coordinate the responses, together with their molecular bases, are not well defined. Estrogens upregulate the expressions of Bcl-2, BMP-2, and OPG in osteoblasts, reduce the expression of cathepsin K in osteoclasts, and suppress the levels of pro-osteoclastogenic cytokines (review: [233]).

β-Adrenergic Signaling Promotes Osteoclastogenesis

In addition to its anti-appetite effect, leptin suppresses bone formation via a hypothalamic relay that activates the sympathetic nervous system [234]. In the periphery, β_2-adrenergic receptors on osteoblasts suppress proliferation and promote the expression of RANK-L and, thus, induce osteoclastogenesis and bone resorption ([235]; review: [201]). The full physiological significance of this sympathetic nervous system mechanism and the nature of its primary sensing modalities are currently unknown.

Bone Formation and Local Regulation of Bone Mineralization

Bone formation, including expansion of the bone matrix and mineralization, is dependent upon the actions of mature, differentiated osteoblasts that align to the bone surface. Osteoblast maturation is under the control of signals arising from apoptotic osteocytes including withdrawal of sclerostin, a key inhibitor (review: [213]), together with various systemic signals as noted above.

Mature osteoblasts produce the osteoid collagen scaffold, initiate mineralization by seeding calcium-phosphate-containing matrix vesicles, and promote its nucleation via tissue nonspecific alkaline phosphatase (TNAP), which hydrolyses key local inhibitors including pyrophosphate (review: [236]) and polyphosphates [237]. Inactivating mutants of TNAP underlie the human inherited disorder, hypophosphatasia [238] and TNAP-null mice exhibit similar phenotypic features including rickets due to developmental arrest in epiphyses, as well as osteomalacia [239]. Although matrix vesicle-dependent calcium phosphate seeding occurs normally, extension of nascent hydroxyapatite crystals is arrested in the absence of TNAP (review: [240]).

Whether localized to the intracortical or endochondral surfaces of cortical bone, or to the trabeculae of cancellous bone, mineralization requires net transfers of calcium and phosphate ions from the plasma to the surfaces of growing hydroxyapatite crystals. Under steady-state conditions in adults around 8 mmol of calcium and 5 mmol of phosphate are transferred to hydroxyapatite per day and are balanced by similar fluxes of calcium and phosphate arising from bone resorption (Fig. 2.2; [207, 208]).

Control of Mineralization

Critical to the targeting of mineralization is its restriction to discrete sites that support bone integrity with avoidance of joint capsules and joint spaces. Thus, molecular mechanisms for suppressing inappropriate mineralization and for selectively deactivating them in a spatially and temporally appropriate manner are critical to effective growth and/or repair of bone. In addition to TNAP, the pyrophosphate exporter Ank, which is expressed by chondrocytes [241, 242] and osteoblasts [243] and exports pyrophosphate into the extracellular space, is an important contributor to the local inhibitory mechanism. Interestingly, pyrophosphate appears to have multiple inhibitory effects on mineralization that arise from mineral binding, upregulated expression of osteopontin, and suppressed TNAP activity [244].

Osteoblasts also modulate hydroxyapatite expansion by releasing SIBLINGs that bind to Ca^{2+} ions at the crystal surface [236]. They include DMP-1, bone sialoprotein, osteopontin, and MEPE. While these proteins typically act as inhibitors of hydroxyapatite formation in their full-length forms, phosphorylation and proteolytic processing yields peptides, which (1) promote mineralization, (2) yield more potent inhibitors of mineralization, and/or (3) enter the circulation to modify phosphate metabolism. Dmp1 provides an example of such an inhibitor, which in an intact phosphorylated form binds to hydroxyapatite and suppresses mineralization [245]. However, upon dephosphorylation and proteolytic processing, a 57-kDa C-terminal peptide is generated that promotes mineralization [245, 246].

SIBLING proteins are also modified by limited proteolysis to generate intensely acidic (i.e., negatively charged) peptides. These so-called ASARM peptides negatively modulate hydroxyapatite crystal growth [247] and upon their release into the blood, promote renal phosphate excretion to lower serum phosphate levels by downregulating the expression of Npt2a (review: [236]). An example of potential clinical importance arises in the context of the cleavage of osteopontin-derived ASARM peptides by the integral membrane endopeptidase, PHEX. Inactivating mutations of PHEX underlie X-linked hypophosphatemic rickets (review: [41]) and failure of PHEX cleavage of phosphorylated osteopontin results in the accumulation of a potent phosphopeptide inhibitor of mineralization [248]. Whether this, or a related, peptide promotes phosphate wasting, another key element of the phenotype, is currently unknown.

Rickets and Osteomalacia: Impact of Low Serum Phosphate

Rickets arises from impaired apoptosis of hypertrophic chondrocytes in the growth plate [249] resulting in a failure of vascularization and ossification. The serum phosphate concentration is critical to the process and hypophosphatemia induces the persistent survival of hypertrophic chondrocytes suggesting the existence of a phosphate-sensing mechanism coupled to the activation of apoptosis (review: [105]).

Osteomalacia arises from impaired mineralization of osteoblast- or osteocyte-derived osteoid and is also highly sensitive to the serum phosphate concentration [250]. In addition to its inhibitory effect on mineralization arising from the lowering of the calcium-phosphate solubility product, low serum phosphate concentration suppresses the maturation of osteoblasts as revealed by reduced expression of osteocalcin and osteopontin (review: [105]).

Hypophosphatemic Rickets

Several human inherited disorders feature hypophosphatemia and rickets. These include X-linked hypophosphatemic rickets (XLH), ADHR, and various forms of autosomal recessive hypophosphatemic rickets (ARHR). Hypophosphatemia has been causally linked to abnormalities of the growth plate and bone in all of these disorders. In part, it arises from impaired proteolytic processing and/or enhanced expression of FGF-23.

ADHR arises typically from gain-of-function mutations in the FGF-23 gene that disable a critical RXXR proteolytic cleavage site (residues 176–179; [63, 251]). Serum FGF-23 levels are elevated and hypophosphatemia results from renal phosphate wasting and an inadequate intestinal absorption response secondary to suppressed serum calcitriol levels. In addition to persistence of the active, full-length form of FGF-23, impaired processing interferes with the production of a potent C-terminal peptide antagonist of full-length FGF-23 [252].

XLH arises from inactivating mutations in the *PHEX* gene [253–255] and is also associated with elevations of the serum FGF-23 concentration [64]. The *Hyp* mouse, which has an inactivating mutation of the PHEX gene, exhibits a comparable phenotype to human XLH including elevated serum FGF-23 levels [256]. These phenotypes were initially ascribed to a failure of FGF-23 processing by defective PHEX [64] but PHEX does not cleave FGF-23 and instead appears to negatively modulate its expression [257]. Possibly via the processing of SIBLINGs as described above. Consistent with the notion that enhanced serum FGF-23 levels mediate hypophosphatemia in the Hyp mouse, *fgf23/Hyp* double null mice, in which FGF-23 production is ablated, exhibit renal phosphate retention and hyperphosphatemia, i.e., a reversal of the Hyp phenotype [258, 259].

ARHR arises from homozygous or compound heterozygous mutations of several genes in humans. These include inactivating mutations of the Npt2c or Npt2a genes (review: [260]) as noted above, as well as inactivating mutations of the Dmp1 gene, which exhibit hypophosphatemic rickets and enhanced serum FGF-23 levels ([189]; review: [261]). Consistent with this, Dmp1 null mice exhibit hypophosphatemic rickets associated with elevated serum FGF-23 levels and renal phosphate wasting [262]. The significance of elevated FGF-23 levels and attendant suppression of the serum phosphate level is underscored by the findings that FGF-23 neutralizing antibodies or a high phosphate diet rescues key features of the phenotype. These include rickets, osteomalacia, and delayed marrow cavity formation, as well as impaired osteoblast to osteocyte differentiation as reported by enhanced expression of *Osterix (OSX)* and *Col-I*, and reduced expression of *SOST*, which encodes the key inhibitory regulator of osteoblast differentiation, sclerostin [263]. Taken together, the results suggest that Dmp1, like PHEX, is a negative regulator of FGF-23 expression. The nature of the interactions between key regulators of osteoblast maturation and mineralization, on the one hand, and enzymes responsible for their proteolytic processing, on the other, remain to be determined. Nevertheless, it seems clear that limited proteolysis of Dmp1 like that of other SIBLING proteins is critical to its actions in bone [246].

Modulation of Bone Formation and Resorption by the Calcium-Sensing Receptor

Early cellular and transgenic mouse studies aimed at exploring a possible role of the CaSR in bone cell biology led to considerable confusion (review: [15]). More recent analyses based on tissue-specific deletion of CaSR exon-7, which encodes the receptor's heptahelical signaling domain [264] rather than global deletion of CaSR exon-5, which encodes a C-terminal fragment of the receptor's VFT nutrient-sensing domain [265], has led to a new appreciation of the roles played by the CaSR expressed in the osteoblast, chondrocyte, and monocyte–macrophage–osteoclast lineages with developmental implications for bone and cartilage as well as functional implications for bone remodeling. With respect to bone, homozygous deletion of CaSR exon-7 in osteoblasts under the control of either the *Col-I* or *OSX* promoters induced growth retardation and impaired mineralization associated with defective expression of type-I collagen, alkaline phosphatase, and osteocalcin [264]. Consistent with these findings, the CaSR inhibitor (calcilytic) NPS 89636 prevented extracellular Ca^{2+}-dependent upregulation of key markers of osteoblast function in cultured fetal rat calvarial cells [266]. The results indicate that the CaSR, in the presence of physiologically relevant extracellular Ca^{2+} concentrations, promotes the differentiation of osteoblast progenitors. Furthermore, examination of neonatal global CaSR/PTH double null mice indicates that the CaSR is required for dietary calcium-dependent stimulation of bone turnover [267]. Thus, the CaSR may mediate key nutritional influences on bone development and bone mass (review: [104]). Surprisingly, expression of a constitutively active CaSR under the osteocalcin promoter induced cancellous bone loss in transgenic mice associated with increased osteoclast number and increased osteoclast surface [268]. The physiological significance of these findings requires further study.

The CaSR is also expressed in osteoclasts and their monocyte precursors. Although its significance in osteoclast biology is less well understood, it promotes monocyte differentiation and chemotaxis and provides a mechanism whereby elevated Ca^{2+} concentrations in the proximity of the bone resorption pit may negatively modulate further bone resorption prior to the recruitment, proliferation, and maturation of osteoblasts in support of bone formation (review: [93]).

Conclusion

When the author agreed to write this chapter, he thought he had undertaken to write an account of the regulation of calcium metabolism alone. That would have simplified life somewhat but would also have been a shame, since this story is really only complete when the metabolisms of both calcium and phosphate are considered together in detail. The story is necessarily complex and involves multiple small intestinal and renal tubular segments, as well as the development and homeostasis of bone and cartilage, together with hormonal and more local molecular signals, some yet undiscovered, that precisely control the functions of these tissues and their interactions. Much of the story points to the roles of micronutrient sensors including the CaSR, which has pluripotent roles in the gut, kidney, bone, and cartilage as well as other sensors, such as those for inorganic phosphate, not yet identified. Ultimately, it provides a picture of an asymmetric economy in which calcium and phosphate are common treated very differently from one another. The positive impact of PTH on serum calcium levels and its neutral or negative impact on serum phosphate levels provides one example. In addition, when their plasma levels are disturbed, calcium and phosphate provoke quite distinct outcomes on bone turnover. The cases of hypocalcemia and hypophosphatemia are particularly striking since the former provokes bone resorption and the latter arrests bone mineralization. There are notable exceptions: the intestinal absorptions of calcium and phosphate are both positively modulated by calcitriol; and calcium and phosphate belong together in the hydroxyapatite crystals in bone. Consideration of all these effects ultimately points to vitamin D and its active metabolites 25-hydroxyvitamin D and calcitriol as central regulators of calcium and phosphate metabolism. The metabolism of calcitriol, in particular, is salutary since it is subject to sensitive and potentially competitive control by all other key players including calcium, phosphate, PTH, and FGF-23. This places the regulation of intestinal calcium and phosphate absorption with its implications for bone mineralization at the very heart of the metabolic web. Clearly, however, there is much still to learn. What are the molecular identities of the phosphate sensors? How does the proteolytic processing of hydroxyapatite binding proteins control phosphate metabolism? What are the mechanisms that underlie the macronutrient modulation of calcium and, perhaps, phosphate transport? How do osteocytes coordinate the actions of bone remodeling cells and participate themselves in the processes of bone turnover? How does the nutritional modulator, 25-hydroxyvitamin D, interact with key control points in calcium and phosphate metabolism? And how can all of the context-specific variations that perturb calcium and phosphate metabolism independently of one another be explained?

Acknowledgments The author wishes to thank his colleague Prof. Rebecca Mason for critical comments on the manuscript and the National Health and Medical Research Council of Australia for project grant support in the areas of bone and mineral metabolism and its interactions with macronutrient-sensing mechanisms.

References

1. Aylward GH, Findlay TJV. Dissociation constants of acids and hydrated metal ions. SI chemical data. Australasia: John Wiley and Sons; 1974. p. 122–4.
2. Wagner C, Devuyst O, Bourgeois S, Mohebbi N. Regulated acid–base transport in the collecting duct. Pflugers Arch. 2009;458:137–56.
3. Jovancicevic V, Bauer B. Calcium phosphate deposition on iron in oxygen-containing neutral aqueous solutions: an electrochemical approach. Langmuir. 1989;5:261–7.
4. Verbeeck RMH, Bruyne PAMD, Driessens FCM, Verbeek F. Solubility of magnesium hydrogen phosphate trihydrate and ion-pair formation in the system magnesium hydroxide-phosphoric acid-water at 25 degree C. Inorg Chem. 1984;23:1922–6.
5. Brown EM, MacLeod RJ. Extracellular calcium sensing and extracellular calcium signaling. Physiol Rev. 2001;81:239–97.
6. Kantham L, Quinn S, Egbuna O, Baxi K, Butters R, Pang J, Pollak M, Goltzman D, Brown E. The calcium-sensing receptor (CaSR) defends against hypercalcemia independently of its regulation of parathyroid hormone secretion. Am J Physiol Endocrinol Metab. 2009;297:E915–23.
7. Brown A, Zhong M, Finch J, Ritter C, McCracken R, Morrissey J, Slatopolsky E. Rat calcium-sensing receptor is regulated by vitamin D but not by calcium. Am J Physiol. 1996;270:F454–60.
8. Silver J, Russell J, Sherwood LM. Regulation by vitamin D metabolites of messenger ribonucleic acid for preproparathyroid hormone in isolated bovine parathyroid cells. Proc Natl Acad Sci USA. 1985;82:4270.
9. Silver J, Naveh-Many T, Mayer H, Schmelzer H, Popovtzer M. Regulation by vitamin D metabolites of parathyroid hormone gene transcription in vivo in the rat. J Clin Invest. 1986;78:1296–301.
10. Ben-Dov I, Galitzer H, Lavi-Moshayoff V, Goetz R, Kuro-o M, Mohammadi M, Sirkis R, Naveh-Many T, Silver J. The parathyroid is a target organ for FGF23 in rats. J Clin Invest. 2007;117:4003–8.
11. Ritter C, Armbrecht H, Slatopolsky E, Brown A. 25-Hydroxyvitamin D(3) suppresses PTH synthesis and secretion by bovine parathyroid cells. Kidney Int. 2006;70:654–9.
12. Laroche M. Phosphate, the renal tubule, and the musculoskeletal system. Joint Bone Spine. 2001;68: 211–5.
13. Conigrave AD, Mun H-C, Delbridge L, Quinn SJ, Wilkinson M, Brown EM. L-Amino acids regulate parathyroid hormone secretion. J Biol Chem. 2004;279:38151–9.
14. Conigrave AD, Quinn SJ, Brown EM. Cooperative multi-modal sensing and therapeutic implications of the extracellular Ca^{2+}-sensing receptor. Trends Pharm Sci. 2000;21:401–7.
15. Conigrave AD, Hampson DR. Broad-spectrum amino acid-sensing class C G-protein coupled receptors: molecular mechanisms, physiological significance and options for drug development. Pharmacol Ther. 2010;127:252–60.
16. Hendy G, Goltzman D. Does calcitriol have actions independent from the vitamin D receptor in maintaining skeletal and mineral homeostasis? Curr Opin Nephrol Hypertens. 2005;14:350–4.
17. Slatopolsky E. The intact nephron hypothesis: the concept and its implications for phosphate management in CKD-related mineral and bone disorder. Kidney Int. 2011;121:S3–8.
18. Imura A, Tsuji Y, Murata M, Maeda R, Kubota K, Iwano A, Obuse C, Togashi K, Tominaga M, Kita N, Tomiyama K, Iijima J, Nabeshima Y, Fujioka M, Asato R, Tanaka S, Kojima K, Ito J, Nozaki K, Hashimoto N, Ito T, Nishio T, Uchiyama T, Fujimori T, Nabeshima Y. alpha-Klotho as a regulator of calcium homeostasis. Science. 2007;316:1615–8.
19. Tawfeek H, Bedi B, Li J, Adams J, Kobayashi T, Weitzmann M, Kronenberg H, Pacifici R. Disruption of PTH receptor 1 in T cells protects against PTH-induced bone loss. PLoS One. 2010;5:e12290.
20. Samadfam R, Xia Q, Miao D, Hendy G, Goltzman D. Exogenous PTH and endogenous 1,25-dihydroxyvitamin D are complementary in inducing an anabolic effect on bone. J Bone Miner Res. 2008;23:1257–66.
21. Lee M, Partridge N. Parathyroid hormone signaling in bone and kidney. Curr Opin Nephrol Hypertens. 2009;18:298–302.

22. Boros S, Bindels R, Hoenderop J. Active Ca(2+) reabsorption in the connecting tubule. Pflugers Arch. 2009;458:99–109.
23. Stewart A, Broadus A. The regulation of renal calcium excretion: an approach to hypercalciuria. Annu Rev Med. 1981;32:457–73.
24. Picard N, Capuano P, Stange G, Mihailova M, Kaissling B, Murer H, Biber J, Wagner C. Acute parathyroid hormone differentially regulates renal brush border membrane phosphate cotransporters. Pflugers Arch. 2010;460:677–87.
25. Popovtzer M, Massry S, Villamil M, Kleeman C. Renal handling of phosphorus in oliguric and nonoliguric mercury-induced acute renal failure in rats. J Clin Invest. 1971;50:2347–54.
26. Lavi-Moshayoff V, Wasserman G, Meir T, Silver J, Naveh-Many T. PTH increases FGF23 gene expression and mediates the high-FGF23 levels of experimental kidney failure: a bone parathyroid feedback loop. Am J Physiol Renal Physiol. 2010;299: F882–9.
27. Kolek O, Hines E, Jones M, LeSueur L, Lipko M, Kiela P, Collins J, Haussler M, Ghishan F. 1alpha,25-Dihydroxyvitamin D3 upregulates FGF23 gene expression in bone: the final link in a renal-gastrointestinal-skeletal axis that controls phosphate transport. Am J Physiol Gastrointest Liver Physiol. 2005;289:G1036–42.
28. Girotra M, Rubin M, Bilezikian J. The use of parathyroid hormone in the treatment of osteoporosis. Rev Endocr Metab Disord. 2006;7:113–21.
29. Goltzman D. Studies on the mechanisms of the skeletal anabolic action of endogenous and exogenous parathyroid hormone. Arch Biochem Biophys. 2008;473:218–24.
30. Parsons J, Neer R, Potts JJ. Initial fall of plasma calcium after intravenous injection of parathyroid hormone. Endocrinology. 1971;89:735–40.
31. Parsons J, Robinson C. Calcium shift into bone causing transient hypocalcaemia after injection of parathyroid hormone. Nature. 1971;230:581–2.
32. Kronenberg F. Emerging risk factors and markers of chronic kidney disease progression. Nat Rev Nephrol. 2009;5:677–89.
33. Bouillon R, Carmeiet G, Verlinden L, van Etten E, Verstuyf A, Luderer HF, Lieben L, Mathieu C, Demay M. Vitamin D and human health: lessons from vitamin D receptor null mice. Endocr Rev. 2008;29:726–76.
34. Masuda M, Yamamoto H, Kozai M, Tanaka S, Ishiguro M, Takei Y, Nakahashi O, Ikeda S, Uebanso T, Taketani Y, Segawa H, Miyamoto K, Takeda E. Regulation of renal sodium-dependent phosphate co-transporter genes (Npt2a and Npt2c) by all-trans-retinoic acid and its receptors. Biochem J. 2010; 429:583–92.
35. Goltzman D, Miao D, Panda D, Hendy G. Effects of calcium and of the vitamin D system on skeletal and calcium homeostasis: lessons from genetic models. J Steroid Biochem Mol Biol. 2004;2004:485–9.
36. Willett A. Vitamin D status and its relationship with parathyroid hormone and bone mineral status in older adolescents. Proc Nutr Soc. 2005;64:193–203.
37. Rowling M, Gliniak C, Welsh J, Fleet J. High dietary vitamin D prevents hypocalcemia and osteomalacia in CYP27B1 knockout mice. J Nutr. 2007;137:2608–15.
38. Yoshizawa T, Handa Y, Uematsu Y, Takeda S, Sekine K, Yoshihara Y, Kawakami T, Arioka K, Sato H, Uchiyama Y, Masushige S, Fukamizu A, Matsumoto T, Kato S. Mice lacking the vitamin D receptor exhibit impaired bone formation, uterine hypoplasia and growth retardation after weaning. Nat Genet. 1997;16:391–6.
39. Panda D, Miao D, Tremblay M, Sirois J, Farookhi R, Hendy G, Goltzman D. Targeted ablation of the 25-hydroxyvitamin D 1alpha-hydroxylase enzyme: evidence for skeletal, reproductive, and immune dysfunction. Proc Natl Acad Sci USA. 2001;98: 7498–503.
40. Dardenne O, Prud'homme J, Glorieux F, St-Arnaud R. Rescue of the phenotype of CYP27B1 (1alpha-hydroxylase)-deficient mice. J Steroid Biochem Mol Biol. 2004;89–90:327–30.
41. Bergwitz C, Jüppner H. Regulation of phosphate homeostasis by PTH, vitamin D, and FGF23. Annu Rev Med. 2010;61:91–104.
42. Heaney R, Dowell M, Hale C, Bendich A. Calcium absorption varies within the reference range for serum 25-hydroxyvitamin D. J Am Coll Nutr. 2003;22:142–6.
43. Whiting S, Calvo M. Correcting poor vitamin D status: do older adults need higher repletion doses of vitamin D3 than younger adults? Mol Nutr Food Res. 2010;54:1077–84.
44. Aloia J, Bojadzievski T, Yusupov E, Shahzad G, Pollack S, Mikhail M, Yeh J. The relative influence of calcium intake and vitamin D status on serum parathyroid hormone and bone turnover biomarkers in a double-blind, placebo-controlled parallel group, longitudinal factorial design. J Clin Endocrinol Metab. 2010;95:3216–24.
45. Björkman M, Sorva A, Tilvis R. Responses of parathyroid hormone to vitamin D supplementation: a systematic review of clinical trials. Arch Gerontol Geriatr. 2009;48:160–6.
46. Morris HA, Anderson PH. Autocrine and paracrine actions of vitamin D. Clin Biochem Rev. 2010; 31:129–38.
47. Nesbitt T, Drezner M. Insulin-like growth factor-I regulation of renal 25-hydroxyvitamin D-1-hydroxylase activity. Endocrinology. 1993;132:133–8.
48. Menaa C, Vrtovsnik F, Friedlander G, Corvol M, Garabédian M. Insulin-like growth factor I, a unique calcium-dependent stimulator of 1,25-dihydroxyvitamin D3 production. Studies in cultured mouse kidney cells. J Biol Chem. 1995;270:25461–7.
49. Bianda T, Hussain M, Glatz Y, Bouillon R, Froesch E, Schmid C. Effects of short-term insulin-like growth factor-I or growth hormone treatment on

bone turnover, renal phosphate reabsorption and 1,25 dihydroxyvitamin D3 production in healthy man. J Intern Med. 1997;241:143–5.
50. Zierold C, Darwish H, DeLuca H. Two Vitamin D Response Elements Function in the Rat 1,25-Dihydroxyvitamin D 24-Hydroxylase Promoter. J Biol Chem. 1995;270:1675–8.
51. Meyer M, Goetsch P, Pike J. A downstream intergenic cluster of regulatory enhancers contributes to the induction of CYP24A1 expression by 1alpha,25-dihydroxyvitamin D3. J Biol Chem. 2010;285: 15599–610.
52. Lou Y-R, Molnar F, Perakyla M, Qiao A, Kalueff AV, St-Arnaud R, Carlberg C, Tuohimaa P. 25-Hydroxyvitamin D3 is an agonistic vitamin D receptor ligand. J Steroid Biochem Mol Biol. 2010;118:162–70.
53. St-Arnaud R, Arabian A, Travers R, Barletta F, Raval-Pandya M, Chapin K, Depovere J, Mathieu C, Christakos S, Demay M, Glorieux F. Deficient mineralization of intramembranous bone in vitamin D-24-hydroxylase-ablated mice is due to elevated 1,25-dihydroxyvitamin D and not to the absence of 24,25-dihydroxyvitamin D. Endocrinology. 2000; 141:2658–66.
54. Nykjaer A, Dragun D, Walther D, Vorum H, Jacobsen C, Herz J, Melsen F, Christensen E, Willnow T. An endocytic pathway essential for renal uptake and activation of the steroid 25-(OH) vitamin D3. Cell. 1999;96:507–15.
55. Leheste J, Melsen F, Wellner M, Jansen P, Schlichting U, Renner-Müller I, Andreassen T, Wolf E, Bachmann S, Nykjaer A, Willnow T. Hypocalcemia and osteopathy in mice with kidney-specific megalin gene defect. FASEB J. 2003;17:247–9.
56. Nykjaer A, Fyfe JC, Kozyraki R, Leheste J-R, Jacobsen C, Nielsen MS, Verroust P, Aminoff M, de la Chapelle A, Moestrup SK, Ray R, Gliemann J, Willnow TE, Christensen EI. Cubilin dysfunction causes abnormal metabolism of the steroid hormone 25(OH) vitamin D3. Proc Natl Acad Sci USA. 2001;98:13895–900.
57. Safadi F, Thornton P, Magiera H, Hollis B, Gentile M, Haddad J, Liebhaber S, Cooke N. Osteopathy and resistance to vitamin D toxicity in mice null for vitamin D binding protein. J Clin Invest. 1999;103:239–51.
58. Christakos S, Dhawan P, Liu Y, Peng X, Porta A. New insights into the mechanisms of vitamin D action. J Cell Biochem. 2003;88:695–705.
59. Dardenne O, Prudhomme J, Hacking S, Glorieux F, St-Arnaud R. Rescue of the pseudo-vitamin D deficiency rickets phenotype of CYP27B1-deficient mice by treatment with 1,25-dihydroxyvitamin D3: biochemical, histomorphometric, and biomechanical analyses. J Bone Miner Res. 2003;18:637–43.
60. Xue Y, Fleet J. Intestinal vitamin D receptor is required for normal calcium and bone metabolism in mice. Gastroenterology. 2009;136:1317–27.
61. Hori M, Shimizu Y, Fukumoto S. Minireview: fibroblast growth factor 23 in phosphate homeostasis and bone metabolism. Endocrinology. 2011;152:4–10.
62. Jüppner H. Phosphate and FGF-23. Kidney Int. 2011;79 Suppl 121:S1–4.
63. ADHR-Consortium. Autosomal dominant hypophosphataemic rickets is associated with mutations in FGF23. Nat Genet. 2000;26:345–8.
64. Jonsson K, Zahradnik R, Larsson T, White K, Sugimoto T, Imanishi Y, Yamamoto T, Hampson G, Koshiyama H, Ljunggren O, Oba K, Yang I, Miyauchi A, Econs M, Lavigne J, Jüppner H. Fibroblast growth factor 23 in oncogenic osteomalacia and X-linked hypophosphatemia. N Engl J Med. 2003;348:1656–63.
65. Garringer H, Malekpour M, Esteghamat F, Mortazavi S, Davis S, Farrow E, Yu X, Arking D, Dietz H, White K. Molecular genetic and biochemical analyses of FGF23 mutations in familial tumoral calcinosis. Am J Physiol Endocrinol Metab. 2008;295: E929–37.
66. Chefetz I, Sprecher E. Familial tumoral calcinosis and the role of O-glycosylation in the maintenance of phosphate homeostasis. Biochim Biophys Acta. 2009;1792:847–52.
67. Shimada T, Kakitani M, Yamazaki Y, Hasegawa H, Takeuchi Y, Fujita T, Fukumoto S, Tomizuka K, Yamashita T. Targeted ablation of Fgf23 demonstrates an essential physiological role of FGF23 in phosphate and vitamin D metabolism. J Clin Invest. 2004;113:561–8.
68. Razzaque M, Sitara D, Taguchi T, St-Arnaud R, Lanske B. Premature aging-like phenotype in fibroblast growth factor 23 null mice is a vitamin D-mediated process. FASEB J. 2006;20:720–2.
69. Shimada T, Hasegawa H, Yamazaki Y, Muto T, Hino R, Takeuchi Y, Fujita T, Nakahara K, Fukumoto S, Yamashita T. FGF-23 is a potent regulator of vitamin D metabolism and phosphate homeostasis. J Bone Miner Res. 2004;19:429–35.
70. Gattineni J, Bates C, Twombley K, Dwarakanath V, Robinson M, Goetz R, Mohammadi M, Baum M. FGF23 decreases renal NaPi-2a and NaPi-2c expression and induces hypophosphatemia in vivo predominantly via FGF receptor 1. Am J Physiol Renal Physiol. 2009;297:F282–91.
71. Jüppner H, Wolf M, Salusky I. FGF-23: more than a regulator of renal phosphate handling? J Bone Miner Res. 2010;25:2091–7.
72. Tomoe Y, Segawa H, Shiozawa K, Kaneko I, Tominaga R, Hanabusa E, Aranami F, Furutani J, Kuwahara S, Tatsumi S, Matsumoto M, Ito M, Miyamoto K. Phosphaturic action of fibroblast growth factor 23 in Npt2 null mice. Am J Physiol Renal Physiol. 2010;298:F1341–50.
73. Saito H, Maeda A, Ohtomo S, Hirata M, Kusano K, Kato S, Ogata E, Segawa H, Miyamoto K, Fukushima N. Circulating FGF-23 is regulated by 1alpha,25-dihydroxyvitamin D3 and phosphorus in vivo. J Biol Chem. 2005;280:2543–9.

74. Saji F, Shigematsu T, Sakaguchi T, Ohya M, Orita H, Maeda Y, Ooura M, Mima T, Negi S. Fibroblast growth factor 23 production in bone is directly regulated by 1{alpha}, 25-dihydroxyvitamin D, but not PTH. Am J Physiol Renal Physiol. 2010;299: F1212–7.
75. Rejnmark L, Vestergaard P, Heickendorff L, Andreasen F, Mosekilde L. Loop diuretics alter the diurnal rhythm of endogenous parathyroid hormone secretion. A randomized-controlled study on the effects of loop- and thiazide-diuretics on the diurnal rhythms of calcitropic hormones and biochemical bone markers in postmenopausal women. Eur J Clin Invest. 2001;31:764–72.
76. Carpenter T, Insogna K, Zhang J, Ellis B, Nieman S, Simpson C, Olear E, Gundberg C. Circulating levels of soluble klotho and FGF23 in X-linked hypophosphatemia: circadian variance, effects of treatment, and relationship to parathyroid status. J Clin Endocrinol Metab. 2010;95:E352–7.
77. Perwad F, Azam N, Zhang M, Yamashita T, Tenenhouse H, Portale A. Dietary and serum phosphorus regulate fibroblast growth factor 23 expression and 1,25-dihydroxyvitamin D metabolism in mice. Endocrinology. 2005;146:5358–64.
78. Antoniucci D, Yamashita T, Portale A. Dietary phosphorus regulates serum fibroblast growth factor-23 concentrations in healthy men. J Clin Endocrinol Metab. 2006;91:3144–9.
79. Nishida Y, Taketani Y, Yamanaka-Okumura H, Imamura F, Taniguchi A, Sato T, Shuto E, Nashiki K, Arai H, Yamamoto H, Takeda E. Acute effect of oral phosphate loading on serum fibroblast growth factor 23 levels in healthy men. Kidney Int. 2006;70: 2141–7.
80. Ito N, Fukumoto S, Takeuchi Y, Takeda S, Suzuki H, Yamashita T, Fujita T. Effect of acute changes of serum phosphate on fibroblast growth factor (FGF)23 levels in humans. J Bone Miner Metab. 2007;25: 419–22.
81. Vervloet M, van Ittersum F, Büttler R, Heijboer A, Blankenstein M, ter Wee P. Effects of dietary phosphate and calcium intake on fibroblast growth factor-23. Clin J Am Soc Nephrol. 2011;6:383–9.
82. Burnett-Bowie S, Henao M, Dere M, Lee H, Leder B. Effects of hPTH(1–34) infusion on circulating serum phosphate, 1,25-dihydroxyvitamin D, and FGF23 levels in healthy men. J Bone Miner Res. 2009;24:1681–5.
83. Kurosu H, Ogawa Y, Miyoshi M, Yamamoto M, Nandi A, Rosenblatt K, Baum M, Schiavi S, Hu M, Moe O, Kuro-o M. Regulation of fibroblast growth factor-23 signaling by klotho. J Biol Chem. 2006;281:6120–3.
84. Nakatani T, Sarraj B, Ohnishi M, Densmore M, Taguchi T, Goetz R, Mohammadi M, Lanske B, Razzaque M. In vivo genetic evidence for klotho-dependent, fibroblast growth factor 23 (Fgf23)-mediated regulation of systemic phosphate homeostasis. FASEB J. 2009;23:433–41.
85. Urakawa I, Yamazaki Y, Shimada T, Ijima K, Hasegawa H, Okawa K, Fujita T, Fukumoto S, Yamashita T. Klotho converts canonical FGF receptor into a specific receptor for FGF23. Nature. 2006;444:770–4.
86. Chang Q, Hoefs S, van der Kemp A, Topala C, Bindels R, Hoenderop J. The beta-glucuronidase klotho hydrolyzes and activates the TRPV5 channel. Science. 2005;310:490–3.
87. Cha S, Ortega B, Kurosu H, Rosenblatt K, Kuro-O M, Huang C. Removal of sialic acid involving Klotho causes cell-surface retention of TRPV5 channel via binding to galectin-1. Proc Natl Acad Sci USA. 2008;105:9805–10.
88. de Groot T, Bindels R, Hoenderop J. TRPV5: an ingeniously controlled calcium channel. Kidney Int. 2008;74:1241–6.
89. Tsuruoka S, Nishiki K, Ioka T, Ando H, Saito Y, Kurabayashi M, Nagai R, Fujimura A. Defect in parathyroid-hormone-induced luminal calcium absorption in connecting tubules of Klotho mice. Nephrol Dial Transplant. 2006;21:2762–7.
90. Brown EM, Gamba G, Riccardi D, Lombardi M, Butters R, Kifor O, Sun A, Hediger MA, Lytton J, Hebert SC. Cloning and characterization of an extracellular Ca^{2+}–sensing receptor from bovine parathyroid. Nature. 1993;366:575–80.
91. Riccardi D, Park J, Lee W, Gamba G, Brown EM, Hebert SC. Cloning and functional expression of a rat kidney extracellular calcium/polyvalent cation receptor. Proc Natl Acad Sci USA. 1995;92:131–5.
92. Riccardi D, Brown E. Physiology and pathophysiology of the calcium-sensing receptor in the kidney. Am J Physiol Renal Physiol. 2010;298:F485–99.
93. Yamaguchi T. The calcium-sensing receptor in bone. J Bone Miner Metab. 2008;26:301–11.
94. Conigrave AD, Franks AH, Brown EM, Quinn SJ. L-Amino acid sensing by the calcium-sensing receptor: a general mechanism for coupling protein and calcium metabolism? Eur J Clin Nutr. 2002;56:1072–80.
95. Pollak MR, Brown EM, Chou YW, Hebert SC, Marx SJ, Steinmann B, Levi T, Seidman CE, Seidman JG. Mutations in the human Ca^{2+}-sensing receptor gene cause familial hypocalciuric hypercalcemia and neonatal severe hyperparathyroidism. Cell. 1993;75: 1297–303.
96. Gamba G, Friedman PA. Thick ascending limb: the Na^+: K^+: $2Cl^-$ co-transporter, NKCC2, and the calcium-sensing receptor. Pflugers Arch. 2009;458: 61–76.
97. Brown EM. Clincal lessons from the calcium-sensing receptor. Nat Clin Pract Endocrinol Metab. 2007;3:122–33.
98. Pollak MR, Chou YW, Marx SJ, Steinmann B, Cole DEC, Brandi ML, Papdopoulos SE, Menko FH, Hendy GN, Brown EM, Seidman CE, Seidman JG. Familial hypocalciuric hypercalcemia and neonatal severe hyperparathyroidism. Effects of mutant gene dosage on phenotype. J Clin Invest. 1994;93:1108–12.

99. Conigrave AD, Brown EM. L-Amino acid-sensing by calcium-sensing receptors: implications for GI physiology. Am J Physiol. 2006;291:G753–61.
100. Conigrave AD, Hampson DR. Broad-spectrum amino acid sensing by class 3 G-protein coupled receptors. Trends Endocrinol Metab. 2006;17: 398–407.
101. Hira T, Nakajima S, Eto Y, Hara H. Calcium-sensing receptor mediates phenylalanine-induced cholecystokinin secretion in enteroendocrine STC-1 cells. FEBS J. 2008;275:4620–6.
102. Wang Y, Chandra R, Samsa L, Gooch B, Fee B, Cook J, Vigna S, Grant A, Liddle R. Amino acids stimulate cholecystokinin release through the calcium-sensing receptor. Am J Physiol Gastrointest Liver Physiol. 2010;300:G528–37.
103. Liou A, Sei Y, Zhao X, Feng J, Lu X, Thomas C, Pechhold S, Raybould H, Wank S. The extracellular calcium sensing receptor is required for cholecystokinin secretion in response to L-phenylalanine in acutely isolated intestinal I cells. Am J Physiol Gastrointest Liver Physiol. 2011;300:G538–46.
104. Conigrave AD, Brown EM, Rizzoli R. Dietary protein and bone health: roles of amino acid-sensing receptors in the control of calcium metabolism and bone homeostasis. Annu Rev Nutr. 2008;28: 131–55.
105. Tiosano D, Hochberg Z. Hypophosphatemia: the common denominator of all rickets. J Bone Miner Metab. 2009;27:392–401.
106. Khoshniat S, Bourgine A, Julien M, Weiss P, Guicheux J, Beck L. The emergence of phosphate as a specific signaling molecule in bone and other cell types in mammals. Cell Mol Life Sci. 2011;68:205–18.
107. Peng JB, Chen XZ, Berger UV, Vassilev PM, Tsukaguchi H, Brown EM, Hediger MA. Molecular cloning and characterization of a channel-like transporter mediating intestinal calcium absorption. J Biol Chem. 1999;274:22739–46.
108. Hoenderop JG, van der Kemp AW, Hartog A, van de Graaf SF, van Os CH, Willems PH, Bindels RJ. Molecular identification of the apical Ca^{2+} channel in 1, 25-dihydroxyvitamin D3-responsive epithelia. J Biol Chem. 1999;274:8375–8.
109. Hoenderop J, Nilius B, Bindels R. Calcium absorption across epithelia. Physiol Rev. 2005;85:373–422.
110. Suzuki Y, Landowski C, Hediger M. Mechanisms and regulation of epithelial Ca^{2+} absorption in health and disease. Annu Rev Physiol. 2008;70: 257–71.
111. Angelow S, Ahlstrom R, Yu A. Biology of claudins. Am J Physiol Renal Physiol. 2008;295:F867–76.
112. Biber J, Hernando N, Forster I, Murer H. Regulation of phosphate transport in proximal tubules. Pflugers Arch. 2009;458:39–52.
113. Murer H, Forster I, Biber J. The sodium phosphate cotransporter family SLC34. Pflugers Arch. 2004; 447:763–7.
114. Marks J, Debnam ES, Unwin RJ. Phosphate homeostasis and the renal-gastrointestinal axis. Am J Physiol Renal Physiol. 2010;299:F285–96.
115. Yamaguchi T, Kimoto E. Inhibition of phosphate transport across the human erythrocyte membrane by chemical modification of sulfhydryl groups. Biochemistry. 1992;31:1968–73.
116. Palmieri F. The mitochondrial transporter family (SLC25): physiological and pathological implications. Pflugers Arch. 2004;447:689–709.
117. Kerstetter JE, O'Brien KO, Caseria DM, Wall DE, Insogna KL. The impact of dietary protein on calcium absorption and kinetic measures of bone turnover in women. J Clin Endocrinol Metab. 2005;90:26–31.
118. Kerstetter JE, O'Brien KO, Insogna KL. Dietary protein affects intestinal calcium absorption. Am J Clin Nutr. 1998;68:859–65.
119. Mace OJ, Lister N, Morgan E, Shepherd E, Affleck J, Helliwell P, Bronk JR, Kellett GL, Meredith D, Boyd R, Pieri M, Bailey PD, Pettcrew R, Foley D. An energy supply network of nutrient absorption coordinated by calcium and T1R taste receptors in rat small intestine. J Physiol. 2009;587:195–210.
120. Dardenne O, Prud'homme J, Hacking S, Glorieux F, St-Arnaud R. Correction of the abnormal mineral ion homeostasis with a high-calcium, high-phosphorus, high-lactose diet rescues the PDDR phenotype of mice deficient for the 25-hydroxyvitamin D-1alpha-hydroxylase (CYP27B1). Bone. 2003;32: 332–40.
121. O'Loughlin P, Morris H. Oestrogen deficiency impairs intestinal calcium absorption in the rat. J Physiol. 1998;511:313–22.
122. Colin E, Van Den Bemd G, Van Aken M, Christakos S, De Jonge H, Deluca H, Prahl J, Birkenhäger J, Buurman C, Pols H, Van Leeuwen J. Evidence for involvement of 17beta-estradiol in intestinal calcium absorption independent of 1,25-dihydroxyvitamin D3 level in the rat. J Bone Miner Res. 1999;14:57–64.
123. Ten Bolscher M, Netelenbos J, Barto R, Van Buuren L, Van der vijgh W. Estrogen regulation of intestinal calcium absorption in the intact and ovariectomized adult rat. J Bone Miner Res. 1999;14:1197–202.
124. Pahuja D, DeLuca H. Stimulation of intestinal calcium transport and bone calcium mobilization by prolactin in vitamin D-deficient rats. Science. 1981;214:1038–9.
125. Charoenphandhu N, Wongdee K, Krishnamra N. Is prolactin the cardinal calciotropic maternal hormone? Trends Endocrinol Metab. 2010;21:395–401.
126. Takeuchi K, Morikawa H, Ueda Y, Mochizuki M. Studies on the effects of placental lactogen on calcium metabolism during pregnancy. Nippon Naibunpi Gakkai Zasshi. 1988;64:1175–86.
127. Bronner F. Recent developments in intestinal calcium absorption. Nutr Rev. 2009;67:109–13.
128. Nordin BE. Calcium and osteoporosis. Nutrition. 1997;13:664–86.
129. Fudge N, Kovacs C. Pregnancy up-regulates intestinal calcium absorption and skeletal mineralization independently of the vitamin D receptor. Endocrinology. 2010;151:886–95.

130. Ajibade D, Dhawan P, Fechner A, Meyer M, Pike J, Christakos S. Evidence for a role of prolactin in calcium homeostasis: regulation of intestinal transient receptor potential vanilloid type 6, intestinal calcium absorption, and the 25-hydroxyvitamin D(3) 1alpha hydroxylase gene by prolactin. Endocrinology. 2010;151:2974–84.
131. Wasserman R, Kallfelz F, Comar C. Active transport of calcium by rat duodenum in vivo. Science. 1961;133:883–4.
132. Van Cromphaut S, Dewerchin M, Hoenderop J, Stockmans I, Van Herck E, Kato S, Bindels R, Collen D, Carmeliet P, Bouillon R, Carmeliet G. Duodenal calcium absorption in vitamin D receptor-knockout mice: functional and molecular aspects. Proc Natl Acad Sci USA. 2001;98:13324–9.
133. Chang Y, Hegsted D. Lactose and calcium transport in gut sacs. J Nutr. 1964;82:297–300.
134. Morgan E, Mace O, Affleck J, Kellett G. Apical GLUT2 and Cav1.3: regulation of rat intestinal glucose and calcium absorption. J Physiol. 2007;580: 593–604.
135. Akhter S, Kutuzova G, Christakos S, DeLuca H. Calbindin D9k is not required for 1,25-dihydroxyvitamin D3-mediated Ca^{2+} absorption in small intestine. Arch Biochem Biophys. 2007;460:227–32.
136. Kutuzova G, Sundersingh F, Vaughan J, Tadi B, Ansay S, Christakos S, Deluca H. TRPV6 is not required for 1alpha,25-dihydroxyvitamin D3-induced intestinal calcium absorption in vivo. Proc Natl Acad Sci USA. 2008;105:19655–9.
137. Benn B, Ajibade D, Porta A, Dhawan P, Hediger M, Peng J, Jiang Y, Oh G, Jeung E, Lieben L, Bouillon R, Carmeliet G, Christakos S. Active intestinal calcium transport in the absence of transient receptor potential vanilloid type 6 and calbindin-D9k. Endocrinology. 2008;149:3196–205.
138. Christakos S, Dhawan P, Ajibade D, Benn B, Feng J, Joshi S. Mechanisms involved in vitamin D mediated intestinal calcium absorption and in non-classical actions of vitamin D. J Steroid Biochem Mol Biol. 2010;121:183–7.
139. Gaffney-Stomberg E, Sun B, Cucchi C, Simpson C, Gundberg C, Kerstetter J, Insogna K. The effect of dietary protein on intestinal calcium absorption in rats. Endocrinology. 2010;151:1071–8.
140. Wright M, Sullivan R, Gaffney-Stomberg E, Caseria D, O'Brien K, Proctor D, Simpson C, Kerstetter J, Insogna K. Inhibiting gastric acid production does not affect intestinal calcium absorption in young, healthy individuals: a randomized, crossover, controlled clinical trial. J Bone Miner Res. 2010;25:2205–11.
141. Marks J, Srai SK, Biber J, Murer H, Unwin RJ, Debnam ES. Intestinal phosphate absorption and the effect of vitamin D: a comparison of rats with mice. Exp Physiol. 2006;91:531–7.
142. Rizzoli R, Fleisch H, Bonjour J. Role of 1,25-dihydroxyvitamin D3 on intestinal phosphate absorption in rats with a normal vitamin D supply. J Clin Invest. 1977;60:639–47.
143. Jones G, Strugnell S, DeLuca H. Current understanding of the molecular actions of vitamin D. Physiol Rev. 1998;78:1193–231.
144. Cross HS, Debiec H, Peterlik M. Mechanism and regulation of intestinal phosphate absorption. Miner Electrolyte Metab. 1990;16:115–24.
145. Williams KB, DeLuca HF. Characterization of intestinal phosphate absorption using a novel method. Am J Physiol Endocrinol Metab. 2007;292: E1917–21.
146. Katai K, Miyamoto K, Kishida S, Segawa H, Nii T, Tanaka H, Tani Y, Arai H, Tatsumi S, Morita K, Taketani Y, Takeda E. Regulation of intestinal Na^+–dependent phosphate co-transporters by a low-phosphate diet and 1,25-dihydroxyvitamin D_3. Biochem J. 1999;343:705–12.
147. Hattenhauer O, Traebert M, Murer H, Biber J. Regulation of small intestinal Na-P(i) type IIb cotransporter by dietary phosphate intake. Am J Physiol. 1999;277:G756–62.
148. Capuano P, Radanovic T, Wagner CA, Bacic D, Kato S, Uchiyama Y, St-Arnoud R, Murer H, Biber J. Intestinal and renal adaptation to a low-Pi diet of type II NaPi cotransporters in vitamin D receptor- and 1αOHase-deficient mice. Am J Physiol Cell Physiol. 2005;288:C429–34.
149. Xu H, Uno J, Inouye M, Xu L, Drees J, Collins J, Ghishan F. Regulation of intestinal NaPi-IIb cotransporter gene expression by estrogen. Am J Physiol Gastrointest Liver Physiol. 2003;285:G1317–24.
150. Heaney R. Phosphorus nutrition and the treatment of osteoporosis. Mayo Clin Proc. 2004;79:91–7.
151. Xu H, Collins J, Bai L, Kiela P, Ghishan F. Regulation of the human sodium-phosphate cotransporter NaP(i)-IIb gene promoter by epidermal growth factor. Am J Physiol Cell Physiol. 2001;280:C628–36.
152. Borowitz S, Granrud G. Glucocorticoids inhibit intestinal phosphate absorption in developing rabbits. J Nutr. 1992;122:1273–9.
153. Arima K, Hines E, Kiela P, Drees J, Collins J, Ghishan F. Glucocorticoid regulation and glycosylation of mouse intestinal type IIb Na-P(i) cotransporter during ontogeny. Am J Physiol Gastrointest Liver Physiol. 2002;283:G426–34.
154. Chen H, Xua H, Duong J, Li J, Ghishan FK. Tumor necrosis factor-alpha impairs intestinal phosphate absorption in colitis. Am J Physiol Gastrointest Liver Physiol. 2009;296:G775–81.
155. Dimke H, Hoenderop HJ, Bindels RJ. Hereditary tubular transport disorders: implications for renal handling of Ca^{2+} and Mg^{2+}. Clin Sci (Lond). 2010;118:1–18.
156. Markadieu N, Bindels R, Hoenderop J. The renal connecting tubule: resolved and unresolved issues in Ca(2+) transport. Int J Biochem Cell Biol. 2011;43: 1–4.

157. van de Graaf SF, Boullart I, Hoenderop JG, Bindels RJ. Regulation of the epithelial Ca^{2+} channels TRPV5 and TRPV6 by 1alpha, 25-dihydroxy Vitamin D_3 and dietary Ca^{2+}. J Steroid Biochem Mol Biol. 2004;89–90:303–8.
158. Hsu Y, Dimke H, Hoenderop J, Bindels R. Calcitonin-stimulated renal Ca^{2+} reabsorption occurs independently of TRPV5. Nephrol Dial Transplant. 2010;25:1428–35.
159. Unwin R, Capasso G, Shirley D. An overview of divalent cation and citrate handling by the kidney. Nephron Physiol. 2004;98:15–20.
160. Shirley D, Walter S, Folkerd E, Unwin R, Bailey M. Transepithelial electrochemical gradients in the proximal convoluted tubule during potassium depletion in the rat. J Physiol. 1998;513:551–7.
161. Hemmingsen C. Regulation of renal calbindin-D28K. Pharmacol Toxicol. 2007;87 Suppl 3:5–30.
162. Koster H, Hartog A, Van Os C, Bindels R. Calbindin-D28K facilitates cytosolic calcium diffusion without interfering with calcium signaling. Cell Calcium. 1995;18:187–96.
163. Hoenderop J, Dardenne O, Van Abel M, Van Der Kemp A, Van Os C, St-Arnaud R, Bindels R. Modulation of renal Ca^{2+} transport protein genes by dietary Ca^{2+} and 1,25-dihydroxyvitamin D_3 in 25-hydroxyvitamin D_3-1alpha-hydroxylase knockout mice. FASEB J. 2002;16:1398–406.
164. Cao L, Bolt M, Wei M, Sitrin M, Chun LY. Regulation of calbindin-D9k expression by 1,25-dihydroxyvitamin D(3) and parathyroid hormone in mouse primary renal tubular cells. Arch Biochem Biophys. 2002;400:118–24.
165. van Abel M, Hoenderop J, van der Kemp A, Friedlaender M, van Leeuwen J, Bindels R. Coordinated control of renal Ca(2+) transport proteins by parathyroid hormone. Kidney Int. 2005;68(4):1708–21.
166. Suki W, Rouse D, Ng R, Kokko J. Calcium transport in the thick ascending limb of Henle. Heterogeneity of function in the medullary and cortical segments. J Clin Invest. 1980;66:1004–9.
167. Günzel D, Yu A. Function and regulation of claudins in the thick ascending limb of Henle. Pflugers Arch. 2009;458:77–88.
168. Simon D, Lu Y, Choate K, Velazquez H, Al-Sabban E, Praga M, Casari G, Bettinelli A, Colussi G, Rodriguez-Soriano J, McCredie D, Milford D, Sanjad S, Lifton R. Paracellin-1, a renal tight junction protein required for paracellular Mg^{2+} resorption Science. 1999;285:103–6.
169. Ikari A, Matsumoto S, Harada H, Takagi K, Hayashi H, Suzuki Y, Degawa M, Miwa M. Phosphorylation of paracellin-1 at Ser217 by protein kinase A is essential for localization in tight junctions. J Cell Sci. 2006;119:1781–9.
170. Müller D, Hoenderop J, Meij I, van den Heuvel L, Knoers N, den Hollander A, Eggert P, García-Nieto V, Claverie-Martín F, Bindels R. Molecular cloning, tissue distribution, and chromosomal mapping of the human epithelial Ca^{2+} channel (ECAC1). Genomics. 2000;67:48–53.
171. Lambers T, Bindels R, Hoenderop J. Coordinated control of renal Ca^{2+} handling. Kidney Int. 2006;69:650–4.
172. Lajeunesse D, Bouhtiauy I, Brunette M. Parathyroid hormone and hydrochlorothiazide increase calcium transport by the luminal membrane of rabbit distal nephron segments through different pathways. Endocrinology. 1994;134:35–41.
173. de Groot T, Lee K, Langeslag M, Xi Q, Jalink K, Bindels R, Hoenderop J. Parathyroid hormone activates TRPV5 via PKA-dependent phosphorylation. J Am Soc Nephrol. 2009;20:1693–704.
174. Li Y, Bolt M, Cao L, Sitrin M. Effects of vitamin D receptor inactivation on the expression of calbindins and calcium metabolism. Am J Physiol Endocrinol Metab. 2001;281:E558–64.
175. Davey R, Turner A, McManus J, Chiu W, Tjahyono F, Moore A, Atkins G, Anderson P, Ma C, Glatt V, MacLean H, Vincent C, Bouxsein M, Morris H, Findlay D, Zajac J. Calcitonin receptor plays a physiological role to protect against hypercalcemia in mice. J Bone Miner Res. 2008;23:1182–93.
176. Turner A, Tjahyono F, Chiu W, Skinner J, Sawyer R, Moore A, Morris H, Findlay D, Zajac J, Davey R. The role of the calcitonin receptor in protecting against induced hypercalcemia is mediated via its actions in osteoclasts to inhibit bone resorption. Bone. 2011;48:354–61.
177. Li S, Watanabe M, Yamada H, Nagai A, Kinuta M, Takei K. Immunohistochemical localization of Klotho protein in brain, kidney, and reproductive organs of mice. Cell Struct Funct. 2004;29:91–9.
178. Hu M, Shi M, Zhang J, Pastor J, Nakatani T, Lanske B, Razzaque M, Rosenblatt K, Baum M, Kuro-o M, Moe O. Klotho: a novel phosphaturic substance acting as an autocrine enzyme in the renal proximal tubule. FASEB J. 2010;24:3438–50.
179. Alexander R, Woudenberg-Vrenken T, Buurman J, Dijkman H, van der Eerden B, van Leeuwen J, Bindels R, Hoenderop J. Klotho prevents renal calcium loss. J Am Soc Nephrol. 2009;20:2371–9.
180. Riccardi D, Traebert M, Ward DT, Kaissling B, Biber J, Hebert SC, Murer H. Dietary phosphate and parathyroid hormone alter the expression of the calcium-sensing receptor (CaR) and the Na^+–dependent Pi transporter (NaPi-2) in the rat proximal tubule. Pflugers Arch. 2000;441:379–87.
181. Ba J, Brown D, Friedman PA. Calcium-sensing receptor regulation of PTH-inhibitable proximal tubule phosphate transport. Am J Physiol. 2003;285:F1233–43.
182. Riccardi D, Hall AE, Chattopadhyay N, Xu JZ, Brown EM, Hebert SC. Localization of the extracellular Ca^{2+}/polyvalent cation-sensing protein in rat kidney. Am J Physiol. 1998;274:F611–22.

183. Escalante B, Erlij D, Falck J, McGiff J. Effect of cytochrome P450 arachidonate metabolites on ion transport in rabbit kidney loop of Henle. Science. 1991;251:799–802.
184. Ikari A, Okude C, Sawada H, Sasaki Y, Yamazaki Y, Sugatani J, Degawa M, Miwa M. Activation of a polyvalent cation-sensing receptor decreases magnesium transport via claudin-16. Biochim Biophys Acta. 2008;1778:283–90.
185. Takaichi K, Kurokawa K. High Ca2+ inhibits peptide hormone-dependent cAMP production specifically in thick ascending limbs of Henle. Miner Electrolyte Metab. 1986;12:342–6.
186. Beck L, Karaplis A, Amizuka N, Hewson A, Ozawa H, Tenenhouse H. Targeted inactivation of Npt2 in mice leads to severe renal phosphate wasting, hypercalciuria, and skeletal abnormalities. Proc Natl Acad Sci USA. 1998;95:5372–7.
187. Segawa H, Onitsuka A, Kuwahata M, Hanabusa E, Furutani J, Kaneko I, Tomoe Y, Aranami F, Matsumoto N, Ito M, Matsumoto M, Li M, Amizuka N, Miyamoto K. Type IIc sodium-dependent phosphate transporter regulates calcium metabolism. J Am Soc Nephrol. 2009;20:104–13.
188. Segawa H, Onitsuka A, Furutani J, Kaneko I, Aranami F, Matsumoto N, Tomoe Y, Kuwahata M, Ito M, Matsumoto M, Li M, Amizuka N, Miyamoto K. Npt2a and Npt2c in mice play distinct and synergistic roles in inorganic phosphate metabolism and skeletal development. Am J Physiol Renal Physiol. 2009;297:F671–8.
189. Lorenz-Depiereux B, Benet-Pages A, Eckstein G, Tenenbaum-Rakover Y, Wagenstaller J, Tiosano D, Gershoni-Baruch R, Albers N, Lichtner P, Schnabel D, Hochberg Z, Strom T. Hereditary hypophosphatemic rickets with hypercalciuria is caused by mutations in the sodium-phosphate cotransporter gene SLC34A3. Am J Hum Genet. 2006;78: 193–201.
190. Bergwitz C, Roslin N, Tieder M, Loredo-Osti J, Bastepe M, Abu-Zahra H, Frappier D, Burkett K, Carpenter T, Anderson D, Garabedian M, Sermet I, Fujiwara T, Morgan K, Tenenhouse H, Juppner H. SLC34A3 mutations in patients with hereditary hypophosphatemic rickets with hypercalciuria predict a key role for the sodium-phosphate cotransporter NaPi-IIc in maintaining phosphate homeostasis. Am J Hum Genet. 2006;78:179–92.
191. Magen D, Berger L, Coady M, Ilivitzki A, Militianu D, Tieder M, Selig S, Lapointe J, Zelikovic I, Skorecki K. A loss-of-function mutation in NaPi-IIa and renal Fanconi's syndrome. N Engl J Med. 2010;362:1102–9.
192. Miyamoto K, Segawa H, Ito M, Kuwahata M. Physiological regulation of renal sodium-dependent phosphate cotransporters. Jpn J Physiol. 2004;54: 93–102.
193. Segawa H, Yamanaka S, Onitsuka A, Tomoe Y, Kuwahata M, Ito M, Taketani Y, Miyamoto K. Parathyroid hormone-dependent endocytosis of renal type IIc Na-Pi cotransporter. Am J Physiol Renal Physiol. 2007;292:F395–403.
194. Shenolikar S, Voltz J, Minkoff C, Wade J, Weinman E. Targeted disruption of the mouse NHERF-1 gene promotes internalization of proximal tubule sodium-phosphate cotransporter type IIa and renal phosphate wasting. Proc Natl Acad Sci USA. 2002;99: 11470–5.
195. Capuano P, Bacic D, Roos M, Gisler S, Stange G, Biber J, Kaissling B, Weinman E, Shenolikar S, Wagner C, Murer H. Defective coupling of apical PTH receptors to phospholipase C prevents internalization of the Na^+–phosphate cotransporter NaPi-IIa in Nherf1-deficient mice. Am J Physiol Cell Physiol. 2007;292:C927–34.
196. Villa-Bellosta R, Barac-Nieto M, Breusegem S, Barry N, Levi M, Sorribas V. Interactions of the growth-related, type IIc renal sodium/phosphate cotransporter with PDZ proteins. Kidney Int. 2008; 73:456–64.
197. Farrow E, Davis S, Summers L, White K. Initial FGF23-mediated signaling occurs in the distal convoluted tubule. J Am Soc Nephrol. 2009;20: 955–60.
198. Berndt T, Thomas L, Craig T, Sommer S, Li X, Bergstralh E, Kumar R. Evidence for a signaling axis by which intestinal phosphate rapidly modulates renal phosphate reabsorption. Proc Natl Acad Sci USA. 2007;104:11085–90.
199. Sabbagh Y, O'Brien S, Song W, Boulanger J, Stockmann A, Arbeeny C, Schiavi S. Intestinal npt2b plays a major role in phosphate absorption and homeostasis. J Am Soc Nephrol. 2009;20: 2348–58.
200. Karsenty G, Yadav VK. Regulation of bone mass by serotonin: molecular biology and therapeutic implications. Annu Rev Med. 2011;62:323–31.
201. Bonnet N, Pierroz DD, Ferrari S. Adrenergic control of bone remodeling and its implications for the treatment of osteoporosis. J Musculoskelet Neuronal Interact. 2008;8:94–104.
202. Carpinteri R, Porcelli T, Mejia C, Patelli I, Bilezikian J, Canalis E, Angeli A, Giustina A, Mazziotti G. Glucocorticoid-induced osteoporosis and parathyroid hormone. J Endocrinol Invest. 2010;33(7 Suppl):16–21.
203. Kronenberg H. PTHrP and skeletal development. Ann N Y Acad Sci. 2006;1068:1–13.
204. Kousteni S, Bilezikian J. The cell biology of parathyroid hormone in osteoblasts. Curr Osteoporos Rep. 2008;6:72–6.
205. Yakar S, Courtland H, Clemmons D. IGF-1 and bone: new discoveries from mouse models. J Bone Miner Res. 2010;25:2543–5.
206. Wang Y, Nishida S, Boudignon B, Burghardt A, Elalieh H, Hamilton M, Majumdar S, Halloran B, Clemens T, Bikle D. IGF-I receptor is required for the anabolic actions of parathyroid hormone on bone. J Bone Miner Res. 2007;22:1329–37.

207. Parfitt AM. Misconceptions (3): calcium leaves bone only by resorption and enters only by formation. Bone. 2003;33:259–63.
208. Rizzoli R, Bonjour J-P. Physiology of calcium and phosphate homeostasis. In: Seibel MJ, Robins SP, Bilezikian JP, editors. Dynamics of bone and cartilage metabolism. San Diego: Academic Press; 1999. p. 247–60.
209. Papapetrou P. Bisphosphonate-associated adverse events. Hormones (Athens). 2009;8:96–110.
210. Stopeck A, Lipton A, Body J, Steger G, Tonkin K, de Boer R, Lichinitser M, Fujiwara Y, Yardley D, Viniegra M, Fan M, Jiang Q, Dansey R, Jun S, Braun A. Denosumab compared with zoledronic acid for the treatment of bone metastases in patients with advanced breast cancer: a randomized, double-blind study. J Clin Oncol. 2010;28:5132–9.
211. Zhao W, Byrne M, Boyce B, Krane S. Bone resorption induced by parathyroid hormone is strikingly diminished in collagenase-resistant mutant mice. J Clin Invest. 1999;103:517–24.
212. Lee R, Weber TJ. Disorders of phosphorus homeostasis. Curr Opin Endocrinol Diabet Obes. 2010;17: 561–7.
213. Martin T, Seeman E. Bone remodelling: its local regulation and the emergence of bone fragility. Best Pract Res Clin Endocrinol Metab. 2008;22:701–22.
214. Matsuo K, Irie N. Osteoclast–osteoblast communication. Arch Biochem Biophys. 2008;473:201–9.
215. Chiusaroli R, Maier A, Knight M, Byrne M, Calvi L, Baron R, Krane S, Schipani E. Collagenase cleavage of type I collagen is essential for both basal and parathyroid hormone (PTH)/PTH-related peptide receptor-induced osteoclast activation and has differential effects on discrete bone compartments. Endocrinology. 2003;144:4106–16.
216. Nakayamada S, Okada Y, Saito K, Tamura M, Tanaka Y. Beta1 integrin/focal adhesion kinase-mediated signaling induces intercellular adhesion molecule 1 and receptor activator of nuclear factor kappaB ligand on osteoblasts and osteoclast maturation. J Biol Chem. 2003;278:45368–74.
217. Henriksen K, Tanko LB, Qvist P, Delmas PD, Christiansen C, Karsdal MA. Assessment of osteoclast number and function: application in the development of new and improved treatment modalities for bone diseases. Osteoporos Int. 2007;18:681–5.
218. Hedgecock N, Hadi T, Chen A, Curtiss S, Martin R, Hazelwood S. Quantitative regional associations between remodeling, modeling, and osteocyte apoptosis and density in rabbit tibial midshafts. Bone. 2007;40:627–37.
219. Lotinun S, Evans G, Bronk J, Bolander M, Wronski T, Ritman E, Turner R. Continuous parathyroid hormone induces cortical porosity in the rat: effects on bone turnover and mechanical properties. J Bone Miner Res. 2004;19:1165–71.
220. Iida-Klein A, Lu S, Kapadia R, Burkhart M, Moreno A, Dempster D, Lindsay R. Short-term continuous infusion of human parathyroid hormone 1–34 fragment is catabolic with decreased trabecular connectivity density accompanied by hypercalcemia in C57BL/J6 mice. J Endocrinol. 2005;186:549–57.
221. Ma Y, Cain R, Halladay D, Yang X, Zeng Q, Miles R, Chandrasekhar S, Martin T, Onyia J. Catabolic effects of continuous human PTH (1–38) in vivo is associated with sustained stimulation of RANKL and inhibition of osteoprotegerin and gene-associated bone formation. Endocrinology. 2001;142:4047–54.
222. Qin L, Raggatt L, Partridge N. Parathyroid hormone: a double-edged sword for bone metabolism. Trends Endocrinol Metab. 2004;15:60–5.
223. Panda D, Miao D, Bolivar I, Li J, Huo R, Hendy G, Goltzman D. Inactivation of the 25-hydroxyvitamin D 1alpha-hydroxylase and vitamin D receptor demonstrates independent and interdependent effects of calcium and vitamin D on skeletal and mineral homeostasis. J Biol Chem. 2004;279:16754–66.
224. Xue Y, Karaplis A, Hendy G, Goltzman D, Miao D. Genetic models show that parathyroid hormone and 1,25-dihydroxyvitamin D_3 play distinct and synergistic roles in postnatal mineral ion homeostasis and skeletal development. Hum Mol Genet. 2005;14:1515–28.
225. Gardiner EM, Baldock PA, Thomas GP, Sims NA, Henderson NK, Hollis B, White CP, Sunn KL, Morrison NA, Walsh WR, Eisman JA. Increased formation and decreased resorption of bone in mice with elevated vitamin D receptor in mature cells of the osteoblastic lineage. FASEB J. 2000;14:1908–16.
226. Rhee Y, Allen M, Condon K, Lezcano V, Ronda A, Galli C, Olivos N, Passeri G, O'Brien C, Bivi N, Plotkin L, Bellido T. PTH receptor signaling in osteocytes governs periosteal bone formation and intra-cortical remodeling. J Bone Miner Res. 2011;26(5):1035–46.
227. Teti A, Zallone A. Do osteocytes contribute to bone mineral homeostasis? Osteocytic osteolysis revisited. Bone. 2009;44:11–6.
228. Bonewald LF. The amazing osteocyte. J Bone Miner Res. 2011;26:229–38.
229. Parthier C, Reedtz-Runge S, Rudolph R, Stubbs M. Passing the baton in class B GPCRs: peptide hormone activation via helix induction? Trends Biochem Sci. 2009;34:303–10.
230. Lee S, Goldring S, Lorenzo J. Expression of the calcitonin receptor in bone marrow cell cultures and in bone: a specific marker of the differentiated osteoclast that is regulated by calcitonin. Endocrinology. 1995;136:4572–81.
231. Garrett JE, Tamir H, Kifor O, Simin RT, Rogers KV, Mithal A, Gagel RF, Brown EM. Calcitonin-secreting cells of the thyroid gland express an extracellular calcium-sensing receptor gene. Endocrinology. 1995;136:5202–11.
232. Bolognese M. SERMs and SERMs with estrogen for postmenopausal osteoporosis. Rev Endocr Metab Disord. 2010;11:253–9.
233. Krum S. Direct transcriptional targets of sex steroid hormones in bone. J Cell Biochem. 2011;112:401–8.

234. Takeda S, Elefteriou F, Levasseur R, Liu X, Zhao L, Parker K, Armstrong D, Ducy P, Karsenty G. Leptin regulates bone formation via the sympathetic nervous system. Cell. 2002;111:305–17.
235. Elefteriou F, Ahn J, Takeda S, Starbuck M, Yang X, Liu X, Kondo H, Richards W, Bannon T, Noda M, Clement K, Vaisse C, Karsenty G. Leptin regulation of bone resorption by the sympathetic nervous system and CART. Nature. 2005;434:514–20.
236. Murshed M, McKee M. Molecular determinants of extracellular matrix mineralization in bone and blood vessels. Curr Opin Nephrol Hypertens. 2010;19:359–65.
237. Omelon S, Georgiou J, Henneman Z, Wise L, Sukhu B, Hunt T, Wynnyckyj C, Holmyard D, Bielecki R, Grynpas M. Control of vertebrate skeletal mineralization by polyphosphates. PLoS One. 2009;4:e5634.
238. Whyte M. Physiological role of alkaline phosphatase explored in hypophosphatasia. Ann N Y Acad Sci. 2010;1192:190–200.
239. Fedde K, Blair L, Silverstein J, Coburn S, Ryan L, Weinstein R, Waymire K, Narisawa S, Millán J, MacGregor G, Whyte M. Alkaline phosphatase knock-out mice recapitulate the metabolic and skeletal defects of infantile hypophosphatasia. J Bone Miner Res. 1999;14:2015–26.
240. Orimo H. The mechanism of mineralization and the role of alkaline phosphatase in health and disease. J Nippon Med Sch. 2010;77:4–12.
241. Ho A, Johnson M, Kingsley D. Role of the mouse ank gene in control of tissue calcification and arthritis. Science. 2000;289:265–70.
242. Zaka R, Williams CJ. Role of the progressive ankylosis gene in cartilage minerlization. Curr Opin Rheumatol. 2006;18:181–6.
243. Kim H, Minashima T, McCarthy E, Winkles J, Kirsch T. Progressive ankylosis protein (ANK) in osteoblasts and osteoclasts controls bone formation and bone remodeling. J Bone Miner Res. 2010;25:1771–83.
244. Addison W, Azari F, Sørensen E, Kaartinen M, McKee M. Pyrophosphate inhibits mineralization of osteoblast cultures by binding to mineral, up-regulating osteopontin, and inhibiting alkaline phosphatase activity. J Biol Chem. 2007;282:15872–83.
245. Tartaix P, Doulaverakis M, George A, Fisher L, Butler W, Qin C, Salih E, Tan M, Fujimoto Y, Spevak L, Boskey A. In vitro effects of dentin matrix protein-1 on hydroxyapatite formation provide insights into in vivo functions. J Biol Chem. 2004;279:18115–20.
246. Sun Y, Prasad M, Gao T, Wang X, Zhu Q, D'Souza R, Feng J, Qin C. Failure to process dentin matrix protein 1 (DMP1) into fragments leads to its loss of function in osteogenesis. J Biol Chem. 2010;285:31713–22.
247. Addison W, Nakano Y, Loisel T, Crine P, McKee M. MEPE-ASARM peptides control extracellular matrix mineralization by binding to hydroxyapatite: an inhibition regulated by PHEX cleavage of ASARM. J Bone Miner Res. 2008;23:1638–49.
248. Addison W, Masica D, Gray J, McKee M. Phosphorylation-dependent inhibition of mineralization by osteopontin ASARM peptides is regulated by PHEX cleavage. J Bone Miner Res. 2010;25:695–705.
249. Sabbagh Y, Carpenter T, Demay M. Hypophosphatemia leads to rickets by impairing caspase-mediated apoptosis of hypertrophic chondrocytes. Proc Natl Acad Sci USA. 2005;102:9637–42.
250. Kumar R. New insights into phosphate homeostasis: fibroblast growth factor 23 and frizzled-related protein-4 are phosphaturic factors derived from tumors associated with osteomalacia. Curr Opin Nephrol Hypertens. 2002;11:547–53.
251. White K, Carn G, Lorenz-Depiereux B, Benet-Pages A, Strom T, Econs M. Autosomal-dominant hypophosphatemic rickets (ADHR) mutations stabilize FGF-23. Kidney Int. 2001;60:2079–86.
252. Goetz R, Nakada Y, Hu M, Kurosu H, Wang L, Nakatani T, Shi M, Eliseenkova A, Razzaque M, Moe O, Kuro-o M, Mohammadi M. Isolated C-terminal tail of FGF23 alleviates hypophosphatemia by inhibiting FGF23-FGFR-Klotho complex formation. Proc Natl Acad Sci USA. 2010;107:407–12.
253. HYP-Consortium. A gene (PEX) with homologies to endopeptidases is mutated in patients with X-linked hypophosphatemic rickets. Nat Genet. 1995;11: 130–6.
254. Holm I, Huang X, Kunkel L. Mutational analysis of the PEX gene in patients with X-linked hypophosphatemic rickets. Am J Hum Genet. 1997;60:790–7.
255. Dixon P, Christie P, Wooding C, Trump D, Grieff M, Holm I, Gertner J, Schmidtke J, Shah B, Shaw N, Smith C, Tau C, Schlessinger D, Whyte M, Thakker R. Mutational analysis of PHEX gene in X-linked hypophosphatemia. J Clin Endocrinol Metab. 1998;83:3615–23.
256. Beck L, Soumounou Y, Martel J, Krishnamurthy G, Gauthier C, Goodyer C, Tenenhouse H. Pex/PEX tissue distribution and evidence for a deletion in the 3′ region of the Pex gene in X-linked hypophosphatemic mice. J Clin Invest. 1997;99:1200–9.
257. Liu S, Guo R, Simpson L, Xiao Z, Burnham C, Quarles L. Regulation of fibroblastic growth factor 23 expression but not degradation by PHEX. J Biol Chem. 2003;278:37419–26.
258. Sitara D, Razzaque M, Hesse M, Yoganathan S, Taguchi T, Erben R, Jüppner H, Lanske B. Homozygous ablation of fibroblast growth factor-23 results in hyperphosphatemia and impaired skeletogenesis, and reverses hypophosphatemia in Phex-deficient mice. Matrix Biol. 2004;23:421–32.
259. Liu S, Zhou J, Tang W, Jiang X, Rowe D, Quarles L. Pathogenic role of Fgf23 in Hyp mice. Am J Physiol Endocrinol Metab. 2006;291:E38–49.
260. Segawa H, Aranami F, Kaneko I, Tomoe Y, Miyamoto K. The roles of Na/Pi-II transporters in phosphate metabolism. Bone. 2009;45 Suppl 1:S2–7.
261. Qin C, D'Souza R, Feng J. Dentin matrix protein 1 (DMP1): new and important roles for biomineraliza-

tion and phosphate homeostasis. J Dent Res. 2007;86:1134–41.
262. Feng JQ, Ward LM, Liu S, Lu Y, Xie Y, Yuan B, Yu X, Rauch F, Davis SI, Zhang S, Rios H, Drezner MK, Quarles LD, Bonewald LF, White KE. Loss of DMP1 causes rickets and osteomalacia and identifies a role for osteocytes in mineral metabolism. Nat Genet. 2006;38:1310–5.
263. Zhang R, Lu Y, Ye L, Yuan B, Yu S, Qin C, Xie Y, Gao T, Drezner M, Bonewald L, Feng J. Unique roles of phosphorus in endochondral bone formation and osteocyte maturation. J Bone Miner Res. 2010;26:1047–56.
264. Chang W, Tu C, Chen TH, Bikle D, Shoback D. The extracellular calcium-sensing receptor (CaSR) is a critical modulator of skeletal development. Sci Signal. 2008;1:1.
265. Tu Q, Pi M, Karsenty G, Simpson L, Liu S, Quarles LD. Rescue of the skeletal phenotype in CasR-deficient mice by transfer onto the Gcm2 null background. J Clin Invest. 2003;111:1029–37.
266. Dvorak MM, Siddiqua A, Ward DT, Carter DH, Dallas SL, Nemeth EF, Riccardi D. Physiological changes in extracellular calcium concentration directly control osteoblast function in the absence of calciotropic hormones. Proc Natl Acad Sci USA. 2004;101:5140–5.
267. Shu L, Ji J, Zhu Q, Cao G, Karaplis A, Pollak M, Brown E, Goltzman D, Miao D. The calcium sensing receptor mediates bone turnover induced by dietary calcium and parathyroid hormone in neonates. J Bone Miner Res. 2011;62(5):1057–71.
268. Dvorak MM, Chen TH, Orwoll B, Garvey C, Chang W, Bikle DD, Shoback DM. Constitutive activity of the osteoblast Ca^{2+}–sensing receptor promotes loss of cancellous bone. Endocrinology. 2007;148: 3156–63.
269. Mathew M, Takagi S. Structures of biological minerals in dental research. J Res Natl Inst Stand Technol. 2001;106:1035–44.
270. Uribarri J. Phosphorus homeostasis in normal health and in chronic kidney disease patients with special emphasis on dietary phosphorus intake. Semin Dial. 2007;20:295–301.

Diagnosis and Treatment of the Patient with Abnormal Calcium

3

Elizabeth H. Holt

Abstract

The author describes normal physiology of calcium and phosphorus metabolism and the chemistries associated with their pathophysiology in adults. Extensive discussions are presented about abnormalities of body chemistry in the hypercalcemic and hypocalcemic conditions. The clinical signs and symptoms of patients with these abnormalities are highlighted and provide a framework for diagnosing them. Treatment options for these conditions are given with extensive orientation towards medical therapies.

Keywords

Calcium homeostasis • Serum calcium levels • Cholecalciferol • Hydroxylation • Vitamin D3 • Calcitriol • Ionized calcium • Calcium-sensing receptor • CaSR • Bone resorption • Calcium resorption • Distal nephron • Laboratory measurement • Hypercalcemia • Signs • Symptoms • Etiology • History • Phsyical examination • Dehydration • Polyuria • Polydypsia • Disorientation • Primary hyperparathyroidism • Nephrolithiasis • Medications • Sarcoidosis • Multiple endocrine neoplasia • Malignanacy • Orthostasis • Band keratopathy • Granulomatous • Kyphosis • Costovertebral • Diagnostic evaluation • Plasma protein • Multiple myeloma • Chronic hepatitis • HIV infection • Renal function • Intact PTH • Immunochemiluminometric assay • ICMA • 25(OH) vitamin D • 1,25(OH)2 vitamin D • Nephrocalcinosis • Alkaline phosphatase • Hypercalciuria • Electrocardiography • QTc interval • Atriventricular block • DEXA • Dual energy X-ray absorptiometry • Radiographs • Normocalcemia • Renal failure • Osteitis fibrosa cystica • MEN I • MEN II • Lithium • Familial

E.H. Holt, MD, PhD (✉)
Section of Endocrinology and Metabolism,
Department of Internal Medicine, Yale University
of Medicine, New Haven, CT, USA
e-mail: elizabeth.holt@yale.edu

A.A. Licata and E.V. Lerma (eds.), *Diseases of the Parathyroid Glands*,
DOI 10.1007/978-1-4419-5550-0_3, © Springer Science+Business Media, LLC 2012

hypocalciuric hypercalcemia • Tertiary hyperparathyroidism • Intestinal malabsorption • Hyperphosphatemia • Bicarbonate reabsorption • Hypophosphatemia • Markers of bone turnover • Pheochromocytoma • Thyroid cancer • PTH-independent hypercalcemia • Humoral hypercalcemia of malignancy • Local osteolytic hypercalcemia • PTHrP • B cell lymphomas • Tuberculosis • Saline hydration • Bisphosphonate • Pamidronate • Zoledronic acid • Parathyroidectomy • Calcitonin • Tachyphylaxix • Hemodialysis • Immobilization • Calcimimetic • Cinacalcet • Neuromuscular • Tremor • Muscle spasm • Paresthesias • Hypoparathyroidism • Autoimmune disease • Tumor lysis syndrome • Transfusion therapy • Rhabdomyolysis • Shvostek sign • Trousseau sign • Tetany • Seizure • Hemodilution • Albumin serum • Protein malnutrition • Nephrotic symdrome • Hungry bone syndrome • Mucocutaneous candidiasis • Hypmagnesemia • Pseudohypoparathyroidism • Calcium infusion • Calcium gluconate

Serum Calcium in Normal Conditions

Precise regulation of calcium homeostasis in the body is essential for the following reasons: calcium is the main mineral component of the skeleton, calcium plays major roles in neuronal transmission, muscle contraction, and blood clotting, and calcium is an important intracellular signal that controls countless processes throughout the body.

Normal Serum Calcium Levels

A typical laboratory range for serum total calcium concentration is between 8.8 and 10.5 mg/dl. Of this calcium, 50–60% of the calcium is bound to plasma proteins or is complexed with anions such as citrate and phosphate. The remaining ionized or so-called free calcium controls physiologic actions. The normal concentration of ionized calcium is maintained in a very narrow range: 4.5–5.3 mg/dl.

Regulation of Normal Calcium Homeostasis

The body regulates serum calcium by controlling its entry through the intestine, its exit via the kidney, and its storage in bone. These processes are regulated by parathyroid hormone (PTH) and 1,25-dihydroxyvitamin D_3 [1,25-$(OH)_2D_3$]. PTH, secreted by the parathyroid glands, is a peptide hormone with a very brief half-life in plasma (2–4 min). 1,25-$(OH)_2D_3$ is made by a sequence of events beginning when cholecalciferol (vitamin D_3) is generated by exposure of the skin to ultraviolet light; it is also supplied by dietary sources or nutritional supplements. In the liver, vitamin D_3 is hydroxylated to 25-(OH) vitamin D_3, which is in turn hydroxylated in the kidney to the active form, 1,25-$(OH)_2D_3$ (calcitriol). The net effect of PTH and 1,25-$(OH)_2D_3$ is to maintain plasma ionized calcium concentrations under extremely tight control, despite significant variations in calcium supply. In a healthy adult under equilibrium conditions, net calcium absorption from the gastrointestinal tract averages about 150–200 mg/day and the kidneys excrete an equivalent amount of calcium. Bone remodeling also consumes and releases a balanced amount of calcium each day. Thus, net calcium levels in the body do not change from day to day.

Changes in plasma ionized calcium concentration are registered by parathyroid cells via the cell membrane calcium-sensing receptor (CaSR) [1]. Interaction of calcium ions with the extracellular domain of the CaSR triggers a series of intracellular signaling events, which ultimately control PTH secretion. As circulating concentrations of calcium rise, CaSR signaling is activated and causes PTH secretion to fall, and as circulating concentrations of calcium fall, CaSR signaling shuts off and PTH secretion increases.

When serum calcium levels are low, PTH increases bone resorption and distal nephron calcium resorption. PTH also stimulates renal production of calcitriol, which increases calcium absorption by the small intestine. If plasma calcium levels rise above normal, PTH secretion declines, leading to greater renal calcium losses, reduced calcitriol production and thus decreased calcium absorption by the gut. In this fashion, the plasma ionized calcium concentration is maintained in a narrow range, although sometimes at the expense of skeletal calcium stores.

Laboratory Measurement of Blood Calcium

Diagnosis of a calcium disorder is based on measurement of serum or ionized calcium. Serum measurements may be performed by spectrophotometry or by atomic absorption spectrophotometry; the latter yields more accurate measurements. Spurious high readings may occur if the tourniquet is in place too long before the blood is drawn, which can increase measured serum calcium values by up to 0.4 mg/dl [2]. Dilution of blood by drawing samples from a central venous catheter is a common error that leads to spuriously low calcium readings. Accurate measurement of ionized calcium requires that the samples are collected under anaerobic conditions (i.e., in a blood gas syringe) and placed on ice, with immediate analysis.

Hypercalcemia

Hypercalcemia is a common metabolic abnormality. Signs and symptoms of hypercalcemia may be absent or subtle, except in cases where calcium is significantly elevated or has increased rapidly. The diagnostic workup of hypercalcemia is straightforward (Fig. 3.1) [3]. Identification of the etiology of hypercalcemia requires a comprehensive history, physical examination, laboratory tests, and, occasionally, diagnostic imaging studies [4].

History and Physical Examination

Presenting Symptoms

Many individuals with mild hypercalcemia (serum calcium level <11 mg/dl) are asymptomatic, although some may report mild fatigue, vague changes in cognitive function, depression, or constipation. Typical manifestations of hypercalcemia are seen more commonly with serum calcium values between 12 and 14 mg/dl. These symptoms include anorexia, nausea, abdominal pain, muscle weakness, and depressed mental status. Dehydration is common, caused by polyuria and polydipsia (from decreased urine concentrating ability caused by high urinary calcium levels). At calcium levels above 14 mg/dl there may be progressive lethargy, disorientation, and even coma.

In addition to the severity of the serum calcium elevation, the rate of increase in serum calcium may also affect the seriousness of the symptoms. Individuals who are chronically hypercalcemic may have few symptoms even with serum calcium values up to 15–16 mg/dl. In contrast, those whose calcium level has risen abruptly may have symptoms at less severe calcium elevations. Elderly or debilitated patients are more likely to be symptomatic even with mild hypercalcemia.

A common cause of hypercalcemia is primary hyperparathyroidism. Patients with hyperparathyroidism classically have fractures, bone pain, or nephrolithiasis. Currently, however, most cases of primary hyperparathyroidism are discovered incidentally on routine blood chemistry before the patient becomes symptomatic.

Additional History

It may be helpful to review the medical record to determine the duration of the hypercalcemia and its course. Prescription medications (Table 3.1), foods, and nutritional supplements should be considered possible culprits. A careful family history should be performed to identify inherited

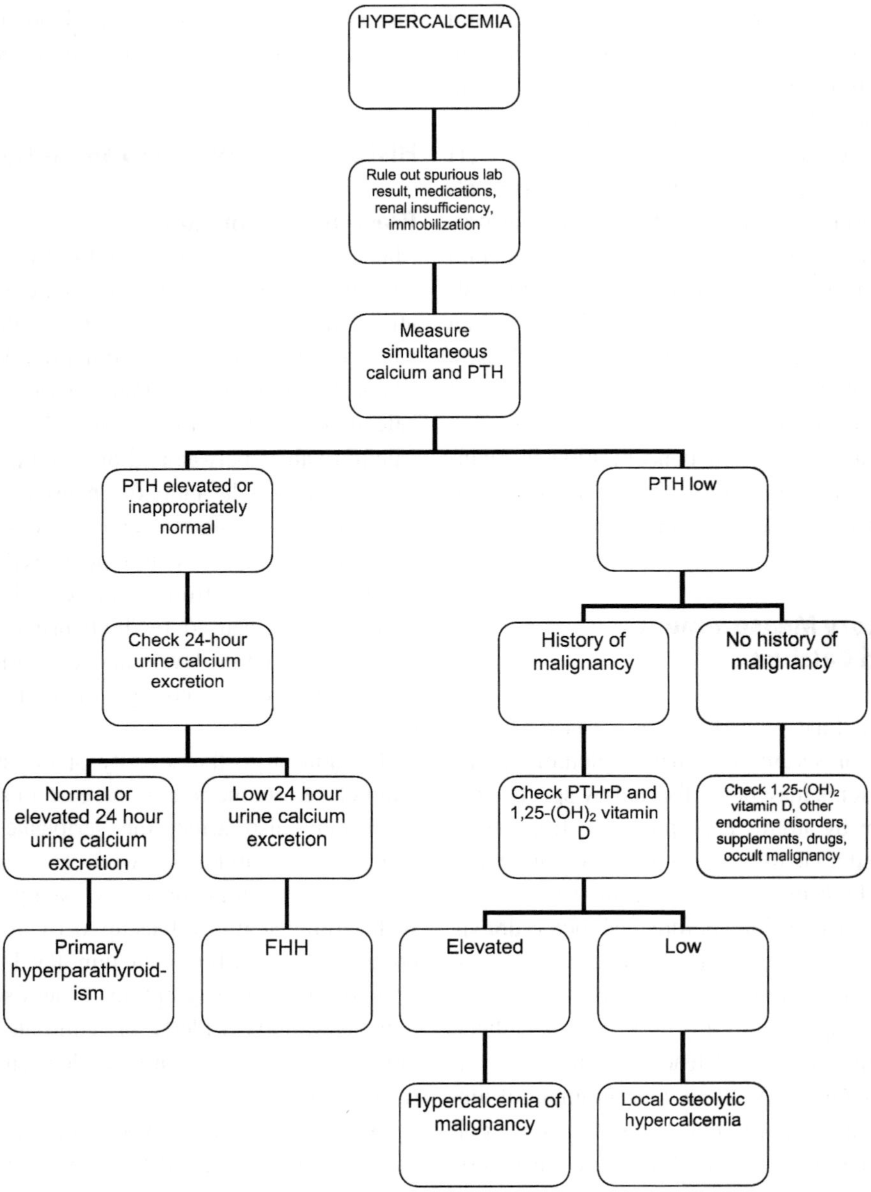

Fig. 3.1 Diagnostic approach to hypercalcemia. *FHH* familial hypocalciuric hypercalcemia, *PTH* parathyroid hormone, *PTHrP* parathyroid hormone-related protein

disorders of calcium metabolism, nephrolithiasis, low-trauma fractures, and evidence of any related endocrinopathies, such as tumors of the pituitary, adrenal, thyroid, or pancreatic islets. Patients who have hyperparathyroidism associated with multiple endocrine neoplasia (MEN) syndromes may have specific manifestations of the other conditions that are part of these syndromes. Patients with sarcoidosis may present with fever, lymphadenopathy, skin rashes, or pulmonary symptoms. Hypercalcemia of malignancy typically develops only when a substantial tumor burden is present; consequently, most of these patients already have an established cancer diagnosis and clinical features associated with the specific tumor type and extent of disease.

Table 3.1 Causes of hypercalcemia

PTH-mediated hypercalcemia	Primary hyperparathyroidism
	Parathyroid adenoma
	Parathyroid hyperplasia
	Parathyroid carcinoma
	Tertiary hyperparathyroidism
	Familial hypocalciuric hypocalcemia (FHH)
	Lithium
PTH-independent hypercalcemia	HHM: PTHrP-mediated
	Squamous carcinoma of the lung, oropharynx, nasopharynx, larynx, and esophagus
	Gynecologic (cervical and ovarian)
	Urologic (renal, transitional cell of bladder)
	Pheochromocytoma
	Pancreatic islet cell tumors
	T-cell lymphoma
	Others
	HHM: 1,25-$(OH)_2$-D_3 mediated
	B-cell lymphoma
	Local osteolytic hypercalcemia
	Multiple myeloma
	Breast carcinoma metastatic to bone
	Lymphoma
	Others
	Medications/supplements
	Vitamin D
	Vitamin A
	Thiazide diuretics
	Calcium-containing antacids (in milk-alkali syndrome)
	Granulomatous diseases
	Sarcoidosis
	Tuberculosis
	Histoplasmosis
	Leprosy
	Other conditions
	Factitious hypercalcemia (due to increased plasma protein levels)
	Acute renal failure
	Severe thyrotoxicosis
	Adrenal insufficiency
	Immobilization

Physical Findings

The physical examination should be directed at identifying signs or symptoms of hypercalcemia. Evidence for dehydration such as orthostasis or dry mucous membranes should be sought. Aside from depressed mental status and signs of dehydration, physical examination findings are generally normal in patients with hypercalcemia, especially if calcium levels are only modestly elevated. Rarely, severe and prolonged hypercalcemia may produce a visible horizontal deposit of calcium salts on the cornea, a finding called band keratopathy.

Effort should be made during the initial examination to identify signs of common causes of hypercalcemia such as malignancy and granulomatous diseases. Hyperparathyroidism associated with a palpable neck mass should raise concern for parathyroid cancer since benign parathyroid conditions typically do not produce a palpable mass. Evidence of complications, such as osteoporosis (manifest as kyphosis) or renal stones (which may cause costovertebral angle tenderness), should also be sought. Other signs and symptoms depend on the etiology of the elevation (see Table 3.1).

Diagnostic Evaluation

Laboratory Studies

The first step in evaluating hypercalcemia is to exclude factitious hypercalcemia, which may result from an increase in circulating concentrations of the plasma proteins that bind calcium. About 50–60% of serum calcium is bound to these proteins, so an elevation in their concentrations (as may occur in HIV infection, chronic hepatitis, and multiple myeloma) will produce a rise in the total serum calcium concentration. The ionized calcium concentration in these settings remains normal. To adjust the measured serum calcium for elevations in plasma protein, the serum calcium level should be lowered by 0.8 mg/dl for every 1 g/dl of albumin above the normal range. When performed under optimal conditions (above), ionized calcium measurement is more accurate than adjusted total serum calcium. Acute renal failure may occasionally lead to hypercalcemia, so renal function should also be assessed early in the workup.

If hypercalcemia is confirmed, the next step is measurement of the serum PTH concentration simultaneous with the serum or ionized calcium. This is the most important test for determining the cause of hypercalcemia [4]. The most common PTH assay today is the two-site immunochemiluminometric assay (ICMA, or so-called intact PTH). The ICMA measures only the intact PTH molecule and is therefore the preferred test in most instances, especially in patients whose renal function is impaired, where inactive fragments of PTH may accumulate in serum.

The results of PTH measurement indicate whether hypercalcemia is mediated by PTH and thus help identify the cause of hypercalcemia (see Table 3.1). In the setting of normally functioning parathyroid glands, hypercalcemia should cause PTH levels to be suppressed. The hypercalcemia is said to be PTH-mediated if serum calcium is elevated and the PTH level is high or inappropriately normal. PTH-mediated hypercalcemia is commonly referred to as hyperparathyroidism. When PTH levels are low in the face of high serum calcium, the hypercalcemia is said to be non-PTH mediated, or PTH independent. This distinction guides subsequent steps in patient evaluation.

Other recommended tests include measurement of serum creatinine and an electrolyte panel. Vitamin D studies are essential. Levels of 25-(OH) vitamin D should be measured to rule out supplemental vitamin D intoxication. High 1,25-$(OH)_2$D levels may be seen in granulomatous disease or certain lymphomas. Inorganic phosphorus measurement may be helpful as low serum phosphate is often seen in primary hyperparathyroidism, while high phosphate may occur in vitamin D intoxication. Serum creatinine may be acutely elevated in individuals who are dehydrated and chronically elevated in patients with nephrocalcinosis (deposition of calcium salts in the renal parenchyma secondary to prolonged hypercalcemia and resultant hypercalciuria). The alkaline phosphatase level may be elevated in patients with hypercalcemic states if there is elevated bone turnover. Patients with hypercalcemia due to malignancy may demonstrate biochemical or hematologic findings consistent with the site of neoplasia and its metastases. Most forms of hypercalcemia can be accompanied by hypercalciuria (24-h urine calcium excretion >4 mg/kg/24 h), which should be recognized and treated as it may lead to nephrocalcinosis or renal stone formation.

Additional Tests

Other diagnostic studies may be dictated by clinical circumstances. Electrocardiography is recommended for patients with severe hypercalcemia to detect shortening of the QT_c interval or atrioventricular block. In addition, many hypercalcemic conditions are associated with low bone mass, which may be noted on plain X-rays but is best assessed by measurement of bone mineral density by dual energy X-ray absorptiometry (DEXA). Abdominal imaging studies may identify renal stones or nephrocalcinosis. Bone radiographs are unlikely to aid in identification of the cause of hypercalcemia: bony abnormalities in individuals with primary hyperparathyroidism are now rare, thanks to early detection of hypercalcemia.

Causes of Hypercalcemia

PTH-Mediated Hypercalcemia

Primary Hyperparathyroidism

Elevation of both the serum calcium and the PTH concentrations (in the absence of lithium use or low urinary calcium excretion as seen in FHH) supports a diagnosis of primary hyperparathyroidism. PTH levels are usually increased to no more than five times the upper limit of normal. More significant elevations should raise suspicion for parathyroid carcinoma. In certain mild cases, the calcium level is only slightly high, and the PTH is mildly elevated or inappropriately normal. Rarely, patients with primary hyperparathyroidism have serum calcium levels in the upper-normal range. In fact, most of these patients will have elevated ionized calcium values and therefore are not actually normocalcemic. A firm diagnosis of primary hyperparathyroidism in such patients can be challenging, and longitudinal monitoring for disease progression may be appropriate.

Primary hyperparathyroidism is the most common cause of hypercalcemia diagnosed in the outpatient setting. The annual incidence of primary hyperparathyroidism is approximately 4/100,000 individuals. The incidence peaks in the fifth–sixth decade of life, and there is a female-to-male ratio of 3:2 [5]. The clinical manifestations of hyperparathyroidism depend, in part, on the severity of the hypercalcemia. When hyperparathyroidism was first described more than 50 years ago, most patients presented with late-stage complications of prolonged and severe hypercalcemia, such as abnormalities of bone (osteitis fibrosa cystica) [6] or kidneys (nephrocalcinosis, renal failure). Since the introduction, more than 30 years ago, of automated multichannel auto-analyzers for measuring serum chemistry, hyperparathyroidism is often diagnosed by routine blood testing, before the development of symptoms. It also may be uncovered during the evaluation of osteoporosis or during the workup of renal stone disease. The most common clinical presentation today is that of asymptomatic mild hypercalcemia discovered incidentally on a blood chemistry panel. In 75–80% of cases a solitary parathyroid adenoma is present, hyperplasia involving multiple parathyroid glands is found in 15–20% of cases, and parathyroid carcinoma is present in less than 1%. On occasion, double adenomas are found [7]. Patients with MEN type I or MEN II usually have parathyroid hyperplasia involving all parathyroid glands [8].

Lithium therapy can change the set point for the CaSR on the parathyroid gland so that a higher serum calcium concentration is needed to inhibit PTH secretion. This can lead to mild biochemical abnormalities (i.e., high levels of calcium and high-normal to elevated PTH levels) that mimic primary hyperparathyroidism but do not require medical intervention.

Familial Hypocalciuric Hypercalcemia

Familial hypocalciuric hypercalcemia (FHH), also referred to as benign familial hypercalcemia, is a rare genetic condition caused by inactivating mutations in the CaSR. This results in insensitivity of the parathyroid cell to serum calcium, a higher set point for the extracellular ionized calcium concentration and inappropriately normal to mildly elevated PTH levels. Patients with FHH have chronic asymptomatic hypercalcemia associated with relatively low urinary calcium excretion. This is usually a benign condition with no complications and thus requires no treatment.

When the PTH level is normal or mildly elevated and the 24-h urinary calcium level is low, consideration should be given to the possibility of FHH [9]. The relatively low urinary calcium output seen in FHH may help distinguish this condition from primary hyperparathyroidism, although low urinary calcium excretion may also occur in individuals with hyperparathyroidism who are taking thiazide diuretics and in those taking lithium. The possibility of FHH is raised when there is a strong family history of asymptomatic, stable, mild hypercalcemia, especially in individuals younger than 40 years, when family members have undergone non-curative parathyroidectomy for a diagnosis of primary hyperparathyroidism, or when the patient's urinary calcium to creatinine clearance ratio is very low (<0.01). When this diagnosis is suspected, further evaluation is necessary, such as the screening of other family members for hypercalcemia. Genetic testing for FHH is available at select centers and may be appropriate in some cases. In some cases, FHH cannot be distinguished confidently from primary hyperparathyroidism. However, in patients where FHH is suspected, hypercalcemia is typically mild, so expectant management is safe and avoids unnecessary parathyroid surgery.

Tertiary Hyperparathyroidism

Conditions that cause a low serum calcium or a high serum phosphate typically will be associated with a rise in PTH secretion as an appropriate corrective measure. This increase of PTH secretion is termed secondary hyperparathyroidism. The rise in PTH may be sufficient to return the serum calcium to normal or the calcium may remain low. Common causes of secondary hyperparathyroidism include vitamin D deficiency, intestinal malabsorption of calcium and/or vitamin D, renal calcium losses, severe dietary calcium inadequacy, and hyperphosphatemia due to chronic renal insufficiency. Correction of the causative abnormality, if possible, will return serum PTH concentrations to normal.

Secondary hyperparathyroidism is typically associated with low or normal serum calcium. However, in patients with long-term secondary hyperparathyroidism, hyperplasia, or neoplasia of the parathyroid glands may develop. As a result the parathyroids function autonomously, producing excess PTH at all times, resulting in hypercalcemia. This is most often seen in patients with chronic kidney disease. All of the parathyroid glands are usually affected.

Further Investigation

Most patients with primary hyperparathyroidism will have a serum calcium concentration below 12 mg/dl (unless coexisting dehydration is present), and they may have mild to moderate hypophosphatemia and a non-anion gap metabolic acidosis (from a PTH-induced defect in bicarbonate resorption). Urinary calcium excretion is often increased: although the high PTH will reduce the fractional calcium excretion, this effect is overcome by the high filtered calcium load, resulting in hypercalciuria. Hypercalciuria may predispose to renal stones in patients with hyperparathyroidism, which are calcium-containing and often occur bilaterally, especially when urinary calcium excretion is high. Rarely, nephrocalcinosis and renal insufficiency develop, usually in those with the most severe and prolonged hypercalcemia, and especially if dehydration or other renal injury is superimposed. Because PTH increases bone turnover, there will be increases in serum and urinary biochemical markers of bone turnover, including bone-specific alkaline phosphatase.

Once the diagnosis of primary hyperparathyroidism is made, additional testing may be necessary to determine whether the condition is severe enough to warrant parathyroidectomy. Consideration should also be given to the possibility of one of the MEN syndromes, particularly if the patient is young or has a personal or family history of a related endocrinopathy [8]. This information is essential to elucidate prior to surgery, because the patient with primary hyperparathyroidism in the setting of an MEN syndrome usually has multigland parathyroid hyperplasia, and in such patients a neck exploration to evaluate all parathyroid glands should be planned. If MEN II is suspected, medullary thyroid cancer should be considered, and pheochromocytoma must be ruled out before the patient can safely go to surgery.

PTH-Independent Hypercalcemia

If the serum calcium concentration is elevated but the PTH level is appropriately very low, the patient has PTH-independent hypercalcemia. Cancer is the most common cause of significant PTH-independent hypercalcemia and is most frequently to blame when an acutely elevated calcium level is discovered in a hospitalized patient. When the PTH is low and the patient is not known to have a malignancy, diagnostic considerations should include thyrotoxicosis, vitamin D intoxication, sarcoidosis, immobilization, certain endocrine disorders, and various drugs and supplements. These conditions require further laboratory assessment, with the choice of tests depending on the clinical situation.

Malignancy-Associated Hypercalcemia

Hypercalcemia of malignancy has two forms: humoral hypercalcemia of malignancy (HHM) and local osteolytic hypercalcemia (LOH). In malignancy-associated hypercalcemia the calcium elevation is usually moderate or severe, and PTH will be low or undetectable. Evidence of significant dehydration and generalized debility will be evident, along with other cancer-related symptoms. Usually, the diagnosis of malignancy has already been established.

HHM results from production by the tumor of a circulating factor that has systemic effects on calcium metabolism, acting at the level of skeletal calcium release, renal calcium handling, or intestinal calcium absorption. Rarely, it can be caused by the unregulated production of calcitriol (usually by B-cell lymphomas) or other mediators that interfere with calcium homeostasis. However, the best-recognized cause of HHM is parathyroid hormone-related protein (PTHrP) [10]. Normally, PTHrP serves as a paracrine factor in a variety of tissues (e.g., bone, skin, breast, uterus, placenta, and blood vessels) where it is involved in cellular calcium handling, smooth muscle contraction, and growth and development [10]. The amino terminus of the PTHrP peptide is homologous with PTH, and they share a common receptor. When PTHrP circulates at supraphysiologic concentrations, it induces similar metabolic effects to PTH, activating osteoclasts to resorb bone, decreasing renal calcium output, and increasing renal phosphate clearance [10].

Tumors that produce HHM by secreting PTHrP are typically squamous carcinomas (e.g., lung, esophageal, laryngeal, oropharyngeal, nasopharyngeal, or cervical carcinomas) [11]. Other tumors that may elaborate PTHrP include adenocarcinoma of the breast or ovary, renal carcinoma, transitional cell carcinoma of the bladder, islet cell tumors of the pancreas, T cell lymphoma, and pheochromocytoma. All tumors that produce PTHrP do so in relatively small amounts, thus the syndrome typically develops in patients with a large tumor burden. It is therefore unusual for HHM to be the presenting feature of a cancer. Radioimmunoassay for PTHrP is commercially available; a high serum PTHrP level will essentially confirm the diagnosis of most cases of HHM. Care should be taken to ensure that blood for PTHrP levels is drawn and handled correctly to avoid spurious low results.

LOH occurs when a tumor growing in bone causes release of calcium through the production of cytokines or other factors that activate bone resorption by osteoclasts. In local osteolytic disease, PTHrP and calcitriol are within normal limits, and there is evidence of bony metastases by symptoms and/or imaging studies. The classic tumor associated with this syndrome is multiple myeloma, although other neoplasms, such as adenocarcinomas of the breast and certain lymphomas, may also cause LOH. Local factors produced by bone cells may in turn promote the growth and survival of the metastases. This results in a positive feedback loop where the tumor induces the bone cells to produce factors that promote tumor growth, bone resorption and hypercalcemia. Interruption of this positive feedback loop is the basis for the use of bisphosphonates in the treatment of multiple myeloma [12].

Other Causes of PTH-Independent Hypercalcemia

PTH-independent hypercalcemia may occur in sarcoidosis, tuberculosis, and other granulomatous diseases, where granulomas produce excessive amounts of calcitriol. Elevation of serum 25-hydroxyvitamin D suggests excessive vitamin D intake, while elevation of serum 1,25-dihydroxyvitamin D occurs in granulomatous diseases. Endocrine conditions that may occasionally lead to hypercalcemia include severe hyperthyroidism (which stimulates bone resorption) and Addison's disease (where volume depletion reduces calcium clearance). Immobilization is a stimulus for bone resorption and may increase serum calcium levels, particularly in bedbound hospitalized patients. This is usually seen in persons with high bone turnover, such as adolescents or those with unrecognized hyperparathyroidism or Paget's disease of bone. Use of drugs and dietary supplements may be associated with hypercalcemia. Vitamin D intoxication and excessive intake of vitamin A (which activates bone resorption) are culprits. Thiazide diuretics may cause hypercalcemia due to enhanced retention of calcium by the kidney. In many cases this develops in individuals with underlying mild primary hyperparathyroidism [13]. Rarely encountered today is the so-called milk-alkali syndrome which results from the long-term consumption of large quantities of vitamin D-fortified milk and calcium-containing antacids. In the days before the development of H_2 receptor blockers and proton pump inhibitors, milk and antacids were the standard treatment of peptic ulcers and milk-alkalai syndrome was seen more frequently.

If investigation of these diagnoses proves fruitless, the very rare possibility of unrecognized malignancy should be considered, especially if PTHrP is elevated. Further imaging studies would then be needed to locate the culprit tumor, including a plain chest radiograph or a computed tomographic scan of the thorax to rule out lung malignancy. If these results are unrevealing, consideration should be given to otolaryngoscopic examination, esophagoscopy, or CT of the abdomen followed by radiographic or endoscopic evaluation of the genitourinary tract if necessary.

Treatment of Hypercalcemia

A nonparathyroid disorder, often a malignancy, is usually responsible for acute hypercalcemia (Table 3.1). When the serum calcium level is substantially elevated, treatment should include

Table 3.2 Treatment of hypercalcemia

Intravenous fluids
0.9% NaCl
Loop diuretic
Furosemide intravenous (titrated to response)
Medications
Bisphosphonates
Pamidronate (60–90 mg IV)
Zoledronic acid (4 mg IV)
Calcitonin (4 IU/kg SC, every 12 h)
Prednisone (20–100 mg PO QD or equivalent)
Other interventions
Decrease calcium and vitamin D intake (if causative)
Maintain adequate oral hydration
Primary therapy directed at tumor
Chemotherapy
Radiation
Surgery

rehydration, as well as efforts to increase renal calcium excretion while simultaneously reducing bone resorption and/or intestinal calcium absorption, depending on which is the main source of excess calcium.

Saline Hydration

Most patients with acute hypercalcemia have some degree of volume contraction, which further exacerbates their inability to excrete calcium, so the first intervention must be restoration of the intravascular volume with intravenous infusion of normal saline (Table 3.2). The use of normal saline is essential as delivery of sodium and water to the distal nephron will enhance urinary calcium excretion. Only once the intravascular volume is replenished should a loop diuretic such as furosemide be started to allow additional aggressive saline hydration and further enhance calcium excretion. A serum calcium–phosphate product greater than 70 indicates the patient is at risk for calciphylaxis, and efforts to reduce the serum phosphate level (e.g., with phosphate binders) should be considered along with the interventions to lower serum calcium.

Bisphosphonate Therapy

If the serum calcium concentration does not return to a safe level quickly with intravenous fluid and diuresis, then pharmacologic therapy is indicated [14]. Nearly all causes of severe hypercalcemia involve some degree of increased osteoclast activity, so drugs that inhibit bone resorption are useful. The treatment of choice is a bisphosphonate, such as pamidronate or zoledronic acid, both of which are administered by intravenous infusion. Pamidronate is given in a dosage of 60–90 mg intravenously over several hours and is generally well tolerated. Typically, serum calcium levels begin to decline within 24–48 h following the infusion, although the maximal effect may not be evident for several days. The actions of pamidronate may persist for several weeks, but treatment may be repeated as needed if renal function will allow. Zoledronic acid is given at a dosage of 4 mg intravenously over no less than 15 min [15]. It appears to have a greater potency and a longer duration of action than pamidronate. A repeat dose may be provided after 7 days if renal function allows. Use of intravenous bisphophonates, particularly zoledronic acid, is often followed immediately by an acute-phase response to the first dose, with flulike symptoms. Caution should be employed with these agents in the setting of renal dysfunction. Reduction in dosage of zoledronic acid is recommended for creatinine clearance below 60 ml/min, and its use in patients with creatinine clearance below 30 ml/min is not recommended [15]. In addition, if parathyroidectomy is planned, administration of bisphosphonates should be considered carefully, because they may make management of any postoperative hypocalcemia more difficult.

Other Treatments for Hypercalcemia

When more rapid reduction in serum calcium is necessary, subcutaneous injection of calcitonin can be employed, either alone or simultaneous with a bisphosphonate. Calcitonin is given at a starting dosage of 4 U/kg every 12 h. Calcitonin is a relatively weak hypocalcemic agent. Tachyphylaxis to the actions of calcitonin usually limits its effectiveness to a few days. Other possible therapies are plicamycin and gallium nitrate, although toxicities limit their use as first-line agents. In severe or refractory cases, hemodialysis against a low-calcium bath may be required.

When hypercalcemia results from an increase in intestinal calcium absorption, as occurs in vitamin D intoxication or granulomatous diseases, glucocorticoid therapy has an integral role. Glucocorticoids directly impair intestinal calcium transport and also inhibit the renal or granulomatous 1α-hydroxylase activity, resulting in a decrease in production of calcitriol. In patients with lymphoma, treatment with steroids may also indirectly reduce hypercalcemia due to their antineoplastic effect.

Contributing factors to hypercalcemia, such as the use of calcium or vitamin D supplements, thiazide diuretic therapy, or immobilization, should be eliminated, if possible.

In malignancy-associated hypercalcemia, surgery, chemotherapy, or radiotherapy targeted at the tumor itself may also reduce the hypercalcemia. However, because hypercalcemia is often an end-stage complication of malignancy, further interventions such as these may not be appropriate.

Treatment of the patient with primary hyperparathyroidism must take into account the degree of the hypercalcemia, the presence of symptoms, and the severity of any end-organ damage and the risk of future complications [16]. Understandably, it is widely agreed that patients with symptoms clearly attributable to hypercalcemia should undergo surgery. Controversy exists over which asymptomatic patients with primary hyperparathyroidism require surgical intervention. Some individuals without symptoms or complications clearly related to hyperparathyroidism can be followed safely for long periods without surgery. Guidelines for surgical intervention in patients with asymptomatic primary hyperparathyroidism were most recently updated at a National Institutes of Health workshop in 2009 [17].

Although there is as yet no widely recognized medical therapy for primary hyperparathyroidism, patients whose mild disease does not meet criteria for surgical intervention or who refuse surgery can be followed expectantly. Drugs that have a tendency to raise serum calcium levels, such as oral calcium supplements, thiazide diuretics, and lithium, should be avoided. Dietary calcium should not be restricted, because such restriction may promote further elevation of PTH and may possibly have adverse effects on bone mass. Any vitamin D deficiency should be treated with gentle supplementation, because vitamin D deficiency will enhance the adverse effects of hyperparathyroidism on bone. Patients should be encouraged to maintain good hydration to avoid the development of renal insufficiency and renal stones, especially in those with hypercalciuria. In patients with low BMD, a bisphosphonate will help to slow bone loss but will not control hypercalcemia [18]. In patients who are very hypercalcemic but cannot or will not have surgery, the calcimimetic agent cinacalcet has been used to control hypercalcemia. Calcimimetic agents such as cinacalcet activate the CaSR and thus diminish PTH production. The drug is FDA-approved for patients with hyperparathyroidism who have chronic renal disease and are on dialysis, patients with hypercalcemia from parathyroid carcinoma, and patients with hyperparathyroidism and severe hypercalcemia who cannot undergo parathyroidectomy. The high cost of these agents and the relative ease and safety of parathyroid surgery make their widespread use in the future unlikely [19]. However, generic equivalent drugs are in the evaluation process and may change the landscape of therapy.

Hypocalcemia

Hypocalcemia is defined as a serum calcium level below the normal range for the laboratory. As with hypercalcemia, an ionized calcium determination on a correctly collected sample will confirm hypocalcemia.

History and Physical Examination

Presenting Symptoms

Chronic mild to moderate hypocalcemia is usually asymptomatic. However, when the serum calcium level falls below 7.5–8 mg/dl (assuming that plasma protein levels are normal), the patient may develop symptoms of neuromuscular irritability, including tremor, muscle spasms, or paresthesias.

Additional History

As with hypercalcemia, the cause of hypocalcemia can usually be identified after a careful history. Dietary calcium and vitamin D intake, lack of sun exposure, and alcohol intake should be discussed. Prior head and neck surgery or irradiation is a risk factor for hypoparathyroidism. Risk for more rare conditions, such as autoimmune disease and iron overload states should be elucidated. Concomitant diseases or conditions such as pancreatitis, rhabdomyolysis, tumor lysis syndrome, or ongoing transfusion therapy should also be considered potential causes of hypocalcemia.

Physical Findings

On examination, Chvostek and Trousseau signs may be present. If the serum calcium level drops further, tetany or seizures may appear. Prolongation of the QT_c interval may be evident on electrocardiogram, indicating the patient is at risk for cardiac arrhythmias.

Diagnostic Evaluation

Laboratory Studies

A low level of serum calcium on laboratory testing is often factitious, due to low plasma calcium binding protein concentration caused by hemodilution or low protein synthetic function. Because circulating calcium is so highly protein bound, decreases in serum albumin concentrations—such as that occurring with protein malnourishment, severe liver disease, or in the nephrotic syndrome—produce proportionate reductions in total serum calcium. In these situations, the measured serum calcium level may be corrected by adding 0.8 mg/dl for each 1 g/dl the patient's serum albumin level falls below 4 g/dl. An accurate ionized calcium measurement will circumvent these pitfalls.

Once true hypocalcemia is confirmed, efforts to identify the cause should be undertaken. Guided by clues from the history and physical exam, the levels of phosphorus, magnesium, creatinine, PTH, and 25-(OH)D_3 should be measured. Measurement of 1,25-(OH)D_3 is typically not very helpful as levels may be normal even in the setting of significant vitamin D deficiency.

Differential Diagnosis

True hypocalcemia is most often related to vitamin D deficiency or parathyroid gland hypofunction (Table 3.3). Removal of or injury to the parathyroid glands during thyroidectomy surgery can result in hypoparathyroidism, which is manifested by hypocalcemia accompanied by inappropriately low serum PTH. However, unless all four parathyroid glands are removed or their blood supply is severely damaged, hypocalcemia after thyroidectomy is usually a mild and transient phenomenon. Normal parathyroid function typically returns after a period of several days to weeks. Patients who have had prolonged, severe primary hyperparathyroidism accompanied by significant bone turnover may experience protracted hypocalcemia after parathyroidectomy as a result of the rapid deposition of large quantities of calcium into the unmineralized matrix of the skeleton. This is referred to as the "hungry bone syndrome."

Automimmune destruction of the parathyroid glands may occur in certain conditions, including autoimmune polyglandular syndrome type 1, a condition marked by hypoparathyroidism, premature ovarian failure, Addison's disease, and mucocutaneous candidiasis [20]. Certain infiltrative diseases, such as hemochromatosis, may adversely affect parathyroid function, as may external-beam irradiation of the neck. Congenital absence of the parathyroid glands may be seen in DiGeorge syndrome. Functional hypoparathyroidism may result from hypomagnesemia, because magnesium is necessary for both PTH release and PTH action. This is commonly seen in hospitalized alcoholic patients who are often hypomagnesemic. Pseudohypoparathyroidism is caused by inherited PTH resistance, resulting in hypocalcemia accompanied by marked elevations of PTH.

Because vitamin D ultimately controls intestinal calcium absorption, disorders of vitamin D supply, production, or activation may lead to hypocalcemia. In vitamin D deficiency, serum calcium concentrations are usually not severely affected, thanks to compensatory increases in

Table 3.3 Causes of hypocalcemia

PTH-associated • Low PTH production • PTH resistance	Hypoparathyroidism Post-surgical External beam radiation (to neck) Autoimmune Polyendocrine syndromes Magnesium deficiency Congenital DiGeorge syndrome Infiltrative Hemochromatosis Thalassemia Wilson disease PTH resistance Pseudohypoparathyroidism Nutritional deficiency (includes vitamin D-dependent rickets and osteomalacia) Insufficient dietary intake of vitamin D Malabsorption Altered vitamin D metabolism Anticonvulsant medications (increased vitamin D metabolism)
Vitamin D-associated • Vitamin D deficiency • Vitamin D resistance	Renal failure Vitamin D pseudodeficiency (VDDR I) Abnormal vitamin D receptor (VDDR II) Vitamin D-resistant hypophosphatemic rickets/osteomalacia Oncogenic osteomalacia
Iatrogenic	Phosphate supplements Calcitonin Bisphosphonates (mainly seen with intravenous preparations) Plicamycin
Miscellaneous conditions	Hypoalbuminemia (factitious) Calcium malabsorption Hyperphosphatemia Acute pancreatitis Rhabdomyolysis Multiple transfusions of citrate-containing blood products Osteoblastic metastases (prostate or breast carcinoma)

PTH and its downstream efforts to keep serum calcium normal. Indeed, the primary clinical manifestations of vitamin D deficiency are in the skeleton (e.g., rickets in children and osteomalacia in adults). Dietary vitamin D deficiency in the elderly is common, but it is often overlooked [21]. Other adults at risk for vitamin D deficiency include persons with darker complexion or those with little sun exposure, combined with low dietary vitamin D intake. Recent reports suggest that vitamin D deficiency may be more prevalent than traditionally considered, even in individuals not previously thought to be at risk [22].

Hypocalcemia may occur in acute pancreatitis, when fatty acids released through the action of pancreatic enzymes complex with calcium. Hypocalcemia due to the formation of calcium phosphate complexes occurs in severe hyperphosphatemic states, such as renal failure, rhabdomyolysis, and the tumor lysis syndrome: formation of these complexes results in a decrease in serum calcium concentrations. Hypocalcemia may also be seen in patients given multiple red blood cell transfusions using cells to which calcium chelators have been added to prevent clotting.

Treatment of Hypocalcemia

In patients with symptoms of marked hypocalcemia (e.g., those with evidence of neuromuscular irritability), calcium (e.g., as calcium gluconate) should be delivered by slow continuous intravenous infusion to raise the serum calcium level until symptoms are relieved. Single boluses of intravenous calcium are not recommended as they have only a transient effect on serum calcium. A typical calcium infusion is prepared with 10 ampules (100 ml) of 10% calcium gluconate in 1 L of D_5W and administered at 50 cc/h. Serum calcium should be tested frequently and the rate of infusion adjusted accordingly to maintain levels in the low-normal range. Concurrently, any deficiency in magnesium and/or vitamin D stores should be corrected. In severe cases, hypocalcemia may recur quickly after discontinuation of the calcium infusion, so oral calcium should be administered concurrent with tapering the infusion. In less severe cases, calcium infusion will not be necessary and calcium can be administered orally as calcium carbonate or calcium citrate in doses starting at 1,000–1,500 mg of elemental calcium daily in divided doses with meals. Note that the elderly and individuals who are taking proton pump inhibitors may malabsorb calcium, so higher doses may be needed to achieve the desired effect. If appropriate, vitamin D also should be provided. If dietary deficiency of vitamin D is suspected, cholecalciferol (vitamin D_3) should be given, or, if cholecalciferol is unavailable, ergocalciferol (vitamin D_2), may be adequate. The recommended daily dose of vitamin D for adults 50 years and older is 400–600 IU/day according to current Institute of Medicine Dietary Reference Intake (DRI) guidelines [23], although many experts recommend a daily dose of 800–1,000 IU [24]. Patients who are deficient in this fat-soluble vitamin may require replenishment of their vitamin D stores with a brief course of prescription-strength ergocalciferol, e.g., 50,000 IU once weekly for 6–8 doses before starting a standard daily dose. Cholecalciferol is currently unavailable by prescription in the United States in this high-dose form. Hydroxylation of vitamin D to its active metabolite may take several days, so a brief course of calcitriol 0.25 μg or more daily may also be necessary to help maintain normal serum calcium while the vitamin D is being activated.

In cases of chronic hypoparathyroidism, long-term administration of calcitriol is needed, because renal 1α-hydroxylase will not be active in the absence of PTH. In hypoparathyroid patients, it is important to avoid fully normalizing the serum calcium level, because this often results in hypercalciuria and hyperphosphaturia, increasing the risk of nephrocalcinosis or renal stones. Instead, serum calcium should be kept at the lower limit of the normal range, at a level sufficient to relieve symptoms and reverse tetanic signs (e.g., Chvostek sign). Periodic monitoring for hypercalciuria and nephrocalcinosis in these patients may be appropriate. In the future, patients may be treated with synthetic human PTH, which has been evaluated in clinical trials as therapy for hypoparathyroidism.

References

1. Brown EM. Physiology and pathophysiology of the extracellular calcium-sensing receptor. Am J Med. 1999;106:238.
2. Lippi G, Salvagno GL, Montagnana M, et al. Influence of short-term venous stasis on clinical chemistry testing. Clin Chem Lab Med. 2005;43:869.
3. Marx SJ. Hyperparathyroid and hypoparathyroid disorders. N Engl J Med. 2000;343:1863.
4. Inzucchi SE. Management of hypercalcemia: diagnostic workup, therapeutic options for hyperparathyroidism and other common causes. Postgrad Med. 2004;115:27.
5. Wermers RA, Khosla S, Atkinson EJ, et al. The rise and fall of primary hyperparathyroidism: a population-based study in Rochester, Minnesota, 1965–1992. Ann Intern Med. 1997;126:433.
6. Khan A, Bilezikian J. Primary hyperparathyroidism: pathophysiology and impact on bone. Can Med Assoc J. 2000;163:184.
7. Kebebew E, Hwang J, Reiff E, et al. Predictors of single-gland vs multigland parathyroid disease in primary hyperparathyroidism: a simple and accurate scoring model. Arch Surg. 2006;141:777.
8. Brandi ML, Gagel RF, Angeli A, et al. Guidelines for diagnosis and therapy of MEN type 1 and type 2. J Clin Endocrinol Metab. 2001;86:5658.
9. Brown EM. Familial hypocalciuric hypercalcemia and other disorders with resistance to extracellular calcium. Endocrinol Clin North Am. 2000; 29:503.
10. Dunbar ME, Wysolmerski JJ, Broadus AE. Parathyroid hormone-related protein: from hypercalcemia of malignancy to developmental regulatory molecule. Am J Med Sci. 1996;312:287.
11. Rankin W, Grill V, Martin TJ. Parathyroid hormone-related protein and hypercalcemia. Cancer. 1997;80 Suppl 8:1564.
12. Corso A, Ferretti E, Lazzarino M. Zoledronic acid exerts its antitumor effect in multiple myeloma interfering with the bone marrow microenvironment. Hematology. 2005;10:215.
13. Wermers RA, Kearns AE, Jenkins GD, et al. Incidence and clinical spectrum of thiazide-associated hypercalcemia. Am J Med. 2007; 120:911.
14. Ziegler R. Hypercalcemic crisis. J Am Soc Nephrol. 2001;12 Suppl 17:S3.
15. Zometa (zoledronic acid) prescribing information. http://www.pharma.us.novartis.com/product/pi/pdf/Zometa.pdf.
16. Silverberg SJ, Shane E, Jacobs TP, et al. A 10-year prospective study of primary hyperparathyroidism with or without parathyroid surgery. N Engl J Med. 1999;341:1249.
17. Bilezikian JP, Khan AA, Potts Jr JT. Guidelines for the management of asymptomatic primary hyperparathyroidism: summary statement from the

third international workshop. J Clin Endocrinol Metab. 2009;94:335.
18. Khan AA, Bilezikian JP, Kung AW, et al. Alendronate in primary hyperparathyroidism: a double-blind, randomized, placebo-controlled trial. J Clin Endocrinol Metab. 2004;89:3319.
19. Peacock M, Bilezikian JP, Klassen PS, et al. Cinacalcet hydrochloride maintains long-term normocalcemia in patients with primary hyperparathyroidism. J Clin Endocrinol Metab. 2005;90:135.
20. Betterle C, Greggio NA, Volpato M. Clinical review 93: autoimmune polyglandular syndrome type 1. J Clin Endocrinol Metab. 1998;83:1049.
21. Thomas MK, Lloyd-Jones DM, Thadhani RI, et al. Hypovitaminosis D in medical inpatients. N Engl J Med. 1998;338:777.
22. Meyer C. Scientists probe role of vitamin D: deficiency a significant problem, experts say. JAMA. 2004;292:1416.
23. Bischoff-Ferrari HA, Giovannucci E, Willett WC, et al. Estimation of optimal serum concentrations of 25-hydroxyvitamin D for multiple health outcomes. Am J Clin Nutr. 2006;84:18.
24. NIH, Office of Dietary Supplements. Dietary supplement fact sheet: vitamin D. 2009. http://dietary-supplements.info.nih.gov/factsheets/vitamind.asp. Accessed 25 Nov 2009.

4 The Calcium-Sensing Receptor: Physiology and Pathophysiology

Friedhelm Raue and Christine Haag

Abstract

The complex control of calcium by the calcium-sensing receptor is the substance of this chapter. It describes the role of this critical receptor at the parathyroid glands and kidneys and focuses on the molecular abnormalities of the receptor and its role in the causation of hypocalcemic and hypercalcemic disorders. It describes how activating and inactivating mutations of the receptor lead to the problems such as familial hypocalciuric hypercalcemia, neonatal severe primary hyperparathyroidism, and other clinical states. It notes the use of genetic analysis of the calcium sensing receptor gene in the diagnosis of these complex problems and provides some therapeutic options for treatment.

Keywords

Calcium-sensing receptor • CaSR • Calcium homeostasis • Parathyroid hormone • Hypercalcemic • Loss-of-function mutations • Autosomal dominant • Hypocalcemia • Hypercalciuria • Bartter's syndrome type V • Hypoparathyroidism • Calcimimetic drug • 1,25-Dihydroxy vitamin D • G-protein receptor • Reabsorption • Proximal tubular cells • Cations • L-Amino acids • Calcilytics • Aminoglycosides • Nephron • Polyamines • Parathyroid adenomas • Calcitonin • FHH • Osteoblasts • Osteoclastogenesis • Apoptosis • Familial hypocalciuric hypercalcemia • Gain-of-function mutations • Hypokalemic metabolic alkalosis • Hyperreninemia • Hyperaldosteronism • Hyperparathyroidism • Chromosomes 3q21.1 • 19p13.3, 19p13 • Hypermagnesemia • Pancreatitis • Nephrolithiasis •

F. Raue, MD (✉)
Endocrine Practice, Bruckenstr. 21, Heidelberg 69120, Germany
e-mail: friedhelm.raue@raue-endokrinologie.de

C. Haag, PhD
Endocrine Practice, Laboratory of Molecular Genetics, Im Weiher 12, Heidelberg 61921, Germany

A.A. Licata and E.V. Lerma (eds.), *Diseases of the Parathyroid Glands*,
DOI 10.1007/978-1-4419-5550-0_4,

Chondrocalcinosis • Neonatal severe primary hyperparathyroidism • Hypotonia • Constipation • Homozygous mutations • Heterozygous mutations • Allele • Autosomal dominant hypocalcemia • Polymorphic variants • Cincalcet hydrochloride

Introduction

Calcium is essential for numerous bodily processes, i.e., as a cofactor for clotting, for modulating neuronal excitability as well as intracellular functions like hormonal secretion, cardiac contraction, neurotransmission, and memory. The maintenance of a constant level of the extracellular calcium within a narrow range is essential to fulfill these physiological roles. The extracellular calcium-sensing receptor (CaSR), which is predominantly expressed in the parathyroids and kidney, has a key role in extracellular calcium homeostasis, regulating the secretion of parathyroid hormone (PTH) and the reabsorption of urinary calcium in a negative feedback manner to the prevailing eucalcemic environment. Molecular abnormalities of the CaSR are responsible for different hypo- or hypercalcemic disorders depending on activating or inactivating mutations of the receptor (Table 4.1). Loss-of-function CaSR mutations have been reported in the hypercalcemic disorders of familial benign hypocalciuric hypercalcemia (FHH) and neonatal severe primary hyperparathyroidism (NSHPT). Gain-of-function CaSR mutations have been shown to result in autosomal dominant hypocalcemia with hypercalciuria (ADH) and Bartter's syndrome type V. Molecular genetic analysis of the CaSR gene facilitates the sometimes difficult diagnosis. CaSR autoantibodies have been found in FHH patients who did not have loss-of-function CaSR mutations, and in patients with acquired form (i.e., autoimmune) of hypoparathyroidism. Therapeutic compounds that modulate CaSR function have a role in the medical management of hyperparathyroidism (calcimimetic drugs).

Overview of Calcium Homeostasis: Role of CaSR

In health, the serum calcium concentration is tightly regulated within the normal range, 2.20–2.65 mmol/l by the action of the major calcitropic hormones, PTH, and 1,25-dihydroxyvitamin D (1,25(OH)2D) acting on kidney, gastrointestinal tract, and bone [1]. The calcium homeostasis is the balance within the body between the ingestion and absorption of calcium by the gastrointestinal tract, circulating calcium, and excretion of calcium by the kidney, as well as the movement of calcium into and out of bone (Fig. 4.1). The CaSR enables the parathyroid glands, the kidney, and bone, to sense alterations in the level of serum Ca and to respond with changes in function that are directed at normalizing the serum calcium concentration. Any decrease in the extracellular calcium ion concentration leads to an inactivation of the CaSR on the parathyroid chief cells, which in

Table 4.1 Diseases of the Calcium-sensing receptor (CaSR)

Disease	CaSR functional activity	CaSR genotype
Familial hypocalciuric hypercalcemia (FHH)	Loss of function	Heterozygous mutation
Neonatal severe primary hyperparathyroidism (NSHPT)	Loss of function	Homozygous mutation
Autosomal dominant hypocalcemia (ADH)	Gain of function	Heterozygous mutation
Bartter syndrome type V	Gain of function	Heterozygous mutation
Autoimmune hypocalciuric hypercalcemia	Loss of function by antibodies	Homozygous normal
Autoimmune hypoparathyroidism	Gain of function by antibodies	Homozygous normal

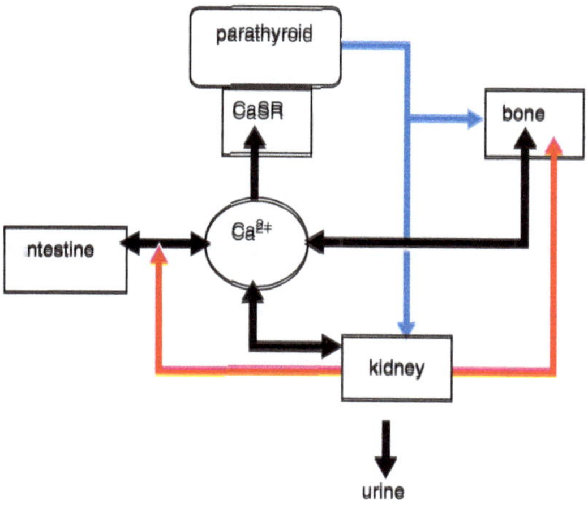

Fig. 4.1 Extracellular calcium homeostasis. *Black arrows* calcium, *blue arrows* PTH, *red arrows* 1,25(OH)2D, *ECF* extracellular fluid, *CaSR* calcium sensing receptor

term increases the rate of PTH release within minutes. When serum calcium levels fall, increased PTH secretion occurs (inverse relationship). PTH acts via its specific G-protein coupled receptor to increase the distal renal tubular reabsorption of calcium, within minutes (short term adjustment). This leads to a rapid increase in serum calcium, activating the CaSR, and inhibiting further PTH release once a normal calcium level has been restored. This rapid feedback loop depends on the fast and accurate sensing of the serum calcium level by the CaSR on the parathyroid cells. The CaSR on tubular cells of the kidney itself directly regulates calcium excretion by (1) diminishing PTH effects, (2) inhibition of calcium reabsorption, and (3) reducing the urinary concentrating ability. PTH, in addition, enhances the activity of osteoclasts and other bone cells, causing calcium release from the skeleton within 1–2 h. A more prolonged PTH release stimulates 1α-hydroxylase activity in the proximal tubular cells which leads to 1,25(OH)2D production. The latter has a long-term effect, regulating both intestinal calcium absorption and skeletal calcium turnover over days to weeks. A slower regulation of the PTH secretion occurs over a period of hours as a result of cellular changes in PTH mRNA. 1,25(OH)2D acting through vitamin D receptors decreases the level of PTH mRNA [2]. The slowest regulation of PTH secretion occurs over days or even months and reflects changes in the growth of the parathyroid glands. All these mechanisms, regulation of PTH secretion, PTH gene expression, and parathyroid cell proliferation, act to produce an increase in the serum calcium concentration correcting it towards the baseline value, which then completes the "feedback loop" by inhibiting PTH release. The feedback relationships between serum calcium and the secretion of the calcium regulatory hormones are appropriate to ensure that the response of their target tissue produces changes in serum calcium that reduces that hormone blood levels, e.g., a self-limiting, negative feedback relationship. The CaSR has the key role in calcium homeostasis, it regulates the synthesis and secretion of PTH as well as parathyroid cellular proliferation; the CaSR serves as the body's "calciostat" [3].

Structure and Function of the CaSR

The CaSR gene is located on chromosome 3q21.1 and has six exons (exons 2–7) encoding the CaSR protein of 1,078 amino acids. It is a cell surface protein with three structural domains: a large extracellular domain, seven transmembrane domains, and an intracellular tail (Fig. 4.2). The first CaSR identified was cloned from a bovine parathyroid gland cDNA library [4], the human CaSR equivalent was cloned from an adenomatous parathyroid gland [5]. It is a member of Family C of the superfamily of seven transmembrane, G-protein-coupled receptors. Other members of this family are so-called metabotrophic receptors for glutamate, receptors for gamma-aminobutyric acid, and for sensing pheromones, taste and odorants in fish [6]. The characteristic of this subfamily is the very large extracellular domain. This extracellular region has a bi-lobed "Venus fly-trap" domain, which is thought to be responsible for ligand binding, and a cysteine-rich region for dimerization. Three to five Ca2+ ions can bind cooperatively to the CaSR [7]. The CaSR functions as a dimer on the cell-surface and undergoes conformational changes after binding of Ca2+. The extracellular cysteine residues are critical for dimerization [8] and the

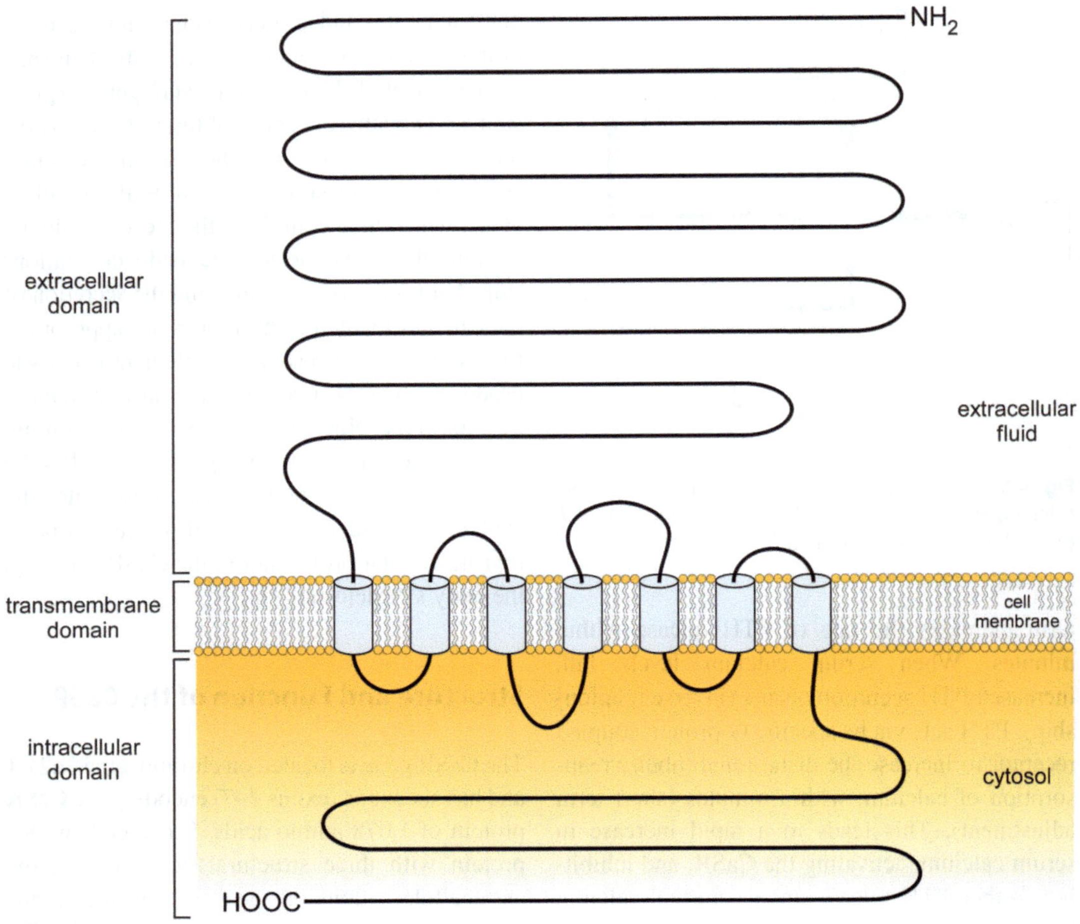

Fig. 4.2 Calcium-sensing receptor protein

majority of naturally occurring mutations identified in subjects with calcium homeostatic disorders are located in this domain. The homodimer of the CaSR is capable of coupling to several G-proteins, for example, Gi, Gq/11, G12/13. The CaSR signals after ligand binding and dimerization through multiple pathways, it stimulates phospholipase A2, C, and D as well as various MAP kinases and inhibits adenylate cyclase.

Although extracellular Ca2+ is considered the primary physiological agonist of the CaSR, there are a host of different stimuli to which the receptor is responsive, like the cations in the rank order of potency :La3+>Gd3+>Be2+>Ba2+=Ca2+>Sr2+>Mg2+ [9] and aromatic L-amino acids in the rank order of potency: L-Phe=L-Trp>LiHis>L-Ala>L-Glu>L-Arg=L-Leu [10]. The binding site of amino acid is believed to be distinct from the Ca2+ binding site [11]. In addition, a number of endogenous polyamines like spermine or polypeptides like polyarginine, polylysine, protamine, and amyloid-ß peptide act through the CaSR. Gamma-glutamyl peptides, known as taste-enhancing substances, stimulate CaSR on taste cells. The CaSR may have a role in the cellular response to changes in other constituents of the extracellular environment than Ca2+.

Pharmacological substances like aminoglycoside antibiotics mimic the effect of extracellular Ca2+ stimulation, and two compounds designed to act on the CaSR, the calcimimetics, which enhance the sensitivity of the CaSR to extracellular Ca2+, and the calcilytics, which act as CaR antagonists (see below).

The CaSR is not only expressed at high levels on the surface of the parathyroid chief cells, but also in the kidney along the whole nephron with different roles in different parts of the nephron. It is an important regulator of urinary calcium excretion. The CaSR is also expressed in bone-cells, osteoblasts, and osteoclasts, as well as in brain, skin, lens epithelium, pancreas, lung, and heart cells, where its function remains to be defined [12].

CaSR in the Parathyroid and C-Cells

The CaSR density on the surface of the parathyroid chief cells is the highest in the body. The expression of the CaSR on the cell surface may be upregulated by extracellular calcium and 1,25(OH)2D3 as shown in rat and avian experiments [13, 14]. CaSR's role is the mediator of the high calcium induced inhibition of PTH secretion. Chronic hypocalcemia increases PTH gene expression and stimulates parathyroid cellular proliferation via the inactivated CaSR. The link between the induction of the different intracellular signals by the CaSR and the inhibition of secretion of PTH in hypercalcemia is still largely unknown. It might be in part induced by decreasing and degradation of PTH mRNA by increase in cytosolic Ca2+ levels [15, 16]. The CaSR is also hypothesized to negatively regulate the proliferation of parathyroid cells based on the evidence of reduced expression in parathyroid adenomas [17] or developing marked parathyroid cellular hyperplasia in CaSR knockout mice [18].

The CaSR is found in the calcitonin-secreting C-cell of the thyroid. Calcitonin secretion is stimulated by increasing serum calcium mediated by the CaSR [19]. Calcitonin inhibits bone resorption and stimulates renal calcium excretion, defending against hypercalcemia and retaining calcium to the body, although many consider calcitonin to play a minor role in calcium homeostasis.

The CaSR in the Kidney

The CaSR is an important regulator of urinary calcium excretion. In the kidney, CaSR is expressed along the whole nephron with different roles in different parts of the nephron:

(1) Diminishing the inhibitory effect of PTH on renal phosphate reabsorption in the proximal tubule [20].
(2) Inhibiting renal tubular reabsorption of calcium by PTH in the cortical thick ascending limb by interference with sodium chloride reabsorption directly impairing generation of the medullary osmotic gradient that is essential for urinary concentration [21].
(3) Reducing urinary concentrating ability in the inner medullary collecting duct by antagonizing the action of vasopressin [22]. Chronically, it may be responsible for the nephrogenic diabetes insipidus associated with chronic hypercalcemia.

In patients with inactivating mutations of the CaSR (FHH), PTH oversecretion occurs with hypercalcemia and PTH-induced reabsorption of calcium from the loop of Henle is no longer inhibited by the CaSR, resulting in a hypocalciuria [3]. The CaSR in the kidney demonstrate the multifaceted nature of the receptor depending on different localizations and functions in various cell types within a single organ.

The CaSR in the Bone

Elevated calcium levels inhibit bone resorption and stimulate bone formation by inhibition of osteoclastogenesis and proliferation of osteoblasts. Some studies have identified the CaSR in osteoblasts, osteoclasts, and some osteocytes, but it is unclear whether the CaSR has functional importance there [23]. It was demonstrated that stimulation of the CaSR expressed in osteoblasts of mouse, rat, and bovine origin led to an increase in proliferation [24]. CaSR activity has been shown to promote both differentiation and apoptosis within osteoclasts. Experiments in CaSR knockout mice suggest that the CaSR plays a role in the embryonic development of the skeleton, postnatal bone formation, and osteoblast differentiation [25]. Additional studies are required to further clarify the role of the CaSR in skeletal homeostasis, including how it relates to mineral ion homeostasis.

The CaSR in Other Organs

Although the CaSR plays a vital role in calcium homeostasis, the receptor has been detected in a host of tissues unrelated to calcium homeostasis, including gastrointestinal tract, skin, heart, brain, and breast. In these cells, the CaSR regulates a multitude of cellular processes including secretion, differentiation, proliferation, apoptosis, and gene expression. This highlights the diversity of the CaSR regulating a variety of biological processes in a range of tissues.

Inherited CaSR Dysfunction

Several inherited disorders of calcium homeostasis are linked to functional abnormalities of the CaSR (Table 4.1). Over 170 CaSR mutations have been identified to interfere with the function of the receptor (Tables 4.2 and 4.3). A summary of CaSR mutations is maintained at the calcium-sensing receptor database [CASRdb] at McGill University (www.casrdb.mcgill.ca):

1. The loss-of-function mutation on one single allele of the CaSR associated with the autosomal dominant disease, familial hypocalciuric hypercalcemia (FHH), characterized by a mild to moderate hypercalcemia, inappropriately normal PTH level, and low rates of urinary calcium excretion;
2. Inactivating mutations on both alleles, a more serious condition known as neonatal severe hyperparathyroidism (NSHPT), characterized by a life-threatening severe hypercalcemia.
3. The gain-of-function CaSR mutations result in autosomal dominant hypocalcemia (ADH) with a generally mild asymptomatic hypocalcemia.
4. Bartter syndrome V is a rare disease with hypocalcemia, hypokalemic metabolic alkalosis, hyperreninemia, and hyperaldosteronism due to activating CaSR mutations.

Similar clinical and biochemical diseases without CaSR mutations are observed, related to circulating activating or inactivating antibodies against the extracellular domain of the CaSR often associated with other autoimmune diseases.

Table 4.2 Inactivating mutations of the CaSR (loss-of-function mutations)

Nucleotide change	Protein change	Disease	Reference
c.-10acg>atg	Regulatory	FHH	[85]
c.2 T>G	p.Met1Arg	FHH/NSHPT	[86]
c.19_20dupT	p.Cys7Leufs*41	FHH	[87]
c.32T>C	p.Leu11Ser	FHH	[88]
c.38T>C	p.Leu13Pro	FHH/NSHPT	[89]
c.61G>A	p.Gly21Arg	FHH	[44]
c.73C>T	p.Arg25Term	FHH/NSHPT	[47]
c.80A>G	p.Gln27Arg	NSHPT	[90]
c.115C>G	p.Pro39Ala	FHH	[91]
c.118A>T	p.Ile40Phe	FHH	[92]
c.157T>C	p.Ser53Pro	FHH	[93]
c.164C>T	p.Pro55Leu	FHH	[35]
c.179G>T	p.Cys60Phe	NSHPT	[94]
c.185G>T	p.Arg62Met	FHH/NSHPT	[34]
c.196C>T	p.Arg66Cys	FHH/NSHPT	[34]
c.197G>A	p.Arg66His	NSHPT	[95]
c.280G>T	p.Gly94Term	NSHPT	[96]
c.299C>T	p.Thr100Ile	FHH	[97]
c.392G>T	p.Cys131Phe	FHH	[98]
c.409T>C	p.Ser137Pro	FHH	[99]
c.413C>T	p.Thr138Met	FHH	[34]

(continued)

Table 4.2 (continued)

Nucleotide change	Protein change	Disease	Reference
c.428G>A	p.Gly143Glu	FHH	[34]
c.476T>C	p.Leu159Pro	FIHP	[100]
c.482A>G	p.Tyr161Cys	NSHPT	[101]
c.488C>G	p.Pro163Arg	TCP	[102]
c.490C>T	p.Gln164Term	NSHPT	[94]
c.492+1G>C	Splicing IVS2	FHH	[103]
c.493-1G>T	Splicing IVS2	FHH/NSHPT	[104]
c.495_499delGTCAG	p.Ser166Cysfs*23	NSHPT	[105]
c.496A>G	p.Ser166Gly	FHH	[106]
c.512G>A	p.Ser171Asn	FHH	[44]
c.514A>G	p.Arg172Gly	FHH	[107]
c.518T>C	p.Leu173Pro	FHH	[108]
c.521T>G	p.Leu174Arg	FHH	[109]
c.532A>G	p.Asn178Asp	FHH	[110]
c.539T>G	p.Phe180Cys	FHH	[111]
c.553C>T	p.Arg185Term	FHH/NSHPT	[50]
c.554G>A	p.Arg185Gln	FHH/NSHPT	[32]
c.570delT	p.Asp190Glufs*67	NSHPT	[112]
c.623G>C	p.Trp208Ser	FHH	[113]
c.635T>G	p.Ile212Ser	NSHPT	[85]
c.635T>C	p.Ile212Thr	FHH	[114]
c.644A>G	p.Asp215Gly	FHH	[93]
c.653A>C	p.Tyr218Ser	FHH	[35]
c.653A>G	p.Tyr218Cys	FHH	[115]
c.658C>T	p.Arg220Trp	FHH/NSHPT	[116]
c.659G>A	p.Arg220Gln	FHH	[110]
c.661C>T	p.Pro221Ser	FHH	[110]
c.662C>A	p.Pro221Gln	FHH	[44]
c.674A>C	p.Lys225Thr	FHH	[44]
c.680G>A	p.Arg227Gln	FHH	[34]
c.680G>T	p.Arg227Leu	FHH/NSHPT	[35]
c.748G>A	p.Glu250Lys	FIHP	[100]
c.788C>T	p.Thr263Met	FHH	[117]
c.801_812del	p.Val268delfs*273	FIHP	[100]
c.812C>T	p.Ser271Phe	FHH	[44]
c.848T>C	p.Ile283Thr	PHPT	[117]
c.889G>A	p.Glu297Lys	FHH/NSHPT	[32]
c.961G>C	p.Ala321Pro	FHH	[118]
c.967A>T	p.Lys323Term	FHH	[47]
c.1006_1008del	p.Lys336del	FIHP	[97]
c.1031_1034delinsT	p.Val344_Val1078delins735	NSHPT	[119]
c.1051T>G	p.Phe351Val	FHH	[117]
c.1055G>A	p.Trp352Term	NSHPT	[44]
c.1183T>C	p.Cys395Arg	FHH	[120]
c.1189G>A	p.Gly397Arg	FHH	[44]
c.1280T>G	p.Ile427Ser	TCP	[102]
c.1297G>C	p.Asp433His	TCP	[102]
c.1378-19A>C	Splicing IVS4	FHH	[117]

(continued)

Table 4.2 (continued)

Nucleotide change	Protein change	Disease	Reference
c.1376A>G	p.Gln459Arg	FHH	[54]
c.1393C>T	p.Arg465Trp	FHH	[117]
c.1394G>A	p.Arg465Gln	FHH	[121]
c.1430T>C	p.Val477Ala	TCP	[102]
c.1525G>A	p.Gly509Arg	FHH	[44]
c.1588T>G	p.Trp530Gly	FHH	[49]
c.1645G>A	p.Gly549Arg	FHH	[87]
c.1652G>A	p.Arg551Lys	NSHPT	[53]
c.1657G>A	p.Gly553Arg	FHH/NSHPT	[122]
c.1663A>G	p.Ile555Val	FHH	[44]
c.1670G>A	p.Gly557Glu	FHH	[123]
c.1685G>A	p.Cys562Tyr	FHH	[124]
c.1703G>A	p.Cys568Tyr	FHH	[49]
c.1719T>A	p.Tyr573X	FHH	[44]
c.1745G>A	p.Cys582Tyr	FHH/NSHPT	[35]
c.1745G>T	p.Cys582Phe	FHH	[44]
c.1772C>G	p.Ser591Cys	NSHPT	[125]
c.1783C>T	p.His595Tyr	FHH	[103]
c.1810G>A	p.Glu604Lys	FHH	[126]
c.1820C>A	p.Ser607X	FHH	[35]
c.1868G>A	p.Gly623Asp	FHH	[44]
c.1913G>T	p.Arg638Leu	FHH/NSHPT	[116]
c.1942C>T	p.Arg648X	FHH/NSHPT	[127]
c.1949T>C	p.Leu650Pro	FIHP	[97]
c.1970C>A	p.Ser657Tyr	FHH	[93]
c.1997_1998dupT	p.Phe667Valfs*41	FHH	[44]
c.2008G>A	p.Gly670Arg	FHH	[35]
c.2009G>A	p.Gly670Glu	FHH/NSHPT	[50]
c.2038C>T	p.Arg680Cys	FHH/NSHPT	[33]
c.2039G>A	p.Arg680His	FHH/NSHPT	[128]
c.2045C>T	p.Pro682Leu	FHH	[129]
c.2065G>A	p.Val689Met	FHH	[75]
c.2154G>A	p.Trp718X	FHH	[46]
c.2182G>T	p.Val728Phe	FHH	[42]
c.2201T>G	p.Met734Arg	FHH	[46]
c.2224T>C	p.Trp742Arg	FHH	[42]
c.2240_2241delinsT	p.Pro747Leufs*30	NSHPT	[33]
c.2243C>A	p.Pro748His	FHH	[81]
c.2243C>G	p.Pro748Arg	FHH	[72]
c.2281_2283delATC	p.Ile761del	FHH	[106]
c.2295C>G	p.Cys765Trp	FHH	[81]
c.2333G>A	p.Gly778Asp	FHH	[44]
c.2383C>T	p.Arg795Trp	FHH	[30]
c.2383delC	p.Arg795Glyfs*42	FHH	[42]
c.2411C>A	p.Ala804Asp	FHH/NSHPT	[130]
c.2427C>G	p.Phe809Leu	FHH	[48]
c.2449G>A	p.Val817Ile	FHH	[33]
c.2495T>C	p.Phe832Ser	FHH	[131]
c.2501delC	p.Ser834Leufs*3	FHH	[132]

(continued)

Table 4.2 (continued)

Nucleotide change	Protein change	Disease	Reference
c.2546T>C	p.Leu849Pro	FHH	[46]
c.2550_2551insCCAG	p.Cys851Profs*131	FHH	[66]
c.2627_2628insAlu		FHH/NSHPT	[133]
c.2641T>C	p.Phe881Leu	FHH	[41]
c.2656C>T	p.Arg886Trp	FHH	[42]
c.2657G>C	p.Arg886Pro	FIHP	[78]
c.2687G>A	p.Arg896His	FHH	[134]
c.2777A>G	p.Gln926Arg	FHH	[46]
c.2980C>T	p.His994Tyr	FHH	[85]
c.3013G>A	p.Asp1005Asn	FHH	[46]
c.3193delA	p.Ser1065Valfs*11	FHH	[135]
c.3235T>C	p.*1079Glnext*8	FHH	[94]

FHH familial hypocalciuric hypercalcemia, *NSHPT* neonatal severe hyperparathyroidism, *FIHP* familial isolated hyperparathyroidism, *TCP* tropical chronic pancreatitis

Table 4.3 Activating mutations of the CaSR (gain-of-function mutations)

Nucleotide change	Protein change	Disease	Reference
c.85A>G	p.Lys29Glu	ADH	[136]
c.141A>C	p.Lys47Asn	ADH	[137]
c.346G>A	p.Ala116Thr	ADH	[62]
c.354C>A	p.Asn118Lys	ADH	[58]
c.372C>A	p.Asn124Lys	ADH	[138]
c.374T>C	p.Leu125Pro	ADH	[128]
c.379G>A	p.Glu127Lys	ADH	[139]
c.380A>C	p.Glu127Ala	ADH	[59]
c.382T>C	p.Phe128Leu	ADH	[58]
c.385T>A	p.Cys129Ser	ADH	[140]
c.386G>T	p.Cys129Phe	ADH	[128]
c.386G>A	p.Cys129Tyr	ADH	[141]
c.393C>G	p.Cys131Trp	ADH	[65]
c.452C>G	p.Thr151Arg	ADH	[142]
c.452C>T	p.Thr151Met	ADH	[143]
c.571G>A	p.Glu191Lys	ADH	[58]
c.662C>T	p.Pro221Leu	ADH	[144]
c.682G>C	p.Glu228Gln	ADH	[144]
c.683A>G	p.Glu228Gly	ADH	[145]
c.734A>G	p.Gln245Arg	ADH	[144]
c.1061A>C	p.Glu354Ala	ADH	[146]
c.1765T>C	p.Phe589Leu	ADH	[147]
c.1835T>C	p.Phe612Ser	ADH	[58]
c.1846C>G	p.Leu616Val	ADH	[148]
c.2043G>T	p.Gln681His	ADH	[62]
c.2056A>G	p.Ile686Val	IE	[146]
c.2180T>A	p.Leu727Gln	ADH	[149]
c.2299G>A	p.Glu767Lys	ADH	[150]
c.2318T>G	p.Leu773Arg	ADH	[60]
c.2362T>C	p.Phe788Leu	ADH	[151]

(continued)

Table 4.3 (continued)

Nucleotide change	Protein change	Disease	Reference
c.2363T>G	p.Phe788Cys	ADH	[61]
c.2395G>A	p.Glu799Lys	ADH	[139]
c.2417T>C	p.Phe806Ser	ADH	[62]
c.2431A>G	p.Met811Val	ADH	[152]
c.2459C>T	p.Ser820Phe	ADH	[153]
c.2461T>C	p.Phe821Leu	ADH	[154]
c.2470G>T	p.Ala824Ser	ADH	[155]
c.2503G>A	p.Ala835Thr	ADH	[116]
c.2506G>C	p.Val836Leu	ADH	[156]
c.2528C>A	p.Ala843Glu	ADH	[157]
c.2530G>A	p.Ala844Thr	ADH	[142]
c.2530G>C	p.Ala844Pro	ADH	[145]
c.2551T>A	p.Cys851Ser	ADH	[62]
c.2682_3224del542	p.S895_V1075del	ADH	[158]
c.2691_2692insG	p.Arg898Alafs*83	ADH	[147]
c.2693G>A	p.Arg898Gln	IE	[146]
c.2788delC	p.Gln930Argfs*9	ADH	[85]
c.2963C>G	p.Ala988Gly	IE	[146]
c.2963C>T	p.Ala988Val	IE	[146]

ADH autosomal dominant hypocalcemia, *IE* idiopathic epilepsy

Hypercalcemic Disorders

CaSR abnormalities are associated with three hypercalcemic disorders, two with inactivating mutations in the CaSR (Table 4.2): the FHH and NSHPT and one induced by antibodies against the CaSR: the autoimmune hypocalciuric hypercalcemia [26, 27].

Familial Hypocalciuric Hypercalcemia

FHH (also called familial benign hypercalcemia, OMIM 14598) is an autosomal dominant benign disease with high penetrance characterized by lifelong, mild hypercalcemia. The prevalence of FHH in the west of Scotland has been estimated to be 1 in 78,000 at least [28], while the prevalence of primary hyperparathyroidism is as high as 1 in 1,000 [29]. It accounts for about 2% of asymptomatic hypercalcemics.

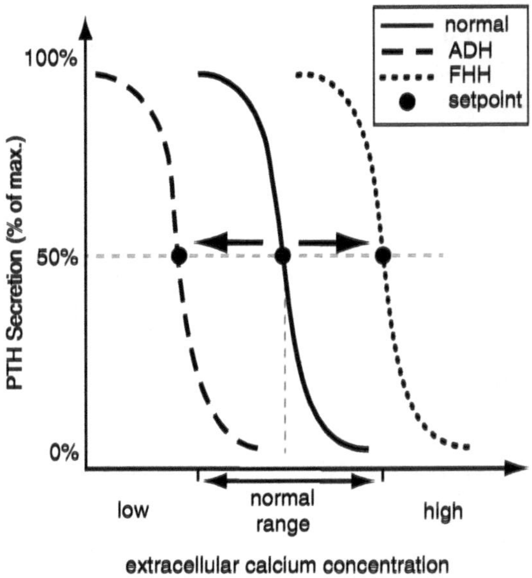

Fig. 4.3 Dose–response curves (*inverse sigmoidal curves*) relating extracelluar calcium and PTH release from parathyroid cells in normal situation, in patients with autosomal dominant hypocalcemia (ADH) and familial hypocalciuric hypercalcemia (FFH)

Etiology, Pathogenesis, and Genetics

Patients with FHH have an abnormality in calcium sensing that is associated with an altered "set-point" for the regulation of PTH by ionic calcium (Fig. 4.3). The mutation in FHH makes the receptor less sensitive to calcium.

Table 4.4 Features of familial hypocalciuric hypercalcemia (FHH), NSHPT, and sporadic primary hyperparathyroidism (pHPT)

Variable	FHH	NSHPT	pHPT
Age of onset	Birth	Birth	Generally >40 years
Serum calcium	Elevated	Marked elevated	Elevated
Serum PTH	Normal to slight elevation	Elevated	Elevated
Serum phosphate	Normal to slight reduction	Normal to low	Low normal to low
Serum magnesium	High normal to elevated		Normal
1,25(OH)2D3	Normal		Normal to elevated
24-h urinary calcium	Low to normal	Low to normal	Normal to high
Ca/Crea. clearance	Generally <0.01		Generally >0.01
Bone mineral density	Normal	Low	Normal to low

In the parathyroid glands, this defect means that a higher than normal serum calcium concentration is required to reduce PTH release, reflecting the presence of a right-shifted set-point for Ca-regulated PTH release [30]. In the kidney, this defect leads to an increase in tubular calcium and magnesium reabsorption [31]. The net effect is hypercalcemia, hypocalciuria, and frequently hypermagnesemia, as well as a normal or very slightly elevated serum PTH concentration despite mild hypercalcemia.

Mutation analyses of the CaSR gene on chromosome 3q21.1 in patients with FHH revealed different missense, nonsense, insertion, deletion, or splice-site mutations that resulted in a loss-of-function [32] (Table 4.2). Over 130 different mutations have been identified, approximately 90% of the FHH kindreds investigated have been found to have unique heterozygous mutations, resulting in less active functioning receptors on the parathyroid or renal cell surface [33–36]. Mutations are scattered throughout all exons of CaSR gene, many of these mutations cluster around the aspartate and glutamate-rich region within the extracellular domain of the receptor with the ligand binding pocket containing negatively charged amino acids. Decreasing affinity of calcium to the changed binding sites results in a loss-of-function with a rightward shift in the dose–response curve, so that the extracellular calcium concentration needed to produce a half-maximal increase in the total intracellular calcium ions (or IP3) is significant higher than that required for the wild-type receptor. Different degree of inactivation of the CaSR by different mutations might be explained in part by the dominant negative effect of the heterodimeric receptors [37].

The remaining FFH families with no CaSR mutation in the coding region of the CaSR gene may have mutations in the noncoding regions or in different loci. By linkage analyses, two different loci have been found on chromosome 19p13.3 and 19q13, referred to as FHH type 2 and FHH type 3 [38, 39]. The classic mutation of the CaSR on chromosome 3q21.1 is called FHH type 1. FHH1 and FHH2 have identical clinical and biochemical features. The type 3 also been referred to as the Oklahoma variant is characterized by different age of onset, higher PTH values, hypophosphatemia, and osteomalacia.

Clinical Features

Affected patients typically present in childhood with the incidental discovery of hypercalcemia, inappropriate hypocalciuria, and mild to moderate hypermagnesemia in more than half of cases [35, 40–42] (Table 4.4). The vast majority of patients with FHH are asymptomatic. Specific CaSR mutations leading to hypercalcemia are associated with a distinct clinical phenotype. These include an association with acute pancreatitis [35]; calcium nephrolithiasis and chondrocalcinosis have also been reported [43]. The normal or slightly elevated serum PTH concentrations may contribute to the benign clinical course of FHH, as compared with primary hyperparathyroidism. Several families, however, have been identified with more marked hypercalcemia, averaging 3 and 3.4 mM without clinical features [44].

Laboratory Findings

FHH is characterized by a mild hypercalcemia, accompanied by a mild hypophosphatemia, and a mild hypermagnesemia. The PTH level is in the upper normal range or slightly elevated, indicating that this is an inappropriately normal or high PTH level in the presence of mild hypercalcemia. The urinary calcium excretion in FFH is generally in the low-normal to reduced range. The 24-h urinary calcium excretion is typically below 200 mg/day (5 mmol/day). The fractional excretion of calcium (calcium clearance to creatinine clearance ratio) is often less than 0.01 in 80% of patients with FHH, indicating that more than 99% of the filtered calcium has been reabsorbed despite the presence of hypercalcemia [40–42, 45]. This can be used to improve the discrimination of FHH from primary hyperparathyroidism [46]. Patients with primary hyperparathyroidism have often hypercalciuria (24-h calcium excretion above 300 mg [7.5 mmol]).

The biochemistry of FHH can vary considerably, and this variability has often been thought to be mutation dependent. Patients with truncation mutants, presumed not to exhibit a dominant-negative effect, had less severe hypercalcemia than patients with missense mutations that result in a dominant-negative effect [47].

Differential Diagnosis

It is sometimes difficult to distinguish FHH from mild and asymptomatic primary hyperparathyroidism (Table 4.4). The differential diagnosis is important, as patients with FHH do not benefit from neck exploration, as hypercalcemia persisted after subtotal parathyroidectomy. Although characteristic of FHH, the fractional excretion of calcium may also be low in primary hyperparathyroidism in which values often range between 0.01 and 0.05. There can be overlap in the clinical presentations of FHH and primary hyperparathyroidism, exemplified by an atypical presentation in an FHH family that exhibited hypercalciuria, hypercalcemia, high PTH levels, and even renal stone formation, but was ultimately proven to harbor an inactivating FHH mutation [43]. In this case, subtotal parathyroidectomy in most affected family members provided long-term remission of their biochemical abnormalities, demonstrating that parathyroid surgery may be appropriate in occasional kindreds and hypocalciuria is not always a diagnostic criterion.

The diagnosis of FHH, particularly, its distinction from primary hyperparathyroidism, is primarily based upon the family history, laboratory findings, and genetic testing. Family screening is recommended. The identification of an inactivating mutation in the CaSR that segregates with the hypercalcemic trait in the family confirms the diagnosis of FHH.

Treatment

Because of the usually benign natural history and subtotal parathyroidectomy does not cure the disorder in most gene carriers, patients with FHH should not undergo neck exploration or any other aggressive intervention [40, 41]. They should not be placed on a low calcium diet. In rare situations with high serum Ca, pancreatitis, or renal stones, when features of typical primary hyperparathyroidism become more prominent, parathyroidectomy may be indicated. Calcimimetics (see below) might be a good alternative treatment [48, 49].

Neonatal Severe Primary Hyperparathyroidism

NSHPT (OMIM 239200) is a life-threatening disorder, manifesting in the first few days of life with failure to thrive, hypotonia, constipation and respiratory distress, dramatic hypercalcemia, elevated PTH, and bony abnormalities, e.g., undermineralization, subperiosteal erosion, multiple fractures of long bones and ribs (Table 4.4). Infants with NSHPT and life-threatening hypercalcemia should be operated by parathyroidectomy as soon as possible.

The NSHPT is usually caused by homozygous mutations in the CaSR gene in children born to consanguineous FHH parents [32] or by compound heterozygous mutation, harboring different mutations from each parent [50] (Table 4.2). The degree of hypercalcemia appears to reflect a gene dosage effect [31, 36, 51]. Heterozygous inactivating mutations leading to FHH with mild hypercalcemia and homozygous or compound heterozygous mutations have more marked disease, presenting with severe neonatal hyperparathyroidism and usually severe hypercalcemia (serum calcium concentration often above 3.75 mmol/l [15 mg/dl]) [32, 36, 51, 52]. In these patients, the more pronounced defect in the parathyroid calcium sensor leads to a greater elevation in the set-point for PTH secretion and more marked hypercalcemia than in heterozygous FHH [36]. The majority of NSHPT children are born to normocalcemic parents and appear to be sporadic, noninherited CaSR mutations [35], due to a spontaneous de novo mutation of one allele of the CaSR which somehow inhibits the function of the normal allele (dominant negative effect) [52]. In the recent years, a milder phenotype has become apparent, who could be managed by conservative therapy, better classified as neonatal primary hyperparathyroidism. Neonatal symptomatic hypercalcemia associated with hyperparathyroid bone disease may spontaneously change to an asymptomatic, benign condition resembling FHH ("self-limited NSHPT") [53]. These patients have heterozygous inactivating mutations in the CaSR with a similar clinical picture like in FHH. An inactivating mutation in the CaSR with mildly reduced sensitivity to calcium presented as an apparent autosomal recessive inheritance. Only the homozygous state has a mild hypercalcemia while heterozygous family members are asymptomatic [54].

Autoimmune Hypocalciuric Hypercalcemia

Some patients, who have the clinical features of FHH but carry no CaSR mutation, may have an autoimmune disorder. Four subjects from two families have been described with acquired hypocalciuric hypercalcemia mediated by autoantibodies against the extracellular domain of CaSR that apparently stimulates PTH release [55]. Three of the four patients with autoimmune hypercalcemia had an additional autoimmune disorder, either hypothyroidism or celiac disease. Hypercalcemia and elevated PTH levels were responsive to corticosteroids [56]. Anti-CaSR antibodies that stimulated the receptor could be confirmed in vitro [57]. A history of autoimmunity should, therefore, be obtained in patients who seem to have FHH but no mutation in the CaSR.

Hypocalcemic Disorders

CaSR abnormalities are associated with three hypocalcemic disorders (Table 4.3): autosomal dominant hypocalcemia (ADH), Bartter syndrome type V, and autoimmune hypoparathyroidism due to blocking autoantibodies against CaSR.

Autosomal Dominant Hypocalcemia

ADH (OMIM 601298) is the mirror image of FHH: familial hypocalcemia with inappropriately high-normal or elevated urinary calcium excretion.

Etiology, Pathogenesis, and Genetics

This disorder is associated with an activating mutation in the CaSR; as a result, a low serum calcium concentration is perceived as normal, leading to a downward resetting of the PTH–calcium relationship [58, 59]. Serum PTH concentrations are within the low normal range or frankly subnormal (inappropriately low given the hypocalcemia) and, in contrast to other causes of hypocalcemia, urinary calcium excretion is normal or elevated, presumably due to increased activation of the CaSR in the loop of Henle.

More than 80% of the reported ADH kindreds have mutations of the CaSR and in vitro studies have confirmed that these mutations produce a gain of function in CaSR (Table 4.3). There is a left shift in the dose–response curve, so that the extracellular calcium concentration needed to produce a half-maximal increase in the total intracellular calcium ions or IP3, is significantly lower than that required for the wild-type receptor (Fig. 4.3). More than 40 different CaSR mutations have been identified in ADH patients, and over 50% of these are in the extracellular domain and the remainder are in the transmembrane domains 5, 6, and 7. Almost every ADH family has its own unique missense heterozygous CaSR mutation.

Clinical Features

These patients are generally asymptomatic despite reductions in the serum calcium concentrations, therefore they are often not diagnosed until adulthood. A few patients, however, have symptomatic hypocalcemia [60], some with low serum PTH concentrations [61]. Some children become symptomatic with spontaneous carpopedal spasms and seizures, some develop basal ganglia calcification and recurrent nephrolithiasis especially after treatment with vitamin D and calcium.

Laboratory Findings

The serum calcium concentration is usually in the range of 1.5–2.0 mmol/l, while serum PTH concentrations are low or inappropriately normal despite the presence of hypocalcemia. In some patients, low serum magnesium concentrations are measured. Urinary calcium excretion is high rather than the expected low excretion.

Differential Diagnosis

About one-third of patients with "idiopathic" hypoparathyroidism have activating mutations in the CaSR. It is important to distinguish this syndrome of ADH from true idiopathic hypoparathyroidism, because subjects with ADH are particularly susceptible to the development of nephrocalcinosis, nephrolithiasis, and renal impairment during treatment with vitamin D and/or calcium. This disorder may be differentiated from true idiopathic hypoparathyroidism or pseudohypoparathyroidism on biochemical grounds: patients with ADH generally have detectable levels of PTH at the time of diagnosis (during treatment with vitamin D and calcium, the PTH levels sometimes become suppressed), they have, on average, a higher pretreatment excretion of urinary calcium and an invariable significant hypomagnesemia. The major clinical clue to this syndrome is its familial nature. The diagnosis can be confirmed by analysis for mutations in the CaSR-gene [58]. Sporadic mutations (de novo) in the CaSR have also been identified [60, 62]. These patients are usually thought to have idiopathic hypoparathyroidism.

Treatment

Once the diagnosis is established, attempts to raise the serum calcium concentration should be considered only in patients who are symptomatic [58]. The aim of treatment should be symptomatic control rather than normocalcemia, because there is a high potential of adverse effects from raising the serum calcium with vitamin D supplementation. As the serum calcium concentration increases, the activating mutation in the CaSR in the kidney will lead to a marked increase in urinary calcium excretion, which can cause renal stones, nephrocalcinosis, and renal insufficiency [58]. Therefore, monitoring of urinary calcium excretion is necessary and if elevated co-administration of a hypocalciuric agent, such as thiazide diuretics is useful. Recombinant PTH has been used to increase serum calcium with little effect on urinary calcium [63]. Alternatively, calcilytics, a class of drugs in development that inhibit the CaSR, may provide a useful therapeutic approach in the future.

Bartter Syndrome Type V

Some patients with an activating mutation of the CaSR have in addition to hypocalcemia potassium wasting, hypokalemia, metabolic alkalosis, hyperreninemic hyperaldosteronism, and increased urinary prostaglandin excretion creating a phenotype similar to classical Bartter's syndrome called Bartter syndrome type V (OMIM 601199.0035) [61, 64]. These patients appear to have a more marked gain-of-function in the CaSR not only with a left shift in the dose–response curve for the receptor, but also a much lower set point than that found in patients with ADH. Three different CaSR mutations are described (Cys131Trp, Ala843Glu, and Leu125Pro) [65]. Severe activation of the CaSR leads to hypokalemia caused by CaSR-mediated inhibition of the apical sodium–potassium-chloride cotransporter in cortical thick ascending limb causing NaCl wasting and resulting in hyperreninemia and hyperaldosteronism.

Autoimmune Acquired Hypoparathyroidism

Twenty percent of patients, who have acquired hypoparathyroidism in association with autoimmune hypothyroidism, were found to have auto-antibodies to the extracellular domain of the CaSR [66]. These antibodies did not persist for long, they diminished often after years. Autoimmune hypoparathyroidism is a common feature of polyglandular autoimmune syndrome type I. One study found that 14 of 25 (56%) of patients with this disorder had autoantibodies directed against the CaSR in the parathyroid glands [67]; the antibodies could decrease PTH secretion if they activated the calcium receptor [68].

Polymorphic Variants of the Extracellular CaSR

Six single nucleotide polymorphisms (SNPs) in the CaSR without any activating and inactivating activity have been described (Table 4.5). Of these, a serine-to-alanine substitution at codon 986 (A986S) has been associated with higher levels of total and ionized serum calcium within the normal range in healthy subjects from several different populations; this could be confirmed in a recent study [69–71]. Other polymorphisms R990G and Q1011E and their haplotypes are also significant predictors of serum calcium [72]. At present, there is little evidence that they are disease-causing; neither impact on bone density in postmenopausal women nor on response to calcium supplementation could be demonstrated for the A986S polymorphism [73, 74]. In a Japanese study, the G990R polymorphism was associated with increased PTH secretion in patients with primary hyperparathyroidism and patients on hemodialysis [75, 76]. The same variant could influence the calcium excretion in stone-forming patients [77].

A special CaSR haplotype, including two of the three polymorphism is significantly associated with PHPT and within the PHPT patient population, another haplotype is significantly associated with kidney stones [78].

Table 4.5 Polymorphisms in the CaSR

Polymorphism	Comments
IVS 5-88t/c	Very common
A826T	16% of normal subjects
C851S	Rare
A986S	24% of normal subjects
R990G	4% of normal subjects
Q1011E	3% of normal subjects

The Extracellular CaSR as a Pharmacological Target

The CaSR can be considered a low-affinity receptor, responding to relatively high concentrations of calcium over 1 mmol/l. The limited selectivity of the receptor is responsible for its activation by numerous divalent or trivalent cations in addition to calcium, such as magnesium, gadolinium, and lanthanum, and by other polycationic compounds such as neomycin, spermine, by extracellular pH, and numerous amino acids. New substances, *calcimimetics*, have been developed to modulate the CaSR, one of this is AMG 073, called cinacalcet, which is able to decrease the PTH secretion from the parathyroids [79]. This substance is completely inactive in the absence of extracellular calcium, it does not interact directly with the calcium-binding site of the CaSR, but with the transmembrane domains, thus causing conformational changes and increasing the calcium sensitivity of the receptor as allosteric modulator. Cinacalcet (Mimpara® in Europe, Sensipar® in USA) is able to lower the PTH concentration in primary and secondary hyperparathyroidism [80, 81]. Cinacalcet is a powerful compound in reducing PTH in patients with poorly controlled secondary hyperparathyroidism (30–180 mg orally once daily), it may also be used in primary hyperparathyroidism especially in parathyroid carcinoma (30 mg up to maximum of 360 mg/day) when operation failed [82]. Cinacalcet hydrochloride maintains long-term normocalcemia in patients with primary hyperparathyroidism [83]. Although not approved for other indications, calcimimetics may prove useful in the treatment of NSHPT and FHH [48, 49].

Another group of substances, called *calcilytics* have been developed with the opposite action, deactivating the CaSR and stimulating PTH secretion. This might have anabolic effects on bone and may become available as treatment for osteoporosis and may also have a role in the treatment of ADH [84].

Conclusion

The CaSR is a critical regulator of normal extracellular calcium homeostasis, particularly concerning to the regulation of PTH secretion and renal calcium reabsorption. The demonstration of mutations in the CaSR gene associated with both hypercalcemic and hypocalcemic disorders has underlined the key role that the CaSR plays in both health and disease and has given us an insight into the pathogenesis of the clinical syndromes described. Gain-of-function mutations are associated with FHH and NSHPT, loss-of-function with ADH. Molecular genetic analyses of the CaSR gene facilitate the sometimes difficult differential diagnosis. Further structure–function studies will allow the design of drugs to target-specific residues of the CaSR to stimulate or suppress PTH secretion. These compounds are used for treatment of secondary hyperparathyroidism, and may become available as treatment for osteoporosis.

References

1. Brown EM, MacLeod RJ. Extracellular calcium sensing and extracellular calcium signaling. Physiol Rev. 2001;81(1):239–97.
2. Silver J, Sela SB, Naveh-Many T. Regulation of parathyroid cell proliferation. Curr Opin Nephrol Hypertens. 1997;6(4):321–6.
3. Brown EM. Editorial: mutant extracellular calcium-sensing receptors and severity of disease. J Clin Endocrinol Metab. 2005;90(2):1246–8.
4. Brown EM, Gamba G, Riccardi D, et al. Cloning and characterization of an extracellular Ca(2+)-sensing receptor from bovine parathyroid. Nature. 1993; 366(6455):575–80.
5. Garrett JE, Capuano IV, Hammerland LG, et al. Molecular cloning and functional expression of human parathyroid calcium receptor cDNAs. J Biol Chem. 1995;270(21):12919–25.
6. Wellendorph P, Brauner-Osborne H. Molecular cloning, expression, and sequence analysis of GPRC6A, a novel family C G-protein-coupled receptor. Gene. 2004;335:37–46.
7. Hu J, Spiegel AM. Structure and function of the human calcium-sensing receptor: insights from natural and engineered mutations and allosteric modulators. J Cell Mol Med. 2007;11(5):908–22.
8. Ray K, Hauschild BC, Steinbach PJ, Goldsmith PK, Hauache O, Spiegel AM. Identification of the cysteine residues in the amino-terminal extracellular domain of the human Ca(2+) receptor critical for dimerization. Implications for function of monomeric Ca(2+) receptor. J Biol Chem. 1999;274(39): 27642–50.
9. Wellcome RD, Lecture P. Cell surface, ion-sensing receptors. Exp Physiol. 2002;87(4):403–11.
10. Conigrave AD, Quinn SJ, Brown EM. L-Amino acid sensing by the extracellular Ca2+-sensing receptor. Proc Natl Acad Sci USA. 2000;97(9):4814–9.
11. Mun HC, Culverston EL, Franks AH, Collyer CA, Clifton-Bligh RJ, Conigrave AD. A double mutation in the extracellular Ca2+-sensing receptor's venus flytrap domain that selectively disables L-amino acid sensing. J Biol Chem. 2005;280(32):29067–72.
12. Hu J, Spiegel AM. Naturally occurring mutations of the extracellular Ca2+-sensing receptor: implications for its structure and function. Trends Endocrinol Metab. 2003;14(6):282–8.
13. Brown AJ, Zhong M, Finch J, et al. Rat calcium-sensing receptor is regulated by vitamin D but not by calcium. Am J Physiol. 1996;270(3 Pt 2):F454–60.
14. Yarden N, Lavelin I, Genina O, et al. Expression of calcium-sensing receptor gene by avian parathyroid gland in vivo: relationship to plasma calcium. Gen Comp Endocrinol. 2000;117(2):173–81.
15. Carrillo-Lopez N, Alvarez-Hernandez D, Gonzalez-Suarez I, et al. Simultaneous changes in the calcium-sensing receptor and the vitamin D receptor under the influence of calcium and calcitriol. Nephrol Dial Transplant. 2008;23(11):3479–84.
16. Ritter CS, Pande S, Krits I, Slatopolsky E, Brown AJ. Destabilization of parathyroid hormone mRNA by extracellular Ca2+ and the calcimimetic R-568 in parathyroid cells: role of cytosolic Ca and requirement for gene transcription. J Mol Endocrinol. 2008;40(1):13–21.
17. Farnebo F, Enberg U, Grimelius L, et al. Tumor-specific decreased expression of calcium sensing receptor messenger ribonucleic acid in sporadic primary hyperparathyroidism. J Clin Endocrinol Metab. 1997;82(10):3481–6.

18. Mun HC, Brennan SC, Delbridge L, Wilkinson M, Brown EM, Conigrave AD. Adenomatous human parathyroid cells exhibit impaired sensitivity to L-amino acids. J Clin Endocrinol Metab. 2009; 94(9):3567–74.
19. Freichel M, Zink-Lorenz A, Holloschi A, Hafner M, Flockerzi V, Raue F. Expression of a calcium-sensing receptor in a human medullary thyroid carcinoma cell line and its contribution to calcitonin secretion. Endocrinology. 1996;137(9):3842–8.
20. Ba J, Brown D, Friedman PA. Calcium-sensing receptor regulation of PTH-inhibitable proximal tubule phosphate transport. Am J Physiol Renal Physiol. 2003;285(6):F1233–43.
21. Motoyama HI, Friedman PA. Calcium-sensing receptor regulation of PTH-dependent calcium absorption by mouse cortical ascending limbs. Am J Physiol Renal Physiol. 2002;283(3):F399–406.
22. Sands JM, Naruse M, Baum M, et al. Apical extracellular calcium/polyvalent cation-sensing receptor regulates vasopressin-elicited water permeability in rat kidney inner medullary collecting duct. J Clin Invest. 1997;99(6):1399–405.
23. Theman TA, Collins MT. The role of the calcium-sensing receptor in bone biology and pathophysiology. Curr Pharm Biotechnol. 2009;10(3):289–301.
24. Dvorak MM, Siddiqua A, Ward DT, et al. Physiological changes in extracellular calcium concentration directly control osteoblast function in the absence of calciotropic hormones. Proc Natl Acad Sci USA. 2004;101(14):5140–5.
25. Garner SC, Pi M, Tu Q, Quarles LD. Rickets in cation-sensing receptor-deficient mice: an unexpected skeletal phenotype. Endocrinology. 2001;142(9): 3996–4005.
26. Thakker RV. Diseases associated with the extracellular calcium-sensing receptor. Cell Calcium. 2004;35(3):275–82.
27. Pearce SH. Clinical disorders of extracellular calcium-sensing and the molecular biology of the calcium-sensing receptor. Ann Med. 2002;34(3): 201–6.
28. Hinnie J, Bell E, McKillop E, Gallacher S. The prevalence of familial hypocalciuric hypercalcemia. Calcif Tissue Int. 2001;68(4):216–8.
29. Boonstra CE, Jackson CE. Serum calcium survey for hyperparathyroidism: results in 50,000 clinic patients. Am J Clin Pathol. 1971;55(5):523–6.
30. Pearce SH, Bai M, Quinn SJ, Kifor O, Brown EM, Thakker RV. Functional characterization of calcium-sensing receptor mutations expressed in human embryonic kidney cells. J Clin Invest. 1996;98(8): 1860–6.
31. Bai M, Janicic N, Trivedi S, et al. Markedly reduced activity of mutant calcium-sensing receptor with an inserted Alu element from a kindred with familial hypocalciuric hypercalcemia and neonatal severe hyperparathyroidism. J Clin Invest. 1997;99(8): 1917–25.
32. Pollak MR, Brown EM, Chou YH, et al. Mutations in the human Ca(2+)-sensing receptor gene cause familial hypocalciuric hypercalcemia and neonatal severe hyperparathyroidism. Cell. 1993;75(7):1297–303.
33. Aida K, Koishi S, Tawata M, Onaya T. Molecular cloning of a putative Ca(2+)-sensing receptor cDNA from human kidney. Biochem Biophys Res Commun. 1995;214(2):524–9.
34. Chou YH, Pollak MR, Brandi ML, et al. Mutations in the human Ca(2+)-sensing-receptor gene that cause familial hypocalciuric hypercalcemia. Am J Hum Genet. 1995;56(5):1075–9.
35. Pearce SH, Trump D, Wooding C, et al. Calcium-sensing receptor mutations in familial benign hypercalcemia and neonatal hyperparathyroidism. J Clin Invest. 1995;96(6):2683–92.
36. Pollak MR, Chou YH, Marx SJ, et al. Familial hypocalciuric hypercalcemia and neonatal severe hyperparathyroidism. Effects of mutant gene dosage on phenotype. J Clin Invest. 1994;93(3):1108–12.
37. Wystrychowski A, Pidasheva S, Canaff L, et al. Functional characterization of calcium-sensing receptor codon 227 mutations presenting as either familial (benign) hypocalciuric hypercalcemia or neonatal hyperparathyroidism. J Clin Endocrinol Metab. 2005;90(2):864–70.
38. Heath 3rd H, Jackson CE, Otterud B, Leppert MF. Genetic linkage analysis in familial benign (hypocalciuric) hypercalcemia: evidence for locus heterogeneity. Am J Hum Genet. 1993;53(1):193–200.
39. Lloyd SE, Pannett AA, Dixon PH, Whyte MP, Thakker RV. Localization of familial benign hypercalcemia, Oklahoma variant (FBHOk), to chromosome 19q13. Am J Hum Genet. 1999;64(1): 189–95.
40. Marx SJ, Attie MF, Levine MA, Spiegel AM, Downs Jr RW, Lasker RD. The hypocalciuric or benign variant of familial hypercalcemia: clinical and biochemical features in fifteen kindreds. Medicine (Baltimore). 1981;60(6):397–412.
41. Law Jr WM, Heath III H. Familial benign hypercalcemia (hypocalciuric hypercalcemia). Clinical and pathogenetic studies in 21 families. Ann Intern Med. 1985;102(4):511–9.
42. Heath III H. Familial benign (hypocalciuric) hypercalcemia. A troublesome mimic of mild primary hyperparathyroidism. Endocrinol Metab Clin North Am. 1989;18(3):723–40.
43. Carling T, Szabo E, Bai M, et al. Familial hypercalcemia and hypercalciuria caused by a novel mutation in the cytoplasmic tail of the calcium receptor. J Clin Endocrinol Metab. 2000;85(5):2042–7.
44. Nissen PH, Christensen SE, Heickendorff L, Brixen K, Mosekilde L. Molecular genetic analysis of the calcium sensing receptor gene in patients clinically suspected to have familial hypocalciuric hypercalcemia: phenotypic variation and mutation spectrum in a Danish population. J Clin Endocrinol Metab. 2007; 92(11):4373–9.

45. Fuleihan Gel H. Familial benign hypocalciuric hypercalcemia. J Bone Miner Res. 2002;17 Suppl 2:N51–6.
46. Christensen SE, Nissen PH, Vestergaard P, Heickendorff L, Brixen K, Mosekilde L. Discriminative power of three indices of renal calcium excretion for the distinction between familial hypocalciuric hypercalcaemia and primary hyperparathyroidism: a follow-up study on methods. Clin Endocrinol (Oxf). 2008;69(5):713–20.
47. Ward BK, Magno AL, Blitvich BJ, et al. Novel mutations in the calcium-sensing receptor gene associated with biochemical and functional differences in familial hypocalciuric hypercalcaemia. Clin Endocrinol (Oxf). 2006;64(5):580–7.
48. Timmers HJ, Karperien M, Hamdy NA, de Boer H, Hermus AR. Normalization of serum calcium by cinacalcet in a patient with hypercalcaemia due to a de novo inactivating mutation of the calcium-sensing receptor. J Intern Med. 2006;260(2):177–82.
49. Rus R, Haag C, Bumke-Vogt C, et al. Novel inactivating mutations of the calcium-sensing receptor: the calcimimetic NPS R-568 improves signal transduction of mutant receptors. J Clin Endocrinol Metab. 2008;93(12):4797–803.
50. Kobayashi M, Tanaka H, Tsuzuki K, et al. Two novel missense mutations in calcium-sensing receptor gene associated with neonatal severe hyperparathyroidism. J Clin Endocrinol Metab. 1997;82(8): 2716–9.
51. Cole DE, Janicic N, Salisbury SR, Hendy GN. Neonatal severe hyperparathyroidism, secondary hyperparathyroidism, and familial hypocalciuric hypercalcemia: multiple different phenotypes associated with an inactivating Alu insertion mutation of the calcium-sensing receptor gene. Am J Med Genet. 1997;71(2):202–10.
52. Bai M, Pearce SH, Kifor O, et al. In vivo and in vitro characterization of neonatal hyperparathyroidism resulting from a de novo, heterozygous mutation in the Ca2+-sensing receptor gene: normal maternal calcium homeostasis as a cause of secondary hyperparathyroidism in familial benign hypocalciuric hypercalcemia. J Clin Invest. 1997;99(1):88–96.
53. Toke J, Czirjak G, Patocs A, et al. Neonatal severe hyperparathyroidism associated with a novel de novo heterozygous R551K inactivating mutation and a heterozygous A986S polymorphism of the calcium-sensing receptor gene. Clin Endocrinol (Oxf). 2007;67(3):385–92.
54. Lietman SA, Tenenbaum-Rakover Y, Jap TS, et al. A novel loss-of-function mutation, Gln459Arg, of the calcium-sensing receptor gene associated with apparent autosomal recessive inheritance of familial hypocalciuric hypercalcemia. J Clin Endocrinol Metab. 2009;94(11):4372–9.
55. Kifor O, Moore Jr FD, Delaney M, et al. A syndrome of hypocalciuric hypercalcemia caused by autoantibodies directed at the calcium-sensing receptor. J Clin Endocrinol Metab. 2003;88(1):60–72.
56. Pallais JC, Kifor O, Chen YB, Slovik D, Brown EM. Acquired hypocalciuric hypercalcemia due to autoantibodies against the calcium-sensing receptor. N Engl J Med. 2004;351(4):362–9.
57. Kemp EH, Gavalas NG, Krohn KJ, Brown EM, Watson PF, Weetman AP. Activating autoantibodies against the calcium-sensing receptor detected in two patients with autoimmune polyendocrine syndrome type 1. J Clin Endocrinol Metab. 2009;94(12): 4749–56.
58. Pearce SH, Williamson C, Kifor O, et al. A familial syndrome of hypocalcemia with hypercalciuria due to mutations in the calcium-sensing receptor. N Engl J Med. 1996;335(15):1115–22.
59. Pollak MR, Brown EM, Estep HL, et al. Autosomal dominant hypocalcaemia caused by a Ca(2+)-sensing receptor gene mutation. Nat Genet. 1994;8(3):303–7.
60. De Luca F, Ray K, Mancilla EE, et al. Sporadic hypoparathyroidism caused by de Novo gain-of-function mutations of the Ca(2+)-sensing receptor. J Clin Endocrinol Metab. 1997;82(8):2710–5.
61. Watanabe T, Bai M, Lane CR, et al. Familial hypoparathyroidism: identification of a novel gain of function mutation in transmembrane domain 5 of the calcium-sensing receptor. J Clin Endocrinol Metab. 1998;83(7):2497–502.
62. Baron J, Winer KK, Yanovski JA, et al. Mutations in the Ca(2+)-sensing receptor gene cause autosomal dominant and sporadic hypoparathyroidism. Hum Mol Genet. 1996;5(5):601–6.
63. Theman TA, Collins MT, Dempster DW, et al. PTH (1-34) replacement therapy in a child with hypoparathyroidism caused by a sporadic calcium receptor mutation. J Bone Miner Res. 2009;24(5):964–73.
64. Konrad M, Weber S. Recent advances in molecular genetics of hereditary magnesium-losing disorders. J Am Soc Nephrol. 2003;14(1):249–60.
65. Watanabe S, Fukumoto S, Chang H, et al. Association between activating mutations of calcium-sensing receptor and Bartter's syndrome. Lancet. 2002; 360(9334):692–4.
66. Gavalas NG, Kemp EH, Krohn KJ, Brown EM, Watson PF, Weetman AP. The calcium-sensing receptor is a target of autoantibodies in patients with autoimmune polyendocrine syndrome type 1. J Clin Endocrinol Metab. 2007;92(6):2107–14.
67. Li Y, Song YH, Rais N, et al. Autoantibodies to the extracellular domain of the calcium sensing receptor in patients with acquired hypoparathyroidism. J Clin Invest. 1996;97(4):910–4.
68. Kifor O, McElduff A, LeBoff MS, et al. Activating antibodies to the calcium-sensing receptor in two patients with autoimmune hypoparathyroidism. J Clin Endocrinol Metab. 2004;89(2):548–56.
69. Kapur K, Johnson T, Beckmann ND, et al. Genome-wide meta-analysis for serum calcium identifies significantly associated SNPs near the calcium-sensing receptor (CASR) gene. PLoS Genet. 2010;6(7): e1001035.

70. Cole DE, Peltekova VD, Rubin LA, et al. A986S polymorphism of the calcium-sensing receptor and circulating calcium concentrations. Lancet. 1999;353(9147):112–5.
71. Cole DE, Vieth R, Trang HM, Wong BY, Hendy GN, Rubin LA. Association between total serum calcium and the A986S polymorphism of the calcium-sensing receptor gene. Mol Genet Metab. 2001;72(2): 168–74.
72. Scillitani A, Guarnieri V, De Geronimo S, et al. Blood ionized calcium is associated with clustered polymorphisms in the carboxyl-terminal tail of the calcium-sensing receptor. J Clin Endocrinol Metab. 2004;89(11):5634–8.
73. Young R, Wu F, Van de Water N, Ames R, Gamble G, Reid IR. Calcium sensing receptor gene A986S polymorphism and responsiveness to calcium supplementation in postmenopausal women. J Clin Endocrinol Metab. 2003;88(2):697–700.
74. Takacs I, Speer G, Bajnok E, et al. Lack of association between calcium-sensing receptor gene "A986S" polymorphism and bone mineral density in Hungarian postmenopausal women. Bone. 2002; 30(6):849–52.
75. Yamauchi M, Sugimoto T, Yamaguchi T, et al. Association of polymorphic alleles of the calcium-sensing receptor gene with the clinical severity of primary hyperparathyroidism. Clin Endocrinol (Oxf). 2001;55(3):373–9.
76. Yano S, Sugimoto T, Kanzawa M, et al. Association of polymorphic alleles of the calcium-sensing receptor gene with parathyroid hormone secretion in hemodialysis patients. Nephron. 2000;85(4): 317–23.
77. Vezzoli G, Tanini A, Ferrucci L, et al. Influence of calcium-sensing receptor gene on urinary calcium excretion in stone-forming patients. J Am Soc Nephrol. 2002;13(10):2517–23.
78. Scillitani A, Guarnieri V, Battista C, et al. Primary hyperparathyroidism and the presence of kidney stones are associated with different haplotypes of the calcium-sensing receptor. J Clin Endocrinol Metab. 2007;92(1):277–83.
79. Nemeth EF, Steffey ME, Hammerland LG, et al. Calcimimetics with potent and selective activity on the parathyroid calcium receptor. Proc Natl Acad Sci USA. 1998;95(7):4040–5.
80. Block GA, Martin KJ, de Francisco AL, et al. Cinacalcet for secondary hyperparathyroidism in patients receiving hemodialysis. N Engl J Med. 2004;350(15):1516–25.
81. Silverberg SJ, Bone 3rd HG, Marriott TB, et al. Short-term inhibition of parathyroid hormone secretion by a calcium-receptor agonist in patients with primary hyperparathyroidism. N Engl J Med. 1997;337(21):1506–10.
82. Silverberg SJ, Rubin MR, Faiman C, et al. Cinacalcet hydrochloride reduces the serum calcium concentration in inoperable parathyroid carcinoma. J Clin Endocrinol Metab. 2007;92(10):3803–8.
83. Peacock M, Bilezikian JP, Klassen PS, Guo MD, Turner SA, Shoback D. Cinacalcet hydrochloride maintains long-term normocalcemia in patients with primary hyperparathyroidism. J Clin Endocrinol Metab. 2005;90(1):135–41.
84. Letz S, Rus R, Haag C, et al. Novel activating mutations of the calcium-sensing receptor: the calcilytic NPS-2143 mitigates excessive signal transduction of mutant receptors. J Clin Endocrinol Metab. 2010;95(10):E229–33.
85. Christie P, Curley A, Nesbit MA, Harding B, Bowl M, Thakker R. Characterisation of 25 calcium-sensing receptor mutations in disorders of calcium homeostasis. Paper presented at the Society for Endocrinology BES 2007. UK: Birmingham.
86. de Andrade SC, Kohara SK, D'Souza-Li L. Novel mutation of the calcium sensing receptor gene in familial hypocalciuric hypercalcaemia and neonatal severe hyperparathyroidism. Clin Endocrinol (Oxf). 2006;65(6):826–7.
87. D'Souza-Li L, Yang B, Canaff L, et al. Identification and functional characterization of novel calcium-sensing receptor mutations in familial hypocalciuric hypercalcemia and autosomal dominant hypocalcemia. J Clin Endocrinol Metab. 2002;87(3):1309–18.
88. Pidasheva S, Canaff L, Simonds WF, Marx SJ, Hendy GN. Impaired cotranslational processing of the calcium-sensing receptor due to signal peptide missense mutations in familial hypocalciuric hypercalcemia. Hum Mol Genet. 2005;14(12):1679–90.
89. Miyashiro K, Kunii I, Manna TD, et al. Severe hypercalcemia in a 9-year-old Brazilian girl due to a novel inactivating mutation of the calcium-sensing receptor. J Clin Endocrinol Metab. 2004;89(12): 5936–41.
90. Chikatsu N, Fukumoto S, Suzawa M, et al. An adult patient with severe hypercalcaemia and hypocalciuria due to a novel homozygous inactivating mutation of calcium-sensing receptor. Clin Endocrinol (Oxf). 1999;50(4):537–43.
91. Aida K, Koishi S, Inoue M, Nakazato M, Tawata M, Onaya T. Familial hypocalciuric hypercalcemia associated with mutation in the human Ca(2+)-sensing receptor gene. J Clin Endocrinol Metab. 1995;80(9):2594–8.
92. Vargas-Poussou R, Huang C, Hulin P, et al. Functional characterization of a calcium-sensing receptor mutation in severe autosomal dominant hypocalcemia with a Bartter-like syndrome. J Am Soc Nephrol. 2002;13(9):2259–66.
93. Heath 3rd H, Odelberg S, Jackson CE, et al. Clustered inactivating mutations and benign polymorphisms of the calcium receptor gene in familial benign hypocalciuric hypercalcemia suggest receptor functional domains. J Clin Endocrinol Metab. 1996;81(4): 1312–7.
94. Waller S, Kurzawinski T, Spitz L, et al. Neonatal severe hyperparathyroidism: genotype/phenotype correlation and the use of pamidronate as rescue therapy. Eur J Pediatr. 2004;163(10):589–94.

95. Pidasheva S, Grant M, Canaff L, Ercan O, Kumar U, Hendy GN. Calcium-sensing receptor dimerizes in the endoplasmic reticulum: biochemical and biophysical characterization of CASR mutants retained intracellularly. Hum Mol Genet. 2006;15(14): 2200–9.
96. Ward BK, Magno AL, Davis EA, et al. Functional deletion of the calcium-sensing receptor in a case of neonatal severe hyperparathyroidism. J Clin Endocrinol Metab. 2004;89(8):3721–30.
97. Warner J, Epstein M, Sweet A, et al. Genetic testing in familial isolated hyperparathyroidism: unexpected results and their implications. J Med Genet. 2004;41(3):155–60.
98. Suzuki M, Aso T, Sato T, et al. A case of gain-of-function mutation in calcium-sensing receptor: supplemental hydration is required for renal protection. Clin Nephrol. 2005;63(6):481–6.
99. Soie YL, Karperien M, Bakker B, Breuning MH, Hendy GN, Papapoulos SE. Familial benign hypercalcemia (FBH) with age-associated hypercalciuria and a missense mutation in the calcium-sensing receptor (CaSR) expands the spectrum of the syndrome towards primary hyperparathyroidism. Paper presented at: American Society for Bone and Mineral Research, 21st Annual Meeting1999, St. Louis, MI, USA.
100. Simonds WF, James-Newton LA, Agarwal SK, et al. Familial isolated hyperparathyroidism: clinical and genetic characteristics of 36 kindreds. Medicine (Baltimore). 2002;81(1):1–26.
101. Rajguru M, Bedu A, Magdelaine C, Bai M, Aujuard Y, Lienhardt A. Neonatal primary hyperparathyroidism due to a new calcium sensing receptor mutation. Pediatr Res. 2001;49:P3–294.
102. Murugaian EE, Premkumar RM, Radhakrishnan L, Vallath B. Novel mutations in the calcium sensing receptor gene in tropical chronic pancreatitis in India. Scand J Gastroenterol. 2008;43(1):117–21.
103. Cetani F, Lemmi M, Cervia D, et al. Identification and functional characterization of loss-of-function mutations of the calcium-sensing receptor in four Italian kindreds with familial hypocalciuric hypercalcemia. Eur J Endocrinol. 2009;160(3): 481–9.
104. D'Souza-Li L, Canaff L, Janicic N, Cole DE, Hendy GN. An acceptor splice site mutation in the calcium-sensing receptor (CASR) gene in familial hypocalciuric hypercalcemia and neonatal severe hyperparathyroidism. Hum Mutat. 2001;18(5): 411–21.
105. Ward BK, Cameron FJ, Magno AL, McDonnell CM, Stuckey BG, Ratajczak T. A novel homozygous deletion in the calcium-sensing receptor ligand-binding domain associated with neonatal severe hyperparathyroidism. J Pediatr Endocrinol Metab. 2006;19(1):93–100.
106. Cole DE, Yun FH, Wong BY, et al. Calcium-sensing receptor mutations and denaturing high performance liquid chromatography. J Mol Endocrinol. 2009; 42(4):331–9.
107. Hinnie J, Vass JK, Rolfe E, et al. Two novel mutations causing familial benign hypocalciuric hypercalcaemia in three Scottish families. Scott Med J. 2009; 54(4):11–4.
108. Felderbauer P, Hoffmann P, Einwachter H, et al. A novel mutation of the calcium sensing receptor gene is associated with chronic pancreatitis in a family with heterozygous SPINK1 mutations. BMC Gastroenterol. 2003;3:34.
109. Ward BK, Stuckey BG, Gutteridge DH, Laing NG, Pullan PT, Ratajczak T. A novel mutation (L174R) in the Ca2+-sensing receptor gene associated with familial hypocalciuric hypercalcemia. Hum Mutat. 1997;10(3):233–5.
110. Pearce SH, Wooding C, Davies M, Tollefsen SE, Whyte MP, Thakker RV. Calcium-sensing receptor mutations in familial hypocalciuric hypercalcaemia with recurrent pancreatitis. Clin Endocrinol (Oxf). 1996;45(6):675–80.
111. Zajickova K, Vrbikova J, Canaff L, Pawelek PD, Goltzman D, Hendy GN. Identification and functional characterization of a novel mutation in the calcium-sensing receptor gene in familial hypocalciuric hypercalcemia: modulation of clinical severity by vitamin D status. J Clin Endocrinol Metab. 2007;92(7):2616–23.
112. Webb EA, Allgrove J, Kurzawinski TR, Dattani MT. Did cinacalcet help in the management of neonatal severe hyperparathyroidism secondary to a novel homozygous inactivating mutation of the calcium-sensing receptor? Paper presented at: 5th International Conference on Children's Bone Health2009, Cambridge, UK.
113. Demedts M, Lissens W, Wuyts W, Matthijs G, Thomeer M, Bouillon R. A new missense mutation in the CASR gene in familial interstitial lung disease with hypocalciuric hypercalcemia and defective granulocyte function. Am J Respir Crit Care Med. 2008;177(5):558–9.
114. Marcocci C, Borsari S, Pardi E, et al. Familial hypocalciuric hypercalcemia in a woman with metastatic breast cancer: a case report of mistaken identity. J Clin Endocrinol Metab. 2003;88(11):5132–6.
115. Cetani F, Pardi E, Borsari S, et al. Two Italian kindreds with familial hypocalciuric hypercalcaemia caused by loss-of-function mutations in the calcium-sensing receptor (CaR) gene: functional characterization of a novel CaR missense mutation. Clin Endocrinol (Oxf). 2003;58(2):199–206.
116. D'Souza-Li L, Silva MBD, Grande MT, Carvalho D, Guerra G. Two novel mutations in the calcium-sensing receptor gene in familial hypocalciuric hypercalcemia and neonatal severe hyperparathyroidism. Paper presented at: American Society for Bone and Mineral Research. 24th Annual Meeting 2002, San Antonio, Texas, USA.
117. Guarnieri V, Canaff L, Yun FH, et al. Calcium-sensing receptor (CASR) mutations in hypercalcemic states: studies from a single endocrine clinic over three years. J Clin Endocrinol Metab. 2010;95(4):1819–29.

118. Ono Y, Oda N, Ishihara S, et al. Insulinoma cell calcium-sensing receptor influences insulin secretion in a case with concurrent familial hypocalciuric hypercalcemia and malignant metastatic insulinoma. Eur J Endocrinol. 2008;159(1):81–6.
119. Dong Q, Cheng Z, Chang W, et al. Naturally-occurring mutation in the calcium-sensing receptor (CaSR) reveals the significance of extracellular domain loop III for receptor and signal transduction. Paper presented at the Endocrine Society's 91st Annual Meeting, ENDO 2009, Washington, DC.
120. Vigouroux C, Bourut C, Guerci B, et al. A new missense mutation in the calcium-sensing receptor in familial benign hypercalcaemia associated with partial lipoatrophy and insulin resistant diabetes. Clin Endocrinol (Oxf). 2000;53(3):393–8.
121. Leech C, Lohse P, Stanojevic V, Lechner A, Goke B, Spitzweg C. Identification of a novel inactivating R465Q mutation of the calcium-sensing receptor. Biochem Biophys Res Commun. 2006;342(3): 996–1002.
122. Schwarz P, Larsen NE, Lonborg Friis IM, Lillquist K, Brown EM, Gammeltoft S. Familial hypocalciuric hypercalcemia and neonatal severe hyperparathyroidism associated with mutations in the human Ca2+-sensing receptor gene in three Danish families. Scand J Clin Lab Invest. 2000;60(3):221–7.
123. Nakayama T, Minato M, Nakagawa M, et al. A novel mutation in Ca2+-sensing receptor gene in familial hypocalciuric hypercalcemia. Endocrine. 2001;15(3):277–82.
124. Burski K, Torjussen B, Paulsen AQ, Boman H, Bollerslev J. Parathyroid adenoma in a subject with familial hypocalciuric hypercalcemia: coincidence or causality? J Clin Endocrinol Metab. 2002;87(3):1015–6.
125. Nyweide K, Feldman KW, Gunther DF, Done S, Lewis C, Van Eenwyk C. Hypocalciuric hypercalcemia presenting as neonatal rib fractures: a newly described mutation of the calcium-sensing receptor gene. Pediatr Emerg Care. 2006;22(11):722–4.
126. Tan YM, Cardinal J, Franks AH, et al. Autosomal dominant hypocalcemia: a novel activating mutation (E604K) in the cysteine-rich domain of the calcium-sensing receptor. J Clin Endocrinol Metab. 2003;88(2):605–10.
127. Jap TS, Wu YC, Jenq SF, Won GS. A novel mutation in the calcium-sensing receptor gene in a Chinese subject with persistent hypercalcemia and hypocalciuria. J Clin Endocrinol Metab. 2001;86(1):13–5.
128. Hendy GN, D'Souza-Li L, Yang B, Canaff L, Cole DE. Mutations of the calcium-sensing receptor (CASR) in familial hypocalciuric hypercalcemia, neonatal severe hyperparathyroidism, and autosomal dominant hypocalcemia. Hum Mutat. 2000;16(4):281–96.
129. Baudry C, Rebours V, Houillier P, Hammel P, Ruszniewski P, Levy P. Recurrent acute pancreatitis caused by association of a novel mutation of the calcium-sensing receptor gene and a heterozygous mutation of the SPINK1 gene. Pancreas. 2010;39(3): 420–1.
130. Miyashiro K, Kasamatsu TS, Steinmetz L, et al. Identification and functional analysis of a novel inactivating mutation (A804D) of the calcium-sensing receptor gene. Clin Endocrinol (Oxf). 2004;61(6):780–2.
131. Dreimane D, Hendy GN, Alon U, Geffner ME. Normalization of serum calcium, phosphorus, and magnesium with homeopathic PTH in a child with hypocalcemic hypercalciuria (HCHC) and a mutation of the calcium-sensing receptor gene Paper presented at the Endocrine Society's 83rd Annual Meeting, ENDO 2001, Denver.
132. Ma RC, Lam CW, So WY, Tong PC, Cockram CS, Chow CC. A novel CASR gene mutation in an octogenarian with asymptomatic hypercalcaemia. Hong Kong Med J. 2008;14(3):226–8.
133. Janicic N, Soliman E, Pausova Z, et al. Mapping of the calcium-sensing receptor gene (CASR) to human chromosome 3q13.3-21 by fluorescence in situ hybridization, and localization to rat chromosome 11 and mouse chromosome 16. Mamm Genome. 1995;6(11):798–801.
134. Felderbauer P, Klein W, Bulut K, et al. Mutations in the calcium-sensing receptor: a new genetic risk factor for chronic pancreatitis? Scand J Gastroenterol. 2006;41(3):343–8.
135. Yabuta T, Miyauchi A, Inoue H, Yoshida H, Hirokawa M, Amino N. A patient with primary hyperparathyroidism associated with familial hypocalciuric hypercalcemia induced by a novel germline CaSR gene mutation. Asian J Surg. 2009; 32(2):118–22.
136. Hu J, Mora S, Weber G, Zamproni I, Proverbio MC, Spiegel AM. Autosomal dominant hypocalcemia in monozygotic twins caused by a de novo germline mutation near the amino-terminus of the human calcium receptor. J Bone Miner Res. 2004;19(4): 578–86.
137. Okazaki R, Chikatsu N, Nakatsu M, et al. A novel activating mutation in calcium-sensing receptor gene associated with a family of autosomal dominant hypocalcemia. J Clin Endocrinol Metab. 1999;84(1): 363–6.
138. Hu J, Mora S, Colussi G, et al. Autosomal dominant hypocalcemia caused by a novel mutation in the loop 2 region of the human calcium receptor extracellular domain. J Bone Miner Res. 2002;17(8):1461–9.
139. Lienhardt A, Bai M, Lagarde JP, et al. Activating mutations of the calcium-sensing receptor: management of hypocalcemia. J Clin Endocrinol Metab. 2001;86(11):5313–23.
140. Hirai H, Nakajima S, Miyauchi A, et al. A novel activating mutation (C129S) in the calcium-sensing receptor gene in a Japanese family with autosomal dominant hypocalcemia. J Hum Genet. 2001;46(1):41–4.
141. Burren CP, Curley A, Christie P, Rodda CP, Thakker RV. A family with autosomal dominant hypocalcaemia with hypercalciuria (ADHH): mutational analysis, phenotypic variability and treatment challenges. J Pediatr Endocrinol Metab. 2005;18(7):689–99.

142. Haag C, Schulze E, Lorenz A, Frank-Raue K, Raue F. Novel mutations of the calcium-sensing receptor in familial hypocalciuric hypercalcemia and autosomal dominant hypocalcemia Paper presented at the Endocrine Society's 87th Annual Meeting, ENDO 2005, San Diego, CA.
143. Lovlie R, Eiken HG, Sorheim JI, Boman H. The Ca(2+)-sensing receptor gene (PCAR1) mutation T151M in isolated autosomal dominant hypoparathyroidism. Hum Genet. 1996;98(2):129–33.
144. Conley YP, Finegold DN, Peters DG, Cook JS, Oppenheim DS, Ferrell RE. Three novel activating mutations in the calcium-sensing receptor responsible for autosomal dominant hypocalcemia. Mol Genet Metab. 2000;71(4):591–8.
145. Nakajima K, Yamazaki K, Kimura H, Takano K, Miyoshi H, Sato K. Novel gain of function mutations of the calcium-sensing receptor in two patients with PTH-deficient hypocalcemia. Intern Med. 2009;48(22):1951–6.
146. Kapoor A, Satishchandra P, Ratnapriya R, et al. An idiopathic epilepsy syndrome linked to 3q13.3-q21 and missense mutations in the extracellular calcium sensing receptor gene. Ann Neurol. 2008;64(2): 158–67.
147. Lienhardt A, Bai M, Lagarde J, Kottler M, Farhid N. New mutation of the calcium-sensing receptor gene associated with isolated hypoparathyroidism. Paper presented at the Endocrine Society's 83rd Annual Meeting, ENDO 2001, Denver.
148. Stock JL, Brown RS, Baron J, et al. Autosomal dominant hypoparathyroidism associated with short stature and premature osteoarthritis. J Clin Endocrinol Metab. 1999;84(9):3036–40.
149. Mittelman SD, Hendy GN, Fefferman RA, et al. A hypocalcemic child with a novel activating mutation of the calcium-sensing receptor gene: successful treatment with recombinant human parathyroid hormone. J Clin Endocrinol Metab. 2006;91(7): 2474–9.
150. Uckun-Kitapci A, Underwood LE, Zhang J, Moats-Staats B. A novel mutation (E767K) in the second extracellular loop of the calcium sensing receptor in a family with autosomal dominant hypocalcemia. Am J Med Genet A. 2005;132A(2):125–9.
151. Hendy GN, Minutti C, Canaff L, et al. Recurrent familial hypocalcemia due to germline mosaicism for an activating mutation of the calcium-sensing receptor gene. J Clin Endocrinol Metab. 2003;88(8): 3674–81.
152. Cole DR, Soule S, Raizis A, George P. Hypocalcemia and a novel calcium-sensing receptor activating mutation. Paper presented at the Annual Scientific Meeting of The Royal Australasian College of Physicians 2005, Wellington, New Zealand.
153. Nagase T, Murakami T, Tsukada T, et al. A family of autosomal dominant hypocalcemia with a positive correlation between serum calcium and magnesium: identification of a novel gain of function mutation (Ser(820)Phe) in the calcium-sensing receptor. J Clin Endocrinol Metab. 2002;87(6):2681–7.
154. Shiohara M, Mori T, Mei B, Brown EM, Watanabe T, Yasuda T. A novel gain-of-function mutation (F821L) in the transmembrane domain of calcium-sensing receptor is a cause of severe sporadic hypoparathyroidism. Eur J Pediatr. 2004;163(2): 94–8.
155. Inoue D, Saika M, Ikeda Y, Matsumoto T. Successful treatment of hypoparathyroidism caused by a novel calcium-sensing receptor mutation with thiazide diuretics and low dose alfacalcidol. Paper presented at the Second Joint Meeting of The American Society for Bone and Mineral Research and The International Bone and Mineral Society 1998, Moscone Convention Center San Francisco, California, USA.
156. Hu J, McLarnon SJ, Mora S, et al. A region in the seven-transmembrane domain of the human Ca2+ receptor critical for response to Ca2+. J Biol Chem. 2005;280(6):5113–20.
157. Zhao XM, Hauache O, Goldsmith PK, Collins R, Spiegel AM. A missense mutation in the seventh transmembrane domain constitutively activates the human Ca2+ receptor. FEBS Lett. 1999;448(1): 180–4.
158. Lienhardt A, Garabedian M, Bai M, et al. A large homozygous or heterozygous in-frame deletion within the calcium-sensing receptor's carboxylterminal cytoplasmic tail that causes autosomal dominant hypocalcemia. J Clin Endocrinol Metab. 2000;85(4):1695–702.

New Concepts for Primary and Secondary Hyperparathyroidism

5

Joachim Beige and Peter Lamesch

Abstract

Primary hyperparathyroidism and secondary disease from chronic kidney disease are highlighted in this chapter. Up-to-date descriptions of new pathological mechanisms focus on fibroblastic growth factor 23 and its emergent importance in overall pathology. Historical, clinical, and examination findings are highlighted and compliment data on laboratory techniques, diagnostic imaging, and skeletal histology clinical workup of the patients. Treatment options at the dialysis and pharmacological levels are blended with some of the nutritional elements in phosphorus control. The integration of all elements is summarized at the end of the section to emphasize its influence on bone metabolism.

Keywords

Primary hyperparathyroidism • Insulinoma • Gastrinoma • Pheochromocytoma • Hypercalcemia • RET • HRPT2 • Renal function • 1,25 (OH)2 vitamin D • Glomerular filtration • Homeostasis • J-shaped curve • Chronic kidney disease • FGF 23 • Vitamin D receptor • RANK ligand • Osteoclastogenesis • Renal osteodystrophy • Calciphylaxis • Fetuin • GLA protein • Epitopes • Serum calculation • Ostase (bone alkaline phosphatase) • TRAP-5b • Osteitits fibrosa • Parathyroidectomy • Calcimimetics • Ca × P product • Randomized controlled trial • Vascular calcification • Venous sampling • Parathyroid scanning • Oxyphilic cells • Neoplasia • Osteoprotegerin • Sodium thiosulfate • Sestamibi • Technetium 99m • Osteoclasts • Osteoblasts • Trabecular

J. Beige, MD, PhD (✉)
Department of Nephrology and KfH Renal Unit,
Hospital St. Georg, Delitzscher Strasse 141,
Leipzig 04129, Saxony, Germany
e-mail: joachim.beige@kfh-dialyse.de

P. Lamesch, MD, FACS
Department of Endocrinological Surgery,
Hospital St. Georg, Delitzscher Strasse 141,
Leipzig 04129, Saxony, Germany

A.A. Licata and E.V. Lerma (eds.), *Diseases of the Parathyroid Glands*,
DOI 10.1007/978-1-4419-5550-0_5, © Springer Science+Business Media, LLC 2012

Pathophysiology and Epidemiology

Parathyroid glands are located in close proximity to the thyroid gland on their posterior surface. In normal health, the parathyroids are small (2–5 mm). Normally the four (sometimes more) glands are derived from the neural crest mesenchyme and the brachial pouch endoderm. The glands are composed of two cell types, of which the "chief cells" are the ones that generate parathyroid hormone (PTH). The larger oxyphilic cells are lighter in staining, fewer in number, and have no known physiologic role. A histological picture of an enlarged, proliferated gland is given in Fig. 5.1.

Excessive secretion of PTH is mostly a consequence of adenomatous proliferation of parathyroid glands in which case it is referred to as *primary (p)* hyperparathyroidism (HPT). The causative circumstance of such benign status is not known. However, in about 1% of pHPT, parathyroid carcinoma is the underlying cause [1]. Some genetic risk loci have been identified among which mutations in HRPT2 and RET [2] are the most important ones. Patients inheriting these genes develop parathyroid carcinoma and phaechromocytoma. In some occasions, pHPT may be associated syndromatically with other endocrinological disorders (multiple endocrinological neoplasia, MEN). In these rare conditions, endocrinological symptoms are often combined depending on the type of disease. In MEN type 1, pHPT coincidences with gastrointestinal tumors like insulinoma or gastrinoma. In MEN 2A, pheochromocytoma is the most frequent combination.

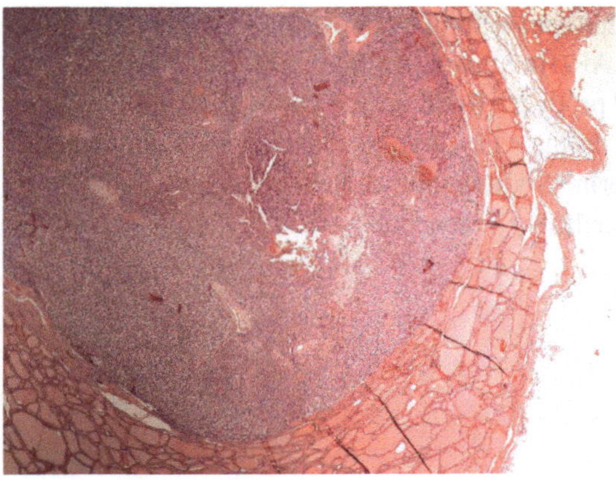

Fig. 5.1 Low magnification of a hyperplastic intrathyreoidal located adenomatous parathyroid gland. Kindly contributed by Andreas Plötner, Pathological Institute, Hospital St. Georg, Leipzig

In pHPT, PTH oversecretion is frequently followed by impaired renal function due to hypercalcemia, which is a harm to healthy kidneys. Hypercalcemia in pHPT is stimulated by increased dietary calcium absorption and calcium mobilization from the bone hydroxyapatite depot. Therefore, in sustained and nontreated pHPT, renal failure due to hypercalcemia is typical sequelae. This condition causes secondary HPT and, therefore, mixes up with the primary problem of pHPT. Following this situation, a pHPT might not be easy to distinguish from secondary forms, if renal injury is already present. The frequency of newly diagnosed pHPT is higher than one might expect: 1 out of 500 women and 1 out 2,000 men were found to be affected among 60-year-old individuals in a population-based registration in Rochester, MN, in 1989 [3].

Functional hyperplasia and hypertrophy of the parathyroid glands due to chronic kidney disease (CKD) are characterized as "secondary" hyperparathyroidism (sHPT). However, following the subsequent pathophysiological considerations, the phrase "functional" hyperparathyroidism is a more appropriate wording. The morphological and imaging aspects of this disease are characterized in a particular chapter. From a functional point of view, sHPT is sequelae of altered mineral metabolism in CKD.

Healthy kidneys coregulate calcium homeostasis by different mechanisms. The major downstream pathway of kidney metabolism in terms of bone and mineral metabolism has been focused to the parathyroids many years ago. However, in such classical reasoning, the renal–parathyroid axis has been thought to be mediated through downregulation of vitamin D activation only. In fact, it is long known, that hydroxylation and activation of inactive vitamin D into the active form, Di-hydroxyl vitamin D (1.25 OH_2D, calcitriol), take place at the tubular-interstitial compartment of kidneys. Already in early forms of CKD, that activation and subsequently the synthesis of 1.25 OH_2D are abolished. The levels of

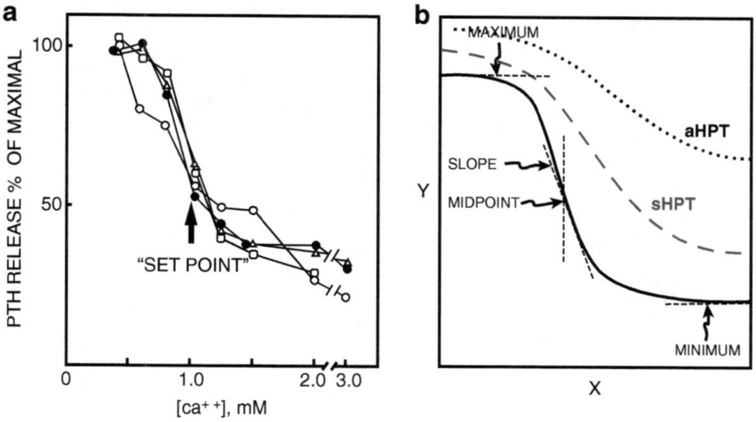

Fig. 5.2 Original (panel **a**, *left*) and schematic (panel **b**, *right*) drawing of the relationship between calcium concentration and PTH response in healthy (**a**) and renal population (**b**) with still functioning response in secondary (s) and autonomous (a) HPT. *Y*-axis PTH concentration, *X*-axis Ca concentration. Response is characterized by slope, midpoint, maximum and minimum which might resemble the functioning status of the Ca–PTH regulation. Adapted from Brown EM, Gardner DG, Brennan MF et al. Calcium-regulated parathyroid hormone release in primary hyperparathyroidism: studies in vitro with dispersed parathyroid cells. Am J Med. 1979;66(6):923–31

1.25 OH_2D in sera of patients with CKD are inversely and linearly correlated with excretory renal function, measured by glomerular filtration rate (GFR) [4].

As this, the classical concept of sHPT reflects the adaptations to decreased 1.25 OH_2D. Since calcium absorption from the bowel wall is mediated by 1.25 OH_2D, a decrease of that hormone results in calcium deficit, particularly present in a reduced level of free serum calcium. In the serum, calcium is partly bound to albumin resulting in a difference between whole and acting/free calcium. Free calcium content of sera is sensed very precisely and tightly by the calcium-sensing receptors (CaR) of the parathyroids [5]. A decrease of free calcium leads to increase of PTH synthesis [6]. PTH increases serum calcium by its action on bowel vitamin D uptake and Ca mobilization from the bone hydroxyapatite depot. By that means, the decrease of 1.25 OH_2D is counter-regulated and the serum-free calcium level, which has much downstream impacts, can be partly maintained through a wide range of renal insufficiency. However, the gross calcium balance including the bone depot is negative and the adaptation maintains serum homeostasis by means of decalcification of bones. During last years, these mechanisms have been discussed more and more as adaptive ones, i.e., in certain sense as a physiological response. A lot of discussion is ongoing concerning the question, if PTH elevation is a pathological process per se, or if the onset of disease-mediating mechanisms has to be determined at a certain PTH threshold. While this is controversial, from a functional viewpoint, an intact calcium–PTH regulation axis could be seen as one aspect of a truly adaptive process [7, 8]. Such classical experiments establishing a J-shaped Ca–PTH response curve [6] have recently been performed in the end-stage renal failure setting using Ca dialysis bath concentration variation and measuring PTH response [9]. The degree of PTH response, measured as relationship between set point and slope of the curve (Fig. 5.2), can be seen as a measure of appropriate regulation.

By note, serum phosphorus elevation comes into play only in later stages of CKD and acts as further stimulus of PTH elevation. Besides a remarkable degree of excretory renal failure in CKD stage 3 and 4, phosphorus (P) levels usually will be found not elevated in these stages [10]. The reason of that difference in time course (P ↑ late, Ca ↓ and PTH ↑ early) has been clarified at least in part during the last few years. Phosphaturia has been demonstrated to be promoted not only

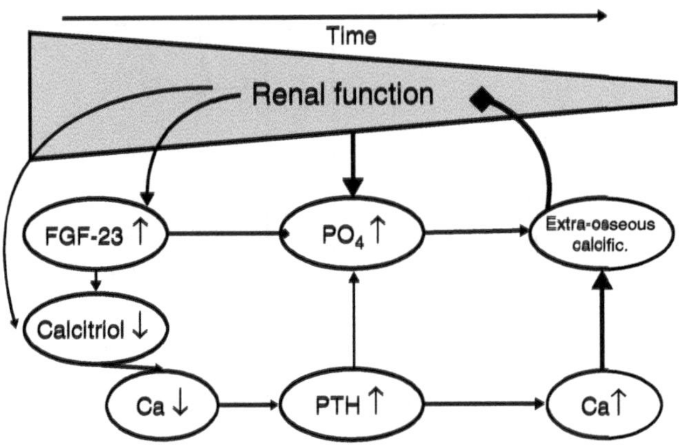

Fig. 5.3 Simplified drawing of time-dependent alterations of mineral metabolism in chronic kidney disease

by PTH but also by fibroblast growth factor 23 (FGF-23), which is secreted mainly from bone-forming osteoblasts [11]. FGF-23 exerts a very strong phosphaturic effect [12–14]. However, it does not only stimulate phosphaturia but also diminish activation of vitamin D by a strong inhibitory effect on 1-α-hydroxylase resulting in 1.25 OH_2D downregulation [14] and does not inhibit HPT [15]. Therefore, FGF-23 is likely to maintain normal phosphate homeostasis in early stages of CKD on the cost of decreased 1.25 OH_2D levels comparable to PTH elevation which is the pay-off to stabilize calcium in early CKD (Fig. 5.3).

In such a concept, looking at PTH and FGF-23, the resulting 1.25 OH_2D deficiency is the key-playing negative regulator in mineral metabolism changes due to CKD. 1.25 OH_2D binds to its receptor (vitamin D receptor, VDR) which is located not only throughout the body, including parathyroids, bowel wall but also in endothelium and immune cells. Like other members of the steroid receptor family, the VDR acts as a ligand-activated transcription factor. Classical down-stream effectors of the 1.25 OH_2D–VDR complex include enhancement of small-bowel calcium absorption and osteoclastogenesis and liberation of calcium from bones. The latter effect is exerted via the regulation of receptor activator of NF-B ligand (RANKL)–receptor activator of NF-B (RANK) interactions and osteoprotegerin interplay through the 1.25 OH_2D–VDR complex. Yet this interaction is complex and altered by PTH. Newer findings suggests that bone forming in the presence of altered 1.25 OH_2D–VDR complex only transforms to bone resorption when PTH increase is paralleled by active vitamin D deficiency [16]. Inactivation of the 25-hydroxyvitamin D 1-hydroxylase and vitamin D receptor demonstrates independent and interdependent effects of calcium and vitamin D on skeletal and mineral homeostasis. This means that if the Ca/1.25 $OH_2D \rightarrow$PTH response is not functional, bone turnover is abolished resulting in bone loss. This condition is characterized as "dead bone disease" but incorporates not only skeletal but also systemic pathological features.

Pathophysiology of Bone Disorder in CKD-MBD

"Dead bone disease" or low *turnover* renal osteodystrophy (ROD) is one of three particular pathologies related to mineral–parathyroid regulation in frame of CKD. While *low-turnover bone disease* is mostly characterized by "arrested" bone metabolism with both inactive osteoblasts and osteoclasts and low PTH, *high-turnover bone disease* is identified by stimulated bone metabolisms and both cell types together with increased PTH.

During recent years, the focus has moved from "bone only" to "bone and vasculature." The hypothesis behind that reasoning is a pathological translocation of calcium salts from bones to vasculature mediated by mechanisms, among which sHPT is one of the best investigated ones. In fact, the presence of ectopic vascular calcification (VC) and the transition of smooth muscle cells (SMC) to osteoblasts represents a cornerstone of vascular risk and an independent risk factor of mortality [17]. Adjusted for age, the risk of death, is elevated up to 100-fold in patients with CKD 5 compared with healthy controls [18]. However, the molecular mechanisms leading to VC and the possible link between bone disease (somewhat mechanistic seen as "calcification minus") and vessel disease ("calcification plus") have not been established until very recent years. During last years, markers of mineral bone metabolism and parathyroid dysregulation have been clearly associated with patient survival [19]. This is true for the serum concentrations of calcium and phosphorus and, in smaller extent with a more J-shaped mortality association curve, for PTH [19]. The role of FGF-23 in terms of survival has to be investigated in future studies. The pathophysiological impacts, which bone disease might execute on vasculature and cardiovascular risk in renal failure, led to the newly inaugurated entity "chronic kidney disease-mineral bone disease" (CKD-MBD). This scenario comprises risks of osteodystrophy like pathological fractures and sequelae of bone decalcification as calcium salt deposition. That deposition may either occur in an elementary form, e.g., in grafted kidneys resulting in earlier transplant loss [20] or in more complex forms together with phosphorus deposition in "brown tumors" of skin and joints, which are already longer known.

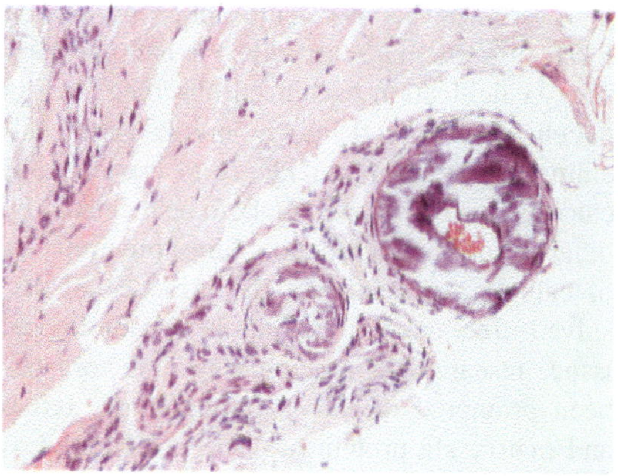

Fig. 5.4 Calcification of intima-media layer of small arteries (→ *arrow*) in calciphylaxis (*von Kossa* staining, ×100 magnification). Kindly contributed by Dr. Jens Plöthner, Pathological Institute, Hospital St. Georg, Leipzig, Germany

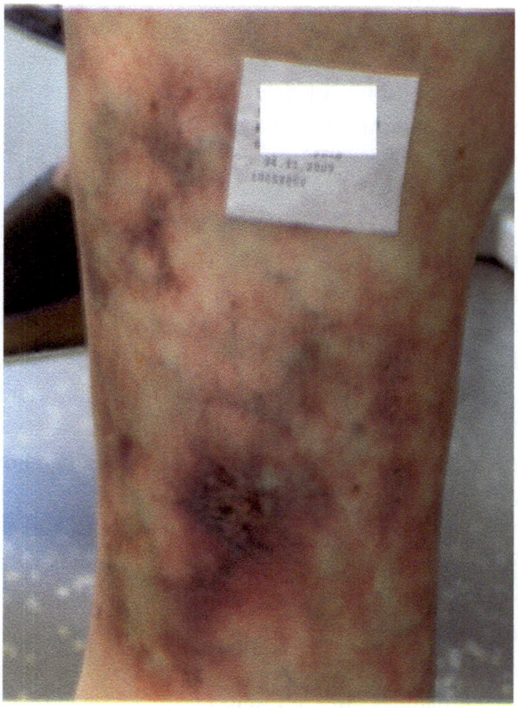

Fig. 5.5 Ulcerated skin surface of the lower leg of a patient with calciphylaxis, concomitant with intima-media arterial calcification seen in Fig. 5.3

Calciphylaxis

In particular, changes of the skin comprising painful ulceration and inflammation and occurring along with calcification of middle and small arteries intima-media-layers (Fig. 5.4) have been defined as calciphylaxis (Fig. 5.5), a condition inheriting 50–80% mortality. At current, there are no evidence-based treatment schemes available for such deleterious complication. However, chelation and excretion of calcium salts with sodium thiosulfate [21–28], lowering calcium concentration by intensified dialysis and pharmaceutical regimes and parathyroidectomy (PTX) yielded beneficial results in single cases and small series [29]. Calcification does not occur only in patients who are subjected to high serum levels of calcium, phosphorus, and PTH. In particular, calciphylaxis and coronary artery calcification have been observed even in patients with normal and low-normal serum calcium. Therefore, the incidence of extraosseous calcification has been thought to be mediated by other factors as calcium, too. Since precipitation of calcium salts and not the presence of dissolved free calcium is the key pathological issue, research on precipitating cofactors has been promoted recently. Among those, fetuin and matrix gla protein have been identified as precipitation inhibitors [30] and a deficiency of these agents has been hypothesized as cofactors of precipitation. In vitro precipitation experiments with fetuin supported that reasoning [30–32]. Since fetuin and matrix gla protein are related to inflammatory activation, a very attractive link has been identified connecting the frequent occurrence of calcification in patients with inflammation. Another important cofactor for precipitation of calcium salts is the inhibition of vitamin K synthesis by warfarin [33], which consequently has to be stopped in calciphylaxis.

Inflammation, particularly subclinical microinflammation, is overrepresented in cohorts with renal disease in general. Without dissecting details, extracorporeal (dialysis) circuits, autoimmune kidney diseases, subclinical transplant rejection, and uremic inflammation are the most important headings pointing to microinflammation in these patients. Taking all recent keys together, to describe a nowadays comprehensive picture of "diseases of parathyroids" in renal patients, hyperplasia and hypertrophy of parathyroid glands with subsequent PTH oversecretion is only one aspect of a more complex disease described as *CKD-MBD* [34]. This complex focuses more on "end-organ-damage" of PTH in terms of calcification of vasculature, specific calcification disease of the skin (calciphylaxis), and renal bone osteodystrophy. That end-organ-damage is mediated by cofactors apart from the calcium–parathyroid axis like precipitation inhibitors and inflammation.

See Chapter 6 for detailed discussion.

Clinical Course, History, and Physical Findings

In primary HPT, which is sometimes a nondiscovered silent disease, hypocalcemia causes the most important symptoms. Central nervous effects of hypocalcemia, if not abrogated by chronic course, are the leading symptoms. Somnolence, cramps, or in lower grade fatigue together with increased serum calcium (in pHPT) must lead to PTH assessment and enable the diagnosis.

An obstacle to withstand a correct and early diagnosis is the later renal effects of hypocalcemia. If pHPT is not diagnosed early, renal calcinosis is a frequent late squeal. In such a situation, as in any CKD, sHPT due to vitamin D deficiency decreases serum calcium and mixes up with the pHPT being the underlying disease in such cases. In general, in more chronic cases of any HPT, clinical symptoms are not very characteristic but must be evaluated by biochemical studies. A summary of symptoms with most observed frequencies is listed in Table 5.1 [35, 36].

Diagnostic Techniques

Imaging

The role of preoperative imaging in HPT is controversial due to varying success rates reported in studies [37]. In the more recent years, ultrasound

Table 5.1 Clinical symptoms of hyperparathyroidism

Symptoms	Frequency (%)
Left ventricular hypertrophy	80
Dullness	70
Arterial hypertension	50
Extraosseous calcification	40
Fatigue	40
Hyperuricemia	30
Joint calcification	20
Obesity	20
Depression	15
Anxiety	10
Cognitive dysfunction	5

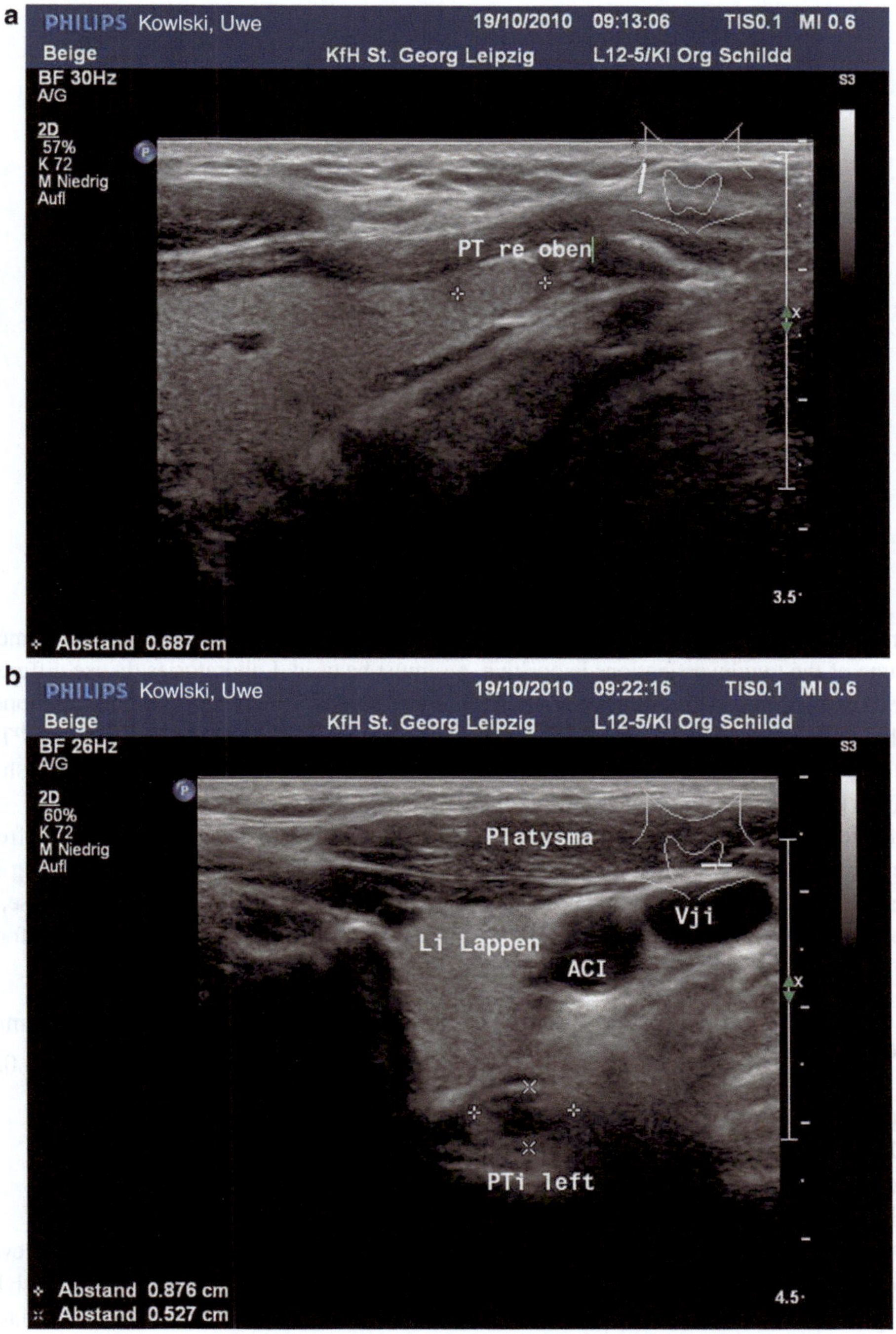

Fig. 5.6 (**a**) Ultrasonography of right adenomatous parathyroid gland (+ picture marks of enlarged gland). (**b**) Ultrasonography of left adenomatous parathyroid gland, note central inhomogenous structure (+ picture marks of enlarged gland, ACI = internal carotid artery, VJi = internal jugular vene, Li Lappen = left thyroid lobe)

(US) and technetium 99m-*methoxyisobutylisonitrile* (sestamibi) scintigraphy scan has been used most frequently. Mihai et al. [38] found in an evidence-based analysis, that sestamibi is a recommended primary test, but ultrasound in experienced hands turned out to be a valuable alternative (see example in Fig. 5.6). The authors concluded, that if both investigations are concordant,

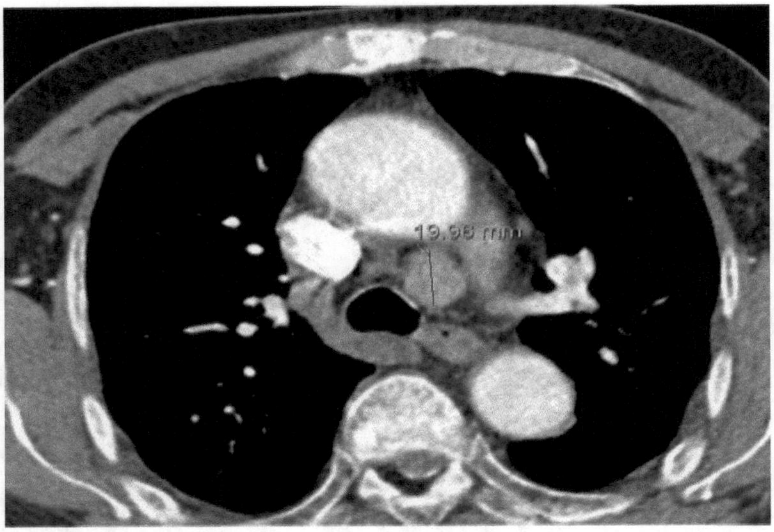

Fig. 5.7 CT scan of atypical localization of parathyroidal glands (between trachea and vena cava)

a minimal invasive surgical approach is indicated, if only one of the two investigations is positive, a unilateral exploration with intraoperative PTH assay should be performed. In case of two negative investigations, a bilateral exploration should be planned [38]. The technological development of US devices (resolution down to 1 mm) currently contributes to use of such methodology. If glands are located atypically, CT scans (Fig. 5.7) might be helpful.

Laboratory Techniques

Most optimal, patients suffering from sHPT and or CKD-MBD should be diagnosed by screening measures during the course of CKD. One of the most discussed issues was establishing thresholds, from which sHPT should be regarded or even treated. Recent guidelines of the Kidney disease global outcome initiative KDIGO [39] discarded further CKD stage-dependent PTH limits and use threshold of up to ninefold "normal" PTH, where normal refers to local reference. This is meaningful, since PTH assays are yet not standardized between different systems and laboratories.

PTH secretion underlies a both short frequent and circadian rhythm. Therefore, for diagnostic studies, standardized assessment time points must be used. Laboratories do use different assay techniques, which target different epitopes of the 84-amino acid protein. The level of PTH compared to baseline can be used to establish surgical success (Table 5.2).

Serum calcium can be measured as free serum calcium or as whole calcium including its albumin-bound proportion. In the latter case, for correct assessment, it must be corrected for plasma albumin concentration

$$\text{Calcium}_{\text{corrected}} = (\text{calcium} / \text{plasma}(\text{mmol} / \text{l})) + (40 - \text{albumin} / \text{plasma}(\text{g} / \text{l})) \times 0.02.$$

Assessment of Bone Disease

Although no clinical routine method, evaluation of bone status is important to distinguish between conditions of either arrested or stimulated turnover of cellular bone-forming mechanisms. That cellular turnover is denoted by a steady state of activity and number of osteoclasts and osteoblasts at the front of trabecular mineralization. It is meaningful, since therapeutic measures are different in such states. Measuring bone density alone cannot help to distinguish between these entities since it gives only information about

Table 5.2 PTH and calcium thresholds for regarding surgical success, failure, and recurrence

Category	PTH level
Success	Normal or below normal PTH later than 6 months after surgery
Failure	Higher than normal PTH and/or hypercalcemia within 6 months after surgery
Recurrence	Higher than normal PTH and/or hypercalcemia later than 6 months after surgery after initial success criteria fulfilled
Multigland disease	Removal of two or more hyperfunctioning glands during surgery in pHPT evidenced by intraoperative PTH test

Table 5.3 Histomorphological classification of renal osteodystrophy (ROD)

ROD notation	ROD type	Key pathophysiology
High turnover	1	Elevated cell turnover by PTH stimulation
Mixed uremic osteodystrophy (osteitis fibrosa)	3	Disturbed salt mineralization and PTH stimulation
Low turnover		
Osteomalacia	2	Accumulation of nonmineralized bone matrix
Adynamic renal bone disease	4	Decreased volume of bone matrix along with suppressed cellular turnover

content of mineral salts. The histomorphometric approach is based on standardized parameters, which were described in 1987 [40]. Bone histology must be processed following certain procedures both in harvesting, transfer and preparation of the samples. Prior to biopsy, patients should be given tetracycline 250 mg bid at day minus 20 and minus 5 before biopsy. That substance accumulates at the endosteal mineralization front and allows quantification by spontaneous fluorescence. Bone sample biopsy is usually done using a mechanical-driven drill device. Since such approach includes relevant patients discomfort and pain, we use a 4-mm diameter bone marrow biopsy trochar (Pajunk™), which allows a safe and uncomplicated biopsy with satisfying biopsy samples. As biopsy site, we use the posterior upper iliac spine. Samples must be transferred to acetone solution (using mineral glassware) and can be shipped without cooling to bone histology. For embedding, methyl-*methacrylate* will be used. Pathologists use different staining procedures, with *Masson-Goldner* and *Giemsa* being the most important ones. Quantitative histomorphometry is usually done by manual methods of *Merz and Schenk* [41] or semiautomatically following *Malluche* [42]. A pathological bone status in CKD is considered from a histopathological point of view as ROD (Table 5.3, Figs. 5.8–5.11). However in recent years, with advanced understanding of systemic implications of pathological bone state, the more comprehensive term CKD-MBD has been used for clinical perception.

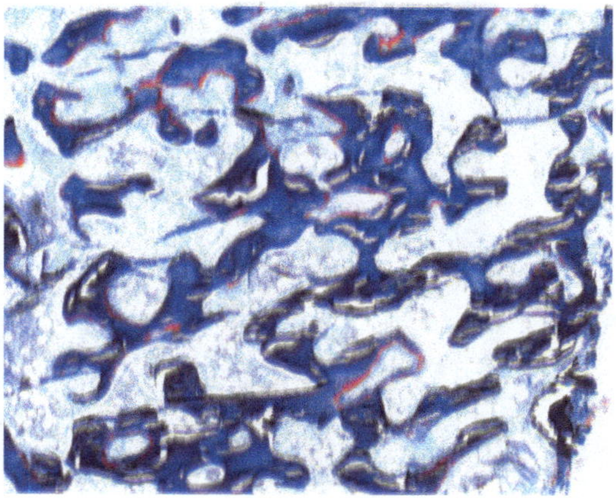

Fig. 5.8 Type 1 ROD. High-turnover variant of osteitis fibrosa with massive osteoclastogenesis (→), high resorptive activity, Masson-Goldner. Kindly contributed by Dr. Gabriele Lehmann, University Hospital Jena, Germany

Biochemical markers of bone status have been studied widely. Although none of these markers have been shown to fit perfectly with the gold standard bone histomorphometry, measuring the bone alkaline phosphatase (ostase) is the most used surrogate. Combination with PTH yielded about 60% fit with histology [43]. Other bone markers include urine cross-links, i.e., fragmentation products of bone collagen. The diagnostic value of these markers is not

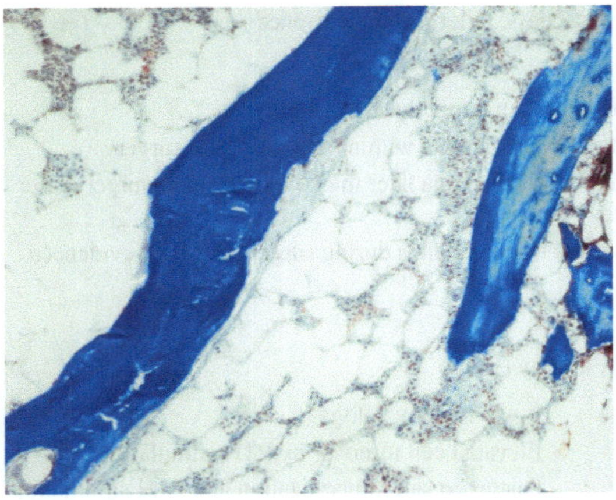

Fig. 5.9 Type 3 ROD mixed osteitis fibrosa, peritrabecular fibrosis (→) and osteoclastic activity (→), Masson-Goldner. Kindly contributed by Dr. Gabriele Lehmann, University Hospital Jena, Germany

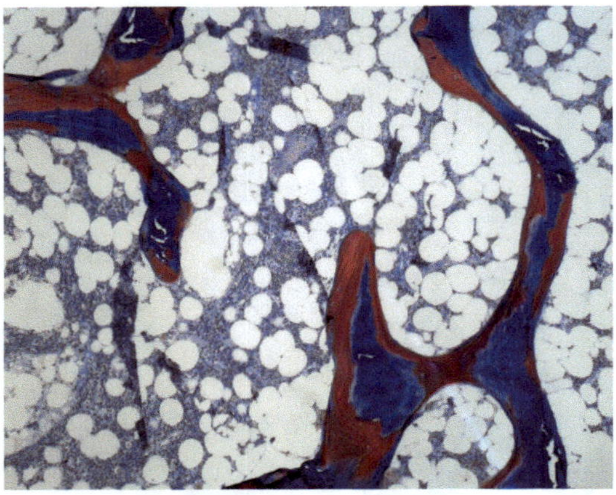

Fig. 5.10 Osteomalacia, intratrabecular disturbed mineralization (→), Masson-Goldner. Kindly contributed by Dr. Gabriele Lehmann, University Hospital Jena, Germany

completely accepted by all. Following trends maybe more helpful than a single-point measurement in time. Therefore, they are promising but must be handled with caution.

Alternative Diagnostic Tools

Biochemical Fine Needle Aspiration

A biochemical fine needle aspiration with PTH measurement allows differentiation of parathyroid tissue from lymph nodes and thyroid tissue with a specificity of 100%. The sample is drawn

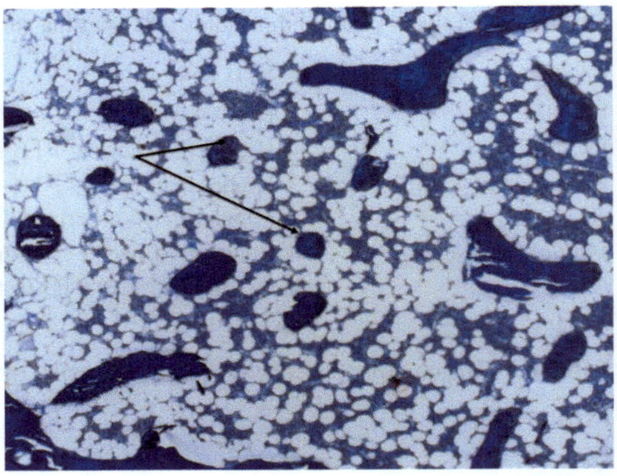

Fig. 5.11 Adynamic bone disease, only small osteoid volume (→) detectable; decreased cellular activity, Masson-Goldner. Kindly contributed by Dr. Gabriele Lehmann, University Hospital Jena, Germany

through a 25-gauge needle, the aspirate is diluted with 1 ml saline solution; after centrifugation for 10 min, the supernatant is used for the PTH measurement [44]. This technique allows prompt tissue identification without frozen section, thereby limiting the preparation of nonparathyroid tissue. It has been proposed for preoperative procedures although with a weak level of evidence but recommendations at grade B [38].

Differential Internal Jugular Venous Sampling

When the preoperative localization techniques are equivocal, a venous sampling may guide the surgeon to the side harboring the hyperfunctioning gland. It has been proposed to analyze simultaneously samples from both jugular veins and from a peripheral vein. In most cases, indirect regionalization, however, should be reserved for preoperative procedures particularly after an extended previous exploration.

Treatment

Therapeutic intervention in dysbalanced mineral-metabolic pathways should consider multiple pathways as outlined in the pathophysiology chapter. In brief and principle, intervention can be done at subsequent levels. Vitamin D replacement in "hormonal doses" acknowledges the central role of that hormone in CKD-MBD. Abolishment of the activity of the parathyroid can be performed by either excision of the glands totally or in parts, by pharmacological intervention in PTH secretion by means of calcimimetics or by "pharmacological vitamin D dose intervention" with the active, double hydroxylated form of vitamin D (calcitriol or analogs/derivatives). Not very acknowledged, but helpful, is treating CKD-MBD by modified dialysis conditions, which will be considered first.

Impact of Dialysis Techniques

Both hemo (HD) and peritoneal dialysis (PD) fluids do use external solute conditions which have been based on a positive net calcium balance to suppress PTH secretion of patients in earlier era. In hemodialysis, calcium bath has been set to 1.5 or 1.75 mEq/l, in PD to 1.2 mEq/l. Nowadays, with the focus on avoidance of PTH oversuppression along with low turnover ROD, calcium baths will be fixed at 1.0–1.5 mEq/l in HD or at 0.9–1.2 mEq/l in PD targeting a neutral calcium balance. That goal, however, is influenced by further dialysis conditions and might be difficult to accomplish. Since patients exhibit different bone status, individualization with regard to clinical condition is a necessary tool to consider [45].

Vitamin D Analogues

Prospective studies have shown that pharmacological doses of Calcitriol and other active vitamin D derivatives suppress parathyroid function and lower PTH levels in CKD and reduced even mortality in retrospective data analysis [46]. Osseous effects include a reduction in bone turnover, improvement of osteitits fibrosa, and stimulation of bone mineralization. Side effects comprise hypercalcemia and hyperphosphatemia. Oral and intravenous forms are on the market, which can be adapted to the kind of treatment, to which patients are subjected (Table 5.4).

The correction of vitamin D deficiency (as assessed by low 25 vitamin D 1-25 OH_2D) in CKD patients has not yet been proven to result in better clinical outcomes. However in routine clinical practice, a vitamin D 1-25 OH_2D level of 45 ng/ml is currently considered optimal and can be reached by daily or weekly application of 1,000 or 10,000 international units, respectively. Hypocalcemia, which is on the other hand a frequent side effect of active vitamin D (i.e., calcitriol), is not common with low inactive vitamin D 1-25 OH_2D (i.e., low 25 vitamin D) and the therapy is not costly. Therefore, many nephrologists treat their patients routinely with vitamin D_2 or D_3 during European and American winter seasons with low light conditions.

Table 5.4 Indication for parathyroidectomy in primary HPT

Increase of serum calcium	>0.26 mEq/l above upper reference
Calcium excretion/24 h	>400 mg
eGFR	<60 ml/min
Bone density *t*-score	<2.5
Age	<50 years

Table 5.5 Indication for parathyroidectomy in secondary HPT

Serum calcium × phosphorus product	>5.5 mEq^2/l^2
Serum calcium	>2.8 mEq/l
Bone pain, pruritus of no other cause	Any
ROD type 1 and 3	Any
Interstitial calcifications, calciphylaxis	Any
Patient awaiting renal transplantation	Need of cinacalcet >30 micg daily

Parathyroidectomy

In primary HPT due to adenoma, surgery is the primary therapy of choice to avoid secondary end-organ damage with renal calcinosis being the first line (indications in Table 5.5). Indications were defined by a 2002 National Institute's of Health summary statement [47]. A clear indication is given along with high-turnover ROD (types 1 and 3) refractory to active vitamin D and calcimimetics. In non- or oligosymptomatic patients, particularly with psychiatric symptoms, decision-making has to incorporate individual aspects of the patients (Table 5.6).

Table 5.6 Active vitamin D analogs

Generic name	Biochemistry	Dosage intravenous (micg)	Dosage oral
Calcitriol	1,25-Dihydroxyvitamin D_3	1–2 micg three times per week	0.25–0.5 micg once daily (up to 2 μg after PTx)
Alfacalcidol	1-Hydroxycholecalciferol	No data	0.25–1 micg once daily (up to 3 μg after PTx)
Doxecalciferol	Synthetic derivative of 1-hydroxycholecalciferol	4 micg three times per week	10 micg three times per week
Paricalcitol	Synthetic derivative of 1,25-dihydroxyvitamin D_3	2–6 micg three times per week	1–5 micg three times per week

These "nonspecific" symptoms, however, can be sufficiently treated by PTX. Furthermore, reduction of blood pressure, left ventricular hypertrophy after PTX have been reported [48–53]. In young patients with established but not sufficient effective conservative therapy, indication for surgery should be established more liberally compared to older and multimorbid patients.

Despite the introduction of new therapeutics like calcimimetics or vitamin D derivatives, these classical indications are still valid in the presence of drug resistance [54]. A recent study has shown the increased mortality due to cardiovascular events in chronic renal failure patients [55].

HPT can resolve after kidney transplantation, but persistent disease may occur in 10–50% of the patients [56]. Recently, the consequences of abnormal mineral metabolism after kidney transplantation have been evaluated in a retrospective study. 11–25% of patients showed abnormal serum calcium or an increased Ca × P product within the first year after kidney transplantation. A calcium >10.5 mg/dl at 3 months was identified as an independent risk factor for recipient death (OR 3.0; 95% CI: 1.2–7.4); a Ca >10.5 mg/dl at 12 months was an independent risk factor for death censored graft loss (OR 4.0; 95% CI: 1.2–14) [57]. Other retrospective studies showed reduced graft survival after PTX following kidney transplantation [58], and was augmented by another German [59] but contradicted by Dutch study [49, 60]

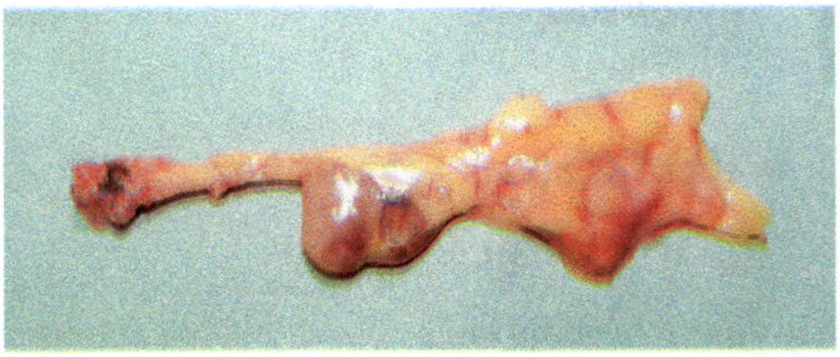

Fig. 5.12 Operative figure of an adenomatous parathyroid gland within the thyreothymic ligament

Operative Technique

In case of a conventional surgical procedure, a *Kocher's* incision is the standard approach to the thyroid and the parathyroids. The strap muscles are divided in the midline, the parathyroids can then be approached on either side. A precise anatomic knowledge is the key for a rapid and safe exploration (Fig. 5.12).

In case of a positive preoperative localization in one or two investigations, a unilateral preparation is justified. After the removal of one enlarged gland, an intraoperative PTH allows to decide whether or not a further neck exploration is required. In contrast to a systematic bilateral exploration, an adequate drop of the PTH in the PTH assay after extirpation of one enlarged gland allows to finish the operation. However the interpretation of the results remains controversial in some details, the success rates of parathyroid surgery using this technique reach 96–98%.

In case of secondary HPT, a bilateral exploration is mandatory in every case. There have been some controversial debates whether to perform a total or a subtotal PTX. Lorenz et al. evaluated the results of total versus subtotal PTX in renal hyperparathyroidism. They showed that measurable PTH following total PTX is the consequence of isolated cell nests that may be responsible for recurrences with time. The authors favored in their conclusions the advantage of total PTX and

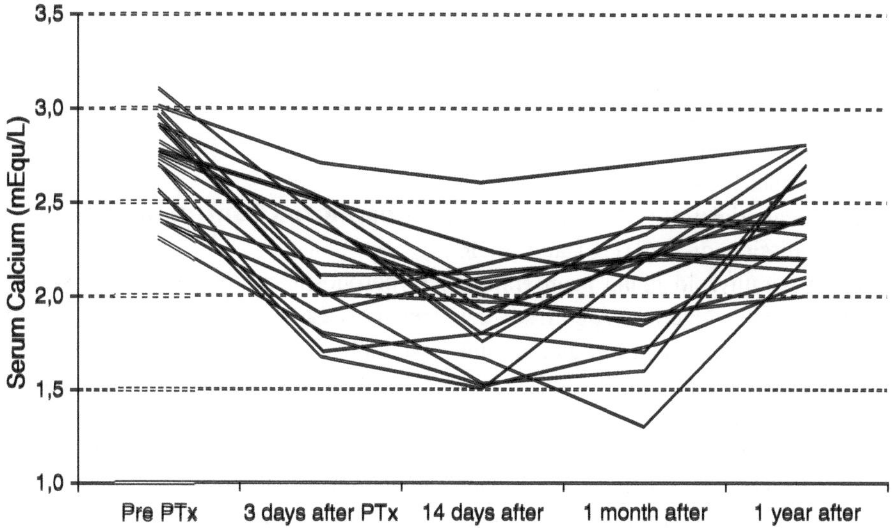

Fig. 5.13 Course of serum calcium after parathyroidectomy in renal transplant patients

cryopreservation with regard to the prevention of recurrence [61].

Follow-up of surgical removal must include close monitoring of serum calcium. Serum calcium level decreases due to recalcification of bones ("hungry bone syndrome") in a typical course within first days and weeks after surgery with the frequent sequela of symptomatic hypocalcemia (Fig. 5.13). Typical symptoms include diathesis and muscular cramps, i.e., the clinical picture of tetanus. Therefore, calcium must be supported orally or even intravenously, necessitating a central venous line. Intravenous calcium infusion raises the danger of cardiac arrhythmia and must not be avoided by using infusion rates less than 5 me/h. Oral calcium frequently causes nausea and vomiting. To overcome these shortcomings, active vitamin D beginning with a (high) daily dose of 2 micg is the therapy of best choice and should be titrated to low-to-normal serum calcium concentration. Since "hungry bone" resolves after weeks to months, that active D therapy has to be adapted following laboratory controls every 1–4 weeks.

Cryopreservation of Parathyroid Tissue

In 1975, S.A. Wells reported his first experiences in autotransplantation of parathyroid tissue [62]. In 29 patients, Wells et al. demonstrated the functional status of the glands 1 year after transplantation. The technique of immediate transplantation of parathyroid tissue during total thyroidectomy of cancer has been proposed in 1977 [63]. The risk of recurrent hyperparathyroidism following transplantation of parathyroid tissue from a parathyroid adenoma has been shown first by Brennan et al. [64]. One case report has shown the occurrence of HPT after transplantation of a normal parathyroid [65].

Questions about the use of cryopreserved tissue and the viability after long-term storage are still matter of debate [66]. Brennan et al. first described viable grafted parathyroids after as long as 18 months of cryopreservation [67].

Independent of the surgical approach, a cryopreservation of parathyroid tissue should be planned in every case of secondary and sporadic or hereditary multiglandular hyperparathyroidism. A frozen section of the parathyroids to be cryopreserved is recommended. The tissue is placed in ice-cold physiologic saline solution, thereafter it is placed into a Petri dish with RPMI 1640 culture medium (RPMI: Roswell Park Memorial Institute). With a sharp scalpel, fragments of 1–2 mm are prepared, 5–8 pieces are stored in one tube, several tubes may be used [68].

Calcimimetics

Calcimimetics interact with the CaR and increase its sensitivity to calcium to lower PTH secretion without increasing calcium serum concentration, which was significantly shown in a controlled, randomized clinical trial [69]. They, moreover, enhance the expression of CaR [70] and VDR [71] and inhibit parathyroid gland proliferation [72]. This differentiates calcimimetics from the vitamin D analogs, which enhance calcium and phosphate resorption from the intestinal tract and increase serum calcium and serum phosphate. The EVOLVE study, a randomized placebo-controlled outcome trial of 3,883 patients to evaluate the influence of cinacalcet on mortality is ongoing and results are expected at the end of 2011 [73]. In a meta-analysis of already conducted studies, the frequency of bone fractures and cardiovascular morbidity (hospital admissions) was reported to be reduced [74]. The KDIGO guidelines [39] give recommendations for using calcimimetics to lower PTH levels.

Calcimimetics after Renal Transplantation

After renal transplantation with a sufficient kidney graft, in the vast majority of cases, sHPT resolves together with reductions of serum calcium and phosphorus. In a few cases that process does not occur appropriately, since parathyroid glands have been proliferated due to long lasting stimulation. That process is comparable to primary HPT with low phosphorus and high calcium both in opposite to sHPT. That condition is called transplant-persistent HPT and should be treated thoroughly since grafts are in danger due to interstitial calcification. Therapy must consider specific pathophysiological features of such state, what usually makes active vitamin D inappropriate due to related hypercalcemia. Cinacalcet has been applied successfully [75–79] but is yet not approved in most European countries and the USA. PTX, in particular, in patients with already injured renal function boosts the risk of graft loss [58] but must be considered anyway in some cases. To overcome the pitfalls, it must be recommended to work-up sHPT in patients awaiting renal transplantation. Patients in need of intensive medical therapy (active vitamin D and cinacalcet >30 mg/day) should be treated with PTX and cryoconservation of glands for later autologous retransplantation.

Phosphorus Control in CKD

Hyperphosphatemia is a key issue in chronic renal disease as outlined in the introductory pathophysiology chapter. Since 50% uptake from the intestine is passive and uncontrolled, renal excretion is of crucial impact for phosphate homeostasis. However, while normophosphatemia is maintained through a wide range of renal failure presumably by the early exert of FGF-23, the association of increased phosphate levels with mortality is out of any doubt. This was shown in dialysis-dependent patients [80], in renal transplantation [57], and even in healthy subjects like the Framingham population [81, 82]. On the other hand, no randomized controlled trial (RCT) has ever been conducted comparing phosphate lowering versus no measure in terms of hard endpoint (mortality). There were, however, numerous efforts to decrease phosphate levels by means of both nonpharmaceutical and pharmaceutical measures.

As for nonpharmaceutical action taking, it is important to recognize that modification of diet with avoidance of phosphate intake is crucial to help patients maintain their phosphate homeostasis. Physicians should convey detailed information to their patients displaying the phosphorus content of daily nutrients. Of note, convenience and preconditioned food is stabilized with phosphate-containing ingredients. Gross amounts of phosphate are carried with Coke (soft drink) of any manufacturer, tinned food and softened cheese, to mention (not comprehensively) the most important ones. Phosphorus can hardly be avoided completely since it comes along with protein-rich food in general. A list of phosphate content of nutrients can be retrieved at a list of the NIH [83]. Patients in stage 5 CKD necessitating dialysis do benefit from formalized nutrition programs which declare phosphorus content and aim to reduce nutritional intake [84]. Phosphate control is of particular importance in patients undergoing peritoneal dialysis compared to hemodialysis. The overall phosphorus excretion is higher in HD compared to PD [85] and can be increased further by choosing convective procedure modalities like hemodiafiltration and usage of larger dialysis filters. However, the best measure to increase phosphorus elimination is prolongation of dialysis time, e.g., use of nocturnal dialysis three times per week for 8 h [86].

Following the need of protein-rich nutrition in hemodialysis, in a majority of patients, nutritional intake must exceed excretion capability and therefore must be coped by measures to decrease intestinal absorption. Historically (until the mid-1980s), aluminum was the cornerstone of phosphate binding. However, oral administration was complicated by systemic toxicity, which was mainly related to accumulation in brain, bone, and joints. Therefore, aluminum is nowadays mostly excluded from clinical use and clinical research, too. If such neglect is fully justified can only be speculated [87] since the poisonous properties were largely interlinked with covariates like nonsterile dialysis water or bone turnover oversuppression, which have changed significantly in recent times. The first substitute of aluminum, introduced in the late 1980s years, was calcium-based binders [88], namely calcium carbonate and calcium acetate. These drugs have medium phosphate-binding capacity compared to aluminum and were never tested for outcome in RCT. However, they are the most applied binders until recent times. Along with the discussion of extraosseous calcification in frame of CKD-MBD, calcium-containing phosphate binders have been incriminated to promote calcification-related morbidity and mortality [89, 90]. In a small RCT ($n=27$) comparing calcium carbonate and a calcium-free alternative (sevelamer), attenuation of vascular calcification has been reported [91]. Sevelamer was introduced in 1997 and acts through its anion-exchange capabilities within the bowel. Their phosphate-binding capacity is smaller compared to calcium salts and aluminum, and moderate gastrointestinal side effects are common. However, sevelamer showed in RCTs and retrospective studies slowing of calcification and amelioration of bone disease [92–96]. One RCT exploring mortality could not show a significant effect of sevelamer versus calcium salts [97].

A further calcium and aluminum-free compound is lanthanum carbonate. As aluminum, lanthanum is a triple charged metal and has been therefore discussed widely envisioning cerebral and bone accumulation and toxicity. In fact it deposits in bones, but not at the mineralization front. In animal toxicological experiments, with multiplies of human dosage, it could be detected in rat brains [98, 99] while no human central nervous system toxicity was reported so far [99, 100]. Phosphate-binding capacity is high, so the substance is in principle highly needed nonaluminum, noncalcium choice. RCTs resulted in substantial phosphate lowering capacity and showed no severe side effects [101] but a high incidence of substance discontinuation in verum groups. No RCT was targeted and powered to demonstrate mortality benefit.

Taking these issues together, there is currently no "ideal" phosphate binder available. Our current practice is summarized in Table 5.7 and can be appreciated further in a current comprehensive review from Tonelli et al. [102].

Research on new substances does focus on iron-based binders, niacin, and chitosan chewing gums while no such substances are being currently available on the market. In a phase 1 study, an iron-containing compound (SBR 759) showed phosphate reduction into the KDIGO target using a dose between 3.5 and 15 g [103], which translates into a pill burden of up to 20 tablets per day. Niacin, in opposite to direct intestinal binding of all other substances, inhibits the phosphate uptake into the bowel wall by inhibiting the small bowel phosphate cotransporter [104]. Chewing gums containing chitosan [105, 106] have experimentally shown to absorb phosphate already with salivation in the mouth.

Influencing Bone Metabolism

Serum parameters of mineral metabolism do not depict the whole complexity of CKD-MBD, in particular, the bone features end the vascular

Table 5.7 Phosphate binders, before and together with ordination consider nonpharmaceutical measures

Generic substance	Binding capacity	Indication	Side effects, caveats
Aluminum hydroxide	↑↑↑	Short-term application (2–4 weeks) for critical phosphorus levels without concomitant calcium intake	Accumulation, *brain toxicity*, aluminum osteopathy
Calcium carbonate	↑↑	Cost-effective phosphate decrease in earlier CKD stages in patients with low-to-normal serum calcium	Calcium intake, extraosseous *calcification*
Calcium acetate	↑↑↑	Cost-effective phosphate decrease in earlier CKD stages in patients with low-to-normal serum calcium, with higher binding capacity	Calcium intake, extraosseous *calcification*, plus gastrointestinal (gi) side effects
Sevelamer	↑	Phosphate decrease with no calcium intake, e.g., renal transplant setting	Gi side effects
Lanthanum carbonate	↑↑↑	Phosphate decrease with no calcium intake, e.g., renal transplant setting with higher binding capacity vs. sevelamer	Bone accumulation, CNS toxicity not principally excluded

injury permitted by such disease. To target these aspects, influencing bone turnover has come into scope during recent years again after two decades of neglect along with diminished use of bone biopsy. While having information's about ROD type, influence on bone turnover, i.e., activity of osteoclasts or osteoblasts might be a sufficient choice to treat patients with CKD-MBD.

In low-turnover ROD (type 4), osteo-arresting therapies like bisphosphonates, convey enhancement of bone disease. They are, however, currently widely applied in postmature osteoporosis even in CKD without information on bone status. Bisphosphonates might be helpful in ROD type 1 or 3, which should be established initially by bone histomorphometry. In two studies, alendronat has been proved to influence bone diseases effectively in patients with *primary* HPT [107, 108]. In a clinical analog, pHPT could be translated in sHPT without low-turnover aspects and with high HPT and therefore be treated with bisphosphonates, although no RCT for such reasoning is available

In low-turnover ROD type 4, arrest of osteoblasts must be resolved. In patients with CKD 4 or 5, most frequently, oversuppression of PTH by active vitamin D and/or positive calcium intake by phosphate binders and/or inadequately high calcium dialysis bath concentration (down to 1.0 mEq/l) must be stopped or adopted, respectively. Teriparatide, i.e., synthetic PTH, resembles a pharmaceutical alternative for enhancing bone turnover. The substance has been used for fracture-prone osteoporosis [109] and could be considered in CKD-MBD associated with abolished PTH secretion as, for instance, after PTX. In a small open-label study in seven patients undergoing chronic hemodialysis with low-turnover ROD, bone mineral density but not coronary calcification scores were improved [110].

Integrative CKD-MBD Therapy

In summary, treatment of secondary hyperparathyroidism must not target PTH levels above certain numerical thresholds alone but has to envision the concept of parathyroid function as a variable of complex regulation of the endocrine–vasculature–bone axis in CKD. A schematic proposal of integrative therapy is given in Fig. 5.14. To conduct such time-dependent and multiple-level approach, continuous monitoring of parameters of CKD-MBD is mandatory. According to recent KDIG guidelines, monthly laboratory monitoring of serum calcium and phosphorus levels in patients dependent from renal replacement therapy is recommended. PTH should be regarded at least every 3 months. Although not directly included in the guidelines, we would recommend additional monitoring of "bone markers" like Ostase every 3 months. Bone biopsy and histomorphometry should be done, when differentiation between high and low-turnover bone

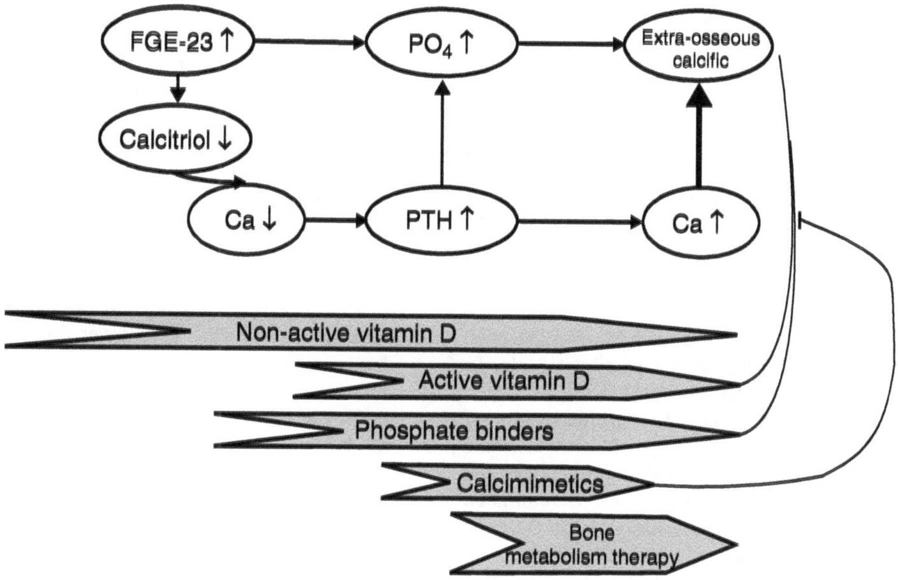

Fig. 5.14 Schematic drawing of integrative therapeutic approach in secondary HPT

disease cannot be done clinically and sufficient therapy choice can be considered. PTX is the therapy of choice in irreversible, autonomous parathyroid hypersecretion along with high-turnover bone disease with a particular regard to patients awaiting renal transplantation.

Overall, the field evolves very rapidly and further implication, e.g., of adipose and muscle tissue can be awaited during the near future. With regard to the excess mortality in CKD, physicians must make any effort, to overcome or at least lighten such disease burden in their patients.

Acknowledgments The authors want to thank Dr. Gabriele Lehmann (Jena), for critical review of the bone section and gratification of histological pictures as well as Andreas Plötner, MD (Leipzig), for gratification of Fig. 5.1.

My wife (J.B.), Karin Kaori Beige, bolstered this work by fine grasp and patience.

References

1. Marcocci C, Cetani F, Rubin MR, Silverberg SJ, Pinchera A, Bilezikian JP. Parathyroid carcinoma. J Bone Miner Res. 2008;23(12):1869–80.
2. Kouvaraki MA, Shapiro SE, Perrier ND, et al. RET proto-oncogene: a review and update of genotype-phenotype correlations in hereditary medullary thyroid cancer and associated endocrine tumors. Thyroid. 2005;15(6):531–44.
3. Heath III H, Hodgson SF, Kennedy MA. Primary hyperparathyroidism. Incidence, morbidity, and potential economic impact in a community. N Engl J Med. 1980;302(4):189–93.
4. Mak RH, Wong JH. The vitamin D/parathyroid hormone axis in the pathogenesis of hypertension and insulin resistance in uremia. Miner Electrolyte Metab. 1992;18(2–5):156–9.
5. Brown EM. PTH secretion in vivo and in vitro. Regulation by calcium and other secretagogues. Miner Electrolyte Metab. 1982;8(3–4):130–50.
6. Brown EM, Wilson RE, Eastman RC, Pallotta J, Marynick SP. Abnormal regulation of parathyroid hormone release by calcium in secondary hyperparathyroidism due to chronic renal failure. J Clin Endocrinol Metab. 1982;54(1):172–9.
7. Rodriguez M, Canalejo A, Garfia B, Aguilera E, Almaden Y. Pathogenesis of refractory secondary hyperparathyroidism. Kidney Int Suppl. 2002;80: 155–60.
8. Felsenfeld AJ, Rodriguez M, guilera-Tejero E. Dynamics of parathyroid hormone secretion in health and secondary hyperparathyroidism. Clin J Am Soc Nephrol. 2007;2(6):1283–305.
9. Holgado R, Haire H, Ross D, et al. Effect of a low calcium dialysate on parathyroid hormone secretion in diabetic patients on maintenance hemodialysis. J Bone Miner Res. 2000;15(5):927–35.
10. Gutierrez O, Isakova T, Rhee E, et al. Fibroblast growth factor-23 mitigates hyperphosphatemia but accentuates calcitriol deficiency in chronic kidney disease. J Am Soc Nephrol. 2005;16(7): 2205–15.
11. Benet-Pages A, Lorenz-Depiereux B, Zischka H, White KE, Econs MJ, Strom TM. FGF23 is processed

by proprotein convertases but not by PHEX. Bone. 2004;35(2):455–62.
12. Rodriguez M, Felsenfeld AJ. PTH, FGF-23 and early CKD. Nephrol Dial Transplant. 2008;23(11): 3391–3.
13. Quarles LD. FGF23, PHEX, and MEPE regulation of phosphate homeostasis and skeletal mineralization. Am J Physiol Endocrinol Metab. 2003;285(1): E1–9.
14. Yu X, White KE. FGF23 and disorders of phosphate homeostasis. Cytokine Growth Factor Rev. 2005;16(2):221–32.
15. Canalejo R, Canalejo A, Martinez-Moreno JM, et al. FGF23 fails to inhibit uremic parathyroid glands. J Am Soc Nephrol. 2010;21(7):1125–35.
16. Panda DK, Miao D, Bolivar I, et al. Inactivation of the 25-hydroxyvitamin D 1alpha-hydroxylase and vitamin D receptor demonstrates independent and interdependent effects of calcium and vitamin D on skeletal and mineral homeostasis. J Biol Chem. 2004;279(16):16754–66.
17. Wang AY, Ho SS, Wang M, et al. Cardiac valvular calcification as a marker of atherosclerosis and arterial calcification in end-stage renal disease. Arch Intern Med. 2005;165(3):327–32.
18. Foley RN, Parfrey PS. Cardiovascular disease and mortality in ESRD. J Nephrol. 1998;11(5):239–45.
19. Block GA, Hulbert-Shearon TE, Levin NW, Port FK. Association of serum phosphorus and calcium x phosphate product with mortality risk in chronic hemodialysis patients: a national study. Am J Kidney Dis. 1998;31(4):607–17.
20. Schwarz A, Mengel M, Gwinner W, et al. Risk factors for chronic allograft nephropathy after renal transplantation: a protocol biopsy study. Kidney Int. 2005;67(1):341–8.
21. Cicone JS, Petronis JB, Embert CD, Spector DA. Successful treatment of calciphylaxis with intravenous sodium thiosulfate. Am J Kidney Dis. 2004;43(6):1104–8.
22. Araya CE, Fennell RS, Neiberger RE, Dharnidharka VR. Sodium thiosulfate treatment for calcific uremic arteriolopathy in children and young adults. Clin J Am Soc Nephrol. 2006;1(6):1161–6.
23. Tokashiki K, Ishida A, Kouchi M, et al. Successful management of critical limb ischemia with intravenous sodium thiosulfate in a chronic hemodialysis patient. Clin Nephrol. 2006;66(2):140–3.
24. Meissner M, Bauer R, Beier C, et al. Sodium thiosulphate as a promising therapeutic option to treat calciphylaxis. Dermatology. 2006;212(4):373–6.
25. Ackermann F, Levy A, Daugas E, et al. Sodium thiosulfate as first-line treatment for calciphylaxis. Arch Dermatol. 2007;143(10):1336–7.
26. Pasch A, Schaffner T, Huynh-Do U, Frey BM, Frey FJ, Farese S. Sodium thiosulfate prevents vascular calcifications in uremic rats. Kidney Int. 2008;74(11): 1444–53.
27. Musso CG, Enz P, Vidal F, et al. Oral sodium thiosulfate solution as a secondary preventive treatment for calciphylaxis in dialysis patients. Saudi J Kidney Dis Transpl. 2008;19(5):820–1.
28. Hayden MR, Goldsmith DJ. Sodium thiosulfate: new hope for the treatment of calciphylaxis. Semin Dial. 2010;23(3):258–62.
29. Velasco N, MacGregor MS, Innes A, MacKay IG. Successful treatment of calciphylaxis with cinacalcet-an alternative to parathyroidectomy? Nephrol Dial Transplant. 2006;21(7):1999–2004.
30. Hermans MM, Brandenburg V, Ketteler M, et al. Association of serum fetuin-A levels with mortality in dialysis patients. Kidney Int. 2007;72(2):202–7.
31. Kuzniar J, Porazko T, Klinger M. Relationship between fetuin-A concentration, elevated levels of inflammatory markers, and arterial wall stiffness in end-stage kidney disease. J Ren Nutr. 2008;18(1): 83–6.
32. Schafer C, Heiss A, Schwarz A, et al. The serum protein alpha 2-Heremans-Schmid glycoprotein/fetuin-A is a systemically acting inhibitor of ectopic calcification. J Clin Invest. 2003;112(3): 357–66.
33. Koos R, Krueger T, Westenfeld R, et al. Relation of circulating Matrix Gla-Protein and anticoagulation status in patients with aortic valve calcification. Thromb Haemost. 2009;101(4):706–13.
34. Moe SM, Chen NX. Pathophysiology of vascular calcification in chronic kidney disease. Circ Res. 2004;95(6):560–7.
35. Bilezikian JP, Rubin M, Silverberg SJ. Asymptomatic primary hyperparathyroidism. Arq Bras Endocrinol Metabol. 2006;50(4):647–56.
36. Bilezikian JP, Silverberg SJ. Clinical spectrum of primary hyperparathyroidism. Rev Endocr Metab Disord. 2000;1(4):237–45.
37. Gayed IW, Kim EE, Broussard WF, et al. The value of 99mTc-sestamibi SPECT/CT over conventional SPECT in the evaluation of parathyroid adenomas or hyperplasia. J Nucl Med. 2005;46(2):248–52.
38. Mihai R, Simon D, Hellman P. Imaging for primary hyperparathyroidism—an evidence-based analysis. Langenbecks Arch Surg. 2009;394(5):765–84.
39. Kidney Disease: Improving Global Outcomes (KDIGO) CKD-MBD Work Group. KDIGO clinical practice guideline for the diagnosis, evaluation, prevention, and treatment of Chronic Kidney Disease-Mineral and Bone Disorder (CKD-MBD). Kidney Int Suppl. 2009;113:S1–130.
40. Klein KB, Orwoll ES, Lieberman DA, Meier DE, McClung MR, Parfitt AM. Metabolic bone disease in asymptomatic men after partial gastrectomy with Billroth II anastomosis. Gastroenterology. 1987;92: 608–16.
41. Merz WA, Schenk RK. Quantitative structural analysis of human cancellous bone. Acta Anat (Basel). 1970;75(1):54–66.
42. Malluche HH, Sherman D, Meyer W, Massry SG. A new semiautomatic method for quantitative static and dynamic bone histology. Calcif Tissue Int. 1982;34(5):439–48.

43. Lehmann G, Ott U, Kaemmerer D, Schuetze J, Wolf G. Bone histomorphometry and biochemical markers of bone turnover in patients with chronic kidney disease Stages 3–5. Clin Nephrol. 2008;70(4):296–305.
44. Irvin III GL, Carneiro D. Parathyroid hyperplasia: parathyroidectomy. Philadelphia: Elsevier Saunders (Textbook of Endocrine Surgery); 2005. p. 472–80. Ref Type: Serial (Book,Monograph).
45. Gotch F, Levin NW, Kotanko P. Calcium balance in dialysis is best managed by adjusting dialysate calcium guided by kinetic modeling of the interrelationship between calcium intake, dose of vitamin D analogues and the dialysate calcium concentration. Blood Purif. 2010;29(2):163–76.
46. Teng M, Wolf M, Lowrie E, Ofsthun N, Lazarus JM, Thadhani R. Survival of patients undergoing hemodialysis with paricalcitol or calcitriol therapy. N Engl J Med. 2003;349(5):446–56.
47. Bilezikian JP, Khan AA, Potts Jr JT. Guidelines for the management of asymptomatic primary hyperparathyroidism: summary statement from the third international workshop. J Clin Endocrinol Metab. 2009;94(2):335–9.
48. Al-Hilali N, Hussain N, Ataia AI, Al-Azmi M, Al-Helal B, Johny KV. Hypertension and hyperparathyroidism are associated with left ventricular hypertrophy in patients on hemodialysis. Indian J Nephrol. 2009;19(4):153–7.
49. Evenepoel P, Claes K, Kuypers D, Maes B, Vanrenterghem Y. Impact of parathyroidectomy on renal graft function, blood pressure and serum lipids in kidney transplant recipients: a single centre study. Nephrol Dial Transplant. 2005;20(8):1714–20.
50. Nasri H, Baradaran A, Naderi AS. Close association between parathyroid hormone and left ventricular function and structure in end-stage renal failure patients under maintenance hemodialysis. Acta Med Austriaca. 2004;31(3):67–72.
51. Piovesan A, Molineri N, Casasso F, et al. Left ventricular hypertrophy in primary hyperparathyroidism. Effects of successful parathyroidectomy. Clin Endocrinol (Oxf). 1999;50(3):321–8.
52. Rosenthal FD, Roy S. Hypertension and hyperparathyroidism. Br Med J. 1972;4(837):396–7.
53. Rubin MR, Maurer MS, McMahon DJ, Bilezikian JP, Silverberg SJ. Arterial stiffness in mild primary hyperparathyroidism. J Clin Endocrinol Metab. 2005;90(6):3326–30.
54. Dotzenrath C. Indications for parathyroidectomy in renal hyperparathyroidism: comments on the significance of new therapeutics. Chirurg. 2010;81(10):902–8.
55. Costa-Hong V, Jorgetti V, Gowdak LH, Moyses RM, Krieger EM, De Lima JJ. Parathyroidectomy reduces cardiovascular events and mortality in renal hyperparathyroidism. Surgery. 2007;142(5):699–703.
56. Alfrey AC, Jenkins D, Groth CG, Schorr WS, Gecelter L, Ogden DA. Resolution of hyperparathyroidism, renal osteodystrophy and metastatic calcification after renal homotransplantation. N Engl J Med. 1968;279(25):1349–56.
57. Egbuna OI, Taylor JG, Bushinsky DA, Zand MS. Elevated calcium phosphate product after renal transplantation is a risk factor for graft failure. Clin Transplant. 2007;21(4):558–66.
58. Lee PP, Schiffmann L, Offermann G, Beige J. Effects of parathyroidectomy on renal allograft survival. Kidney Blood Press Res. 2004;27(3):191–6.
59. Schwarz A, Rustien G, Merkel S, Radermacher J, Haller H. Decreased renal transplant function after parathyroidectomy. Nephrol Dial Transplant. 2007;22(2):584–91.
60. Evenepoel P, Claes K, Kuypers DR, Debruyne F, Vanrenterghem Y. Parathyroidectomy after successful kidney transplantation: a single centre study. Nephrol Dial Transplant. 2007;22(6):1730–7.
61. Lorenz K, Ukkat J, Sekulla C, Gimm O, Brauckhoff M, Dralle H. Total parathyroidectomy without autotransplantation for renal hyperparathyroidism: experience with a qPTH-controlled protocol. World J Surg. 2006;30(5):743–51.
62. Wells Jr SA, Gunnells JC, Shelburne JD, Schneider AB, Sherwood LM. Transplantation of the parathyroid glands in man: clinical indications and results. Surgery. 1975;78(1):34–44.
63. Paloyan E, Lawrence AM, Paloyan D. Successful autotransplantation of the parathyroid glands during total thyroidectomy for carcinoma. Surg Gynecol Obstet. 1977;145(3):364–8.
64. Brennan MF, Brown EM, Marx SJ, et al. Recurrent hyperparathyroidism from an autotransplanted parathyroid adenoma. N Engl J Med. 1978;299(19):1057–9.
65. D'Avanzo A, Parangi S, Morita E, Duh QY, Siperstein AE, Clark OH. Hyperparathyroidism after thyroid surgery and autotransplantation of histologically normal parathyroid glands. J Am Coll Surg. 2000;190(5):546–52.
66. de Menezes Montenegro FL, Custodio MR, Arap SS, et al. Successful implant of long-term cryopreserved parathyroid glands after total parathyroidectomy. Head Neck. 2007;29(3):296–300.
67. Brennan MF, Brown EM, Spiegel AM, et al. Autotransplantation of cryopreserved parathyroid tissue in man. Ann Surg. 1979;189(2):139–42.
68. Al-Sobhi SCO. Parathyroid hyperplasia: parathyroidectomy. Philadelphia: Elsevier Saunders (Textbook of Endocrine Surgery); 2005. p. 481–8. Ref Type: Serial (Book, Monograph).
69. Block GA, Martin KJ, de Francisco AL, et al. Cinacalcet for secondary hyperparathyroidism in patients receiving hemodialysis. N Engl J Med. 2004;350(15):1516–25.
70. Mizobuchi M, Hatamura I, Ogata H, et al. Calcimimetic compound upregulates decreased calcium-sensing receptor expression level in parathyroid glands of rats with chronic renal insufficiency. J Am Soc Nephrol. 2004;15(10):2579–87.

71. Rodriguez M, Nemeth E, Martin D. The calcium-sensing receptor: a key factor in the pathogenesis of secondary hyperparathyroidism. Am J Physiol Renal Physiol. 2005;288(2):F253–64.
72. Colloton M, Shatzen E, Miller G, et al. Cinacalcet HCl attenuates parathyroid hyperplasia in a rat model of secondary hyperparathyroidism. Kidney Int. 2005;67(2):467–76.
73. Chertow GM, Pupim LB, Block GA, et al. Evaluation of Cinacalcet Therapy to Lower Cardiovascular Events (EVOLVE): rationale and design overview. Clin J Am Soc Nephrol. 2007;2(5):898–905.
74. Cunningham J, Danese M, Olson K, Klassen P, Chertow GM. Effects of the calcimimetic cinacalcet HCl on cardiovascular disease, fracture, and health-related quality of life in secondary hyperparathyroidism. Kidney Int. 2005;68(4):1793–800.
75. Kruse AE, Eisenberger U, Frey FJ, Mohaupt MG. The calcimimetic cinacalcet normalizes serum calcium in renal transplant patients with persistent hyperparathyroidism. Nephrol Dial Transplant. 2005;20(7):1311–4.
76. Apostolou T, Damianou L, Kotsiev V, Drakopoulos S, Hadjiconstantinou V. Treatment of severe hypocalcaemia due to refractory hyperparathyroidism in renal transplant patients with the calcimimetic agent cinacalcet. Clin Nephrol. 2006;65(5):374–7.
77. Borchhardt KA, Heinzl H, Mayerwoger E, Horl WH, Haas M, Sunder-Plassmann G. Cinacalcet increases calcium excretion in hypercalcemic hyperparathyroidism after kidney transplantation. Transplantation. 2008;86(7):919–24.
78. Lopez V, Toledo R, Sola E, et al. Treatment with cinacalcet in 29 kidney transplant patients with persistent hyperparathyroidism. Transplant Proc. 2009;41(6):2394–5.
79. Serra AL, Savoca R, Huber AR, et al. Effective control of persistent hyperparathyroidism with cinacalcet in renal allograft recipients. Nephrol Dial Transplant. 2007;22(2):577–83.
80. Block GA, Klassen PS, Lazarus JM, Ofsthun N, Lowrie EG, Chertow GM. Mineral metabolism, mortality, and morbidity in maintenance hemodialysis. J Am Soc Nephrol. 2004;15(8):2208–18.
81. Dhingra R, Sullivan LM, Fox CS, et al. Relations of serum phosphorus and calcium levels to the incidence of cardiovascular disease in the community. Arch Intern Med. 2007;167(9):879–85.
82. Dhingra R, Gona P, Benjamin EJ, et al. Relations of serum phosphorus levels to echocardiographic left ventricular mass and incidence of heart failure in the community. Eur J Heart Fail. 2010;12(8):812–8.
83. USDA National Nutrient Database for Standard Reference, Release 17. http://dietarysupplementdatabase.usda.nih.gov/. Accessed at Nov 2nd 2010.
84. Kuhlmann MK. Practical approaches to management of hyperphosphatemia: can we improve the current situation? Blood Purif. 2007;25(1):120–4.
85. Granja CA, Juergensen P, Finkelstein FO. Phosphate balance in peritoneal dialysis patients: role of ultrafiltration. Contrib Nephrol. 2009;163:198–205.
86. Mucsi I, Hercz G, Uldall R, Ouwendyk M, Francoeur R, Pierratos A. Control of serum phosphate without any phosphate binders in patients treated with nocturnal hemodialysis. Kidney Int. 1998;53:1399–404.
87. Jenkins DA, Gouldesbrough D, Smith GD, Cowie JF, Winney RJ. Can low-dosage aluminium hydroxide control the plasma phosphate without bone toxicity? Nephrol Dial Transplant. 1989;4(1):51–6.
88. Nakamura M, Suzuki H, Ohno Y, et al. Oral calcium carbonate administration ameliorates the progression of renal failure in rats with hypertension. Am J Kidney Dis. 1995;25:910–7.
89. Chertow GM, Raggi P, Chasan-Taber S, Bommer J, Holzer H, Burke SK. Determinants of progressive vascular calcification in haemodialysis patients. Nephrol Dial Transplant. 2004;19(6):1489–96.
90. Zacharias JM, Fontaine B, Fine A. Calcium use increases risk of calciphylaxis: a case-control study. Perit Dial Int. 1999;19(3):248–52.
91. Asmus HG, Braun J, Krause R, et al. Two year comparison of sevelamer and calcium carbonate effects on cardiovascular calcification and bone density. Nephrol Dial Transplant. 2005;20(8):1653–61.
92. Ferreira A, Frazao JM, Monier-Faugere MC, et al. Effects of sevelamer hydrochloride and calcium carbonate on renal osteodystrophy in hemodialysis patients. J Am Soc Nephrol. 2008;19(2):405–12.
93. Izumi M, Morita S, Nishian Y, et al. Switching from calcium carbonate to sevelamer hydrochloride has suppressive effects on the progression of aortic calcification in hemodialysis patients: assessment using plain chest X-ray films. Ren Fail. 2008;30(10):952–8.
94. McIntyre CW, Patel V, Taylor GS, Fluck RJ. A prospective study of combination therapy for hyperphosphataemia with calcium-containing phosphate binders and sevelamer in hypercalcaemic haemodialysis patients. Nephrol Dial Transplant. 2002;17(9):1643–8.
95. Nagano N, Miyata S, Abe M, Wakita S, Kobayashi N, Wada M. Effects of intermittent treatment with sevelamer hydrochloride on parathyroid hyperplasia and vascular calcification in rats with chronic kidney disease. Clin Calcium. 2005;15 Suppl 1:35–9. discussion 39–40.
96. Takei T, Otsubo S, Uchida K, et al. Effects of sevelamer on the progression of vascular calcification in patients on chronic haemodialysis. Nephron Clin Pract. 2008;108(4):c278–83.
97. Suki WN, Zabaneh R, Cangiano JL, et al. Effects of sevelamer and calcium-based phosphate binders on mortality in hemodialysis patients. Kidney Int. 2007;72(9):1130–7.
98. Loghman-Adham M. Safety of new phosphate binders for chronic renal failure. Drug Saf. 2003;26(15):1093–115.
99. Feng L, Xiao H, He X, et al. Neurotoxicological consequence of long-term exposure to lanthanum. Toxicol Lett. 2006;165(2):112–20.

100. Finn WF. Lanthanum carbonate versus standard therapy for the treatment of hyperphosphatemia: safety and efficacy in chronic maintenance hemodialysis patients. Clin Nephrol. 2006;65(3):191–202.
101. Albaaj F, Hutchison AJ. Lanthanum carbonate for the treatment of hyperphosphataemia in renal failure and dialysis patients. Expert Opin Pharmacother. 2005;6(2):319–28.
102. Tonelli M, Pannu N, Manns B. Oral phosphate binders in patients with kidney failure. N Engl J Med. 2010;362(14):1312–24.
103. Block GA, Brillhart SL, Persky MS, Amer A, Slade AJ. Efficacy and safety of SBR759, a new iron-based phosphate binder. Kidney Int. 2010;77(10):897–903.
104. Ahmed MH. Niacin as potential treatment for dyslipidemia and hyperphosphatemia associated with chronic renal failure: the need for clinical trials. Ren Fail. 2010;32(5):642–6.
105. Eknoyan G. Salivary phosphorus binding: a novel approach to control hyperphosphatemia. J Am Soc Nephrol. 2009;20(3):460–2.
106. Savica V, Calo LA, Monardo P, et al. Salivary phosphate-binding chewing gum reduces hyperphosphatemia in dialysis patients. J Am Soc Nephrol. 2009;20(3):639–44.
107. Rossini M, Gatti D, Isaia G, Sartori L, Braga V, Adami S. Effects of oral alendronate in elderly patients with osteoporosis and mild primary hyperparathyroidism. J Bone Miner Res. 2001;16(1):113–9.
108. Khan AA, Bilezikian JP, Kung AW, et al. Alendronate in primary hyperparathyroidism: a double-blind, randomized, placebo-controlled trial. J Clin Endocrinol Metab. 2004;89(7):3319–25.
109. Gallacher SJ, Dixon T. Impact of Treatments for postmenopausal osteoporosis (bisphosphonates, parathyroid hormone, strontium ranelate, and denosumab) on bone quality: a systematic review. Calcif Tissue Int. 2010;87(6):469–84.
110. Cejka D, Kodras K, Bader T, Haas M. Treatment of Hemodialysis-Associated Adynamic Bone Disease with Teriparatide (PTH(1-34)): A Pilot Study. Kidney Blood Press Res. 2010;33(3):221–6.

Calcific Uremic Arteriolopathy (Calciphylaxis)

6

Earl H. Rudolph and Edgar V. Lerma

Abstract

Calcific uremic arteriolopathy (CUA), also referred to as calciphylaxis, is a poorly understood syndrome of vascular calcification and cutaneous necrosis first described in 1898 when its presence was associated with uremia. At present, it is believed to be caused by arteriolar calcification and cutaneous plaque formation which causes vascular stenosis which predisposes to thrombotic occlusion causing tissue ischemia and violaceous skin lesions that may progress to nonhealing ulceration and gangrene which may lead to amputation, sepsis, and death. Although there are many reports of calciphylaxis associated with nonuremic causes, the majority of cases occur in patients with end-stage renal disease on dialysis. It is likely that uremia creates a favorable milieu for extraskeletal deposition of hydroxyapatite in soft tissues including small vessels, predisposing to thrombus formation, and the development of calciphylaxis. In this chapter, the authors present a discussion of the basic and clinical aspects of the disease process as well as novel therapeutic options.

Keywords

Calciphylaxis • Calcific uremic arteriolopathy • Hyperparathyroidism • Cutaneous • Calcinosis • Hyperphosphatemia • Parathyroidectomy • Hydroxyapatite • Intimal • Osteoblast • Osteoprotegerin • Fetuin-A • Bone morphogenic protein • Osteopontin • Leptin • Osteomalacia • Sevelamer • Lanthium • Sodium thiosulfate • Cinacalcet

E.H. Rudolph, DO (✉)
Department of Nephrology and Hypertension,
Georgetown University Medical Center, 3800 Reservoir
Road NW—6 PHC, Washington, DC 20007, USA
e-mail: earlrudolph@yahoo.com

E.V. Lerma, MD
Department of Medicine, Section of Nephrology,
University of Illinois at Chicago College of Medicine,
3543 Wisconsin Ave, Berwyn, IL 60402, USA

A.A. Licata and E.V. Lerma (eds.), *Diseases of the Parathyroid Glands*,
DOI 10.1007/978-1-4419-5550-0_6,

Abbreviations

25-(OH)D_3	25-Hydroxyvitamin D_3 (also known as: 25-hydroxycholecalciferol, calcifediol, or calcidiol)
1,25-(OH_2)D_3	1,25-Dihydroxyvitamin D_3 (also known as: 1,25-dihydroxycholecalciferol or calcitriol)
ApoE	Apolipoprotein E
BMP	Bone morphogenic protein
CKD	Chronic kidney disease
CKD-MBD	Chronic kidney disease-mineral and bone disorder (also known as: renal osteodystrophy)
EGFRs	Epidermal growth factor receptors
ESRD	End-stage renal disease
FGF-23	Fibroblast growth factor-23
HPT	Hyperparathyroidism
IL-1, IL-6	Interleukin-1 and -6
LDL	Low-density lipoprotein
MGP	Matrix Gla protein
OPG	Osteoprotegerin
OPN	Osteopontin
PTH	Parathyroid hormone (also known as: parathormone or parathyrin)
TGF-α	Transforming growth factor-alpha
TGF-β	Transforming growth factor-beta
TNF-α	Tumor necrosis factor-alpha
ucMGP	Uncarboxylated matrix Gla protein

Introduction

Historical Perspective

Calcific uremic arteriolopathy (CUA), more commonly known as calciphylaxis, is a poorly understood syndrome of vascular calcification and cutaneous necrosis first described in 1898 by Bryant and White when they noted its association with uremia. This relationship was not widely accepted because while vascular calcification with uremia was relatively common, vascular calcification with cutaneous necrosis was relatively rare. In 1962, Hans Selye developed an experimental model of systemic calcification with similar cutaneous manifestations and introduced the term *calciphylaxis* to describe this uncommon condition [1, 2]. In 1976, Gipstein et al. first described the clinical significance of this syndrome in terms of morbidity and mortality in a case series of 11 patients with late-stage chronic kidney disease (CKD), presumptive secondary hyperparathyroidism (HPT), and severe hyperphosphatemia who developed medial calcinosis of the arteries and painful ischemic ulcers [3]. All but one patient underwent total or subtotal parathyroidectomy with ulcer healing occurring in seven patients. The etiology and pathogenesis of calciphylaxis are still a matter of investigation as are therapeutic strategies to better manage this condition. However, it is now clear that calciphylaxis is caused by arteriolar calcification and cutaneous plaque formation which causes vascular stenosis which predisposes to thrombotic occlusion causing tissue ischemia and violaceous skin lesions that may progress to nonhealing ulceration and gangrene which may lead to amputation, sepsis, and death. Based on these observations, it has recently been proposed that calciphylaxis is the cutaneous equivalent of a myocardial infarction, an analogy that may lead to development of more standardized and rational approaches to disease management [4]. Moreover, the absence of vascular calcification and thrombotic occlusion in the Selye animal model of calciphylaxis and its presence in humans has led to acceptance of the more recently introduced term *calcific uremic arteriolopathy* to describe this condition in humans [1, 2, 5, 6]. Many other terms used or proposed in the literature to describe calciphylaxis are summarized (Table 6.1) [3, 5, 7–23]. However, the term *calciphylaxis* is still widely used to describe this disease in humans and will be utilized in this discussion as a matter of simplicity and convenience.

Prevalence and Mortality

The prevalence of calciphylaxis in the general population is largely unknown; however, a recent German study of the etiology of chronic leg ulcers in 31,169 patients found that venous insufficiency was the dominant cause accounting for 47.6% of cases, whereas calciphylaxis was among the rarer causes accounting for only 1.1% of cases [24].

Table 6.1 Other terms used or proposed to describe calciphylaxis

Calcific uremic arteriolopathy[a]
Uremic gangrene syndrome
Arterial calcification and gangrene
Vascular calcification-cutaneous necrosis syndrome
Obliterative calcific-thrombotic arteriolopathy
Uremic small artery disease
Small-vessel calcification
Ischemic tissue necrosis
Calcifying panniculitis
Uremic necrosis
Necrotizing livedo reticularis
Disseminated ischemic necrosis
Cutaneous pseudovasculitis syndrome

[a]Currently the most widely accepted terminology

From a practical standpoint, calciphylaxis has been estimated to occur in approximately 1–4% of patients with end-stage renal disease (ESRD) on chronic peritoneal or hemodialysis [17, 25, 26]. In a retrospective case–control study, the diagnosis of calciphylaxis in dialysis patients was associated with an eightfold increased risk of mortality [27]. A 6-month mortality rate of 80% has been reported in dialysis patients with calciphylaxis that develop ulcers at any time after initial presentation with 100% of deaths related to calciphylaxis [28]. In a meta-analysis of 155 cases of calciphylaxis reported between 1936 and 1996, mortality rates were also related to the location of calciphylactic lesions [13]. Proximal lesions (thighs, buttocks, and trunk) were associated with a 63% mortality rate compared to distal lesions (calves, forearms, fingers, toes, and penis) which were associated with a 23% mortality rate. Others have also reported increased mortality with proximal lesions [5, 27]. Hence, calciphylaxis should be considered a very poor prognostic indicator.

Etiology and Pathogenesis

Mechanisms of Vascular Calcification in ESRD

Although much of the work on vascular calcification has focused on the intimal calcification of the arteries characteristic of cardiovascular disease, rather than medial calcification of arterioles characteristic of calciphylaxis, the knowledge gained is invaluable to our understanding of this disease as suggested by the proposed analogy that calciphylaxis is the cutaneous equivalent of a myocardial infarction [4]. Therefore, this discussion of the mechanisms of vascular calcification will draw largely from that body of knowledge while focusing on mechanisms of vascular calcification in ESRD and calciphylaxis whenever possible.

There are two distinct patterns of vascular calcification: (1) intimal calcification of arteries, which is usually a focal process often associated with atherosclerotic plaques and (2) medial calcification of arteries, sometimes called Monckeberg's medial sclerosis, which can occur independent of atherosclerosis and is characterized by diffuse medial calcification that includes the internal elastic lamina causing vascular stiffening and arteriosclerosis [29, 30]. Medial calcification and arteriosclerosis are common in the coronary arteries of older patients and especially prevalent among those with diabetes and ESRD. Moreover, intimal and medial calcification can occur independently or together in patients with ESRD [31]. Calciphylaxis is a distinct subtype of medial calcification that is common among dialysis patients which affects cutaneous and subcutaneous arterioles leading to intimal proliferation, vascular stenosis, and predisposing to thrombotic occlusion, all of which can contribute tissue ischemia [4, 29, 30]. Soft tissue calcium deposits in uremia as hydroxylapatite, also called hydroxyapatite or bone mineral, a naturally occurring mineral form of calcium apatite represented by the molecular formula $Ca_5(PO_4)_3(OH)$ [32].

Vascular Calcification Is Actively Regulated

Vascular calcification is no longer simply considered a passive process, rather it is predominantly actively regulated and likely arises as a result of multiple overlapping mechanisms [4, 29, 30, 33]. Four general and overlapping mechanisms for initiating vascular calcification have been proposed: (1) loss of inhibition of vascular mineralization by constitutive circulating inhibitors which allows for extraskeletal mineral deposition, (2) differentiation of vascular smooth muscle or stem cells to osteoblast-like bone-forming cells capable of extraskeletal mineral deposition, (3) circulating nucleation complexes released from actively remodeling bone which can serve as niduses for extraskeletal mineral deposition, and (4) cell death leading to release of apoptotic bodies and/or other necrotic debris that may serve as nucleation complexes for mineral deposition at sites of injury [29, 33]. Moreover, elevated phosphorus and/or calcium can passively promote extraskeletal mineral nucleation and crystal growth, especially in the context of any of these proposed active mechanisms of vascular calcification.

Early Models of Extraskeletal Calcium Deposition in Calciphylaxis

Early studies by Selye suggested that a series of events might be necessary for the development of calciphylaxis in an experimental animal model [1, 2]. He postulated that calciphylaxis is a hypersensitivity reaction induced by exposure to one or more "sensitizing" agents or events followed by exposure to a "challenging" agent. Experimental sensitization included exposure to high levels of parathyroid hormone (PTH), vitamin D, phosphorus, or calcium salts or by inducing ESRD by nephrectomy, followed by challenge with agents such as albumin, metal salts (e.g., iron, aluminum, others), polymyxin, 5-hydroxytryptamine, or trauma. Sensitization followed by exposure resulted in soft tissue calcification, inflammation, and necrosis. However, while calciphylaxis was initially described in this experimental animal model, the absence of vascular calcification and microthrombi and their presence in humans suggests additional factors are involved that lead to development of the arteriolopathy component [1, 2, 5, 6]. Moreover, it has been suggested in retrospect that the syndrome that is most analogous to Selye's experimental model is that of uremic soft tissue calcification [34, 35].

Role of Uremia in Calciphylaxis

Much has been learned about the etiology and pathogenesis of calciphylaxis since the early studies by Selye, however, as much remains unknown. Although there are many reports of calciphylaxis associated with nonuremic causes, the majority of cases occur in patients with ESRD on dialysis, hence its designation as a uremic arteriolopathy. It is likely that uremia creates a favorable milieu for extraskeletal deposition of hydroxyapatite in soft tissues including small vessels, predisposing to thrombus formation, and the development of calciphylaxis. Secondary HPT with elevated PTH is common among uremic patients and likely further enhances this environment making it more favorable for the development of calciphylaxis, especially via its strong influence on bone metabolism making phosphorus and calcium more readily available, thereby promoting active vascular calcification and mineralization of other soft tissues.

Role of HPT in Calciphylaxis

HPT is due to overactivity of the parathyroid glands resulting in excess production of PTH which regulates calcium and phosphorus homeostasis [36]. Primary HPT results from hyperfunctioning of the parathyroid glands themselves with oversecretion of PTH due to adenoma, hyperplasia, or rarely carcinoma of the parathyroid glands. Secondary HPT results from excessive secretion of PTH in response to hypocalcemia and is associated with hypertrophy of the parathyroid glands. Secondary HPT is most common among patients with late-stage CKD (stage 4 or 5) or ESRD and is due to failure of renal 1α-hydroxylase (also known as 25-(OH)D-1α-hydroxylase) to convert enough of the hepatic prehormone 25-hydroxyvitamin D_3 (25-hydroxycholecalciferol, abbreviated 25-(OH) D_3) to the active hormone 1,25-dihydroxyvitamin D_3 (1,25-dihydroxycholecalciferol, abbreviated 1,25-$(OH_2)D_3$) in the kidney. Decreased serum 1,25-$(OH_2)D_3$ levels impair intestinal calcium absorption and induce a state of skeletal PTH-resistance. Late-stage CKD or ESRD also causes elevated serum phosphorus levels which also inhibits the activity of renal 1α-hydroxylase and consumes circulating calcium forming insoluble hydroxyapatite. Together these processes lead to hypocalcemia and inadequate negative feedback inhibition of the parathyroid glands mediated by calcium-binding to calcium-sensing receptors (CaSRs), thereby resulting in increased PTH secretion in an attempt to restore serum calcium levels. Secondary HPT can also result from malabsorption (chronic pancreatitis, small bowel disease, and other malabsorption syndromes) of fat soluble vitamin D. Moreover, elevated PTH has additional deleterious effects on the immune, nervous, and other body systems that are beyond the scope of this discussion.

Role of Hyperphosphatemia in Calciphylaxis

The main causes of hyperphosphatemia in calciphylaxis are decreased renal excretion, increased dietary intake, and excess bone resorption. Decreased renal excretion of phosphorus is the most important contributor and occurs when the glomerular filtration rate falls below 20 mL/min and dietary intake is sustained. Excess bone resorption is an underrecognized cause and/or contributor to hyperphosphatemia. Several disorders that stimulate bone resorption have been reported to cause hyperphosphatemia although the underlying mechanisms are not completely understood. In the setting of renal failure and uremia, development of secondary HPT is the predominant cause of excess bone reabsorption.

Hyperphosphatemia plays an important role in the development of secondary HPT and chronic kidney disease-mineral and bone disorder (CKD-MBD, also known as renal osteodystrophy) by several mechanisms including hyperphosphatemia-induced hypercalcemia, hyperphosphatemia-associated increased expression of transforming growth factor-alpha (TGF-α) and epidermal growth factor receptors (EGFRs) in parathyroid chief cells causing hyperplasia, increased PTH secretion, inhibition of vitamin D synthesis, and hyperphosphatemia-induced vascular calcification. In advanced renal failure, PTH-mediated osteolysis may become the predominant factor influencing serum phosphorus levels.

Hyperphosphatemia contributes to an increased calcium–phosphorus product ($Ca \times P$, serum calcium multiplied by serum phosphorus) which significantly increases the risk of calcium deposition in soft tissues. Vascular calcification is most often observed in patients with CKD, diabetes, and/or severe atherosclerosis and worsens with age. Calcification of the large blood vessels can cause coronary artery disease, peripheral artery disease, hypertension, heart failure, and myocardial infarction. In fact, both vascular calcification and hyperphosphatemia are independent risk factors for cardiovascular disease and mortality [37–40]. Calcification of smaller peripheral arteries and arterioles can manifest clinically as calciphylaxis. Prolonged hyperphosphatemia and a $Ca \times P$ product >55 mg^2/dL^2 are strongly associated with the development of calciphylaxis.

Role of Oxidative Stress and Inflammation in Calciphylaxis

The uremic milieu also predisposes to and/or promotes multiple metabolic toxicities including oxidative stress and inflammation [37, 38, 41]. Oxidative stress has been clearly shown to influence inflammatory pathways via the nuclear transcription factor NF-κB and is an independent risk factor for cardiovascular disease and mortality [37, 38]. Increased levels of reactive oxygen species and inflammatory mediators promote the development of arteriolopathy by causing endothelial cell dysfunction, which predisposes to thrombus formation, and by influencing vascular smooth muscle cell remodeling [41]. Dysregulation of vascular smooth muscle cells causes intimal hyperplasia, cell differentiation, apoptosis, and fibrosis. The recent understanding that vascular smooth muscle cells can differentiate into osteoblast-like bone-forming cells that promote vascular calcification has greatly enhanced our understanding of this disease and provided new avenues for research [42].

Molecular Factors Involved in Vascular Calcification and/or Calciphylaxis

Molecular factors important to calcium metabolism and regulation of skeletal and extraskeletal mineralization have been identified and are likely involved in the etiology and pathogenesis of vascular calcification, including that of calciphylaxis [4]. Moreover, factors that influence vascular remodeling and vascular smooth muscle cell differentiation into osteoblast-like cells capable of producing bone have been identified. Despite the numerous factors involved in these molecular signaling pathway, it appears that the final common pathway leading to vascular calcification involves activation of the transcription factor NF-κB [4, 43–46]. NF-κB regulates transcription of many factors involved in cell growth, cell differentiation, and inflammatory processes including growth factors, cytokines, and adhesion molecules. Receptor activator of nuclear factor-κB (RANK) and RANK ligand (RANKL) regulate NK-κB and are critical for normal bone development, osteoclast differentiation, and bone mineral reabsorption. Regulators of NF-κB activity, including RANK, RANKL, and other endogenous promoters and inhibitors of vascular calcification, are expressed by vascular smooth muscle cells, endothelial cells, osteoblasts, osteoclasts, and inflammatory cells.

As is the case in many biological systems, homeostasis is maintained by balancing factors that promote and inhibit cellular processes and the same is true for skeletal and extracellular calcification. Dysregulation of factors that promote or inhibit NF-κB activity can lead to vascular calcification. RANKL activates RANK-mediated NF-κB activity which promotes skeletal calcium resorption and extraskeletal vascular calcification, whereas inhibition of RANK-mediated NK-κB activity prevents skeletal calcium resorption and extraskeletal vascular calcification. Moreover, it has been suggested that uremia-induced defects in this system may predispose to development of vascular calcification, including that of calciphylaxis.

Recent evidence suggests that dysregulation or defects of endogenous promoters or inhibitors that affect signaling pathways of skeletal calcium homeostasis can result in extraskeletal calcium deposition that contributes to pathological development of vascular calcification. Several known endogenous promoters and inhibitors involved in vascular calcification are summarized (Table 6.2).

Table 6.2 Molecular factors involved in vascular calcification and/or calciphylaxis

Common final pathway of vascular calcification
NF-κB
RANK
RANKL
Inhibit vascular calcification
OPG
MGP
Fetuin-A (AHSG)
BMPs (e.g., BMP-7)
CIP-α
VEGF
Smad6
Klotho gene product
Carbonic anhydrase
Promote vascular calcification
BMPs (e.g., BMP-2)
Cbfa-1
OPN
Proinflammatory cytokines (TNF-α, IL-1, IL-6, TGF-β)
Inorganic phosphorus
ROS

AHSG α2-Heremans–Schmid glycoprotein, *BMPs* bone morphogenic proteins, *Cbfa-1* core-binding factor alpha-1, *CIP-α* calcification inhibitory protein-alpha, *MGP* matrix Gla protein, *NF-κB* nuclear factor-kappa B, *RANK* receptor activator of NF-κB, *OPG* osteoprotegerin, *OPN* osteopontin, *RANKL* RANK ligand, *ROS* reactive oxygen species, *VEGF* vascular endothelial growth factor

Factors That Inhibit Vascular Calcification

The potential role of factors that inhibit development of vascular calcification (anticalcification proteins) has become an area of great interest. There is evidence that the signaling pathways of osteoprotegerin, matrix Gla protein (MGP), fetuin-A, bone morphogenic proteins (BMPs), and other constitutively expressed anticalcification mediators may be decreased (i.e., loss of inhibition) in the setting of calciphylaxis, allowing for calcium deposition and development of arteriolar medial calcification.

Osteoprotegerin

Osteoprotegerin (OPG) is a soluble antagonist of RANKL that inhibits RANK-mediated NF-κB activity, thereby inhibiting skeletal calcium resorption and extraskeletal vascular calcification [4, 43–47]. Since OPG and RANKL essentially bind to the same receptor, RANK, OPG is one of the most important regulators of RANK-mediated NF-κB activity. Moreover, it is interesting to note that bisphosphonates upregulate OPG expression and RANKL expression, but decrease RANKL activity in most studies possibly suggesting a mechanism to account for reports of healing of calciphylactic lesions in patients treated with bisphosphonates [48–51]. It is likely that the ratio of OPG to RANKL expression may be the important determinant since both bind RANK to mediate NK-κB activity.

Matrix Gla Protein

Matrix Gla protein (MGP) is a member of the Gla protein family, which includes osteocalcin and a number of coagulation factors including factors II, VII, IX, X, and proteins C and S [52–54]. All members of this family have glutamic acid residues that are posttranslationally carboxylated by the enzyme gamma-glutamyl carboxylase in a reaction that requires vitamin K as a cofactor. Carboxylation of Gla proteins confers a high affinity for mineral ions such as calcium, phosphate, and hydroxyapatite crystals, the mineral components of bone.

MGP is an inhibitor of vascular calcification and is expressed at high levels in the heart, lung, and kidney by tissue-specific populations of cells [52–54]. MGP is found in bone along with osteocalcin, both of which are calcium-binding proteins that participate in the organization of bone tissue. MGP is synthesized by vascular smooth muscle cells and chondrocytes, and its expression is upregulated by vitamin D in bone cells. Interestingly, MGP is related to proteins C and S, decreased levels of which are associated with the development of calciphylaxis. Moreover, the mechanism whereby warfarin is believed to induce or aggravate calciphylaxis may also involve this process [55].

Mutations in the human MPG gene have been linked with Keutel syndrome, an autosomal recessive disorder characterized by abnormal cartilage calcification, pulmonary artery stenosis, and midfacial hypoplasia [52]. MGP-deficient mice also exhibit inappropriate calcification of cartilage, including the growth plate, which leads to short stature, osteopenia, and fractures. MGP-deficient mice typically die within 2 months due to accelerated arterial calcification which leads to blood vessel rupture [53].

The circulating inactive uncarboxylated form of MGP (ucMGP) has recently been proposed as a potential biomarker for vascular calcification [56, 57]. Vitamin K deficiency leads to inactive MGP which accumulates at sites of arterial calcification. A recent study found that the circulating fraction of ucMGP is decreased in certain populations at risk for vascular calcification, likely as a result of deposition around sites of arterial calcification [57]. Serum ucMGP levels were decreased nearly in all hemodialysis and calciphylaxis patients studied compared to healthy control subjects. However, patients who underwent angioplasty and in those with aortic stenosis, there was some overlap in serum ucMGP levels with control subjects. Nonetheless, serum ucMGP may prove useful as a biomarker to identify patients at risk for developing vascular calcification, including calciphylaxis, especially in the setting of CKD.

Fetuin-A

Fetuin-A, also known as α2-Heremans–Schmid glycoprotein (AHSG), is an endogenous inhibitor of systemic calcification [58–60]. Reduced serum levels of fetuin-A have been associated with vascular calcification and increased mortality in dialysis patients [60–64]. Both chronic inflammation and uremia appear to contribute to decreased expression of fetuin-A and possibly AHSG gene mutations [64–68]. Mice deficient in fetuin-A were found to have increased expression of osteopontin and widespread extraskeletal calcification of the heart, lungs, and kidneys [69]. Fetuin-A deficiency alone was not associated with disturbances of calcium and phosphorus homeostasis. Although vascular calcification is present in the absence of uremia and hyperphosphatemia, it is severely exaggerated by their presence. Moreover, calcification is severely exaggerated when mice deficient in fetuin-A are combined with the DBA/2 genetic background which is prone to extraskeletal calcification [70]. Mice deficient in fetuin-A were also found to be hyperresponsive to BMP-induced extraskeletal osteogenesis [71]. Mice deficient in fetuin-A and apolipoprotein E (ApoE) with CKD and hyperphosphatemia had a 15-fold increase in vascular calcification, although mostly intimal rather than medial calcification [72]. Finally, recent evidence suggests that elevated fetuin-A levels may be related to insulin resistance, hepatic dysfunction, and the metabolic syndrome [60, 73, 74].

Bone Morphogenic Proteins

BMPs are a group of proteins that are considered cytokines and most are members of the transforming growth factor-beta (TGF-β) superfamily [75]. BMPs are not only known to be involved in bone formation, but are also considered key morphogenic mediators of tissue development throughout the body. For example, BMP-2, -3, -4, and -7 are involved in osteoblast differentiation and/or bone formation [75, 76]. Several BMPs are also involved in extraskeletal calcification, some as promoters and others inhibitors. For example, BMP-2 and -7 have been shown to promote differentiation of vascular smooth muscle cells into osteoblast-like cells capable of extraskeletal mineralization [76]. BMP-7 has also been shown to inhibit vascular calcification in uremic mice deficient in low-density lipoprotein (LDL) receptors [77]. In one study of patients undergoing renal transplantation, vascular calcification of the medial layer of the inferior epigastric artery was found in 44% of patients and was associated with deposition of BMPs [78]. Moreover, BMP-4 was demonstrated at the border of affected arterioles in a biopsy from a patient with calciphylaxis and was thought to be involved in promoting calcification in this patient [79]. Moreover, regulation of BMP expression has been shown to involve the NF-kB pathway, considered the final common pathway of vascular calcification, as well as smad6, a negative regulator of BMP signaling pathways [80, 81].

Factors That Promote Vascular Calcification

The potential role of factors that promote development of vascular calcification has become an area of great interest. There is evidence that the signaling pathways of BMPs, core-binding factor α-1, osteopontin, proinflammatory cytokines (TNF-α, IL-1, IL-6, others), and other calcification mediators are increased in the setting of calciphylaxis, possibly allowing for calcium deposition and development of arteriolar medial calcification. Moreover, inorganic phosphorus, an obvious suspect in the development of calciphylaxis, has also been shown to influence a number of regulatory pathways thought to be involved in the development of vascular calcification and calciphylaxis.

Bone Morphogenic Proteins

As previously discussed, BMPs are known to be involved in bone formation, but are also considered key morphogenic mediators of tissue development throughout the body. BMP-2, -3, -4, and -7 are involved in osteoblast differentiation and/or bone formation [75, 76]. Again, some BMPs are promoters and some are inhibitors of vascular calcification.

Core-Binding Factor α-1

Core-binding factor α-1 (Cbfa-1) is a transcription factor necessary for osteoblast differentiation and function [82–86]. Cbf1-a upregulates expression of RANKL which then activates RANK-mediated NF-κB pathways. Overexpression of Cbf1-a promotes differentiation of vascular smooth muscle cells into osteoblast-like cells capable of extraskeletal mineralization [83, 84, 86]. Mutations in the human Cbfa-1 gene have been linked with cleidocranial dysplasia, an autosomal dominant disorder characterized by defective development of the cranial bones, complete or partial absence of the clavicles, and associated dental and otological abnormalities [87]. Moreover, mice overexpressing Cfb1-a develop osteoporosis, whereas Cfb1-a-deficient mice lack skeletal mineralization and die soon after birth [82, 85].

Osteopontin

Osteopontin (OPN) is an extracellular matrix protein expressed by a variety of tissue types and cells including fibroblasts, osteoblasts, osteoclasts, endothelial cells, and vascular smooth muscle cells [88–91]. OPN is an important factor in bone remodeling where it is thought to stimulate development of osteoclasts, anchor them to the mineral matrix of bone, and promote bone reabsorption [92–95]. OPN expression in bone is stimulated by serum 1,25-$(OH_2)D_3$ (calcitriol) and requires the transcription factors Cbfa-1 and osterix for expression [93]. Under normal circumstances, hypocalcemia and hypophosphatemia stimulate kidney proximal tubule cells to produce 1,25-$(OH_2)D_3$, which in turn increases expression of OPN to promote bone resorption and restore serum levels. PTH, inorganic phosphate, proinflammatory cytokines (TNFα, IL-1, and TGF-β), as well as angiotensin II have also been shown to stimulate OPN expression [89, 93, 94, 96, 97]. In one case–control study of 10 dialysis patients with calciphylaxis, biopsy samples from cutaneous lesions demonstrated substantially increased OPN and decreased α-actin expression by vascular smooth muscle cells in the medial layer of all calcified blood vessels compared to noncalcified vessels [97].

Proinflammatory Cytokines (TNF-α, IL-1, and IL-6)

Chronic inflammation has a significant impact on the development and accelerated progression of vascular calcification, especially with advanced renal disease [98, 99]. The proinflammatory cytokines tumor necrosis factor-α (TNF-α), interleukin-1 (IL-1), and IL-6 are known to promote differentiation of vascular smooth muscle cells into osteoblast-like cells capable of extraskeletal mineralization [4, 98–100]. Expression of these cytokines are common in chronic inflammatory and other diseases including late-stage CKD, ESRD, diabetes, obesity, hepatitis, and malignancies. Strategies focused on modulating immune function are currently under investigation and will likely translate into new therapies to improve clinical outcomes for patients with chronic inflammation associated with vascular disease.

Inorganic Phosphorus

Given the strong association between elevated phosphorus and Ca×P product and the development of calciphylaxis, it is not surprising that phosphorus influences a number of pathways involved in vascular calcification. Phosphorus has also been shown to induce differentiation of vascular smooth muscle cells into osteoblast-like cells capable of extraskeletal mineralization, now recognized as an important process in the development of vascular calcification [29, 101]. Phosphorus is also known to increase expression of Cbfa-1 and OPN [93, 96]. Phosphorus feeding was shown to induce medial calcification in calcification-prone DBA/2 mice that was associated with increased expression of Cbfa-1, OPN, and fibroblast growth factor-23 (FGF-23) [102]. Although the association of elevated phosphorus and development of calciphylaxis was one of the earliest findings associated with development of this disease, the multifaceted role of phosphorus in the molecular pathogenesis of vascular calcification is only beginning to be understood.

Clinical Manifestations

Overview

Calciphylaxis is essentially a manifestation of vascular calcification of arterioles, hence the more recent terminology designating this disease as an arteriolopathy. The proposed analogy that calciphylaxis is the cutaneous equivalent of a myocardial infarction has several instructive implications [4]. First, both calcification and stenosis of arterioles and thrombotic occlusion are necessary for development of full-blown calciphylactic lesions. Second, there is likely a temporal separation between these two distinct processes—the insidious onset of calcification and stenosis of arterioles and the acute manifestations of thrombotic occlusion. Third, the insidious onset of calcification and stenosis of arterioles likely accounts for the absent or mild signs and symptoms reported with early disease, whereas the acute onset of thrombotic occlusion of arterioles likely accounts for the more severe signs and symptoms often reported as the disease progresses, most notably tissue necrosis and severe pain. Lastly, recognizing that calciphylaxis involves the distinct processes of calcification and stenosis of arterioles and thrombotic occlusion has obvious therapeutic implications.

Location and Distribution of Calciphylactic Lesions

Calciphylaxis can cause extensive calcification of the skin, subcutaneous tissues, including muscle and adipose tissue, and in severe cases visceral organs. Lesions can occur in proximal, distal, and acral regions of the body, but are most commonly reported in proximal areas containing a high percentage of adipose tissue including the abdomen, thighs, and breasts, although lesions can occur in essentially any location (Table 6.3; Fig. 6.1) [103]. Lesions have been reported to affect the fingers, toes, penis, tongue, temporal arteries, and visceral organs, including lungs, kidneys, pancreas, stomach, intestines, and pancreas [104–112]. However, underreporting of calciphylaxis due to non- or misdiagnosis and overreporting of unusual cases make it difficult to determine the probability of any specific clinical manifestation. The location and distribution of calciphylactic lesions also has significant clinical consequences as many have reported significantly worse mortality rates associated with proximal (thighs, buttocks, and trunk) lesions [5, 13, 27].

Table 6.3 Distribution and location of calciphylactic lesions

Proximal	Trunk
	Thigh
	Buttocks
	Breast
Distal	Forearm
	Calves
	Fingers
	Toes
Visceral	Lungs
	Kidneys
	Pancreas
	Stomach
	Small and large intestines
Other	Penis
	Tongue
	Temporal arteries

Description of Calciphylactic Lesions

Characteristic cutaneous lesions typically begin as small erythematous patches, often associated with plaques and/or nodules, and tenderness to palpation. Early lesions often progress to full-blown lesions that are commonly described as painful, violaceous, mottled, or reticulated skin patches (livedo reticularis) that may progress to nonhealing ulcerated necrotic tissue that commonly causes eschar formation, gangrene requiring amputation, sepsis, and death (Fig. 6.2a, b) [25]. The time course and progression of calciphylactic lesions likely reflects the distinct processes of insidious calcification and stenosis of arterioles and acute thrombotic occlusion. Calciphylactic lesions initially may be mistaken for infectious cellulitis, treated as such without

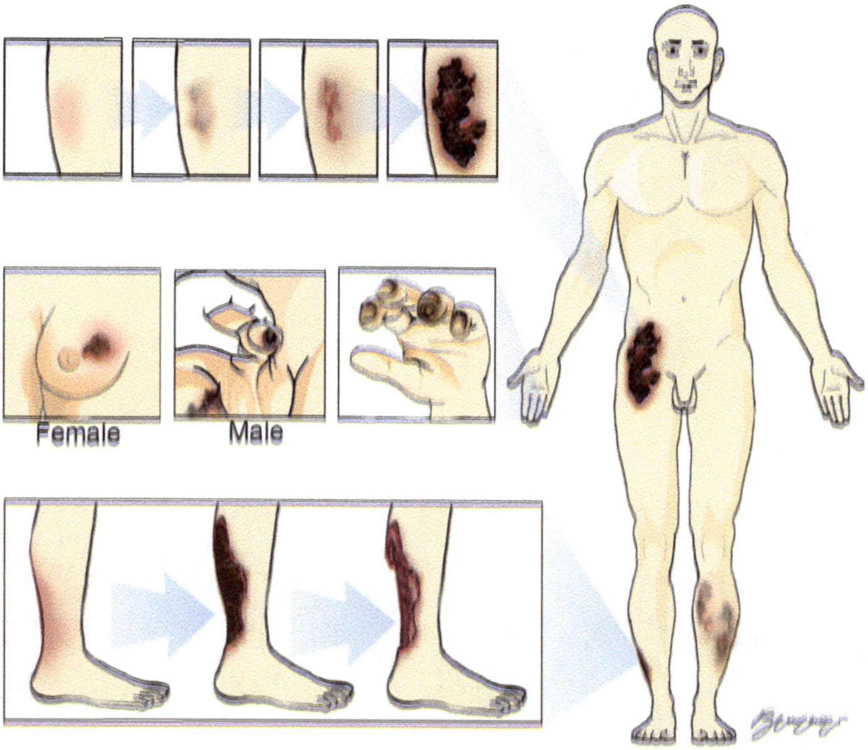

Fig. 6.1 Schematic diagram depicting some commonly reported locations and the progression of calciphylactic lesions. Illustration by Bashar Ericsoussi, M.D

significant resolution, while delaying appropriate treatment [28]. Moreover, lesions may be difficult to identify in African American patients due to darker skin pigmentation which can make erythema and violaceous skin discoloration more difficult to appreciate (Fig. 6.2c, d). Moreover, experience in identifying lesions in African American patients is limited because they occur more commonly in Caucasian patients.

One study found that while the vast majority of published cases presented with characteristic ulceration, the initial presentation was usually nonulcerating, suggesting reporting bias [28]. Of 35 new cases that occurred in a single dialysis unit over a 7-year period, all presented with lesions on the legs, 80% with tender indurated subcutaneous plaques only, 17% with painful ulceration only, and 3% with plaques and ulceration. Subcutaneous plaques were associated with erythema, warmth, and tenderness, and most commonly occurred 2–5 cm above the Achilles' tendon (Fig. 6.1, bottom left panel), ranging in diameter from a few to many centimeters. Moreover, approximately one-third of patients who presented with plaques only developed ulceration, suggesting that plaque formation likely reflects early disease due to insidious calcification and stenosis of arterioles, whereas ulceration likely reflects disease progression due to acute thrombotic occlusion of arterioles. The time course of lesion progression also varied between individuals, likely reflecting the temporal separation of calcification and stenosis of arterioles and thrombotic occlusion, and progression was rapid in the absence of timely and aggressive intervention which had a direct impact on morbidity and mortality [28].

Tissue Ischemia and Secondary Infection of Calciphylactic Lesions

Vascular calcification and arteriolar stenosis in calciphylaxis likely predisposes to thrombotic

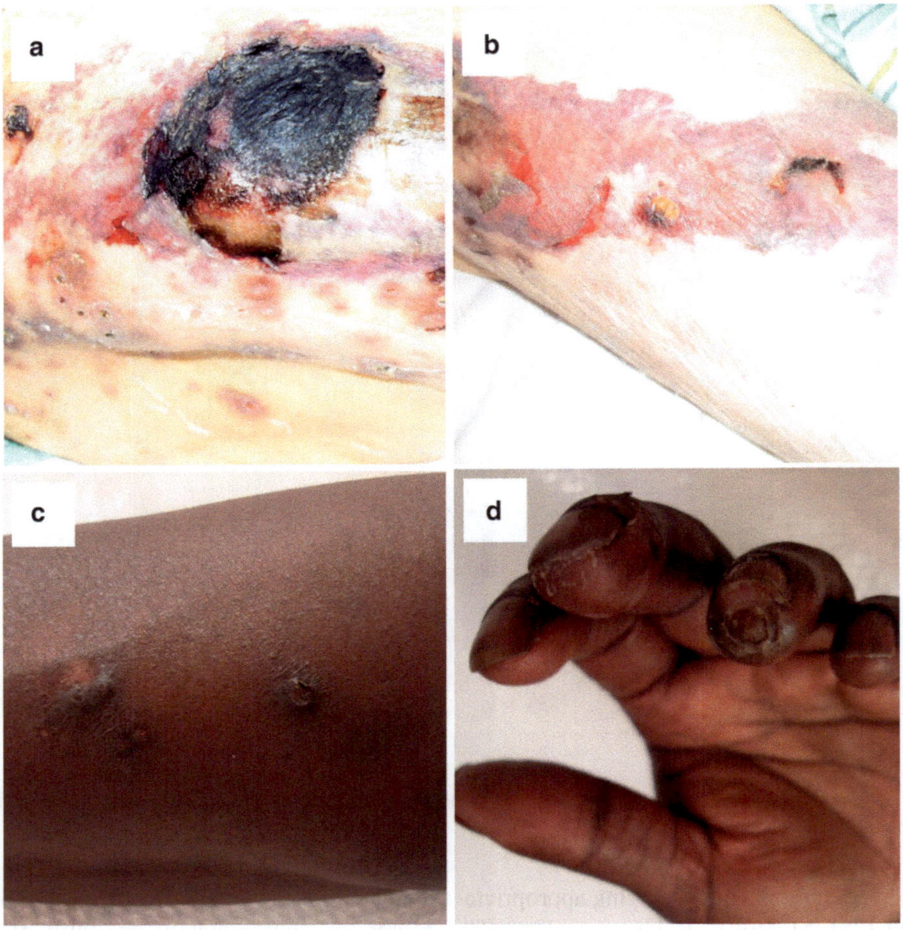

Fig. 6.2 (**a**, **b**) Biopsy-proven calciphylactic lesions in the absence of uremia of the right thigh (**a**) and leg (**b**) of a 55-year-old Caucasian female with a history of diabetes, hypertension, and morbid obesity. These full-blown lesions demonstrate characteristic nonhealing, ulcerated, necrotic tissue with eschars. PTH level was <100 ng/L and calcium–phosphorus product was <40 mg^2/dL^2 at the time of lesion manifestation and biopsy. (**c**, **d**) Subcutaneous nodules of the forearm (**c**) and ischemic necrosis of the fingers (**d**) of biopsy-proven calciphylaxis in a 47-year-old African American male with ESRD on hemodialysis and history of a failed renal transplant. PTH level was >800 ng/L and calcium–phosphorus product was >70 mg^2/dL^2 at the time of lesion manifestation and biopsy

occlusion resulting in tissue ischemia and necrosis. In one study, the transcutaneous oxygen tension was measured in 21 patients with calciphylaxis and compared to age-matched controls [113]. Patients with calciphylaxis had extremely low transcutaneous oxygen tension (<30 mmHg while breathing room air) in 62% of body regions with lesions and 26% of body regions without lesions, compared to <1% in all body regions of control patients, suggesting severe and diffuse skin ischemia exists even in areas without visible lesions. Moreover, while breathing 100% supplemental oxygen, transcutaneous oxygen tension remained relatively low in patients with calciphylaxis, suggesting that the vascular insufficiency may be fixed. However, there was significant improvement in transcutaneous oxygen tension of some patients with calciphylaxis suggesting oxygen therapy may be of some benefit. The differential response to oxygen therapy in some patients may reflect the difference between the presence of vascular calcification and arteriolar stenosis, which may be more responsive to oxygen therapy, and the presence of vascular thrombosis, which may preclude oxygen delivery to affected tissues, as well as the relative severity of each of these distinct components.

Although not primarily infectious in etiology, tissue ischemia, breach of the skin barrier, and the painful debilitating nature of calciphylactic lesions make them highly vulnerable to secondary infection. Moreover, majority of patients are on chronic dialysis and spend a substantial amount of time in a healthcare setting which increases the risk of healthcare-associated multidrug-resistant infections in this highly vulnerable population [114–116].

Factors Associated with Calciphylaxis

Calciphylaxis is most often associated with late-stage CKD or ESRD and uremia, although there are many reports of its presence in the absence of uremia. Given that calciphylaxis is poorly understood, it stands to reason that understanding the factors associated with this disease may help to better understand the etiology and pathogenesis, identify patients at increased risk of developing the disease, and develop better treatment strategies. However, it is important to emphasize that many of these factors are only associated with calciphylaxis, rather than causes or contributors to the disease, and may be analogous to the "sensitizing" and "challenging" agents described in the early studies by Selye [1, 2]. Factors reported to be associated with calciphylaxis are summarized in Table 6.4. Although not necessarily distinct categories and some related factors may appear under more than one heading, for convenience these factors are categorized as general associations, demographic factors, comorbid conditions, laboratory abnormalities, and medications or other agents reported to be associated with calciphylaxis.

Table 6.4 Factors reported to be associated with calciphylaxis

General associations
Uremic causes
Nonuremic causes
Demographic factors
Caucasian race
Female gender
Younger age
Comorbid conditions
Late-stage chronic kidney disease (stage 4 or 5)
End-stage renal disease
Peritoneal or hemodialysis
Postrenal transplant
Hyperparathyroidism
Hyperphosphatemia
Hypercalcemia
Diabetes
Obesity (BMI >30 kg/m^2)
Hypoalbuminemia
Hypercoaguable diseases or states
Inflammatory diseases
Liver disease
POEMS syndrome
Laboratory abnormalities
Increased serum phosphorus levels
Increased serum calcium levels
Calcium–phosphorus (Ca × P) product >55 mg^2/dL^2
Increased serum PTH levels
Increased serum alkaline phosphatase levels
Increased serum aluminum levels
Hypoalbuminemia
Protein S or C deficiency
Increased serum aluminum levels
Medications or other agents
Calcium-containing medications (e.g., phosphorus binders, antacids, others)
High-calcium dialysate
Steroids
Warfarin

BMI body mass index, *POEMS* polyneuropathy, organomegaly, endocrinopathy, monoclonal gammopathy, and skin abnormalities, *PTH* parathyroid hormone

Uremic Calciphylaxis

The vast majority of patients presenting with calciphylaxis have ESRD and are on peritoneal or hemodialysis [13, 25–28, 117]. Some evidence suggests calciphylaxis may be more common among patients on peritoneal dialysis [28, 118]. Calciphylaxis has also been reported to occur after renal transplantation [9, 110, 119–123]. Metabolic abnormalities associated with uremia are speculated to play an important role in the etiology and pathogenesis of calciphylaxis, including secondary HPT, hyperphosphatemia, and hypercalcemia (Fig. 6.3) [26]. However, given the many reports of its presence in nonuremic patients, many of these factors are likely "sensitizers" to the development of calciphylaxis.

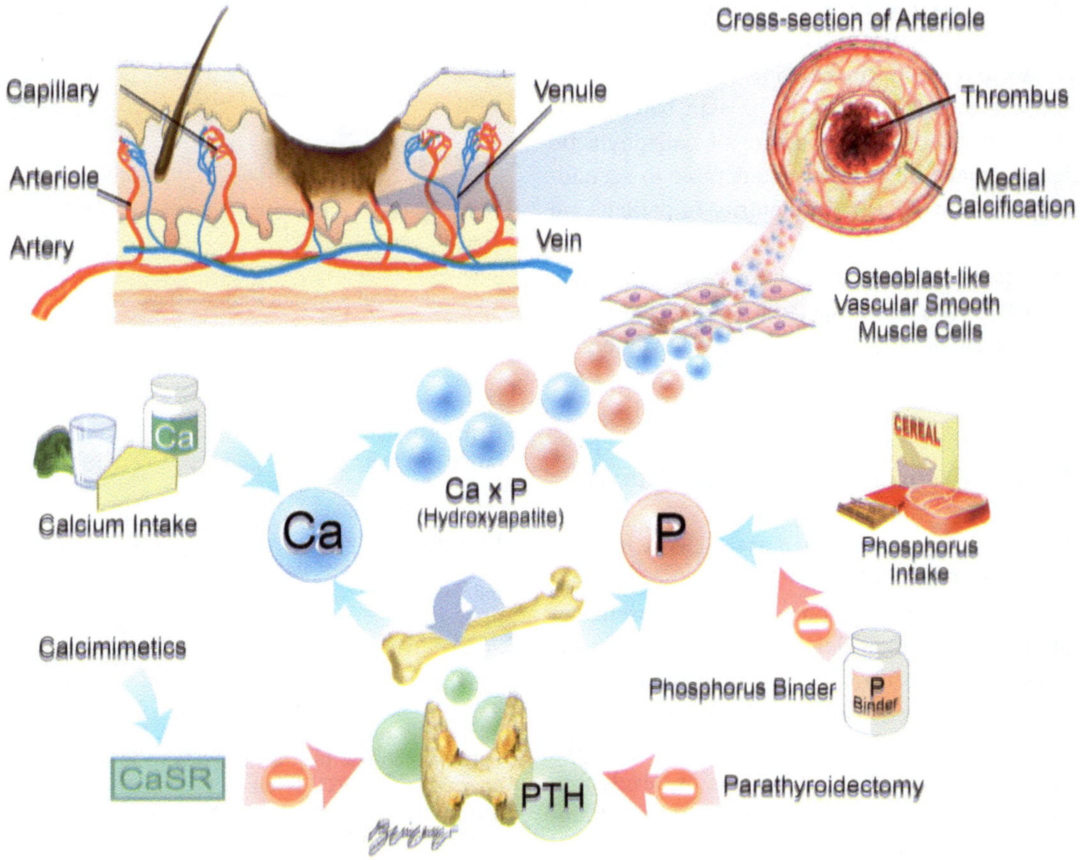

Fig. 6.3 Schematic diagram depicting some of the common factors involved in the etiology and pathogenesis of calciphylaxis. Parathyroid-mediated bone resorption, dietary intake, and medications may contribute to an elevated calcium–phosphorus (Ca×P) product. Vascular smooth muscle cells can be stimulated to differentiate into osteoblast-like cells capable of extraskeletal calcium and phosphorus deposition in the form of hydroxyapatite [$Ca_5(PO_4)_3(OH)$] in the medial wall of arterioles and other small vessels causing vascular stenosis and predisposing to thrombotic occlusion and ischemia that may progress to nonhealing ulceration. While many of these factors are common, likely serving as "sensitizing" or "challenging" agents, it important to note that none are required and calciphylaxis can develop in the absence of many or all of these factors. Illustration by Bashar Ericsoussi, M.D

Demographic Factors Associated with Calciphylaxis

Caucasian Race

The vast majority of patients who develop calciphylaxis are Caucasian [13, 25, 27, 117, 124]. In one case series derived from 347 dialysis patients, nine of nine calciphylaxis cases occurred in Caucasian patients, despite the fact that approximately half of the study population was African American [117].

Female Gender

Female gender has been associated with increased risk of developing calciphylaxis [5, 27, 28, 103, 117, 124–127]. In a retrospective case–control study of 19 patients with calciphylaxis, females had sixfold increased likelihood of developing calciphylaxis [27]. In another study, females were affected five times more frequently than males [128]. Some investigators have suggested this may be related to an increased percentage of adipose tissue in females which may predispose to hypoperfusion of subcutaneous tissues and skin resulting in ischemic necrosis [27]. Moreover, calciphylactic lesions are more common in proximal locations (thighs, buttocks, and trunk) where adipose tissue is more abundant. This hypothesis is also supported by the finding of an association between obesity and calciphylaxis [117, 128, 129]. The association between female gender and calciphylaxis has been speculated to involve estrogen and leptin [4]. Estrogen has been shown to increase the expression of the vascular calcification inhibitor OPG, whereas estrogen deficiency has been associated with osteoporosis and vascular calcification [47]. Similarly, leptin has been shown to influence OPG and RANKL. Leptin is a hormone produced by adipocytes that is thought to have distinct effects by acting via the central nervous system to increase osteoblast activity or via by binding directly to its receptors on osteoblasts to increase activity [130, 131]. Dysregulation of leptin is thought to promote vascular calcification which may contribute to the increased prevalence of calciphylaxis in females.

Younger Age

Younger age has been associated with the development of calciphylaxis. One retrospective study of a single outpatient hemodialysis unit reported that the age at the time of diagnosis was 49 compared to 50 years old for control patients [25]. It has been suggested that younger age may be related to a longer time period on dialysis which also may be associated with the development of calciphylaxis. In fact, it was reported in this same study that the length of time on dialysis at the time of diagnosis was 80 months for calciphylaxis patients compared to 20 months for control patients [25].

Laboratory Abnormalities Associated with Calciphylaxis

Hypercalcemia and Vitamin D Therapy

Hypercalcemia has been associated with the development of calciphylaxis in only a few studies [118, 127, 132]. This is likely because cellular and extracellular calcium levels are tightly regulated within a narrow range and only relatively small deviations can be life-threatening. Vitamin D therapy also has been reported to cause or exacerbate calciphylaxis as it is known to increase absorption of both calcium and phosphorus. Patients on dialysis are generally in a positive calcium balance due to dietary calcium intake, ingestion of calcium-based phosphorus binders, absorption of calcium from dialysate, treatment of secondary HPT with vitamin D, and abnormalities in bone metabolism [133]. Renal transplantation can also exacerbate hypercalcemia, especially before resolution of secondary HPT which may be prolonged in some cases [134].

In one study, the median serum calcium level of 10 dialysis patients diagnosed with calciphylaxis was 9.7 mg/dL at the time of diagnosis compared to 9.2 mg/dL for control patients [25]. High doses of calcium carbonate have been reported to cause calciphylaxis which resolves when discontinued [132]. One case–control study of eight peritoneal dialysis patients over a 3-year period reported a strong trend toward increased risk of calciphylaxis with the use of calcium carbonate [118, 127]. In another study, treatment with both calcium salts and vitamin D increased the likelihood of developing calciphylaxis threefold compared to control patients [28]. Since calcium-based phosphorus binders have been identified as a possible risk factor for the development of calciphylaxis, their use has fallen out of favor. In general, calcium salts of any kind should be avoided in dialysis patients whenever possible, except for patients with clinically significant hypocalcemia. When vitamin D therapy is necessary in patients at risk or with established calciphylaxis, less calcemic analogs should be considered.

Hyperphosphatemia

Calciphylaxis is commonly associated with hyperphosphatemia [3, 25, 27, 28, 117]. Clinically, hyperphosphatemia is often associated with hypocalcemia and tetany, secondary HPT and CKD-MBD, and extraskeletal soft tissue calcification. Soft tissue calcification associated with hyperphosphatemia increases with advancing age in patients with late-stage CKD or ESRD, diabetes, and advanced atherosclerosis. In one study, the median serum phosphorus level of ten dialysis patients diagnosed with calciphylaxis was 8.2 mg/dL at the time of diagnosis compared to 5.7 mg/dL for control patients [25]. The magnitude and importance of the association between serum phosphorus and the development of calciphylaxis is underscored by a case–control study of 19 patients with ESRD and calciphylaxis that found a 3.5-fold increased likelihood of developing calciphylaxis for each 1 mg/dL increase in serum phosphorus over the 12-month period prior to the diagnosis [27]. Hyperphosphatemia has also been reported to increase the risk of sepsis in dialysis patients which may contribute to mortality in those with calciphylaxis [27, 133, 135, 136].

Elevated Calcium–Phosphorus Product (Ca × P)

An elevated calcium–phosphorus (Ca × P) product >55 mg^2/dL^2 is commonly associated with the development of calciphylaxis [28, 128, 137]. In one study, the median Ca × P product of ten dialysis patients diagnosed with calciphylaxis was 81.5 mg/dL at the time of diagnosis compared to 52.9 mg/dL for the control patients [25]. However, several studies did not find an elevated Ca × P product suggesting that its presence is not required for the development of calciphylaxis [117, 127]. While both calcium and phosphorus contribute to the elevated Ca × P product commonly reported with calciphylaxis, hyperphosphatemia is almost always present, whereas hypercalcemia is not. Hypercalcemia alone rarely accounts for the elevated Ca × P product commonly reported with calciphylaxis, except in cases of severe hypercalcemia, often associated with excess calcium salts, vitamin D therapy, and malignancy. In one study of nonuremic calciphylaxis, malignancy was the second most common cause accounting for 22.2% of cases [138].

Elevated Serum PTH

Elevated serum PTH levels are commonly associated with the development of calciphylaxis [3, 25, 124, 139]. In one study, the median serum PTH level of ten dialysis patients diagnosed with calciphylaxis was 1496 pg/mL at the time of diagnosis compared to 138 pg/mL for the control patients [25]. However, increased serum PTH is not required for the development of calciphylaxis [117, 127]. In fact, some patients with calciphylaxis have low or normal PTH levels [127]. Like elevated serum calcium and phosphorus, elevated serum PTH levels likely represent a "sensitizing" agent for the development of calciphylaxis rather than a cause of the disease. When present, elevated serum PTH is usually due to secondary HPT caused by late-stage CKD or ESRD. However, in one study of nonuremic calciphylaxis, primary HPT was the most common cause accounting for 27.8% of cases [138].

Elevated Serum Alkaline Phosphatase

Elevated serum alkaline phosphatase levels have been associated with the development of calciphylaxis [3, 25, 27, 117]. In one study, the median serum alkaline phosphatase level of ten dialysis patients diagnosed with calciphylaxis was 188 IU/L at the time of diagnosis compared to 89 IU/L for the control patients [25]. In a case–control study of 19 patients with calciphylaxis, there was a 19% increase in the likelihood of developing calciphylaxis for each 10 IU/L increase in serum alkaline phosphatase at the time of diagnosis [27]. Some investigators have suggested that increased serum alkaline phosphatase may reflect more advanced bone disease in some patients, especially those with ESRD and severe secondary HPT [27].

Elevated Serum Aluminum

Elevated serum aluminum levels have been associated with the development of calciphylaxis [4, 128]. Aluminum-induced osteomalacia has many features in common with other forms of bone disease associated with vascular calcification; therefore, it has been suggested to potentially be involved in the pathogenesis of calciphylaxis for several reasons [4, 140, 141]. Aluminum-induced osteomalacia was found in some patients with calciphylaxis who underwent bone biopsy [140]. Aluminum also has direct toxic effects on osteoblasts, thereby potentially perturbing the balance between bone resorption and formation [142]. In one study, elevated serum aluminum levels were more common among dialysis patients with calciphylaxis than without [128]. Aluminum deposits have also demonstrated along with medial calcification in biopsy specimens from patients with calciphylaxis [4]. Based on these observations, it has been suggested that aluminum likely represents a "challenging" agent for the development of calciphylaxis rather than a cause of the disease. In fact, aluminum was one of the "challenging" agents described in the early studies by Selye to induce calciphylaxis in "sensitized" animals [1, 2].

However, it is important to note that some studies have reported that serum aluminum levels were not associated with calciphylaxis [27].

Comorbidities Associated with Calciphylaxis

Hyperparathyroidism

Both primary and secondary HPT with elevated serum PTH are commonly associated with the development of calciphylaxis [3, 20, 25, 137–139, 143–145]. The significance of HPT was previously discussed in the context of elevated PTH as a "sensitizing" agent for the development of calciphylaxis [1, 2, 4]. Elevated PTH levels are not always present in patients who develop calciphylaxis; therefore, neither HPT nor elevated PTH levels are necessary for the development of calciphylaxis [138]. However, when HPT and elevated PTH levels are present, they likely represent powerful sensitizers to the development of calciphylaxis as treatment has been reported to cause resolution of lesions in a substantial number of cases.

Diabetes

Diabetes has been associated with the development of calciphylaxis in some studies, while others did not find this association [13, 27, 28, 129]. However, the mechanisms whereby diabetes may be related to the development of calciphylaxis are unknown. Perhaps hyperglycemia or some other metabolic disturbance related to diabetes can act as a "sensitizing" agent predisposing to the development of calciphylaxis.

Obesity

Obesity (BMI, body mass index >30 kg/m^2) has been associated with the development of calciphylaxis is some studies, while others did not find this association [27, 117, 128]. In one study, obesity was approximately four times more common in dialysis patients with calciphylaxis than without [128]. Obesity may be related to development of calciphylaxis in a number of ways. Some investigators have suggested that increased percentage of adipose tissue predisposes to hypoperfusion of subcutaneous tissues and skin resulting in ischemic necrosis [27]. Moreover, calciphylactic lesions are more common in proximal locations (thighs, buttocks, and trunk) where adipose tissue is more abundant. This hypothesis is also supported by the finding of an association between obesity and calciphylaxis [117, 128]. Moreover, obesity is clearly associated with the development of diabetes and the metabolic syndrome, both of which may potentially predispose to the development of calciphylaxis.

Hypoalbuminemia

Hypoalbuminemia has been associated with the development of calciphylaxis [27, 117]. In one case–control study of nine patients with proximal calciphylaxis, there was a 17-fold increased likelihood of developing calciphylaxis for each 1 g/dL decrease in serum albumin [117]. In another study, there was a 21% decrease in the likelihood of developing calciphylaxis for each increase in serum albumin 0.1 g/dL over the 12-month period prior to and at the time of diagnosis [27]. In a case series of 16 patients with calciphylaxis, it was reported that 43% of patients lost >10% of their total body weight over the 6-month period prior to diagnosis [5]. In general, protein malnutrition as reflected by low serum albumin levels likely predisposes patients with calciphylaxis to poor wound healing and increased risk of infection, sepsis, and death [27, 136].

Hypercoaguable States

Hypercoaguable states have been associated with the development of calciphylaxis, especially protein C and/or S deficiency [138, 146–149]. In one review of 36 cases of nonuremic calciphylaxis, protein C and/or S deficiency was present in 11% of patients [138]. In another review of calciphylaxis cases that reported protein C and/or S levels, 38% had decreased protein C and 43% had decreased protein S levels [146]. Other reports of calciphylaxis associated with hypercoaguable states include antiphospholipid syndrome and cryofibrinogenemia [146, 150, 151].

Inflammatory Diseases

Inflammatory diseases, including connective tissue, autoimmune, and other diseases, have also been associated with development of calciphylaxis.

There are several reports of calciphylaxis associated with rheumatoid arthritis, systemic lupus erythematosus, Crohn's disease, temporal arteritis, and various other inflammatory diseases [8, 104, 112, 138, 145, 152–159]. Moreover, calciphylaxis is associated with inflammatory disease and is often reported in the absence of uremia or HPT; therefore, additional triggers are suspected in this context [138, 156, 157]. Moreover, many patients with inflammatory diseases are treated with corticosteroids, which are considered a predisposing or "sensitizing" factor, and various other immune-modulating agents which may further confound these associations.

POEMS Syndrome

POEMS syndrome has recently been associated with the development of calciphylaxis. POEMS syndrome is a rare plasma cell lymphoproliferative disorder associated with *p*olyneuropathy, *o*rganomegaly, *e*ndocrinopathy, *m*onoclonal gammopathy, and *s*kin abnormalities. Multiple cases of POEMS syndrome with skin abnormalities manifesting as calciphylaxis in the absence of renal failure, HPT, or clotting disorders have been reported [160–164]. Although a pathogenic link between POEMS syndrome and calciphylaxis has yet to be elucidated, in one case report the patient was found to have markedly elevated serum vascular endothelial growth factor (VEGF) [161]. This led to the hypothesis that VEGF may play a role in the pathogenesis of calciphylaxis as it is known to influence vascular calcification along with other bone morphogenetic proteins. Moreover, corticosteroids and several proinflammatory cytokines that activate NF-κB, considered the final common pathway of vascular calcification, also may be involved.

Liver Disease

Liver disease has been associated with the development of calciphylaxis [128, 165–167]. In one study of nonuremic calciphylaxis, alcoholic liver disease accounted for 16.7% of cases [138]. Although the relationship between liver disease and development of calciphylaxis is poorly understood, liver disease causes a multitude of metabolic abnormalities many of which may serve as "sensitizing" or "challenging" agents. Liver disease is often associated with renal failure, and liver failure is almost universally associated with hypoalbuminemia, severe malnutrition, and all of their respective associated comorbidities. Therefore, like uremia associated with late-stage CKD and ESRD, chronic liver disease or failure may create a favorable milieu for the development of calciphylaxis.

Medications Associated with Calciphylaxis

Warfarin

Warfarin has been associated with the development of calciphylaxis which has been reported to resolve upon discontinuation in some cases [5, 168, 169]. The association between warfarin and calciphylaxis may potentially be explained by warfarin's ability to inhibit vitamin-K-dependent carboxylation of the vascular calcification inhibitor MGP, thereby locally decreasing its activity allowing for the development of vascular calcification [55]. Low molecular weight heparin has been suggested as an alternative if continuation of anticoagulation is necessary. Moreover, it is important to note that the clinical manifestations of warfarin-induced skin necrosis and calciphylaxis are similar; therefore, the diagnoses are easily confused [168, 170].

Corticosteroids

Corticosteroid use has been associated with the development of calciphylaxis; however, it does not necessarily resolve readily upon discontinuation [112, 128, 152–154]. Corticosteroids are often used to treat autoimmune and inflammatory diseases which also have been associated with the development of calciphylaxis. Steroids likely represent a predisposing or "sensitizing" agent for the development of calciphylaxis, rather than a cause of the disease [138]. Moreover, corticosteroids are often associated with poor wound healing and should be avoided in the presence of ischemic ulcers. By contrast, some studies have reported corticosteroid therapy may be beneficial in some cases in the absence of ischemic ulcers [28]. Indeed, corticosteroid therapy may be necessary for some patients, especially those with autoimmune or connective tissue diseases; therefore, the risks versus benefits must be carefully considered for each individual patient.

Nonuremic Calciphylaxis

Calciphylaxis is usually associated with ESRD and occasionally with renal transplantation, and hence its designation as a uremic arteriolopathy. However, nonuremic causes have also been reported with morphologically similar skin lesions, but often in the absence of some of the major purported associated factors. In a review of 36 cases of nonuremic calciphylaxis reported between 1956 and 2007, defined as a histopathologic diagnosis of calciphylaxis in the absence of ESRD, renal transplantation, or acute kidney injury requiring renal replacement therapy, primary HPT (27.8%), malignancy (22.2%), alcoholic liver disease (16.7%), and connective tissue disease (11.1%), were among the most common causes [138]. Similar to uremic calciphylaxis, majority of patients were Caucasian females, mortality was high (52%), and sepsis was the most common cause of death. In contrast to uremic calciphylaxis, normal serum calcium (58.0%), phosphorus (69.4%), and Ca×P product <55 mg^2/dL^2 (38.9%) were found in a significant number of cases. Moreover, although PTH levels were high in many cases (30.5%), levels were normal in even more cases (38.9%) and low in a significant number of cases (11.1%). Clearly, the metabolic abnormalities associated with uremic calciphylaxis and secondary HPT (hypercalcemia, hyperphosphatemia, Ca×P product >55 mg^2/dL^2, and elevated PTH) do not predominate in nonuremic calciphylaxis despite similar morphologic and histologic disease manifestations suggesting that other mechanisms may contribute significantly to the etiology and pathogenesis of calciphylaxis. Moreover, it is interesting to note that calciphylaxis associated with renal transplantation has been reported with varying degrees of renal function and sometimes without the metabolic abnormalities associated with uremic calciphylaxis [121].

Diagnosis

Clinical Diagnosis vs. Biopsy

In most patients, the diagnosis of calciphylaxis is made only after vascular calcification has caused significant tissue damage. Biopsy is considered the gold standard for definitive diagnosis; however, it has been reported to cause nonhealing ulcers in some cases and is usually unnecessary when clinical manifestations suggest the diagnosis [28]. Clinically, calciphylaxis is the likely diagnosis in ESRD patients on dialysis with hyperphosphatemia, Ca×P product >55 mg^2/dL^2, elevated PTH, and characteristic painful lesions with plaques resembling livedo reticularis, nonhealing ulcerated necrotic tissue with eschars, or some combination of both (Fig. 6.2).

The differential diagnosis of calciphylaxis is extensive as clinical manifestations and lesions can mimic many other disease states, many of which are common in late-stage CKD or ESRD (Table 6.5) [8, 23, 104, 147, 150, 151, 170–172]. Distinguishing between lesions associated with calciphylaxis and those associated with other causes is often difficult. Early calciphylaxis is often mistaken for cellulitis, whereas nonhealing ulcerations in advanced calciphylaxis may resemble ulcerations from other causes. For example, ulcerations of the lower extremities in late-stage CKD or ESRD patients are often caused by peripheral vascular disease (PVD) and are usually associated with significant pain, whereas ulcerations in diabetic patients are often associated with peripheral neuropathy and may be painless.

Histopathology

Calciphylaxis is characterized histopathologically by vascular and extravascular calcification. Extravascular calcification of subcutaneous tissues and skin, along with vascular insufficiency, causes tissue ischemia that may manifests as necrosis and epidermolysis on biopsy (Fig. 6.4a, b). Vascular calcification is characterized by prominent medial calcification, intimal proliferation

Table 6.5 Differential diagnosis of calciphylaxis and calciphylactic lesions

Infectious cellulitis
Peripheral vascular disease
Venous stasis ulceration
Cutaneous vasculitis
Coumadin- or warfarin-induced skin necrosis
Heparin-induced skin necrosis
Nephrogenic systemic fibrosis (nephrogenic fibrosing dermopathy)
Hypercoaguable diseases or states Protein C or S deficiency Antiphospholipid syndrome Cryofibrinogenemia Thromboembolic phenomena Other clotting abnormalities
Erythema nodosum
Bullous pemphigoid
Pyoderma gangrenosum
Necrotizing fasciitis
Temporal arteritis (giant cell arteritis)
Brown recluse spider bite

(hyperplasia), and arteriolar stenosis, often with superimposed thrombotic occlusion causing vascular insufficiency (Fig. 6.4c, d) [143]. However, it is important to note that not all biopsy specimens will demonstrate all of the characteristic findings of calciphylaxis owing to sampling error. In one study, evidence of subcutaneous tissue or skin thrombosis was found in only 38 of 44 (86%) of biopsies [128].

Diagnostic Imaging

^{99m}Tectnetium-methylene diphosphonate (^{99m}Te-MDP) scans have been reported to be useful in supporting the clinical diagnosis of calciphylaxis by demonstrating areas of increased radiotracer activity corresponding to subcutaneous calcified plaques [28, 173]. Moreover, effective treatment of calciphylaxis may result in decreased radiotracer activity corresponding to clinical resolution of calciphylactic lesions [173–175]. While not considered diagnostic, such scans may support the clinical diagnosis and possibly help avoid the risks associated with biopsy of suspicious lesions.

X-ray surveys may demonstrate areas corresponding to subcutaneous calcified plaques, but has been reported to appear normal in up to 30% of patients with confirmed disease [28]. Moreover, false-positive X-ray bone surveys have been reported in a significant percentage of patients without the diagnosis of calciphylaxis [25]. Therefore, while X-ray bone surveys may support the clinical diagnosis when positive, they are neither sensitive nor specific enough to recommend routine clinical use.

Novel techniques for imaging of arteriolar calcification in patients with calciphylaxis have also been reported. A recent report of digital subtraction mammography suggests that it may be a safe and effective technique and is superior to X-ray surveys and computed tomographic scans. Such techniques may prove useful in the future for screening patients at high risk of calciphylaxis [176].

Prevention

Approach to Patients at Risk for Calciphylaxis

Prevention is the mainstay of management for patients at risk for calciphylaxis (e.g., ESRD, primary or secondary HPT with increased PTH, hyperphosphatemia) and strategies should target known risk factors, particularly those that can be modified by lifestyle changes or medication. Serum phosphorus should be <5.5 mg/dL, although levels within the reference range of 2.5–4.5 mg/dL (0.81–1.45 mmol/L) may be more ideal. Corrected serum calcium should be <9.6 mg/dL (corrected calcium [mg/dL] = measured calcium [mg/dL] + 0.8 (4.0-measured serum albumin [g/dL]), where 4.0 represents an normal serum albumin concentration in g/dL), although levels within the reference range of 9.0–10.5 mg/dL (2.2–2.6 mmol/L) may be more ideal. In either case, maintaining a Ca × P product <55 mg^2/dL^2 may decrease the risk of developing calciphylaxis. Although an ideal target has yet to be established, lowering PTH levels to <200 pg/mL has been suggested [133].

Treatment of hyperphosphatemia and maintenance of normocalcemia to avoid an elevated Ca × P product is very important. The approach to achieving these goals should focus primarily on

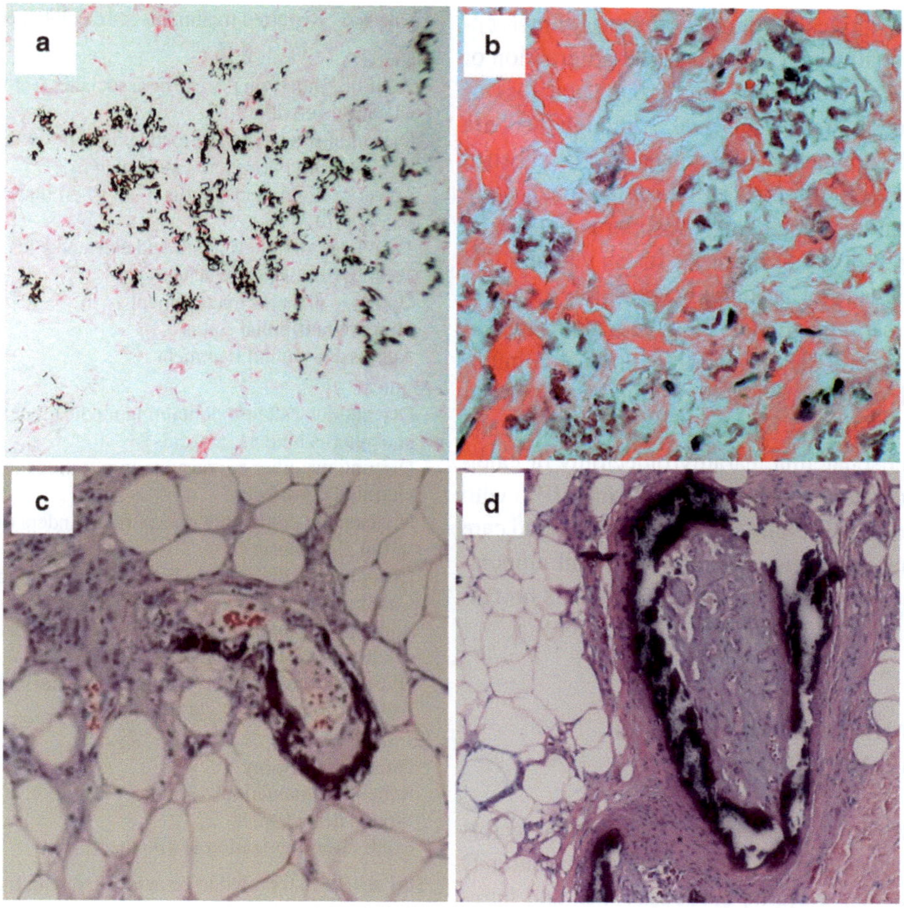

Fig. 6.4 Histopathology of calciphylactic lesions. (**a**, **b**) Skin biopsy of the right thigh of a patient with the clinical diagnosis of calciphylaxis prepared using von Kossa's method for calcium demonstrating extravascular calcium deposition in the subcutaneous tissues and skin consistent with a diagnosis of calciphylaxis. *Magnification* × *40* (***a***) *and* × *100* (***b***). (**c**, **d**) Characteristic prominent medial calcification and intimal proliferation of the arterioles consistent with a diagnosis of calciphylaxis. As is often the case, superimposed thrombotic occlusion causing vascular insufficiency are absent in this tissue section

managing secondary HPT associated with late-stage CKD or ESRD, targeting serum PTH, phosphorus, and calcium levels to improve overall calcium–phosphorus balance which may prevent or delayed the development of calciphylaxis. Since phosphorus is not removed effectively by peritoneal or hemodialysis and most patients who develop calciphylaxis have ESRD, prevention for must focus on limiting or avoiding intake or exposure by dietary modification, use of aluminum- and calcium-free phosphorus binders, and use of low-calcium dialysate. Limiting or avoiding calcium salts (calcium-based phosphorus binders, antacids, supplements, others) and vitamin D supplements are recommended. Other novel therapies for the treatment of calciphylaxis have also been reported in the literature and some will be included in this discussion.

Treatment

Multidisciplinary Approach to Patients with Established Calciphylaxis

Therapeutic strategies are still under investigation, but are mostly supportive. Early recognition and an aggressive multidisciplinary approach including medical, surgical, wound, and dietary intervention may slow, halt, or reverse the progression of the disease, potentially minimizing the loss of limbs and improving survival. Although there are currently no standard treatments for established calciphylaxis, the most effective approaches are those that target calcium–phosphorus homeostasis. Aggressive correction of serum calcium and phosphorus levels as quickly and safely as possible is recommended [177]. The mainstays of treatment are dietary modification, aluminum- and calcium-free phosphorus binders, low-calcium dialysate for hypercalcemia and hyperphosphatemia, parathyroidectomy or calcimimetics for primary or secondary HPT with increased PTH levels, and aggressive wound care including debridement, antibiotics, and amputation when necessary. Reported treatments for calciphylaxis are summarized in Table 6.6.

Table 6.6 Reported treatments for calciphylaxis

General
Treat the underlying cause or associated factors whenever possible
Discontinue aggravating medications or other agents
Lower serum phosphorus and calcium
Lower calcium–phosphorus (Ca × P) product to <55 mg²/dL²
Treat hyperparathyroidism and elevated PTH levels
Treat hypercoaguable states
Optimize diabetes management
Improve nutritional status
Aggressive wound treatment
Medical
Discontinue calcium-containing medications (e.g., phosphorus binders, antacids)
Discontinue other aggravating medications (e.g., vitamin D, warfarin)
Noncalcium containing phosphorus binders to lower serum phosphorus
Low-calcium dialysate to lower serum calcium
Calcimimetics to lower serum PTH (e.g., cinacalcet)
Sodium thiosulfate to solubilize or curtail further calcium deposition
Hyperbaric oxygen to promote wound healing
Antibiotics to treat or curtail infection
Surgical
Parathyroidectomy
Renal transplantation[a]
Wound debridement
Limb revascularization or amputation

[a]Has also been reported to be associated with the development of calciphylaxis

Discontinuation of Potential Aggravating Factors

Discontinuation of potential aggravating factors including calcium salts, aluminum salts, vitamin D supplements, warfarin, corticosteroids, and intravenous iron therapy should be considered [127, 132]. When vitamin D therapy is necessary in patients with established calciphylaxis, less calcemic analogs should be used at the minimum effective dose [133]. Discontinuation of warfarin may allow resolution of calciphylactic lesions and low molecular weight heparin has been suggested as a suitable alternative in patients without contraindication if continuation of anticoagulation is necessary [5, 168]. Argatroban may also be used when contraindication to heparin exists, such as with heparin-induced thrombocytopenia (HIT), which is not uncommon among dialysis patients [178].

Adjustment of Dialysis Therapy

Low-calcium dialysate should be used for patients with calciphylaxis in the absence of hypocalcemia. Peritoneal dialysis has been associated with the development of calciphylaxis and one study reported that conversion to hemodialysis led to marked early improvement of calciphylactic lesions [118]. Some have also suggested that increasing the frequency of hemodialysis may be beneficial, especially for patients with hypercalcemia, hyperphosphatemia, and/or an elevated Ca × P product.

Phosphorus Binders

Phosphorus binders are a mainstay of treatment for calciphylaxis as they decrease intestinal phosphorus absorption when ingested with food [3, 27, 28, 103, 179]. There have been case reports of refractory calciphylaxis responsive to phosphorus binders [179]. Available phosphorus binders include calcium, sevelamer, lanthium, and aluminum.

Calcium-based phosphorus binders (e.g., calcium carbonate, calcium acetate) are effective and inexpensive, but are relatively contraindicated in calciphylaxis because they increase both serum calcium levels and the Ca×P product. Their use is generally be avoided in dialysis patients, except perhaps for patients with hypocalcemia [180].

Sevelamer-based phosphorus binders (e.g., sevelamer hydrochloride, sevelamer carbonate) are effective but expensive; however ,they are not absorbed and therefore cause diarrhea more often [181]. Moreover, sevelamer hydrochloride has been associated with metabolic acidosis, whereas sevelamer carbonate has not. Sevelamer also reduces serum uric acid which may be beneficial to calciphylaxis patients with hyperuricemia, uric acid nephrolithiasis, and gout. Despite these issues, sevelamer-based preparations have become the leading calcium-free binders used to treat hyperphosphatemia.

Lanthium-based phosphorus binders (e.g., lanthium carbonate) are useful in patients who cannot tolerate sevelamer-based phosphorus binders [179]. However, lanthium carbonate is one of the largest pills manufactured and should be chewed, not swallowed whole, to avoid choking which has been reported.

Aluminum-based phosphorus binders (e.g., aluminum hydroxide) are highly effective; however, their long-term use is associated with aluminum toxicity and deposition in the bones, joints, and brain which has limited their use mostly to short-term treatment of severe hyperphosphatemia. Although epidemiological studies have failed to establish an link between aluminum exposure and neurological disorders, there are still concerns that long-term exposure may cause or promote dementia. Moreover, evidence of aluminum deposits in calciphylactic lesions further limits their use.

Phosphorus binders must be ingested with food in order to bind dietary phosphorus. However, gastrointestinal intolerance (bloating, nausea, vomiting, and diarrhea) is common. Moreover, high dietary phosphorus intake requires a high pill burden for some phosphorus binders. These simple issues likely account for a significant portion of the noncompliance commonly associated with phosphorus binders. Route of administration can also be problematic as only certain phosphorus binders are available as liquid or powder formulations. Finally, phosphorus binders cannot be used in patients on total parenteral nutrition, rather the phosphorus content of the nutritional formulation must be adjusted.

Parathyroidectomy

Total or subtotal parathyroidectomy may also be beneficial in the setting of HPT with significantly elevated PTH and has been reported to reverse calciphylaxis in many, but not all, cases [3, 13, 28, 103, 124, 126, 139, 144, 182, 183]. In general, parathyroidectomy for the treatment of calciphylaxis reduces serum PTH, calcium, phosphorus, and the Ca×P product and improves wound healing and overall survival. Once strongly advocated as a reasonable and definitive treatment for calciphylaxis associated with secondary HPT and elevated PTH levels, the overall benefit is still a matter of debate. Many now advocate a more conservative approach and reserve parathyroidectomy for patients with very high PTH levels, high Ca×P product, or rapidly progressive disease [13]. Others argue that parathyroidectomy still offers the highest rate of cure for calciphylaxis associated with secondary HPT and should be considered first-line treatment in some cases. In one observational study of 46 patients with secondary HPT that underwent total parathyroidectomy, there was no evidence of clinical bone disease or pathologic fractures after a median follow-up period of more than 5 years [184]. Parathyroidectomy for the treatment of calciphylaxis associated with primary HPT is usually indicated, especially when due to hyperactive parathyroid adenomas [143]. Medical parathyroidectomy with local injection of parathyroid glands with alcohol has been suggested as an alternative to parathyroidectomy for patients with poor wound healing or that are otherwise poor surgical candidates [181]. Calcimimetics have also been suggested as an alternative to parathyroidectomy for poor surgical candidates.

Calcimimetic Agents

Calcimimetic agents may also be beneficial to treat calciphylaxis in the setting of primary or secondary HPT with significantly elevated PTH [185–189]. Calcimimetics work by increasing the sensitivity of CaSRs to available calcium, thereby decreasing PTH secretion. Cinacalcet is the prototypic drug of this class and some suggest it may offer an alternative to parathyroidectomy for the treatment of calciphylaxis in the setting of secondary HPT and some have also suggested it may be useful as first-line therapy in certain cases [186, 188]. Cinacalcet is currently not approved by the FDA for the treatment of calciphylaxis, nor would it be appropriate in all cases. However, cinacalcet is approved for the treatment of secondary HPT; therefore, it is reasonable to incorporate it into the treatment regimen for secondary HPT in patients at risk or with established calciphylaxis given the high mortality and potential for significant benefit. However, cinacalcet may be inappropriate in the setting of primary HPT, secondary HPT with normal or low PTH levels, or in the presence of hypocalcemia. In any case, more studies are needed to better understand the potential role of calcimimetics for the treatment of calciphylaxis.

Sodium Thiosulfate

Sodium thiosulfate is a colorless crystalline sulfur-containing compound that bears a significant negative charge on its sulfur moiety, can distribute throughout the extracellular fluid compartment, and is excreted in the urine. Sodium thiosulfate is an antioxidant cation chelator that has several medical applications, most notably as an antidote for cyanide poisoning where it acts as a sulfur donor, and more recently as prophylaxis for carboplatin- and cisplatin-induced nephrotoxicity [190, 191]. Sodium thiosulfate has been reported to be beneficial in the treatment of calciphylaxis in recent years. The thiosulfate anion is believed to react directly with calcium forming highly soluble calcium thiosulfate which is then excreted [173, 192]. There is also some evidence that sodium thiosulfate-induced metabolic acidosis may play a role in promoting calcium excretion [192].

Sodium thiosulfate had previously been reported to successfully treat tumoral calcinosis, masses of calcium–phosphate usually occurring in a periarticular distribution in dialysis patients [193–195]. Given the similarities between calciphylaxis and tumoral calcinosis, including the nature of the calcium deposits as hydroxyapatite, sodium thiosulfate was used to successfully used to treat a patient who developed debilitating calciphylactic lesions 4 months after initiating peritoneal dialysis [173]. Intravenous sodium thiosulfate three times weekly resulted in rapid and dramatic improvement in the signs and symptoms of calciphylaxis within 2 weeks of initiating therapy. Since then, others have reported similar results and advocate using sodium thiosulfate alone or in combination with other therapies [123, 196–202].

While the precise mechanism of sodium thiosulfate remains unknown, many believe it increases the solubility of calcium deposits thereby promoting urinary excretion [173, 192–195]. Studies of vascular calcification in uremic rats found that sodium thiosulfate prevented aortic calcification, decreased serum calcium, increased urinary calcium excretion, decreased the calcium content of aortic, heart, and renal tissue, induced metabolic acidosis, increased serum PTH levels, and also increased serum levels of the calcification inhibitor MGP compared to control animals [192]. However, there was evidence of decreased bone strength in treated animals likely related to increased PTH levels and hypercalciuria, associations that have been reported to reduce bone mineral density in humans [203]. Moreover, sodium thiosulfate has been reported to prevent calcium nephrolithiasis in humans, which may be related to decreased urinary excretion of endogenous thiosulfate causing recurrent calcium nephrolithiasis, which also may be related to soft tissue calcium deposition [204–206].

Finally, given that sodium thiosulfate is an antioxidant, it may also have additional benefit in curtailing inflammation and oxidative stress, both known to be involved in vascular calcification [41, 42]. Unfortunately, sodium thiosulfate is currently not approved by the FDA for the treatment of calciphylaxis and the use is considered off-label. Therefore, as the popularity of sodium thiosulfate for the treatment of calciphylaxis increases, outcome studies for this indication are warranted as the long-term effects of chronic administration are unknown, especially as they relate to bone mineral density.

Bisphosphonates

Several bisphosphonates also have been reported to be beneficial in the treatment of calciphylaxis [164, 207–211]. Bisphosphonates are mainly used to inhibit bone resorption in patients with osteoporosis and Paget disease and to treat hypercalcemia associated with malignancy. However, bisphosphonates are also known to inhibit calcium–phosphate crystal formation which is a much more prominent feature of first-generation bisphosphonates such as etidronate. Multiple case reports of successful treatment of calciphylaxis with etidronate, pamidronate, and ibandronate have been reported [164, 207–211]. Ibandronate has also been shown to prevent calciphylaxis in an animal model at doses that inhibit bone resorption [212]. Moreover, it should be noted that the bioavailability of intravenous bisphosphonates is 100%, whereas that of oral preparations is less than 5% which may influence treatment decisions.

Anticoagulation

The potential role of hypercoagulable states in the pathogenesis of calciphylaxis suggests anticoagulation may be beneficial [146]. There are reports of improvement of calciphylactic lesions with low molecular weight heparin, particularly when associated with hypercoaguable states [146, 149]. Healing of calciphylactic lesions has also been reported with low dose tissue plasminogen activator [21, 213]. The use of anticoagulation intuitively makes sense since tissue ischemia and necrosis likely results from thrombotic occlusion of calcified and stenotic arterioles. However, long-term anticoagulation may be problematic given the association of warfarin with development or aggravation of calciphylaxis, a theoretical mechanism by which it may occur, and a relative paucity of reasonable alternatives to warfarin [55, 168, 170].

Corticosteroids

Corticosteroids have been suggested to be beneficial for some patients without ulcerations; however, their use has been identified as a predisposing factor in many cases [28]. Indeed, corticosteroid therapy may be necessary in some cases; therefore, the risks versus benefits must be carefully considered for each individual patient. However, there is no evidence to suggest their routine use in the treatment of calciphylaxis.

Wound Management

Wound infections should be treated aggressively with debridement of necrotic tissue and antibiotics to avoid development of life-threatening sepsis, the most common cause of death among patients with calciphylaxis [13, 27, 124, 128, 133]. Surgical debridement of calciphylactic lesions has been reported to substantially improve 1-year survival [128]. Physicians should be aware of local microbial resistance patterns to guide antibiotic therapy for specific clinical situations. Consider infectious disease consultation when secondary infections fail to respond to antibiotic therapy. In some cases, revascularization for limb salvage may be considered, but only after aggressive management of modifiable risk factors. However, one case series and review of the literature suggested patients with calciphylaxis may not necessarily benefit from revascularization [214]. Limb amputation should also be considered for infected nonhealing lesions to help avoid sepsis, the most common cause of death. For patients with calciphylactic ulcerations that are responding to medical and/or surgical treatment, excision and skin grafting may be beneficial [119, 215].

Hyperbaric Oxygen

Hyperbaric oxygen therapy has been used to treat patients who do not respond to medical and surgical wound treatment, especially those who are hypoxic, and also has been reported to enhance healing of calciphylactic lesions [189, 201, 216–223]. Use of hyperbaric oxygen therapy is supported by the finding of extremely low transcutaneous oxygen tension in body regions of calciphylaxis patients with and without lesions compared to control patients, suggesting severe and diffuse subcutaneous tissue and skin ischemia exists even in areas without visible lesions [113]. Although transcutaneous oxygen tension in calciphylaxis patients breathing 100% supplemental oxygen remains relatively low, suggesting that the vascular insufficiency may be fixed, oxygen tension does increase enough in some patients to suggest there may be clinical benefit. It is thought that increasing the partial pressure of oxygen (PO_2) in tissue to normal or above-normal promotes fibroblast and endothelial cell proliferation, collagen synthesis, angiogenesis, and wound healing [189, 201, 222, 223]. In a retrospective case series of dialysis patients treated for calciphylaxis with hyperbaric oxygen, eight of nine patients responded favorably with significant healing of calciphylactic lesions [218].

Pain Management

Pain management is an important component of any comprehensive treatment plan and can significantly improve quality of life. Unfortunately, the severity of pain causes many patients become dependent on narcotic analgesics for relief. However, neurolytic lumber sympathetic block may offer an alternative for pain associated with calciphylaxis in some patients [224].

Future Therapies

There are currently no standard treatments for calciphylaxis, and outcomes for the aforementioned therapies are unknown as there are no prospective randomized controlled trials. Moreover, there are even fewer treatment options for patients without renal failure associated with hyperphosphatemia and/or without HPT associated with elevated PTH levels. Future therapies are likely to target molecular mechanisms that mediate the development of vascular calcification. Several of the inhibitors of vascular calcification that have been identified may hold promise as potential future treatments.

Prognosis

Prognosis is directly related to the progression and extent of disease. Fine et al. reported in a prospective case–control study of 33 patients with calciphylaxis that the 1-year mortality rate was 41% for patients initially presenting with plaques only, 67% for patients initially presenting with ulcers with or without plaques, and 45% for all patients [28]. Moreover, the 1-year mortality rate was 80% for patients who developed ulcers at any time during the course of their disease, in contrast to 17% for patients who did not develop ulcers at any time. Therefore, calciphylaxis should be considered a very poor prognostic indicator and every effort should be made to halt disease progression, with particular emphasis on preventing the development of ulcers.

Prognosis also may be related to the location of calciphylactic lesions with more proximal lesions (thighs, buttocks, and trunk) associated with a worse prognosis than more distal lesions (calves, forearms, fingers, toes, and penis) [5, 13, 27]. Moreover, 61% of diabetic patients with calciphylaxis and late-stage CKD or ESRD had acral gangrene compared to 34% of nondiabetic patients [13]. In a retrospective study of 64 patients with calciphylaxis (49 on dialysis), the 1-year survival was 61.6% for patients who received surgical debridement compared to 27.4% for those who did not [128].

Parathyroidectomy appears to significantly affect the progression, extent of disease, and survival and may be appropriate for patients who are resistant to medical therapy [13, 103]. Arch-Ferrer et al. reported in a retrospective [more specific] study of 35 calciphylaxis patients treated with total or subtotal parathyroidectomy that surgical patients had significantly improved serum calcium, phosphorus, PTH, calciphylactic lesions, and overall survival rate (80 months) compared to nonsurgical patients (35 months) [103].

Discussion

Calciphylaxis is a poorly understood syndrome of vascular calcification and cutaneous necrosis. Clinically, calciphylaxis is the likely diagnosis in ESRD patients on dialysis with hyperphosphatemia, Ca×P product >55 mg^2/dL^2, elevated PTH, and characteristic painful lesions with plaques resembling livedo reticularis, nonhealing ulcerated necrotic tissue with eschars, or some combination of both. Calciphylaxis appears to result from a number of predisposing factors and/or "sensitizing" events that are commonly present in the uremic milieu. However, many of the metabolic abnormalities common among uremic patients with calciphylaxis may not be present in nonuremic calciphylaxis. Moreover, while the precise etiology and pathogenesis of calciphylaxis have yet to be elucidated, the understanding that vascular calcification is an active, cell-mediated process that results from an imbalance between factors that promote and inhibit extraskeletal mineralization has greatly advanced our understanding of calciphylaxis and will likely lead to the development of more effective treatments.

Identifying the patients at risk and targeting modifiable risk factors are key to prevention. There are currently no standard treatments for established calciphylaxis and many strategies are of unproven benefit. Current treatment strategies are mostly supportive and new approaches are under investigations. Early recognition and aggressive treatment are key to improving the overall prognosis. Comprehensive wound care and antibiotics are key to avoiding life-threatening complications as many patients eventually succumb to wound infection, gangrene and sepsis, the most common cause of death.

Conclusion

The majority of our clinical knowledge is based on individual case reports often of advanced, complicated, or unusual cases and with relatively few controlled studies. Moreover, there is a relative paucity of case reports or studies of early disease, when intervention would likely have the greatest impact in terms of morbidity and mortality. Interestingly, the overwhelming majority of calciphylaxis patients have ESRD and spend an extensive amount of time in dialysis centers which are highly specialized and controlled medical environments which theoretically should make it easier to conduct multicenter prospective randomized controlled trials.

The prevalence of calciphylaxis is currently estimated at approximately 1 in 25 hemodialysis patients; therefore, as the number of patients on hemodialysis increases so too will the need for more effective disease prevention, early recognition, and treatment strategies. Since majority of patients developing calciphylaxis are on dialysis, education programs should be targeted at this patient population, nephrologists, and other healthcare professionals involved in providing dialysis services.

References

1. Selye H. Calciphylaxis. Chicago: University of Chicago Press; 1962.
2. Selye H, Gabbiani G, Strebel R. Sensitization to calciphylaxis by endogenous parathyroid hormone. Endocrinology. 1962;71:554–8.
3. Gipstein RM, Coburn JW, Adams DA, et al. Calciphylaxis in man. A syndrome of tissue necrosis and vascular calcification in 11 patients with chronic renal failure. Arch Intern Med. 1976;136:1273–80.
4. Weenig RH. Pathogenesis of calciphylaxis: Hans Selye to nuclear factor kappa-B. J Am Acad Dermatol. 2008;58:458–71.

5. Coates T, Kirkland GS, Dymock RB, et al. Cutaneous necrosis from calcific uremic arteriolopathy. Am J Kidney Dis. 1998;32:384–91.
6. Janigan DT, Hirsch DJ, Klassen GA, et al. Calcified subcutaneous arterioles with infarcts of the subcutis and skin ("calciphylaxis") in chronic renal failure. Am J Kidney Dis. 2000;35:588–97.
7. Anderson DC, Stewart WK, Piercy DM. Calcifying panniculitis with fat and skin necrosis in a case of uraemia with autonomous hyperparathyroidism. Lancet. 1968;2:323–5.
8. Carlson JA, Chen KR. Cutaneous pseudovasculitis. Am J Dermatopathol. 2007;29:44–55.
9. Conn Jr J, Krumlovsky FA, Del Greco F, et al. Calciphylaxis: etiology of progressive vascular calcification and gangrene? Ann Surg. 1973;177:206–10.
10. Dahl PR, Winkelmann RK, Connolly SM. The vascular calcification-cutaneous necrosis syndrome. J Am Acad Dermatol. 1995;33:53–8.
11. Friedman SA, Novack S, Thomson GE. Arterial calcification and gangrene in uremia. N Engl J Med. 1969;280:1392–4.
12. Grob JJ, Legre R, Bertocchio P, et al. Calcifying panniculitis and kidney failure. Considerations on pathogenesis and treatment of calciphylaxis. Int J Dermatol. 1989;28:129–31.
13. Hafner J, Keusch G, Wahl C, et al. Calciphylaxis: a syndrome of skin necrosis and acral gangrene in chronic renal failure. Vasa. 1998;27:137–43.
14. Henschel A, Dannenberg L, Gobel U, et al. Disseminated ischemic necrosis and livedo racemosa in a chronic dialysis patient with calciphylaxis. Hautarzt. 1999;50:439–44.
15. Kane WJ, Petty PM, Sterioff S, et al. The uremic gangrene syndrome: improved healing in spontaneously forming wounds following subtotal parathyroidectomy. Plast Reconstr Surg. 1996;98:671–8.
16. Kyttaris VC, Timbil S, Kalliabakos D, et al. Calciphylaxis: a pseudo-vasculitis syndrome. Semin Arthritis Rheum. 2007;36:264–7.
17. Levin A, Mehta RL, Goldstein MB. Mathematical formulation to help identify the patient at risk of ischemic tissue necrosis—a potentially lethal complication of chronic renal failure. Am J Nephrol. 1993;13:448–53.
18. Llach F. Calcific uremic arteriolopathy (calciphylaxis): an evolving entity? Am J Kidney Dis. 1998;32:514–8.
19. Lowry LR, Tschen JA, Wolf JE, et al. Calcifying panniculitis and systemic calciphylaxis in an end-stage renal patient. Cutis. 1993;51:245–7.
20. Peterson R. Small vessel calcification and its relationship to secondary hyperparathyroidism in the renal homotransplant patient. Radiology. 1978;126:627–33.
21. Rogers NM, Teubner DJ, Coates PT. Calcific uremic arteriolopathy: advances in pathogenesis and treatment. Semin Dial. 2007;20:150–7.
22. Ross CN, Cassidy MJ, Thompson M, et al. Proximal cutaneous necrosis associated with small vessel calcification in renal failure. Q J Med. 1991;79:443–50.
23. Stout C, Ayoub M. Calcific uremic arteriolopathy. Hosp Physician. 2007;43(1):31–7.
24. Korber A, Klode J, Al-Benna S, et al. Etiology of chronic leg ulcers in 31,619 patients in Germany analyzed by an expert survey. J Dtsch Dermatol Ges. 2011;9(2):116–21.
25. Angelis M, Wong LL, Myers SA, et al. Calciphylaxis in patients on hemodialysis: a prevalence study. Surgery. 1997;122:1083–9. discussion 1089–90.
26. Budisavljevic MN, Cheek D, Ploth DW. Calciphylaxis in chronic renal failure. J Am Soc Nephrol. 1996;7:978–82.
27. Mazhar AR, Johnson RJ, Gillen D, et al. Risk factors and mortality associated with calciphylaxis in end-stage renal disease. Kidney Int. 2001;60:324–32.
28. Fine A, Zacharias J. Calciphylaxis is usually non-ulcerating: risk factors, outcome and therapy. Kidney Int. 2002;61:2210–7.
29. Giachelli CM. Vascular calcification mechanisms. J Am Soc Nephrol. 2004;15:2959–64.
30. Qunibi WY, Nolan CA, Ayus JC. Cardiovascular calcification in patients with end-stage renal disease: a century-old phenomenon. Kidney Int Suppl. 2002;62:S73–80.
31. Schwarz U, Buzello M, Ritz E, et al. Morphology of coronary atherosclerotic lesions in patients with end-stage renal failure. Nephrol Dial Transplant. 2000;15:218–23.
32. Contiguglia SR, Alfrey AC, Miller NL, et al. Nature of soft tissue calcification in uremia. Kidney Int. 1973;4:229–35.
33. Speer MY, Giachelli CM. Regulation of cardiovascular calcification. Cardiovasc Pathol. 2004;13:63–70.
34. Llach F. The evolving pattern of calciphylaxis: therapeutic considerations. Nephrol Dial Transplant. 2001;16:448–51.
35. Llach F. The evolving clinical features of calciphylaxis. Kidney Int Suppl. 2003:S122–4.
36. Fraser WD. Hyperparathyroidism. Lancet. 2009;374:145–58.
37. Cottone S, Lorito MC, Riccobene R, et al. Oxidative stress, inflammation and cardiovascular disease in chronic renal failure. J Nephrol. 2008;21:175–9.
38. Zoccali C, Mallamaci F, Tripepi G. Novel cardiovascular risk factors in end-stage renal disease. J Am Soc Nephrol. 2004;15 Suppl 1:S77–80.
39. Covic A, Kanbay M, Voroneanu L, et al. Vascular calcification in chronic kidney disease. Clin Sci (Lond). 2010;119:111–21.
40. Spasovski G, Massy Z, Vanholder R. Phosphate metabolism in chronic kidney disease: from pathophysiology to clinical management. Semin Dial. 2009;22:357–62.
41. Sowers KM, Hayden MR. Calcific uremic arteriolopathy: pathophysiology, reactive oxygen species and therapeutic approaches. Oxid Med Cell Longev. 2010;3:109–21.
42. Tintut Y, Patel J, Territo M, et al. Monocyte/macrophage regulation of vascular calcification in vitro. Circulation. 2002;105:650–5.

43. Collin-Osdoby P, Rothe L, Anderson F, et al. Receptor activator of NF-kappa B and osteoprotegerin expression by human microvascular endothelial cells, regulation by inflammatory cytokines, and role in human osteoclastogenesis. J Biol Chem. 2001;276:20659–72.
44. Kaden JJ, Bickelhaupt S, Grobholz R, et al. Receptor activator of nuclear factor kappaB ligand and osteoprotegerin regulate aortic valve calcification. J Mol Cell Cardiol. 2004;36:57–66.
45. Schoppet M, Al-Fakhri N, Franke FE, et al. Localization of osteoprotegerin, tumor necrosis factor-related apoptosis-inducing ligand, and receptor activator of nuclear factor-kappaB ligand in Monckeberg's sclerosis and atherosclerosis. J Clin Endocrinol Metab. 2004;89:4104–12.
46. Tintut Y, Abedin M, Cho J, et al. Regulation of RANKL-induced osteoclastic differentiation by vascular cells. J Mol Cell Cardiol. 2005;39:389–93.
47. Jules J, Ashley JW, Feng X. Selective targeting of RANK signaling pathways as new therapeutic strategies for osteoporosis. Expert Opin Ther Targets. 2010;14:923–34.
48. Enjuanes A, Ruiz-Gaspa S, Peris P, et al. The effect of the alendronate on OPG/RANKL system in differentiated primary human osteoblasts. Endocrine. 2010;37:180–6.
49. Giner M, Rios MJ, Montoya MJ, et al. Alendronate and raloxifene affect the osteoprotegerin/RANKL system in human osteoblast primary cultures from patients with osteoporosis and osteoarthritis. Eur J Pharmacol. 2011;650(2–3):682–7.
50. Koch FP, Merkel C, Ziebart T, et al. Influence of bisphosphonates on the osteoblast RANKL and OPG gene expression in vitro. Clin Oral Investig. 2012;16(1):79–86.
51. Neville-Webbe HL, Coleman RE. Bisphosphonates and RANK ligand inhibitors for the treatment and prevention of metastatic bone disease. Eur J Cancer. 2010;46:1211–22.
52. Munroe PB, Olgunturk RO, Fryns JP, et al. Mutations in the gene encoding the human matrix Gla protein cause Keutel syndrome. Nat Genet. 1999;21:142–4.
53. Luo G, Ducy P, McKee MD, et al. Spontaneous calcification of arteries and cartilage in mice lacking matrix GLA protein. Nature. 1997;386:78–81.
54. Cancela L, Hsieh CL, Francke U, et al. Molecular structure, chromosome assignment, and promoter organization of the human matrix Gla protein gene. J Biol Chem. 1990;265:15040–8.
55. Wallin R, Cain D, Sane DC. Matrix Gla protein synthesis and gamma-carboxylation in the aortic vessel wall and proliferating vascular smooth muscle cells—a cell system which resembles the system in bone cells. Thromb Haemost. 1999;82:1764–7.
56. Schurgers LJ, Barreto DV, Barreto FC, et al. The circulating inactive form of matrix gla protein is a surrogate marker for vascular calcification in chronic kidney disease: a preliminary report. Clin J Am Soc Nephrol. 2010;5:568–75.
57. Cranenburg EC, Vermeer C, Koos R, et al. The circulating inactive form of matrix Gla Protein (ucMGP) as a biomarker for cardiovascular calcification. J Vasc Res. 2008;45:427–36.
58. Jahnen-Dechent W, Schafer C, Ketteler M, et al. Mineral chaperones: a role for fetuin-A and osteopontin in the inhibition and regression of pathologic calcification. J Mol Med. 2008;86:379–89.
59. Shroff RC, Shanahan CM. The vascular biology of calcification. Semin Dial. 2007;20:103–9.
60. Suliman ME, Garcia-Lopez E, Anderstam B, et al. Vascular calcification inhibitors in relation to cardiovascular disease with special emphasis on fetuin-A in chronic kidney disease. Adv Clin Chem. 2008;46:217–62.
61. Blaha V, Mistrik E, Dusilova-Sulkova S, et al. Circulating fetuin-A predicts early mortality in chronic hemodialysis patients. Clin Biochem. 2009;42:996–1000.
62. Hermans MM, Brandenburg V, Ketteler M, et al. Association of serum fetuin-A levels with mortality in dialysis patients. Kidney Int. 2007;72:202–7.
63. Ketteler M, Bongartz P, Westenfeld R, et al. Association of low fetuin-A (AHSG) concentrations in serum with cardiovascular mortality in patients on dialysis: a cross-sectional study. Lancet. 2003;361:827–33.
64. Verduijn M, Prein RA, Stenvinkel P, et al. Is fetuin-A a mortality risk factor in dialysis patients or a mere risk marker? A Mendelian randomization approach. Nephrol Dial Transplant. 2011;26(1):239–45.
65. Cozzolino M, Galassi A, Biondi ML, et al. Serum fetuin-A levels link inflammation and cardiovascular calcification in hemodialysis patients. Am J Nephrol. 2006;26:423–9.
66. Cozzolino M, Gallieni M, Brancaccio D. Inflammation and vascular calcification in chronic kidney disease: the role of Fetuin-A. Cytokine. 2009;45:70–1.
67. Wang AY, Lam CW, Chan IH, et al. Long-term mortality and cardiovascular risk stratification of peritoneal dialysis patients using a combination of inflammation and calcification markers. Nephrol Dial Transplant. 2009;24:3826–33.
68. Wang AY, Lam CW, Wang M, et al. Increased circulating inflammatory proteins predict a worse prognosis with valvular calcification in end-stage renal disease: a prospective cohort study. Am J Nephrol. 2008;28:647–53.
69. Westenfeld R, Schafer C, Smeets R, et al. Fetuin-A (AHSG) prevents extraosseous calcification induced by uraemia and phosphate challenge in mice. Nephrol Dial Transplant. 2007;22:1537–46.
70. Schafer C, Heiss A, Schwarz A, et al. The serum protein alpha 2-Heremans-Schmid glycoprotein/fetuin-A is a systemically acting inhibitor of ectopic calcification. J Clin Invest. 2003;112:357–66.
71. Rittenberg B, Partridge E, Baker G, et al. Regulation of BMP-induced ectopic bone formation by Ahsg. J Orthop Res. 2005;23:653–62.

72. Westenfeld R, Schafer C, Kruger T, et al. Fetuin-A protects against atherosclerotic calcification in CKD. J Am Soc Nephrol. 2009;20:1264–74.
73. Reinehr T, Roth CL. Fetuin-A and its relation to metabolic syndrome and fatty liver disease in obese children before and after weight loss. J Clin Endocrinol Metab. 2008;93:4479–85.
74. Yilmaz Y, Yonal O, Kurt R, et al. Serum fetuin A/{alpha}2HS-glycoprotein levels in patients with non-alcoholic fatty liver disease: relation with liver fibrosis. Ann Clin Biochem. 2010;47(Pt 6):549–53.
75. Reddi AH, Reddi A. Bone morphogenetic proteins (BMPs): from morphogens to metabologens. Cytokine Growth Factor Rev. 2009;20:341–2.
76. McCullough PA, Chinnaiyan KM, Agrawal V, et al. Amplification of atherosclerotic calcification and Monckeberg's sclerosis: a spectrum of the same disease process. Adv Chronic Kidney Dis. 2008;15:396–412.
77. Davies MR, Lund RJ, Hruska KA. BMP-7 is an efficacious treatment of vascular calcification in a murine model of atherosclerosis and chronic renal failure. J Am Soc Nephrol. 2003;14:1559–67.
78. Moe SM, O'Neill KD, Duan D, et al. Medial artery calcification in ESRD patients is associated with deposition of bone matrix proteins. Kidney Int. 2002;61:638–47.
79. Griethe W, Schmitt R, Jurgensen JS, et al. Bone morphogenic protein-4 expression in vascular lesions of calciphylaxis. J Nephrol. 2003;16:728–32.
80. Csiszar A, Smith KE, Koller A, et al. Regulation of bone morphogenetic protein-2 expression in endothelial cells: role of nuclear factor-kappaB activation by tumor necrosis factor-alpha, H_2O_2, and high intravascular pressure. Circulation. 2005;111:2364–72.
81. Feng JQ, Xing L, Zhang JH, et al. NF-kappaB specifically activates BMP-2 gene expression in growth plate chondrocytes in vivo and in a chondrocyte cell line in vitro. J Biol Chem. 2003;278:29130–5.
82. Ducy P, Starbuck M, Priemel M, et al. A Cbfa1-dependent genetic pathway controls bone formation beyond embryonic development. Genes Dev. 1999;13:1025–36.
83. Engelse MA, Neele JM, Bronckers AL, et al. Vascular calcification: expression patterns of the osteoblast-specific gene core binding factor alpha-1 and the protective factor matrix gla protein in human atherogenesis. Cardiovasc Res. 2001;52:281–9.
84. Karsenty G, Ducy P, Starbuck M, et al. Cbfa1 as a regulator of osteoblast differentiation and function. Bone. 1999;25:107–8.
85. Komori T, Yagi H, Nomura S, et al. Targeted disruption of Cbfa1 results in a complete lack of bone formation owing to maturational arrest of osteoblasts. Cell. 1997;89:755–64.
86. Steitz SA, Speer MY, Curinga G, et al. Smooth muscle cell phenotypic transition associated with calcification: upregulation of Cbfa1 and downregulation of smooth muscle lineage markers. Circ Res. 2001;89:1147–54.
87. Schroeder TM, Jensen ED, Westendorf JJ. Runx2: a master organizer of gene transcription in developing and maturing osteoblasts. Birth Defects Res C Embryo Today. 2005;75:213–25.
88. Waller AH, Sanchez-Ross M, Kaluski E, et al. Osteopontin in cardiovascular disease: a potential therapeutic target. Cardiol Rev. 2010;18:125–31.
89. Jono S, Shioi A, Ikari Y, et al. Vascular calcification in chronic kidney disease. J Bone Miner Metab. 2006;24:176–81.
90. Rennenberg RJ, Schurgers LJ, Kroon AA, et al. Arterial calcifications. J Cell Mol Med. 2010;14: 2203–10.
91. Ikeda T, Shirasawa T, Esaki Y, et al. Osteopontin mRNA is expressed by smooth muscle-derived foam cells in human atherosclerotic lesions of the aorta. J Clin Invest. 1993;92:2814–20.
92. Reinholt FP, Hultenby K, Oldberg A, et al. Osteopontin—a possible anchor of osteoclasts to bone. Proc Natl Acad Sci USA. 1990;87:4473–5.
93. Ducy P, Zhang R, Geoffroy V, et al. Osf2/Cbfa1: a transcriptional activator of osteoblast differentiation. Cell. 1997;89:747–54.
94. Standal T, Borset M, Sundan A. Role of osteopontin in adhesion, migration, cell survival and bone remodeling. Exp Oncol. 2004;26:179–84.
95. Merry K, Dodds R, Littlewood A, et al. Expression of osteopontin mRNA by osteoclasts and osteoblasts in modelling adult human bone. J Cell Sci. 1993;104(Pt 4):1013–20.
96. Fatherazi S, Matsa-Dunn D, Foster BL, et al. Phosphate regulates osteopontin gene transcription. J Dent Res. 2009;88:39–44.
97. Ahmed S, O'Neill KD, Hood AF, et al. Calciphylaxis is associated with hyperphosphatemia and increased osteopontin expression by vascular smooth muscle cells. Am J Kidney Dis. 2001;37:1267–76.
98. Shao JS, Cheng SL, Sadhu J, et al. Inflammation and the osteogenic regulation of vascular calcification: a review and perspective. Hypertension. 2010; 55:579–92.
99. Stinghen AE, Bucharles S, Riella MC, et al. Immune mechanisms involved in cardiovascular complications of chronic kidney disease. Blood Purif. 2010;29:114–20.
100. Tintut Y, Patel J, Parhami F, et al. Tumor necrosis factor-alpha promotes in vitro calcification of vascular cells via the cAMP pathway. Circulation. 2000;102:2636–42.
101. Moe SM, Chen NX. Pathophysiology of vascular calcification in chronic kidney disease. Circ Res. 2004;95:560–7.
102. El-Abbadi MM, Pai AS, Leaf EM, et al. Phosphate feeding induces arterial medial calcification in uremic mice: role of serum phosphorus, fibroblast growth factor-23, and osteopontin. Kidney Int. 2009;75:1297–307.
103. Arch-Ferrer JE, Beenken SW, Rue LW, et al. Therapy for calciphylaxis: an outcome analysis. Surgery. 2003;134:941–4. discussion 944–5.
104. Awwad ST, Ghosn S, Hogan RN. Calciphylaxis of the temporal artery masquerading as temporal arteritis. Clin Experiment Ophthalmol. 2010;38:511–3.

105. Bedoya RM, Gutierrez JL, Mayorga F. Calciphylaxis causing localized tongue necrosis: a case report. J Oral Maxillofac Surg. 1997;55:193–6.
106. Crippa C, Ferrari S, Drera M, et al. Pulmonary calciphylaxis and metastatic calcification with acute respiratory failure in multiple myeloma. J Clin Oncol. 2010;28:e133–5.
107. Giacobetti R, Feldman SA, Ivanovich P, et al. Sudden fatal pulmonary calcification following renal transplantation. Nephron. 1977;19:295–300.
108. Khafif RA, Delima C, Silverberg A, et al. Acute hyperparathyroidism with systemic calcinosis. Report of a case. Arch Intern Med. 1989;149:681–4.
109. Schmidt H, Creutzfeldt W. Calciphylactic pancreatitis and pancreatitis in hyperparathyroidism. Clin Orthop Relat Res. 1970;69:135–45.
110. Shapiro C, Coco M. Gastric calciphylaxis in a patient with a functioning renal allograft. Clin Nephrol. 2007;67:119–25.
111. Tuthill MH, Stratton J, Warrens AN. Calcific uremic arteriolopathy presenting with small and large bowel involvement. J Nephrol. 2006;19:115–8.
112. Brouns K, Verbeken E, Degreef H, et al. Fatal calciphylaxis in two patients with giant cell arteritis. Clin Rheumatol. 2007;26:836–40.
113. Wilmer WA, Voroshilova O, Singh I, et al. Transcutaneous oxygen tension in patients with calciphylaxis. Am J Kidney Dis. 2001;37:797–806.
114. D'Agata EM, Mount DB, Thayer V, et al. Hospital-acquired infections among chronic hemodialysis patients. Am J Kidney Dis. 2000;35:1083–8.
115 Johnson LB, Venugopal AA, Pawlak J, et al. Emergence of community-associated methicillin-resistant *Staphylococcus aureus* infection among patients with end-stage renal disease. Infect Control Hosp Epidemiol. 2006;27:1057–62.
116. Pop-Vicas A, Strom J, Stanley K, et al. Multidrug-resistant gram-negative bacteria among patients who require chronic hemodialysis. Clin J Am Soc Nephrol. 2008;3:752–8.
117. Bleyer AJ, Choi M, Igwemezie B, et al. A case control study of proximal calciphylaxis. Am J Kidney Dis. 1998;32:376–83.
118. Fine A, Fontaine B. Calciphylaxis: the beginning of the end? Perit Dial Int. 2008;28:268–70.
119. Alikadic N, Kovac D, Krasna M, et al. Review of calciphylaxis and treatment of a severe case after kidney transplantation with iloprost in combination with hyperbaric oxygen and cultured autologous fibrin-based skin substitutes. Clin Transplant. 2009;23:968–74.
120. Brewster UC, Perazella MA. Calcific uremic arteriolopathy in a transplanted kidney. Am J Med Sci. 2005;329:102–3.
121. Hanvesakul R, Silva MA, Hejmadi R, et al. Calciphylaxis following kidney transplantation: a case report. J Med Case Reports. 2009;3:9297.
122. Massry SG, Gordon A, Coburn JW, et al. Vascular calcification and peripheral necrosis in a renal transplant recipient. Reversal of lesions following subtotal parathyroidectomy. Am J Med. 1970;49:416–22.
123. Wenzel-Seifert K, Harwig S, Keller F. Fulminant calcinosis in two patients after kidney transplantation. Am J Nephrol. 1991;11:497–500.
124. Hafner J, Keusch G, Wahl C, et al. Uremic small-artery disease with medial calcification and intimal hyperplasia (so-called calciphylaxis): a complication of chronic renal failure and benefit from parathyroidectomy. J Am Acad Dermatol. 1995;33:954–62.
125. Chan YL, Mahony JF, Turner JJ, et al. The vascular lesions associated with skin necrosis in renal disease. Br J Dermatol. 1983;109:85–95.
126. Kang AS, McCarthy JT, Rowland C, et al. Is calciphylaxis best treated surgically or medically? Surgery. 2000;128:967–71. discussion 971–2.
127. Zacharias JM, Fontaine B, Fine A. Calcium use increases risk of calciphylaxis: a case-control study. Perit Dial Int. 1999;19:248–52.
128. Weenig RH, Sewell LD, Davis MD, et al. Calciphylaxis: natural history, risk factor analysis, and outcome. J Am Acad Dermatol. 2007;56:569–79.
129. Ruggian JC, Maesaka JK, Fishbane S. Proximal calciphylaxis in four insulin-requiring diabetic hemodialysis patients. Am J Kidney Dis. 1996;28:409–14.
130. Caetano-Lopes J, Canhao H, Fonseca JE. Osteoblasts and bone formation. Acta Reumatol Port. 2007;32:103–10.
131. Lamghari M, Tavares L, Camboa N, et al. Leptin effect on RANKL and OPG expression in MC3T3-E1 osteoblasts. J Cell Biochem. 2006;98:1123–9.
132. Campistol JM, Almirall J, Martin E, et al. Calcium-carbonate-induced calciphylaxis. Nephron. 1989;51:549–50.
133. Block GA. Prevalence and clinical consequences of elevated Ca×P product in hemodialysis patients. Clin Nephrol. 2000;54:318–24.
134. Morales E, Gutierrez E, Andres A. Treatment with calcimimetics in kidney transplantation. Transplant Rev (Orlando). 2010;24:79–88.
135. Plantinga LC, Fink NE, Melamed ML, et al. Serum phosphate levels and risk of infection in incident dialysis patients. Clin J Am Soc Nephrol. 2008;3:1398–406.
136. Powe NR, Jaar B, Furth SL, et al. Septicemia in dialysis patients: incidence, risk factors, and prognosis. Kidney Int. 1999;55:1081–90.
137. Torok L, Kozepessy L. Cutaneous gangrene due to hyperparathyroidism secondary to chronic renal failure (uraemic gangrene syndrome). Clin Exp Dermatol. 1996;21:75–7.
138. Nigwekar SU, Wolf M, Sterns RH, et al. Calciphylaxis from nonuremic causes: a systematic review. Clin J Am Soc Nephrol. 2008;3:1139–43.
139. Duh QY, Lim RC, Clark OH. Calciphylaxis in secondary hyperparathyroidism. Diagnosis and parathyroidectomy. Arch Surg. 1991;126:1213–8. discussion 1218–9.
140. Mawad HW, Sawaya BP, Sarin R, et al. Calcific uremic arteriolopathy in association with low turnover uremic bone disease. Clin Nephrol. 1999;52:160–6.
141. Smith AJ, Faugere MC, Abreo K, et al. Aluminum-related bone disease in mild and advanced renal failure: evidence for high prevalence and morbidity and

studies on etiology and diagnosis. Am J Nephrol. 1986;6:275–83.
142. Kasai K, Hori MT, Goodman WG. Transferrin enhances the antiproliferative effect of aluminum on osteoblast-like cells. Am J Physiol. 1991;260:E537–43.
143. Bishop J, Brown E, Podesta A, et al. Surgical management of calciphylaxis associated with primary hyperparathyroidism: a case report and review of the literature. Int J Endocrinol. 2010; 2010. pii 823210.
144. Girotto JA, Harmon JW, Ratner LE, et al. Parathyroidectomy promotes wound healing and prolongs survival in patients with calciphylaxis from secondary hyperparathyroidism. Surgery. 2001;130: 645–50. discussion 650–1.
145. Zechlinski JJ, Angel JR. Calciphylaxis in the absence of renal disease: secondary hyperparathyroidism and systemic lupus erythematosus. J Rheumatol. 2009;36:2370–1.
146. Harris RJ, Cropley TG. Possible role of hypercoagulability in calciphylaxis: review of the literature. J Am Acad Dermatol. 2011;64(2):405–12.
147. Kant KS, Glueck HI, Coots MC, et al. Protein S deficiency and skin necrosis associated with continuous ambulatory peritoneal dialysis. Am J Kidney Dis. 1992;19:264–71.
148. Mehta RL, Scott G, Sloand JA, et al. Skin necrosis associated with acquired protein C deficiency in patients with renal failure and calciphylaxis. Am J Med. 1990;88:252–7.
149. Perez-Mijares R, Guzman-Zamudio JL, Payan-Lopez J, et al. Calciphylaxis in a haemodialysis patient: functional protein S deficiency? Nephrol Dial Transplant. 1996;11:1856–9.
150. Sankarasubbaiyan S, Scott G, Holley JL. Cryofibrinogenemia: an addition to the differential diagnosis of calciphylaxis in end-stage renal disease. Am J Kidney Dis. 1998;32:494–8.
151. Wong JJ, Laumann A, Martinez M. Calciphylaxis and antiphospholipid antibody syndrome. J Am Acad Dermatol. 2000;42:849.
152. Ozbalkan Z, Calguneri M, Onat AM, et al. Development of calciphylaxis after long-term steroid and methotroxate use in a patient with rheumatoid arthritis. Intern Med. 2005;44:1178–81.
153. Korkmaz C, Dundar E, Zubaroglu I. Calciphylaxis in a patient with rheumatoid arthritis without renal failure and hyperparathyroidism: the possible role of long-term steroid use and protein S deficiency. Clin Rheumatol. 2002;21:66–9.
154. Barri YM, Graves GS, Knochel JP. Calciphylaxis in a patient with Crohn's disease in the absence of end-stage renal disease. Am J Kidney Dis. 1997;29:773–6.
155. Al Beladi FI. Catastrophic calciphylaxis in a patient with lupus nephritis and recent onset of end-stage renal disease. Saudi J Kidney Dis Transpl. 2010;21:323–7.
156. Lee JL, Naguwa SM, Cheema G, et al. Recognizing calcific uremic arteriolopathy in autoimmune disease: an emerging mimicker of vasculitis. Autoimmun Rev. 2008;7:638–43.
157. Ortiz A, Ceccato F, Roverano S, et al. Calciphylaxis associated with rheumatoid arthritis: communication of the second case. Clin Rheumatol. 2009;28 Suppl 1:S65–8.
158. Slough S, Servilla KS, Harford AM, et al. Association between calciphylaxis and inflammation in two patients on chronic dialysis. Adv Perit Dial. 2006; 22:171–4.
159. Swanson AM, Desai SR, Jackson JD, et al. Calciphylaxis associated with chronic inflammatory conditions, immunosuppression therapy, and normal renal function: a report of 2 cases. Arch Dermatol. 2009;145:723–5.
160. De Roma I, Filotico R, Cea M, et al. Calciphylaxis in a patient with POEMS syndrome without renal failure and/or hyperparathyroidism. A case report. Ann Ital Med Int. 2004;19:283–7.
161. Hineno A, Kinoshita T, Kinoshita M, et al. Calciphylaxis as a catastrophic complication in a patient with POEMS syndrome. Case Rep Neurol. 2009;1:47–53.
162. Lee FY, Chiu HC. POEMS syndrome with calciphylaxis: a case report. Acta Derm Venereol. 2011; 91(1):96–7.
163. Rossi D, Gaidano G. POEMS and calciphylaxis: a novel association? Ann Ital Med Int. 2004;19:235–7.
164. Yoshikawa M, Uhara H, Arakura F, et al. Calciphylaxis in POEMS syndrome: a case treated with etidronate. Acta Derm Venereol. 2011;91(1):98–9.
165. Fader DJ, Kang S. Calciphylaxis without renal failure. Arch Dermatol. 1996;132:837–8.
166. Ferreres JR, Marcoval J, Bordas X, et al. Calciphylaxis associated with alcoholic cirrhosis. J Eur Acad Dermatol Venereol. 2006;20:599–601.
167. Lim SP, Batta K, Tan BB. Calciphylaxis in a patient with alcoholic liver disease in the absence of renal failure. Clin Exp Dermatol. 2003;28:34–6.
168. Banerjee C, Woller SC, Holm JR, et al. Atypical calciphylaxis in a patient receiving warfarin then resolving with cessation of warfarin and application of hyperbaric oxygen therapy. Clin Appl Thromb Hemost. 2010;16:345–50.
169. Comp PC, Elrod JP, Karzenski S. Warfarin-induced skin necrosis. Semin Thromb Hemost. 1990;16:293–8.
170. Chacon G, Nguyen T, Khan A, et al. Warfarin-induced skin necrosis mimicking calciphylaxis: a case report and review of the literature. J Drugs Dermatol. 2010;9:859–63.
171. Jacobs-Kosmin D, Dehoratius RJ. Calciphylaxis: an important imitator of cutaneous vasculitis. Arthritis Rheum. 2007;57:533–7.
172. Wallace JS, Hall JC. Use of drug therapy to manage acute cutaneous necrosis of the skin. J Drugs Dermatol. 2010;9:341–9.
173. Cicone JS, Petronis JB, Embert CD, et al. Successful treatment of calciphylaxis with intravenous sodium thiosulfate. Am J Kidney Dis. 2004;43:1104–8.
174. Landau D, Krymko H, Shalev H, et al. Transient severe metastatic calcification in acute renal failure. Pediatr Nephrol. 2007;22:607–11.

175. Soni S, Leslie WD. Bone scan findings in metastatic calcification from calciphylaxis. Clin Nucl Med. 2008;33:502–4.
176. Bleibel W, Hazar B, Herman R. A case report comparing various radiological tests in the diagnosis of calcific uremic arteriolopathy. Am J Kidney Dis. 2006;48:659–61.
177. Don BR, Chin AI. A strategy for the treatment of calcific uremic arteriolopathy (calciphylaxis) employing a combination of therapies. Clin Nephrol. 2003;59:463–70.
178. Barginear MF, Donahue L, Allen SL, et al. Heparin-induced thrombocytopenia complicating hemodialysis. Clin Appl Thromb Hemost. 2008;14:105–7.
179. Chan MR, Yevzlin AS, Hinshaw M, et al. Calciphylaxis responsive to lanthanum carbonate (FOSRENOL) therapy. WMJ. 2008;107:335–8.
180. Moe SM, Chertow GM. The case against calcium-based phosphate binders. Clin J Am Soc Nephrol. 2006;1:697–703.
181. Goldberg DI, Dillon MA, Slatopolsky EA, et al. Effect of RenaGel, a non-absorbed, calcium- and aluminium-free phosphate binder, on serum phosphorus, calcium, and intact parathyroid hormone in end-stage renal disease patients. Nephrol Dial Transplant. 1998;13:2303–10.
182. Oikawa S, Osajima A, Tamura M, et al. Development of proximal calciphylaxis with penile involvement after parathyroidectomy in a patient on hemodialysis. Intern Med. 2004;43:63–8.
183. Wang HY, Yu CC, Huang CC. Successful treatment of severe calciphylaxis in a hemodialysis patient using low-calcium dialysate and medical parathyroidectomy: case report and literature review. Ren Fail. 2004;26:77–82.
184. Stracke S, Keller F, Steinbach G, et al. Long-term outcome after total parathyroidectomy for the management of secondary hyperparathyroidism. Nephron Clin Pract. 2009;111:c102–9.
185. Mohammed IA, Sekar V, Bubtana AJ, et al. Proximal calciphylaxis treated with calcimimetic 'Cinacalcet'. Nephrol Dial Transplant. 2008;23:387–9.
186. Pallure V, Comte C, Leray-Mouragues H, et al. Cinacalcet as first-line treatment for calciphylaxis. Acta Derm Venereol. 2008;88:62–3.
187. Robinson MR, Augustine JJ, Korman NJ. Cinacalcet for the treatment of calciphylaxis. Arch Dermatol. 2007;143:152–4.
188. Velasco N, MacGregor MS, Innes A, et al. Successful treatment of calciphylaxis with cinacalcet—an alternative to parathyroidectomy? Nephrol Dial Transplant. 2006;21:1999–2004.
189 Drueke TB, Ritz E. Treatment of secondary hyperparathyroidism in CKD patients with cinacalcet and/or vitamin D derivatives. Clin J Am Soc Nephrol. 2009;4:234–41.
190. Dickey DT, Wu YJ, Muldoon LL, et al. Protection against cisplatin-induced toxicities by *N*-acetylcysteine and sodium thiosulfate as assessed at the molecular, cellular, and in vivo levels. J Pharmacol Exp Ther. 2005;314:1052–8.
191. Hall AH, Dart R, Bogdan G. Sodium thiosulfate or hydroxocobalamin for the empiric treatment of cyanide poisoning? Ann Emerg Med. 2007;49: 806–13.
192. Pasch A, Schaffner T, Huynh-Do U, et al. Sodium thiosulfate prevents vascular calcifications in uremic rats. Kidney Int. 2008;74:1444–53.
193. Kyriakopoulos G, Kontogianni K. Sodium thiosulfate treatment of tumoral calcinosis in patients with end-stage renal disease. Ren Fail. 1990;12:213–9.
194. Papadakis JT, Patrikarea A, Digenis GE, et al. Sodium thiosulfate in the treatment of tumoral calcifications in a hemodialysis patient without hyperparathyroidism. Nephron. 1996;72:308–12.
195. Yatzidis H, Agroyannis B. Sodium thiosulfate treatment of soft-tissue calcifications in patients with end-stage renal disease. Peritoneal Dial Bull. 1987;7:250–2.
196. Guerra G, Shah RC, Ross EA. Rapid resolution of calciphylaxis with intravenous sodium thiosulfate and continuous venovenous haemofiltration using low calcium replacement fluid: case report. Nephrol Dial Transplant. 2005;20:1260–2.
197. Hayden MR, Goldsmith D, Sowers JR, et al. Calciphylaxis: calcific uremic arteriolopathy and the emerging role of sodium thiosulfate. Int Urol Nephrol. 2008;40:443–51.
198. Meissner M, Bauer R, Beier C, et al. Sodium thiosulphate as a promising therapeutic option to treat calciphylaxis. Dermatology. 2006;212:373–6.
199. Meissner M, Kaufmann R, Gille J. Sodium thiosulphate: a new way of treatment for calciphylaxis? Dermatology. 2007;214:278–82.
200. Raymond CB, Wazny LD. Sodium thiosulfate, bisphosphonates, and cinacalcet for treatment of calciphylaxis. Am J Health Syst Pharm. 2008;65:1419–29.
201. Rogers NM, Coates PT. Calcific uraemic arteriolopathy: an update. Curr Opin Nephrol Hypertens. 2008;17:629–34.
202. Schlieper G, Brandenburg V, Ketteler M, et al. Sodium thiosulfate in the treatment of calcific uremic arteriolopathy. Nat Rev Nephrol. 2009;5: 539–43.
203. Heller HJ, Zerwekh JE, Gottschalk FA, et al. Reduced bone formation and relatively increased bone resorption in absorptive hypercalciuria. Kidney Int. 2007;71:808–15.
204. Agroyannis B, Tzanatos H, Vlahakos DV, et al. Does long-term administration of sodium thiosulphate inhibit progression to renal failure in nephrocalcinosis? Nephrol Dial Transplant. 2001;16:2443–4.
205. Yatzidis H. Successful sodium thiosulphate treatment for recurrent calcium urolithiasis. Clin Nephrol. 1985;23:63–7.
206. Yatzidis H. Absence or decreased endogenous thiosulfaturia: a cause of recurrent calcium nephrolithiasis. Int Urol Nephrol. 2004;36:587–9.
207. da Costa JB, da Costa AG, Gomes MM. Pamidronate as a treatment option in calciphylaxis. J Eur Acad Dermatol Venereol. 2008;22:1128–30.

208. Monney P, Nguyen QV, Perroud H, et al. Rapid improvement of calciphylaxis after intravenous pamidronate therapy in a patient with chronic renal failure. Nephrol Dial Transplant. 2004;19:2130–2.
209. Schliep S, Schuler G, Kiesewetter F. Successful treatment of calciphylaxis with pamidronate. Eur J Dermatol. 2008;18:554–6.
210. Shiraishi N, Kitamura K, Miyoshi T, et al. Successful treatment of a patient with severe calcific uremic arteriolopathy (calciphylaxis) by etidronate disodium. Am J Kidney Dis. 2006;48:151–4.
211. Musso CG, Enz PA, Guelman R, et al. Non-ulcerating calcific uremic arteriolopathy skin lesion treated successfully with intravenous ibandronate. Perit Dial Int. 2006;26:717–8.
212. Price PA, Omid N, Than TN, et al. The amino bisphosphonate ibandronate prevents calciphylaxis in the rat at doses that inhibit bone resorption. Calcif Tissue Int. 2002;71:356–63.
213. Sewell LD, Weenig RH, Davis MD, et al. Low-dose tissue plasminogen activator for calciphylaxis. Arch Dermatol. 2004;140:1045–8.
214. Mureebe L, Moy M, Balfour E, et al. Calciphylaxis: a poor prognostic indicator for limb salvage. J Vasc Surg. 2001;33:1275–9.
215. Bronson N, Menon R, Butler J, et al. Parathyroidectomy, excision and skin grafting with topical negative pressure for calciphylactic ulcers. J Wound Care. 2007;16:295–7.
216. Arenas MD, Gil MT, Gutierrez MD, et al. Management of calcific uremic arteriolopathy (calciphylaxis) with a combination of treatments, including hyperbaric oxygen therapy. Clin Nephrol. 2008;70:261–4.
217. Basile C. Hyperbaric oxygen therapy in the treatment of calciphylaxis? Yes, more than hope. Kidney Int. 2002;62:2300. author reply 2300.
218. Basile C, Montanaro A, Masi M, et al. Hyperbaric oxygen therapy for calcific uremic arteriolopathy: a case series. J Nephrol. 2002;15:676–80.
219. Podymow T, Wherrett C, Burns KD. Hyperbaric oxygen in the treatment of calciphylaxis: a case series. Nephrol Dial Transplant. 2001;16: 2176–80.
220. Vassa N, Twardowski ZJ, Campbell J. Hyperbaric oxygen therapy in calciphylaxis-induced skin necrosis in a peritoneal dialysis patient. Am J Kidney Dis. 1994;23:878–81.
221. Dean SM, Werman H. Calciphylaxis: a favorable outcome with hyperbaric oxygen. Vasc Med. 1998;3:115–20.
222. Bishop A. Role of oxygen in wound healing. J Wound Care. 2008;17:399–402.
223. Wu SC, Marston W, Armstrong DG. Wound care: the role of advanced wound healing technologies. J Vasc Surg. 2010;52:59S–66.
224. Green JA, Green CR, Minott SD. Calciphylaxis treated with neurolytic lumbar sympathetic block: case report and review of the literature. Reg Anesth Pain Med. 2000;25:310–2.

Cystic Parathyroid Lesions

7

Jean-François Henry and Maurizio Iacobone

Abstract

Cystic lesions in parathyroid glands are often incidentally discovered, but in general, the cystic component has no clinical significance. This chapter primarily focuses on cystic parathyroid lesions (CPLs) with a predominantly cystic component large enough to be clinically significant. CPLs arise in two different settings: (1) as a true cyst with an epithelial lining, which are usually referred to as nonfunctional parathyroid cysts (NFPCs) and (2) as the cystic degeneration of an adenoma, also referred to as functional parathyroid cysts (FPCs). Whereas the former is usually asymptomatic, the latter is commonly associated with symptoms of hyperparathyroidism.

Keywords

Parathyroid cysts • Functional • Nonfunctional • Hyperparathyroidism

Introduction

Cystic lesions in parathyroid glands are often incidentally noted but generally the cystic component has no clinical significance. This chapter only deals with cystic parathyroid lesions (CPLs) with a predominant cystic component large enough to be clinically significant.

J.-F. Henry, MD, FRCS
Department of Endocrine Surgery, University Hospital La Timone, 264, Rue St. Pierre, Marseilles 13385, France
e-mail: JeanFrancois.HENRY@ap-hm.fr

M. Iacobone, MD, FEBS (✉)
Endocrine Surgery Unit, Department of Surgical, Oncological and Gastroenterological Sciences, University of Padua, Via Giustiniani 2, Padua 35128, Italy
e-mail: maurizio.iacobone@unipd.it

Clinical CPLs are rare lesions of the neck and the superior mediastinum that were first described by Sandstrom in 1880 [1]. The first resection of a cervical CPL was performed by Goris in 1905 [2], and since then only case reports or small series of no more than 50 cases have been reported in the world literature.

CPLs arise in two different settings: (1) as a true cyst with an epithelial lining or (2) as the cystic degeneration of an adenoma or more rarely a hyperplastic gland. True parathyroid cysts are observed without any symptoms of hyperparathyroidism. They have been described as nonfunctional parathyroid cysts (NFPCs). On the other hand, CPLs resulting from the cystic degeneration of an adenoma are associated with symptoms of hyperparathyroidism. They have been described as functional parathyroid cysts (FPCs).

A.A. Licata and E.V. Lerma (eds.), *Diseases of the Parathyroid Glands*,
DOI 10.1007/978-1-4419-5550-0_7, © Springer Science+Business Media, LLC 2012

This division into two groups, namely, functional which cause hyperparathyroidism and nonfunctional which do not, may be challenged, since embryological and histological data suggest that FPCs and NFPCs differ and are likely two separate entities. If the term cystic parathyroid lesion can be used for both lesions, some authors consider that only NFPCs should be considered as true or essential parathyroid cysts.

Nonfunctional Parathyroid Cysts

Clinical Presentation

NFPCs or true parathyroid cysts are very rare lesions. They are reported to occur in 1.5% of parathyroid diseases [3, 4] and represent 1% of all cystic lesions of the neck [5]. The largest series reports 37 cases observed in 22,009 patients (0.17%) operated on for thyroid lesions [4]. Mediastinal localization has been reported in up to 30% of cases [6]. NFPCs present most commonly in middle-aged women, with a female to male ratio of 2.5:1. They are usually asymptomatic and most often discovered on a routine clinical examination. At physical examination, NFPCs tend to be soft, mobile, nontender solitary lumps, moving with deglutition, and usually located in the lower part of the neck where they may be mistaken for a thyroid nodule. There is a disposition for left laterality. They may be partially descended into the anterosuperior mediastinum and may be discovered on a routine chest X-ray. They may occasionally cause compressive symptoms such as dyspnea, hoarseness, dysphagia, or chest pain, especially when localized in the mediastinum. Cases complicated by massive hemorrhage into the neck or the mediastinum have also been reported [7, 8], but these hematomas are more usually related with the cystic degeneration of an adenoma than with a true NFPC.

Diagnosis

Prior to the advent of fine needle aspiration (FNA), NFPCs were most often mistaken for thyroid lesions and diagnosed during surgery. When performed, radionuclide thyroid scanning showed an area of no uptake, simulating an inferior solid thyroid nodule or a thyroid cyst. Today, the diagnosis of NFPCs can be made preoperatively. Ultrasound reveals a thin-walled cystic unilocular structure (Fig. 7.1). Computed tomography (CT) and magnetic resonance imaging (MRI) may also demonstrate the cystic nature of these lesions. Nevertheless, these imaging techniques are not able to determine the exact etiology [9]. FNA is the main diagnostic tool. When intracystic fluid is water-clear and colorless, it is highly suggestive not only of a parathyroid origin but also of a NFPC [3, 4, 10, 11] (Fig. 7.2). According to the characteristics of the aspirate, it is possible to distinguish NFPCs not only from thyroid cysts but also from FPCs. NFPCs typically contain a crystal-clear, colorless fluid, whereas FPCs and thyroid cysts produce an amber or brown, or even hemorrhagic fluid.

The diagnosis is usually confirmed by sending the fluid for chemistry. Detection of high parathormone (PTH) levels on aspirated material confirms that the cyst is of parathyroid origin [3, 4, 10, 11].With NFPCs the PTH concentration in the cyst fluid is elevated many times above serum PTH levels, and thyroglobulin level should be undetectable, in contrast with thyroid cyst fluid that has higher thyroglobulin concentration, with undetectable or low PTH levels [12]. Parathyroid cysts may contain breakdown products rather than the intact PTH molecule itself [5, 13]. Although intact PTH assays are generally used, it has been suggested that the measurement of PTH using a mid-molecule assay may be a more appropriate test since the intact specific assay could be normal or only slightly increased [13]. In a series of 27 patients with NFPCs, mean intracystic C-terminal/mid-region PTH level was 1,900 pg/ml (normal serum level <105 pg/ml) and mean intact PTH level was 552 pg/ml, ranging from 97 to 1,300 pg/ml (normal serum range: 10–65 pg/ml) [4]. However, detection of high PTH levels on aspirated cystic fluid does not indicate that the cyst is functioning. All these 27 patients had normal serum calcium and normal serum PTH levels [4].

Finally, a crystal-clear and colorless fluid is virtually pathognomonic for NFPCs. Parathyroid

a

b

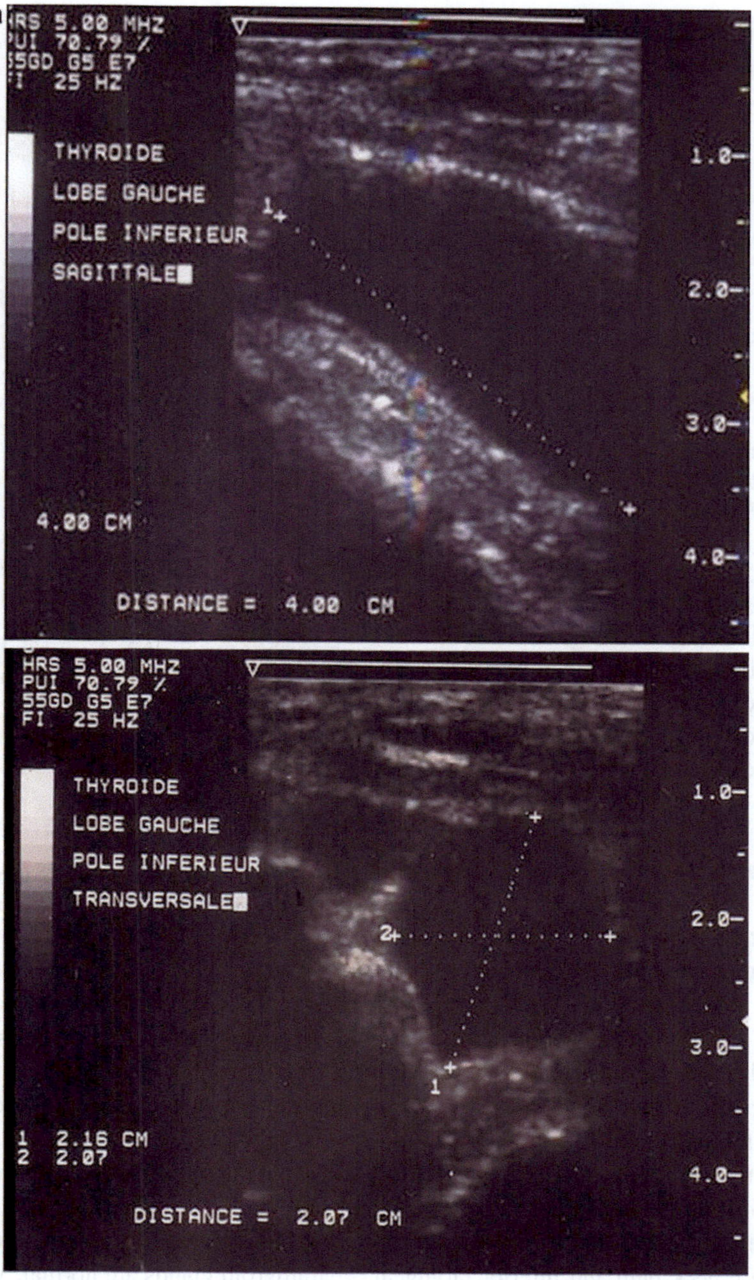

Fig. 7.1 Sagittal (**a**) and transverse (**b**) ultrasound images of a left inferior nonfunctional parathyroid cyst. Ultrasound reveals a thin-walled, cystic, unilocular structure

hormone assay of the cyst fluid can confirm the diagnosis, although it is probably unnecessary.

Mediastinal NFPCs are often unexpectedly discovered in chest radiography. They should be considered in the differential diagnosis of space-occupying cystic lesions in the superior mediastinum such as thymic cysts, bronchogenic cysts, cystic lymphangiomas, cystic strumas. Mediastinal NFPCs can extend very deep into the mediastinum down to the level of the carina, but the location of their superior pole is characteristic always at the level of the inferior pole of the thyroid lobe. Unenhanced CT shows homogeneous areas of water density, and unenhanced

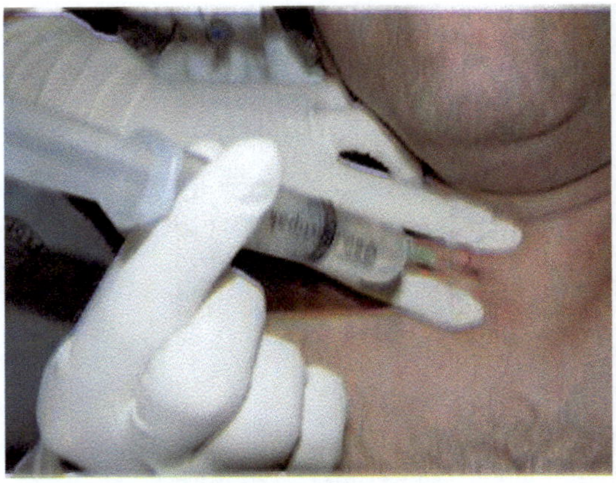

Fig. 7.2 Fine needle aspiration (FNA) of a left inferior nonfunctional parathyroid cyst. Intracystic fluid is water-clear and colorless

MRI shows homogeneous areas isointense to cerebrospinal fluid, reflecting the serous fluid content. Mediastinal NFPCs can be very large, containing more than 200 ml of water-clear fluid. As for cervical NFPCs, diagnosis is made by examining the fluid extracted from the cyst.

Management

The management of NFPCs is a matter of debate. It has been suggested that the optimal treatment for NFPCs is aspiration alone [3, 14]. Successful outcomes of this initial treatment have been reported [4, 15, 16]. However, NFPCs can recur after conservative treatment, and although repeated aspiration may be performed, the effectiveness of this approach is variable. Intracystic tetracycline injection may be used in patients with a recurrence [17, 18]. This treatment may be associated with neck pain and inferior laryngeal nerve palsy due to leakage of the sclerosing agents through the disrupted cyst wall which is particularly thin in NFPCs [19].

Overall, FNA under ultrasound guidance with detection of PTH on aspirated cystic fluid represents the approach of choice for both diagnosis and initial treatment since this is safe, easy and repeatable. The effectiveness of this approach requires long-term follow-up. Repeated recurrence should be treated surgically when compressive symptoms are associated. Nevertheless, surgery is not imperative in all cases, since NFPCs are virtually never cancer. Carcinomas within parathyroid cysts were only observed in patients presenting with FPCs [20, 21].

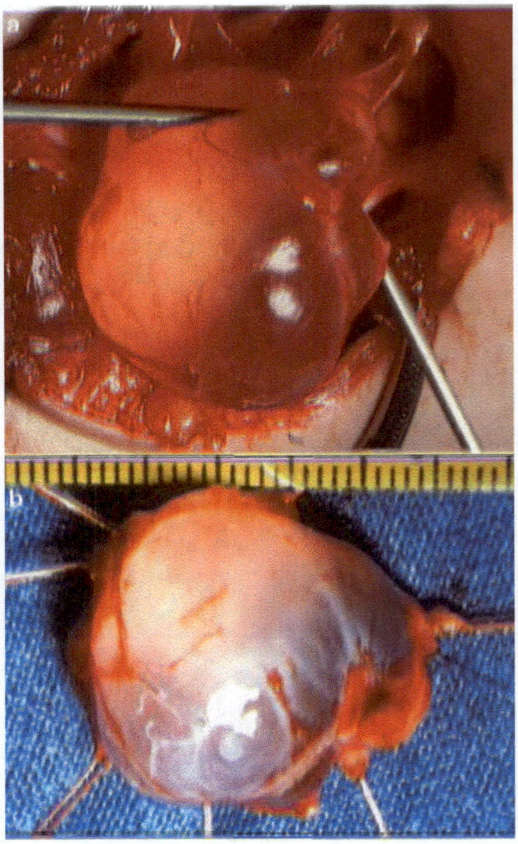

Fig. 7.3 Intraoperative view of a nonfunctional parathyroid cyst (**a**). The cyst is thin-walled, translucent, and unilocular (**b**)

At surgery, NFPCs have a well-defined plane of dissection, with the exception of rare cysts that are intrathyroidal [4]. When examined, other parathyroid glands are normal. Very few patients present with two NFPCs [4]. In most cases, the origin of NFPCs is from inferior parathyroid glands. The literature describes a predominance of left sided NFPCs. Intraoperatively, NFPCs are thin-walled, translucent, and unilocular (Fig. 7.3), with diameters ranging from a few mm to 60 mm, or even more (up to 12 cm) when they are in cervicomediastinal location [6]. Usually, they are loosely attached to the inferior pole of the thyroid gland with a definitive cleavage. Great care should be taken not to rupture these cysts during dissection and mobilization to facilitate complete resection. Despite this, rupture of these very fragile lesions can occur sometimes, but until now, no case of parathyromatosis has been reported.

Etiopathogeny

The etiology of NFPCs is uncertain and there are several theories concerning their origin. Based on histologic assessment, it seems unlikely that NFPCs represent the ultimate evolution of the cystic degeneration of an adenoma or a hyperplastic gland.

Indeed, NFPCs are true cysts with an epithelial lining. Microscopic examination shows the NFPC to be composed of a connective tissue wall lined by a single thin layer of cuboidal cells. Nests of parathyroid cells are found embedded deeply or compressed around the cyst wall without any signs of acute and chronic organization [4, 22, 23].

The microcyst theory suggests that NFPCs originate from an accumulation or retention of secretions, with a gradual enlargement or coalescence of the cysts [24]. In autopsy series, microcysts are common, increase with age, and may be detected in 50% of otherwise normal parathyroid glands [25].While it is conceivable that these cysts could become grossly visible, it remains to be explained why NFPCs are rare and occur in young patients and microcysts are so common particularly in older patients.

NFPCs may be persistent embryological remnants of branchial pouches, and more likely of the third branchial pouches. The inferior parathyroid glands and the thymus arise from the dorsal and the ventral portion of the third branchial pouches, respectively. At the 13–14 mm stage, the parathymus complex separates from the pharyngeal wall and moves toward the caudal and medial region. At 20 mm stage, the inferior parathyroids are normally abandoned by the thymus at the level of the thyrothymic ligaments, vestigial structures indicative of their former connections. A variable number of small epithelial tubules, canal of Kürsteiner, arise intimately related to the thymic tissue [26] and extend into surrounding connective tissue, possibly persisting into postnatal life as vesicular, canalicular or gland-like rudiments, given origin to a NFPC. This theory would explain why NFPCs are typically found in the inferior parathyroids. In a series of 38 NFPCs, all cysts were located in the inferior parathyroid glands [4]. Furthermore, beneath the epithelial lining, various combinations of mesenchymal cells, thymic remnants, salivary gland heterotopia, and adipose, muscular and lymphoid tissue have been also noted. In one case, an immunohistochemical study of the wall was performed, which demonstrated that the lining stained positively for low-molecular-weight keratins (AE1-AE3, CK7, pan-keratin) and mesenchymal markers (HBME1, vimentin). The wall stained negatively for high-molecular-weight keratins (CK 19), chromogranin, and NSE [4]. These findings are also highly suggestive of a branchial origin.

Functional Parathyroid Cysts

Etiopathogeny

The term of FPCs has been proposed to describe CPLs resulting from the cystic degeneration of a parathyroid adenoma. Cystic degeneration is very common in adenomas but the cystic component is rarely large enough to be clinically significant and palpable (Fig. 7.4). This can explain that the

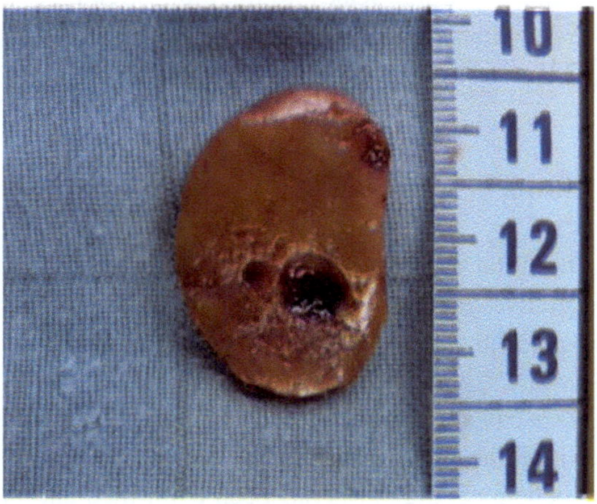

Fig. 7.4 Limited cystic degeneration of a parathyroid adenoma. In this case the cystic component is not large enough to be clinically significant

reported incidence of FPCs in literature is variable according to the criterion used to define these lesions: either parathyroid adenomas with a cystic component more or less predominant, or cystic adenomas clinically palpable.

Moreover, even when the cystic component of the adenoma is predominant the term of FPC is probably inappropriate to define these lesions. In most cystic adenomas, a fragment of the adenoma protrudes from the cyst wall into the lumen. Very rarely, the lesion is cystic in its entirety, the hyperfunctional parathyroid tissue being flattened in the cyst wall. Whether true parathyroid cysts associated with symptoms of hyperparathyroidism exist remains questionable.

When defined as parathyroid adenomas with a cystic component, FPCs are more frequently observed than NFPCs. In a recent reported series of 48 patients with CPLs, 41 (85%) had FPCs and 7 (15%) had NFPCs [11]. These findings differ from data described in other articles in the literature [3, 22] because nearly all patients were referred to surgery for primary hyperparathyroidism. FPCs account for 1–2.5% of all cases of hyperparathyroidism [11, 27].

The pathogenesis of hypercalcemia in patients with FPCs has not been fully elucidated. The hyperfunctional parathyroid tissue flattened in the cyst wall or fragments of the adenoma protruding from the cyst wall into the lumen may secrete PTH directly into the blood circulation. It has also been suggested that PTH from the lumen of the cyst might leak into the bloodstream [28]. In the latter case, it remains to be explained why PTH does not leak from the lumen of NFPCs.

Clinical Presentation

The usual clinical presentation of FPCs is hyperparathyroidism in a patient with a neck lump. This explains that there is a predominance of female sex for FPCs, with a female to male ratio of 2.4:1 [11]. FPCs can arise in two settings: (1) in a patient with symptoms of hyperparathyroidism in whom the biochemical diagnosis has been confirmed and in whom localization studies show a functional cystic parathyroid lesion or, (2) in a patient presenting with a cystic neck lump, initially mistaken for a thyroid cyst, but in whom preoperative serum calcium level is increased and in favor of an associated primary hyperparathyroidism.

Today, few patients with FPCs are misdiagnosed before surgery. In both the above-described settings, the diagnosis of hyperparathyroidism is established before surgery. Overall, all symptoms of primary hyperparathyroidism can be observed. Compressive neck or mediastinal symptoms are less likely to occur in patients with FPCs than in patients with NFPCs because the functional status of FPCs might be expected to lead to earlier clinical presentation [11]. However, the development of spontaneous cervical or cervicomediastinal hematomas or massive extracapsular hemorrhages from FPCs have been reported and can be associated with dysphagia and dyspnea [8]. In addition, massive infarction of FPCs can lead to a hypercalcemic crisis.

In contrast to NFPCs, FPCs have an equal affinity for parathyroid glands arising from the third or fourth branchial pouches and have an even distribution with regard to side. Rarely, they can also be found in ectopic parathyroid glands and therefore be located anywhere from the angle of the mandible to the mediastinum.

At physical examination FPCs do not differ from NFPCs. They present as smooth, nontender, soft, solitary lumps, often mistaken for thyroid lesions. They may be partially developed into the superior mediastinum.

Diagnosis

As for NFPCs, the diagnosis of FPCs can be made preoperatively. The association hyperparathyroidism-cystic mass in the neck is already very suggestive of a FPC. Morphologic imaging studies including ultrasonography, CT and MRI show a lesion with a cystic component predominant. Nevertheless, rarely the lesion is cystic in its entirety, and ultrasonography shows solid fragments in the wall or in the lumen of the cyst. The accuracy rate of parathyroid scintigraphy (99mTc-sestamibi) is considerably lower than that reported for parathyroid lesions overall. False-negative results are observed in approximately one third of FPCs. As for NFPCs, FNA is

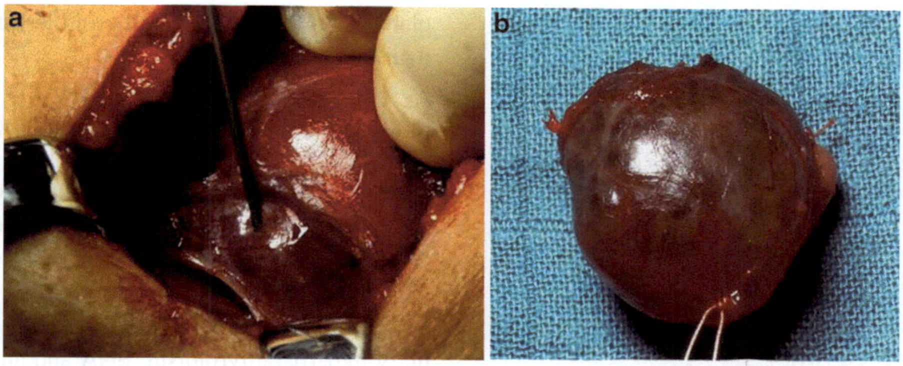

Fig. 7.5 Intraoperative view of a functional parathyroid cyst (**a**). The cyst fluid is not crystal-clear but brown (**b**)

particularly useful to confirm the diagnosis. FPCs produce an amber, brown, or even hemorrhagic fluid. However, the appearance of the fluid is not characteristic and cannot exclude the diagnosis of a thyroid cyst. To further differentiate FPCs from thyroid cysts, aspirated fluid should be analyzed for PTH. As observed with NFPCs, FPCs produce fragments rather than intact PTH.

FNA may be temporarily related to the development of a hypercalcemic crisis [29]. It was postulated that needle tracks made holes in the cyst wall, which allowed fluid rich in PTH to leak into the bloodstream. This is questionable as FNA of NFPCs has not been reported to be associated with hypercalcemia [4]. More probably, the hypercalcemia is related to the mobilization of the solid component of the lesion during FNA.

Management

Patients who have FPCs should be treated in a similar fashion as those who have noncystic parathyroid tumors. In contrast with the management of NFPCs, aspiration alone cannot be proposed as the first-line treatment. Aspiration eliminates the cystic mass, most often temporarily, but above all does not cure hyperparathyroidism. Intracystic injection of tetracycline or alcohol have been proposed but one must be concerned about injury to the adjacent recurrent laryngeal nerve due to leakage of the sclerosing agents through the disrupted thin cyst wall. In addition, although exceptional, cases of parathyroid carcinomas presenting as a cystic neck mass have been reported in the literature [20, 21].

Therefore, FPCs must be surgically removed according to the established guidelines for patients with primary hyperparathyroidism. Identification of four parathyroid glands and resection of those that are enlarged formed the basis of a standard operative approach to primary hyperparathyroidism. Today, with the development of improved localization studies and the introduction of intraoperative quick parathyroid hormone (QPTH) assay, a less extensive exploration, targeted on the FPC, may be proposed. The concept of limited parathyroid surgery is based on the fact that 85% of patients will have a single-gland disease and therefore systematic exploration of all four glands is not mandatory in all cases. This is also observed in patients with FPCs. Very few cases of patients with multiple functioning cytic parathyroid lesions have been described [30].

Nevertheless, in patients with FPCs, intraoperative QPTH level monitoring may be misleading [11]. In some patients, who were considered cured at follow-up, intraoperative postresection QPTH levels did not meet the usual criteria for definitive cure. This was more specifically observed in patients whose cyst was ruptured during the dissection [11].

At surgery, FPCs are loosely attached to the thyroid gland and are easily dissected free from the surrounding tissues. Certain features of their gross appearance help to differentiate them from NFPCs. They are less thin-walled and less translucent than NFPCs. The cyst fluid is not crystal-clear, but usually turbid, amber or brown (Fig. 7.5). Even when the cystic component of the adenoma is largely predominant, fragments of flattened

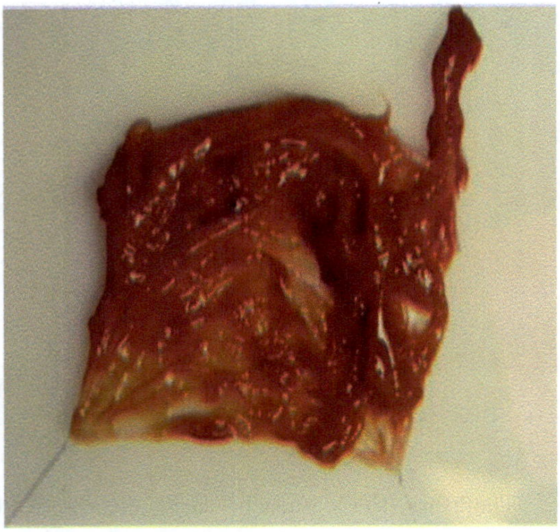

Fig. 7.6 Opened functional parathyroid cyst. Fragments of flattened hyperfunctional parathyroid tissue can be macroscopically identified in the cyst wall

hyperfunctional parathyroid tissue can be macroscopically identified in the cyst wall (Fig. 7.6).

Removing FPCs without perforating the cyst is crucial because, as with any parathyroid tumor, rupture can cause parathyromatosis. Because FPCs are very fragile lesions, great care must be taken not to rupture the cyst wall during dissection. Patients with large FPCs are at higher risk of symptomatic hypocalcemia after surgery [11]. Nevertheless, postoperative hypocalcemia is more probably related with the weight of the solid component of the adenoma than with the size of the cyst itself.

Conclusion

Cystic parathyroid lesions, large enough to be clinically significant and palpable, are rare lesions of the neck and the mediastinum. They have been described as functional, causing hyperparathyroidism, or nonfunctional. This division is questionable, since embryological and histological data suggest that FPCs and NFPCs are likely two separate entities. NFPCs are true cysts with an epithelial lining and are probably of branchial origin. FPCs result from the cystic degeneration of an adenoma or more rarely a hyperplastic gland. FPCs are cystic parathyroid lesions rather than true parathyroid cysts.

NFPCs are very rare lesions found in the inferior parathyroid glands, usually asymptomatic and most often discovered on routine clinical examination. FNA is diagnostic, due to the characteristic of the fluid and high PTH levels on assay, and may be curative. Repeated recurrence may be treated surgically.

FPCs account for 1–2.5% of all cases of primary hyperparathyroidism. FNA and analysis of cyst fluid for PTH is particularly important to confirm the diagnosis of FPCs. Patients with FPCs should be treated surgically according to the established guidelines for patients with primary hyperparathyroidism. Surgical exploration of all four glands is not mandatory in patients with a preoperative diagnosis of solitary FPC. During limited parathyroid exploration, the surgeon must keep in mind that intraoperative QPTH level monitoring may be misleading, in particular after cyst rupture.

References

1. Sandstrom I. Om en Körtel hos menniskan och atskilliga doggdjus. Upsala Lläkarför Forhandl. 1880; 14:441.
2. Goris D. Extirpation de trois nodules parathyroïdiens kystiques. Ann Soc Belg Chir. 1952;5:394.
3. Clark OH. Parathyroid cysts. Am J Surg. 1978;135: 395–402.
4. Ippolito G, Palazzo F, Sebag F, et al. A single-institution 25-year review of true parathyroid cysts. Langenbeck Arch Surg. 2006;91:13–8.
5. Silvermann JF, Khazanie PG, Norris HT, et al. Parathyroid hormone (PTH) assay of parathyroid cysts examined by fine-needle aspiration biopsy. Am J Clin Pathol. 1986;86:776–80.
6. Shields TW, Immerman SC. Mediastinal parathyroid cysts revisited. Ann Thorac Surg. 1999;67:581–90.
7. Taniguchi J, Maeda T, Morimoto K, et al. Spontaneous retropharyngeal hematoma of a parathyroid cyst: report of a case. Surg Today. 2003;33:354–7.
8. Simcic KJ, McDermottt MT, Crawford GJ, et al. Massive extracapsular hemorrhage from a parathyroid cyst. Arch Surg. 1989;124:1347–50.
9. Hughes CR, Kanmaz B, Isitman AT, et al. Misleading imaging results in the diagnosis of parathyroid cysts. Clin Nucl Med. 1994;19:422–5.
10. Pinney SP, Daly PA. Parathyroid cyst: an uncommon cause of a palpable neck mass and hypercalcemia. West J Med. 1999;170:118–20.

11. Mc Coy KL, Yim JH, Zuckerbraun BS, et al. Cystic parathyroid lesions: functional and nonfunctional parathyroid cysts. Arch Surg. 2009;144:52–6.
12. Pacini F, Antonelli A, Lari R, et al. Unsuspected parathyroid cysts diagnosed by measurement of thyroglobulin and parathyroid hormone concentration in fluid aspirates. Ann Intern Med. 1985;102: 793–4.
13. Bimbaum J, Van Herle AJ. Immunoheterogeneity of parathyroid hormone in parathyroid cysts: diagnostic implications. J Endocrinol Invest. 1989;12:831–6.
14. Katz AD, Dunklman D. Needle aspiration of non-functioning parathyroid cysts. Arch Surg. 1984;119: 307–8.
15. Shi B, Guo H, Tang N. Treatment of parathyroid cysts with fine-needle aspiration. Ann Intern Med. 1999; 131:797–8.
16. Prinz RA, Peters JR, Kane JM, Wood J. Needle aspiration of non-functioning parathyroid cysts. Am J Surg. 1990;56:420–2.
17. Okamura K, Ikenoue H, Sato K, et al. Sclerotherapy for benign parathyroid cysts. Am J Surg. 1992;163: 344–5.
18. Akel M, Salti I, Azar ST. Successful treatment of parathyroid cyst using ethanol sclerotherapy. Am J Med Sci. 1999;317:50–2.
19. Sanchez A, Caretto H. Treatment of a nonfunctioning parathyroid cyst with tetracycline injection. Head Neck. 1993;15:263–5.
20. Wright JG, Brangle RW. Carcinoma in a parathyroid cyst. IMG Ill Med J. 1985;168:98–100.
21. Pirundini P, Zarif A, Wibbey JG. A rare manifestation of parathyroid carcinoma presenting as a cystic neck mass. Conn Med. 1998;62:195–7.
22. Rosenberg J, Orlando R, Ludwig M, et al. Parathyroid cysts. Am J Surg. 1982;143:473–80.
23. Miyauchi A, Kakudo K, Fujimoto T, et al. Parathyroid cyst: analysis of the cyst fluid and ultrastructural observations. Arch Pathol Lab Med. 1981;105:497–9.
24. Forsyth D. The parathyroid glands. II. Their pathology in man. Q J Med. 1908;1:287–311.
25. Castelman B, Mallory TB. The pathology of the parathyroid gland in hyperparathyroidism. Am J Pathol. 1935;11:1–80.
26. Kursteiner W. Die epithelkorperchen des herschen in iher beziehung zur thyreoidea und thymus. Anat Hefte. 1899;11:391.
27. Gough IR. Parathyroid cysts. Aust N Z Surg. 1999; 69:404–6.
28. Spitz AF. Management of functioning mediastinal parathyroid cysts. J Clin Endocrinol Metab. 1995;80: 2866–8.
29. Kobayashi A, Kuma K, Matsuzuka F. Exacerbation of hypercalcemia after needle biopsy of a parathyroid cyst. Ann Intern Med. 1989;110:326–7.
30. Ujiki MB, Nayar R, Sturgeon C, et al. Parathyroid cyst: often mistaken for a thyroid cyst. World J Surg. 2006;31:60–4.

Parathyroid Cancer

8

Maurizio Iacobone and Jean-François Henry

Abstract

Parathyroid carcinoma is a rare endocrine malignancy derived from the parenchymal cells of the parathyroid glands. It is usually associated with more severe and profound clinical and laboratory manifestations than its more common benign counterparts. Its course is usually indolent but progressive; unlike other malignancies, most patients die because of metabolic complications of parathormone (PTH)-related hypercalcemia rather than tumor invasion and spread.

The definitive diagnosis of parathyroid carcinoma may be particularly challenging, since the histology of parathyroid tumors may be equivocal or frankly misleading; for this reason, malignancy is often confirmed on a clinical basis only when local or distant metastases occur. Recent advances in the molecular pathogenesis of the disease will lead to the development of more reliable diagnostic markers.

Keywords

Parathyroid carcinoma • Hyperparathyroidism • PTH-dependent hypercalcemia • Jaw tumor syndrome • HRPT2 • Parafibromin • Atypical parathyroid adenoma

Introduction

Parathyroid carcinoma is a rare endocrine malignancy derived from the parenchymal cells of the parathyroid glands. It accounts for 1–5% of all cases of primary hyperparathyroidism [1–5]; it is usually associated with more severe and profound clinical and laboratory manifestations than its more common benign counterparts. Its course is usually indolent but progressive; unlike other malignancies, most patients die

M. Iacobone, MD, FEBS (✉)
Endocrine Surgery Unit, Department of Surgical, Oncological and Gastroenterological Sciences, University of Padua, Via Giustiniani 2, Padua 35128, Italy
e-mail: maurizio.iacobone@unipd.it

J.-F. Henry, MD, FRCS
Department of Endocrine Surgery, University Hospital La Timone 264, Rue St. Pierre, Marseilles 13385, France
e-mail: JeanFrancois.HENRY@ap-hm.fr

A.A. Licata and E.V. Lerma (eds.), *Diseases of the Parathyroid Glands*,
DOI 10.1007/978-1-4419-5550-0_8, © Springer Science+Business Media, LLC 2012

because of metabolic complications of parathormone (PTH)-related hypercalcemia rather than tumor invasion and spread [1, 6–10].

The first case of metastatic parathyroid carcinoma causing manifestations of Recklinghausen's disease was reported in 1933 by Sainton and Millot [11], although the very first description of this malignant neoplasm was probably made by De Quervain in 1904, and, interestingly, it was a nonsecreting parathyroid carcinoma [12]. This report described the case of a 68-year-old man with a large neck mass who died with local recurrences and distant metastases, in the absence of any evident signs and symptoms of hypercalcemia.

The definitive diagnosis of parathyroid carcinoma may be challenging, since the histology of parathyroid tumors may be equivocal or frankly misleading also for experienced pathologists [13, 14]; for this reasons, malignancy is often confirmed on a clinical basis only when local or distant metastases occur [1, 15]. Recent advances in the molecular pathogenesis of the disease will lead to the development of more reliable diagnostic markers [16–25].

To date, surgery remains the most effective therapy for parathyroid carcinoma, since ultimate prognosis depends upon complete successful excision at initial operation [1, 8, 9, 26–28].

Epidemiology

Parathyroid cancer accounts for approximately 1% of cases of PTH-dependent hypercalcemia in most series. Fewer than 1,000 cases have been reported in the entire English-language literature [15]; no single center has ever published data on more than 50 patients, and all such observations are retrospective. A meta-analysis [29] including 20,225 cases of primary hyperparathyroidism revealed only 0.74% of parathyroid carcinoma. The largest series collected by the National Cancer Data Base [2] reported 286 cases in a 10-year period, accounting for 0.005% of all cancer; in this series, no clustering was seen with respect to race or geographic regions. However, the incidence of the disease appears to be higher (approximately 5%) in the Japanese and Italian series [1, 3–5]. It remains unknown if this discrepancy may be related to geographic, environmental, epidemiologic, and genetic reasons or to varying pathological criteria for its diagnosis.

Usually men and women are equally affected by parathyroid carcinoma, differently from benign parathyroid disease in which females predominate over males by 3–4:1 [6–10, 15, 30–33]; the age at diagnosis is approximately a decade earlier (in the mid-40s or 50s) [6, 10, 15, 30, 33], although patients as young as 8 years of age have been reported [34].

Etiopathogenesis

The etiology of parathyroid carcinoma is largely unknown. Several risk conditions have been reported: neck irradiations, chronic stimulation from long-standing hypocalcemia, and familial hyperparathyroidism [7, 15, 35–38].

Prior neck irradiation has been documented in some cases, with a reported latency of more than 20 years [39, 40]. However, its role is less evident than in the development of benign parathyroid disease [31, 38–42].

End-stage renal disease with secondary hyperparathyroidism has been reported in a subset of patients with parathyroid carcinoma [43], with an average latency of 6 years following the start of hemodialysis. In these cases, the clinical course of the disease is more indolent because of the tendency of renal insufficiency to lower serum calcium levels [43, 44]. However, though the increased number of hemodialyzed patients in the recent years, the prevalence of parathyroid carcinoma remains constant, suggesting an uncertain pathogenetic role for this condition [2, 8, 9]. To date, only one case has been reported in a patient with a prolonged secondary hyperparathyroidism due to celiac disease [45].

Although parathyroid carcinoma is usually a sporadic tumor, it has also been reported in associations with hereditary variants of hyperparathyroidism [46–50], especially in

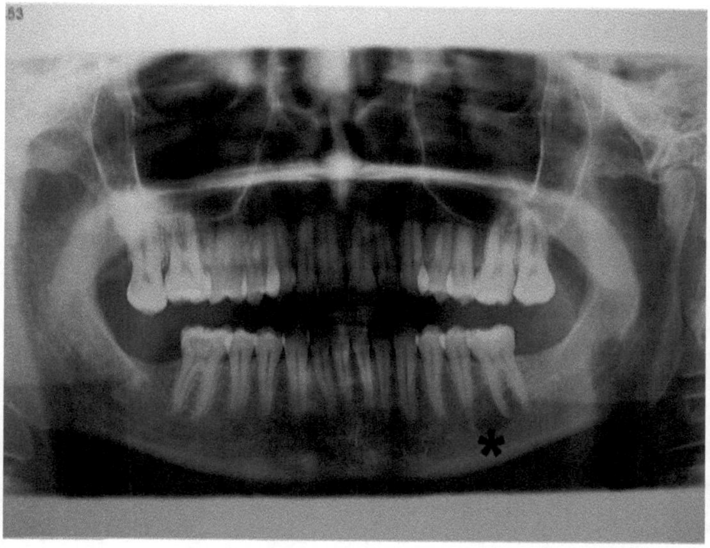

Fig. 8.1 Orthopantomographic X-ray: ossifying fibroma of the left ramus of the mandible (*) in a young patient with hyperparathyroidism–jaw tumor syndrome

hyperparathyroidism–jaw tumor syndrome (HPT-JT; online Mendelian inheritance in man OMIM #145001). HPT-JT syndrome (*please refer to Chapter on Jaw Tumor Syndrome for further discussion*) is an autosomal dominant disease with incomplete penetrance and variable expression, characterized by multiple parathyroid tumors, with a significantly increased prevalence of carcinomas and atypical adenomas (10–25% of cases), ossifying fibromas of mandible and/or maxilla (5–30% of cases) (see Figs. 8.1–8.3), uterine tumors in approximately 60% of cases (leyomiomas, endometrial hyperplasia, adenomyosis, adenosarcomas, and adenofibromas), and a variety of renal lesions in 5–15% of cases (hamartomas, polycystic disease, Wilms tumors, and adenocarcinomas) [16, 51, 52].

HPT-JT is caused by mutations in the tumor suppressor gene HRPT2 (also known as CDC73), located on chromosome 1q25-31, which encodes a protein with antiproliferative properties, named parafibromin [16].

Parafibromin is a nuclear protein evolutionary conserved [37, 53, 54], that is involved in the cell cycle control, with a role in the transcription elongation, in the RNA processing pathways, and in the hystone methylation [55–64]. Parafibromin has been shown to participate in transcription regulation by interacting with the polymerase II-associated factor 1 transcription elongation complex [57]; it may inhibit cell proliferation by inducing cell cycle arrest by blocking cyclin D1 expression [60, 65]; wild type but not mutant parafibromin promotes apoptosis in transfected cells [62].

In HPT-JT patients, inactivating mutations (generally, frameshift mutations, deletions, insertions, and duplications scattered throughout the encoding region of the HRPT2 gene) lead to abnormal hemizygosity; loss of heterozygosity after chromosomial deletions or further inactivating mutations in the remaining copy of the gene cause a biallelic HRPT2 inactivation, with subsequent premature codon stop and/or production of a truncate, inactive, or easily degradable parafibromin [16, 66].

Parafibromin inactivation has been confirmed by immunohistochemical and functional studies, which demonstrated that HRPT2 mutations result in the loss of parafibromin expression [25, 51, 59, 67, 68] or abnormal subcellular localization [62, 63], and subsequent abolition of its antiproliferative activity [60].

The loss of parafibromin expression could be a pivotal step in parathyroid oncogenetic process; in fact, it is considered the distinctive feature in

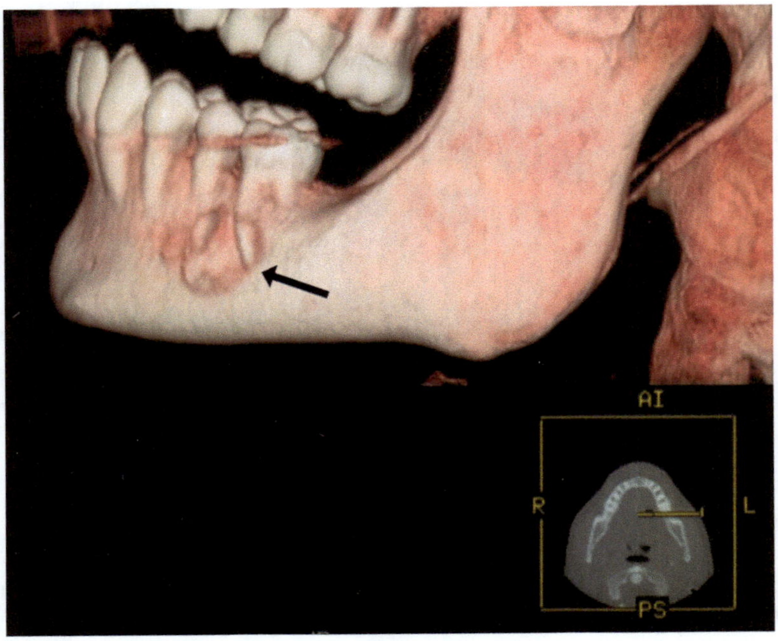

Fig. 8.2 CT scan (reconstruction): ossifying fibroma of the left ramus of the mandible (*arrow*) in a young patient with hyperparathyroidism-jaw tumor syndrome

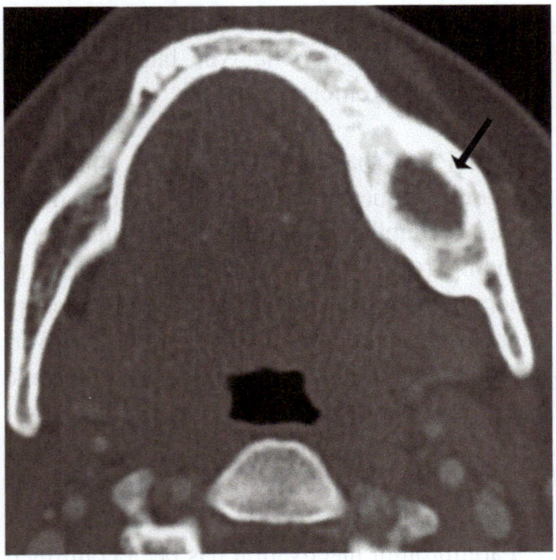

Fig. 8.3 CT scan: ossifying fibroma of the left ramus of the mandible in a young patient with hyperparathyroidism-jaw tumor syndrome

affected parathyroid glands in HPT-JT patients and in sporadic parathyroid carcinoma [21, 25, 51, 52, 68], suggesting also a diagnostic role for this protein.

HRPT2 mutations occur not only in all affected parathyroid glands in HPT-JT patients but also in approximately one third of cases of sporadic carcinoma, while they are rare in sporadic parathyroid adenomas [17–19, 25, 69–72]; this finding supports the hypothesis that a subset of patients with apparently sporadic parathyroid carcinomas may have the HPT-JT syndrome or a variant with altered penetrance of the mutation [6, 13, 19, 37, 69, 73]. For these reasons, every patient with apparently sporadic parathyroid carcinoma should be tested for germ-line HRPT2 mutations.

Few cases of parathyroid carcinoma occurring in an MEN1 setting have been described [74, 75], although these reports should be cautiously considered since recurrences of MEN1-related hyperparathyroidism at the site of previous surgery may simulate parathyroid malignancy. Somatic mutations of the MEN1 gene have been rarely reported in parathyroid carcinoma [55, 76], suggesting a limited role for Menin in the pathogenesis of parathyroid malignancies.

Only one case of parathyroid carcinoma has been observed in patients with MEN2A [77], and none in MEN2B.

Many other tumor suppressor genes and oncogenes have been related to parathyroid cancer, especially those that have a role in the control of the cell cycle as retinoblastoma (Rb), breast carcinoma susceptibility (BRCA2), p53 and cyclin D1/parathyroid adenomatosis gene 1 (PRAD1) genes [6, 10, 15]. However, it is not certain whether these genes may have a primary role in parathyroid carcinoma, although their altered expression may contribute to the process of malignant transformation [6, 7, 15].

Rb is located on chromosome 13; acquired mutations might contribute to the development of parathyroid carcinoma [10]. Rb mutations and loss of Rb nuclear expression have been reported in parathyroid cancer, although these alterations have been also reported (although less frequently) in parathyroid adenomas [6, 13, 37, 70, 78–82]. Also, BRCA2 gene is located on chromosome 13; it has a role in homologous recombination, an important DNA mechanism. Cells that are deficient for BRCA2 accumulate chromosomal aberrations and are sensitive to radiation; this finding may suggest an increased risk of primary hyperparathyroidism in patients subjected to head and neck irradiation [37, 81]. A loss of heterozygosity on chromosome 13, a region including both the Rb and the BRCA2 genes was demonstrated by several investigators in parathyroid cancer [78, 80, 83], although others were not able to demonstrate tumor-specific somatic mutations in either Rb or BRCA2 in a series of parathyroid carcinomas with 13q loss of heterozygosity [69]. However, the role of these genes in the pathogenesis of parathyroid carcinomas needs further investigations.

Cyclin D1 is an oncogene located at chromosome band 11q13 and codify for a cell cycle regulator which plays an important role in transition of cells from the G1 phase of the cell cycle into the S phase [84]. A possible mechanism for the oncogenic activity of cyclin D1/PRAD1 is the inactivation of protein encoded by Rb gene [69]. According to some studies, in 20–40% of patients affected by parathyroid adenoma and in up to 91% of those with parathyroid carcinoma, an overexpression of the oncogene cyclin D1 has been found. However, it is unclear if this feature is causative or only an association [10, 37].

P53 is another important cell cycle regulator which has been considered as a candidate for malignant parathyroid tumors, but the frequency of abnormal p53 expression in parathyroid carcinomas is low [10].

Clinical Presentation

The majority of parathyroid cancers are functioning tumors with indolent tendency to local invasion; therefore, the most frequent symptoms and signs are related to hyperparathyroidism while clinical manifestations from tumor burden occur lately [10, 85, 86]. Metabolic complications subsequent to the increased secretion of PTH and hypercalcemia, rather than tumor invasiveness, are the main causes of death [1, 6, 7].

Generally, manifestations of hyperparathyroidism in parathyroid cancer are virtually indistinguishable from those in patients with benign disease, although they are usually more severe [10, 30].

Hypercalcemia may results in fatigue, malaise, weakness, weight loss, and anemia. Psychiatric manifestations such as depression are also discovered in some patients [6, 15, 33, 37, 82]; lethargy, confusion, and coma may occur in case of severe hypercalcemia [33]. Hypercalcemic crisis, although rare (approximately 10%), are more commonly associated with parathyroid carcinoma than benign tumors [6, 7, 10, 13, 47]. Classic target organs, such as the kidneys and skeleton, are frequently affected. Polyuria, polydipsia, renal colic, nephrolithiasis, nephrocalcinosis, and impaired renal function occur in up to 80% of cases. Bone impairment includes diffuse osteopenia, pathologic fractures, and bone pain that occur in 90% of cases, while in benign hyperparathyroidism renal and bone involvement are present in 20% and 5%, respectively [10, 87–89]; radiologic findings as subperiostal resorption, "salt and pepper" skull and osteitis fibrosa cystic are seen in more than 40% of patients (see Fig. 8.4). Different from benign disease, most patients with parathyroid carcinoma manifest evidence of both renal and skeletal involvement at the time of presentation [8–10]. Digestive

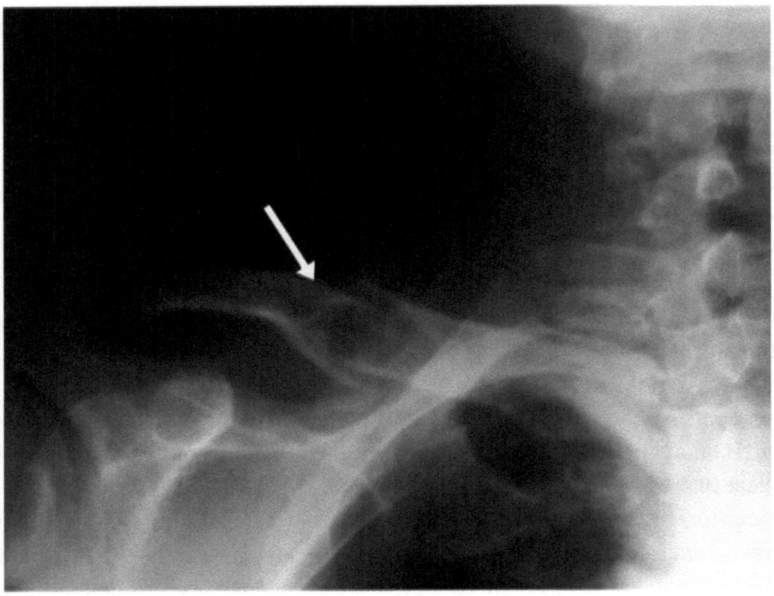

Fig. 8.4 Plain radiographs of the right clavicle: presence of a pathological fracture of a lytic bone lesion (Brown's tumor)

symptoms such as nausea, vomiting abdominal pain, peptic ulcer, recurrent severe pancreatitis, and constipations occur with greater frequency in patients with malignant disease than in those with benign primary hyperparathyroidism. Nonfunctioning carcinomas are extremely rare (2% of all parathyroid malignancies) and usually show only signs and symptoms of local growth and invasion, including neck mass, hoarseness, and dysphagia [90]. As opposed to functional parathyroid cancer, patients with nonfunctional tumors eventually die from invasion to vital organs and systemic spread rather than hypercalcemia [33, 90].

Physical examination in patients with parathyroid carcinoma is generally unrevealing but the presence of a paralyzed vocal cord and a palpable cervical mass may predict the presence of a parathyroid malignancy. In fact, a paralyzed vocal cord in a hyperparathyroid patient not previously subjected to a neck surgery may predict a parathyroid carcinoma on the side of paralysis; a palpable cervical mass is very rare in case of benign parathyroid mass (less than 5%), while it may be found in 15–70% of cases of parathyroid carcinoma [1–5, 8–10, 86, 91–94]; however, these findings have become less frequent in the recent years since the diagnosis is possibly performed earlier [2, 33].

Diagnosis

The diagnosis of parathyroid carcinoma is quite difficult: it may be suspected pre- or intraoperatively but, in practice, it is most often made postoperatively through histological examination. In some equivocal cases, also pathology may be inconclusive, and the diagnosis must be confirmed only by the clinical course at a prolonged follow-up by the occurrence of metastases (Table 8.1) [1, 6, 7, 13, 14].

Preoperative Diagnosis

Parathyroid cancer cannot be diagnosed preoperatively, but only suspected by the mean of a triad of clinical, laboratory, and radiological examinations (Table 8.2) [7–10].

However, these features may be frequently absent and so the preoperative confirmation is very difficult if not impossible. Only the unequivocal presence of local invasion or distant metastases can definitively assess the diagnosis of parathyroid carcinoma, but it is rare at initial presentation, since usually it occur late because of the slow and indolent course of the disease [1, 6, 15, 30, 33, 95]. Usually the clinical features are similar to those of primary hyperparathyroidism but may be more marked [76].

Table 8.1 Criteria of suspicion of parathyroid carcinoma

Preoperative criteria
- Male sex, 40–50-year old
- Severe hypercalcemia (>3, 5 mmol/L)
- Very high PTH levels (>4-fold of normal levels)
- Palpable neck mass associated with unilateral vocal cord paralysis
- Symptomatic hyperparathyroidism (concomitant renal and skeletal disease)

Intraoperative criteria
- Large stonyhard mass (>30 mm if solid), with a fibrous, grayish-white capsule
- Presence of infiltrative aspects with tenacious adhesion to adjacent structures
- Presence of local lymph-node involvement

Postoperative criteria

Pathological criteria
- Uniform sheets of chief cells with lobular pattern of growth
- Presence of dense, thick fibrous trabeculae
- Atypical mitotic figures
- Vascular, capsular, or perineural invasion[a]

Clinical criteria
- Recurrences and distant metastases[a]

[a]Unequivocal criteria

Clinical Features

The clinical suspicion should rise if the patient is an adult male patient, with a palpable neck mass, renal and skeletal disease from hyperparathyroidism, peptic ulcers, pancreatitis, and recurrent laryngeal nerve palsy [6, 10, 14, 32, 76, 96–99]. In fact, in parathyroid carcinoma, men and women are equally affected [6, 7, 10, 15, 30–33]; the average age of patients is approximately 40–50 years, one decade younger than that of patients with benign disease [6, 10, 15, 30, 33]. However, considerations of gender and age are of little help in evaluating the individual patient.

Neck mass are more frequent because parathyroid carcinomas are usually larger than benign disease, but the inadequate predictive value of this finding and the frequent presence of concomitant thyroid nodules limit the diagnostic role of these features. In contrast of benign disease, where the majority of patients are actually asymptomatic, parathyroid cancer patients usually show clinical features of end-organ disease. Renal and bone involvement (and the combination of both) occur more frequently at the presentation in parathyroid carcinoma [6, 10, 15, 30, 31, 33, 99].

Laboratory Studies

The biochemical abnormalities observed in benign primary hyperparathyroidism are usually over-expressed in parathyroid carcinoma. Patients with parathyroid carcinoma have PTH levels

Table 8.2 Clinical features in benign versus malignant parathyroid tumors

	Benign primary hyperparathyroidism	Parathyroid carcinoma
Age at presentation	50–60 years	40–50 years
Women:men ratio	>3:1	1:1
Serum calcium	Mildly elevated	Markedly elevated
Serum PTH	Mildly elevated	Markedly elevated
Palpable neck mass	Very rare	Common (15–70%)
Renal involvement	<20%	>50%
Severe bone involvement	Rare (<5%)	Common (>50%)
Concomitant bone and renal involvement	Rare	Common
Hypercalcemic crisis	Very rare	Very common
Asymptomatic	Very common	Very rare

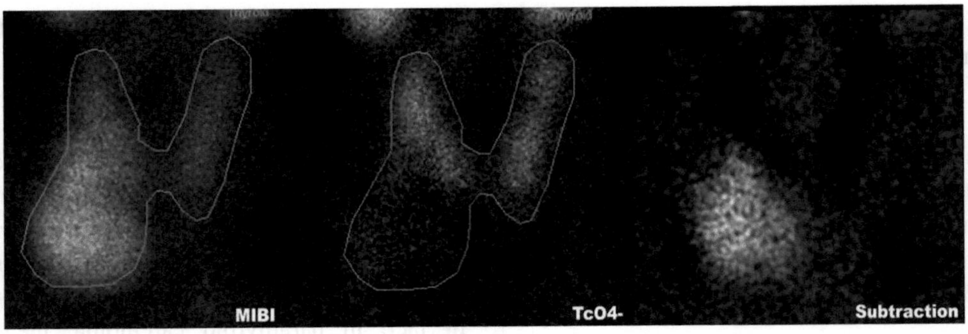

Fig. 8.5 Sestamibi scan (MIBI, Technetium, and subtraction images): large inferior right parathyroid lesion that histologically proved to be parathyroid carcinoma (courtesy of Diego Cecchin, Department of Nuclear Medicine, University of Padua, Italy)

3–10 times above normal values and calcium levels above 3.5 mmol/l; sometimes they show hypercalcemic crisis [6, 7, 36]. On the contrary, in case of benign disease, serum PTH and calcium values are usually only mildly raised, often discovered while being investigated for an unrelated problem, and patients have usually mild symptoms or none [6, 8, 9, 15]. However, no predictive cutoff values may be indicated [100], although the diagnosis of malignancy can be reliably ruled out for PTH increments inferior to four times the upper limit of normal range and tumor weights inferior to 1.9 g [100].

Furthermore, different PTH molecules (other than the usual intact human 1–84 PTH) may be produced by parathyroid carcinoma, especially N-terminal fragments that can be selectively identified by modern laboratory techniques, although the diagnostic value of this finding need to be further assessed [101, 102]. Paraneoplastic production of alfa and beta subunits of human chorionic gonadotropin has also been detected in these patients [102, 103]. Also, alkaline phosphatase activity is higher in patients with parathyroid carcinoma.

Fine-needle aspiration cytology of a suspected parathyroid carcinoma is not recommended: benign and malignant disease cannot be effectively differentiated on cytology; a potential risk of track seeding is present, since a case with cutaneous spread of parathyroid carcinoma after aspiration cytology has been described [104]; furthermore, false negatives and false positive may be caused by sampling errors and by degenerative changes following fine-needle aspiration that closely mimic parathyroid carcinoma at final pathology [105–107].

Imaging Techniques

Various imaging modalities such as ultrasonography, computed tomography (CT), magnetic resonance imaging (MRI), and sestamibi scintigraphy can be used to investigate parathyroid carcinoma. These investigations are rarely diagnostic of malignancy but are effective in assessing the size and localizing the pathological glands. Imaging studies are optional at initial presentation, but mandatory in case of recurrent or metastatic disease before surgery [108, 109].

Ultrasonography and Technetium-99 m sestamibi are the first line investigations [107–110]. Ultrasound is a very useful and noninvasive method for parathyroid tumors located at the neck, providing general information about the structure of the lesion and its rapport with adjacent structures [15]. Parathyroid carcinoma appears as a large hypoechoic soft tissue mass with poorly defined margins and, possibly, signs of local invasion; lymph-node metastases can be also accurately detected [82].

Technetium-99 m sestamibi is a radiopharmaceutical with a high affinity for the mitochondria of parathyroid tissue (see Fig. 8.5). Sestamibi scanning may localize abnormal parathyroid tissue with a reported sensitivity of 85% and specificity of 95% [107–111].

Contrast CT is useful for providing some details on the localization of the lesion; it can also reveal invasion of surrounding structures and enlarged lymph nodes; it is more sensitive in detecting recurrent and metastatic parathyroid carcinoma, especially at mediastinal, pulmonary, hepatic, and bone sites [109]. MRI with gadolinium and fat suppression gives the best details on the soft tissues of the neck; it is the investigation of choice for localizing an ectopic gland in the mediastinum and for characterization of metastatic lesions at specific sites such as liver and bone. Moreover, MRI, during any assessment of recurrence, also avoids the artifacts produced by surgical clips that make interpretation of CT scans difficult [15, 82, 112]. However, ultrasonography, CT, and MRI, although sensitive, have a limited specificity, because they are not able to differentiate between recurrence and non-neoplastic masses (lymph nodes, scar tissue) while sestamibi scan is more sensitive and specific in detecting the sites of recurrent and metastatic disease [108, 109].

Very few reports exist on the use of fluorodeoxyglucose positron emission tomography (FDG-PET) in parathyroid carcinoma. Both primary parathyroid carcinoma and recurrent and metastatic lesions have a mildly increased metabolic activity; it should be remembered that also lytic bone lesions appear hypermetabolic at FDG-PET and can be mistaken as bone metastases [113]. Also, the classical nuclear bone scans show increased bone turnover consistent with metabolic bone disease both in Brown's tumors and metastatic lesions; in these cases, whole-body MIBI scan will help differentiate Brown's tumors from metastatic bone disease [113]. In case of recurrent disease, if noninvasive imaging are inconclusive to identify the lesion, selective venous catheterization with PTH measurements has been recommended, or, in alternative, at least two concordant noninvasive localization studies should be performed before embarking on iterative surgery, in order to avoid negative re-explorations [108, 109].

Intraoperative Diagnosis

Parathyroid carcinoma may be intraoperatively suspected in case of glands particularly large (>30 mm if solid), lobulated, firm to stonyhard mass, whitish-gray, surrounded by a dense, fibrous, grayish-white capsule, with tenacious adhesion to adjacent structures, or if local lymph-node involvement is found (although it occurs rarely) [76, 93, 114, 115]. This is in contrast to normal parathyroid glands which have the color of peanut butter, soft consistency, and a median size of approximately 10–30 mm. However, the surgical appearances of parathyroid cancer may be sometimes indistinguishable from benign parathyroid disease; degenerative changes in parathyroid adenomas may simulate the gross appearance of parathyroid malignancy [14, 116].

Intraoperative frozen section may sometimes suggest the diagnosis (e.g., dense fibrosis, nuclear monotony), but it is usually of little value in distinguishing benign from malignant disease, and may cause artifactual dislodgement that can simulate falsely positive aspects at definitive histology [13].

Postoperative Diagnosis

The histopathological diagnosis of parathyroid carcinoma is sometimes obvious, but—in case of absence of unequivocal features—may be an extremely challenging task. The malignant parathyroid gland is usually particularly large, typically with a weight between 2 and 10 g, firm, solid, whitish-gray, adherent to the adjacent structures (see Fig. 8.6). Several histopathological findings have been described to diagnose parathyroid carcinoma, but, as is the case with many endocrine neoplasms, the histopathological distinction between benign and malignant parathyroid tumors is difficult. The most used criteria have been established by Schantz and Castleman in 1973 [93]. These histological features consist in the presence of uniform sheets of chief cells arranged in a lobular pattern separated by dense, thick fibrous trabeculae that extend into and divide the gland; atypical mitotic figures within tumor cells and vascular or capsular invasion (see Figs. 8.7–8.12).

The epithelial cells of parathyroid carcinoma are larger than normal cells; mitotic activity is present in 80% of carcinomas (but also in 60% of

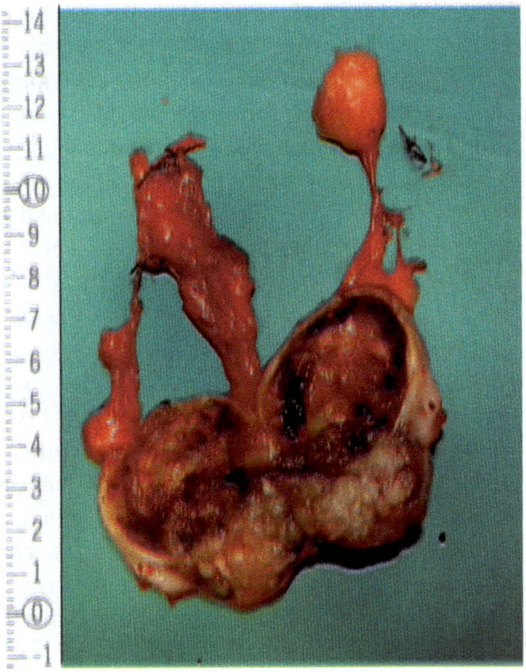

Fig. 8.6 Surgical specimen: parathyroid carcinoma; necrosis and degenerative changes are also present (the specimen has been sectioned longitudinally)

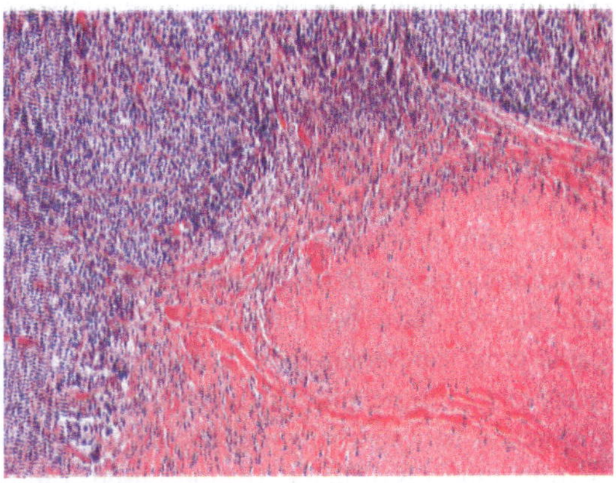

Fig. 8.7 Photomicrograph of a histological section of parathyroid carcinoma. Solid (*sheet-like*) proliferation of monotonous cells with solid architectural growth pattern; focal tumor necrosis and fibrous bands within the tumor are also evident (H&E, 100×) (courtesy of Gianmaria Pennelli, Department of Pathology, University of Padua, Italy)

parathyroid adenomas); furthermore, it should be distinguished from endothelial cell mitoses [117]. However, a high mitotic rate (>5 per 50 high-power fields) and atypical mitoses indicate an increased risk of malignant behavior [118] and

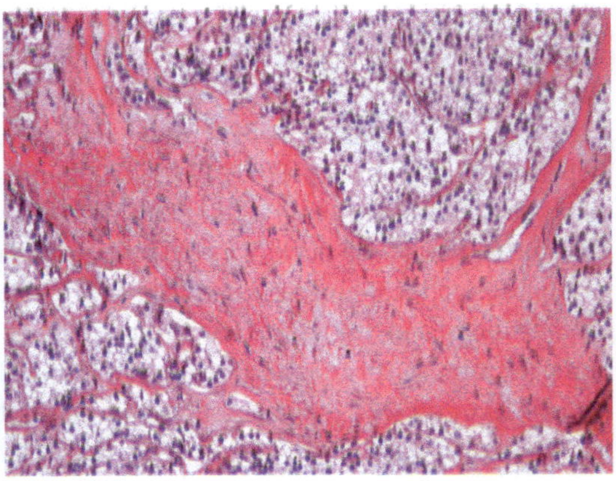

Fig. 8.8 Photomicrograph of a histological section of parathyroid carcinoma. Neoplastic clear cells separated by broad bands of fibrous tissue (H&E 200×) (courtesy of Gianmaria Pennelli, Department of Pathology, University of Padua, Italy)

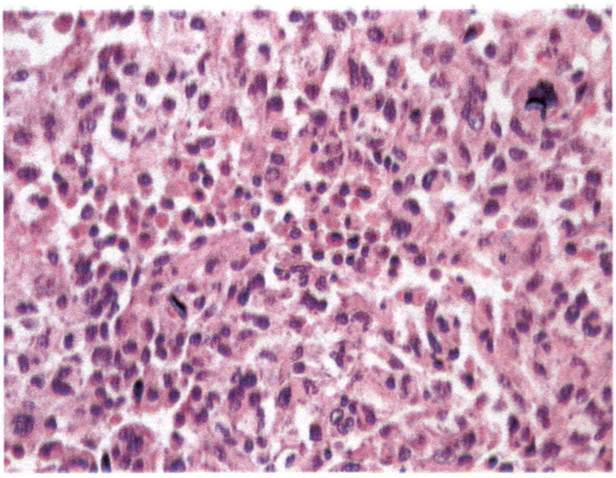

Fig. 8.9 Photomicrograph of a histological section of parathyroid carcinoma. High mitotic activity with atypical figures (H&E, 400×) (courtesy of Gianmaria Pennelli, Department of Pathology, University of Padua, Italy)

should lead to a careful search of other features of disease. Giant cells and/or focal necrosis may also be present [14, 36, 119, 120].

Furthermore, dense fibrous trabeculae and trabecular growth pattern have been found also in parathyroid adenomas, especially, in the presence of degenerative changes [13]. Degenerative changes in a nonmalignant gland that closely mimic the features of a parathyroid carcinoma may be caused also by a preoperative fine-needle aspiration [105, 106].

True capsular invasion is early evident only in a limited portion of cases [81, 91] and should be

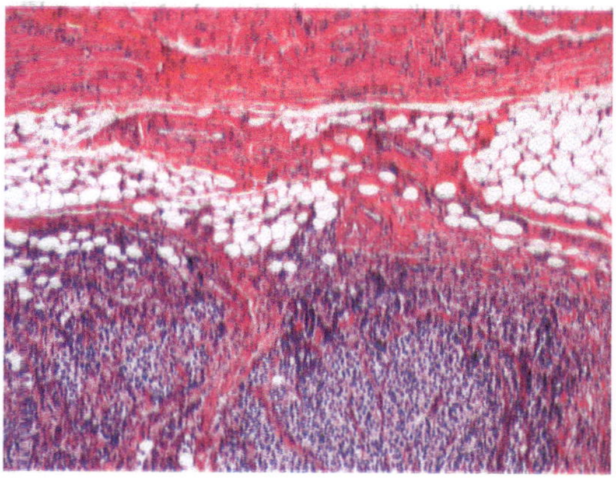

Fig. 8.10 Photomicrograph of a histological section of parathyroid carcinoma. The neoplasm invades the periglandular soft tissue (H&E, 100×) (courtesy of Gianmaria Pennelli, Department of Pathology, University of Padua, Italy)

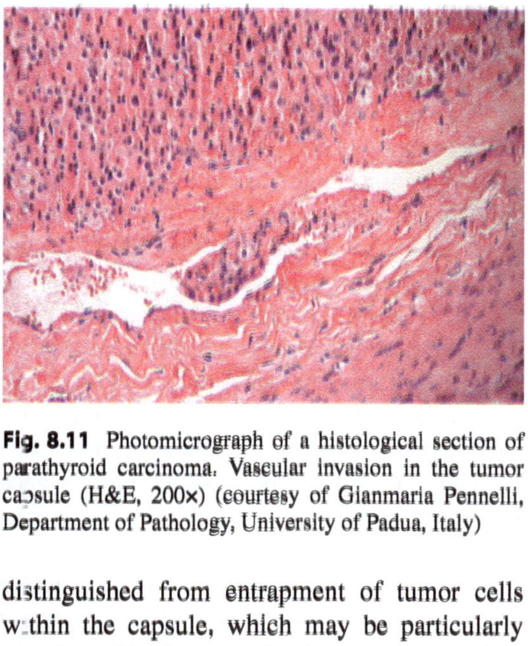

Fig. 8.11 Photomicrograph of a histological section of parathyroid carcinoma. Vascular invasion in the tumor capsule (H&E, 200×) (courtesy of Gianmaria Pennelli, Department of Pathology, University of Padua, Italy)

distinguished from entrapment of tumor cells within the capsule, which may be particularly prominent in adenomas that have undergone cystic regressive transformation.

Vascular invasion is evident even in fewer cases [81, 91] and should be diagnosed only in cases of vessels present within the tumor capsule or in the surrounding soft tissues. The tumor clusters should be surrounded by endothelium or associated with fibrin thrombi. Artifactual dislodgement of tumor cells is characterized by the presence of irregularly shaped cell clusters that are not endothelialized or associated with

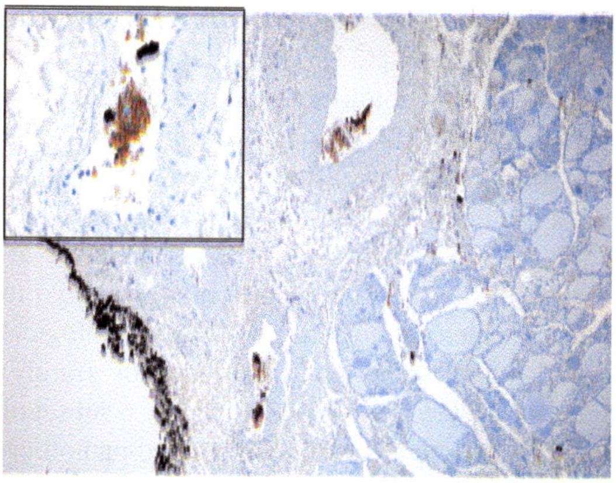

Fig. 8.12 Photomicrograph of a histological section of parathyroid carcinoma. Vascular invasion is present in the soft tissue surrounding the thyroid gland (Chromogranin, 50×). En cartouche: particular of the invaded vessels (Chromogranin, 400×) (courtesy of Gianmaria Pennelli, Department of Pathology, University of Padua, Italy)

thrombus, as it may occur when fresh specimens are handled for intraoperative frozen sections [13, 14].

However, adopting current hystopathological criteria [118], only capsular and adjacent tissue invasion (present in 60% of cases, vascular invasion (10–15%)) and perineural space invasion (rarely present) [81, 91, 121] appear to correlate best with tumor recurrence and metastatic course, and can be considered pathognomonic of malignancy.

True parathyroid carcinoma should be distinguished from parathyromatosis and "atypical parathyroid adenoma." Parathyromatosis may occur in case of implantation of parathyroid tissue following intraoperative capsular rupture or incomplete excision of a parathyroid benign lesion [122]. Differentiation of parathyromatosis from recurrence of a previously excised and possibly underdiagnosed carcinoma is difficult since both may be associated with extensive infiltration of soft tissues and fibrosis. The presence of vascular and perineural space invasion are helpful features to distinguish recurrent parathyroid carcinoma from parathyromatosis.

The "atypical parathyroid adenoma" is an equivocal lesion that share only some of the features of carcinomas (fibrosis, mitoses, eventual capsular invasion), without definitive evidence of invasive growth of the surrounding tissue and vascular invasion [123]. The behavior of atypical adenomas may not differ from that of adenomas of usual type [124], although late recurrences and metastasis have also been reported, thus requiring a prolonged follow-up [13, 33, 82, 116].

In fact, histology alone will not diagnose all cases [115], since a proportion of parathyroid tumors which do not meet the histopathological criteria for carcinoma may recur or (rarely) metastasize [16, 59]. In contrast, only a subset of tumors classified as malignant at histopathological examination demonstrate recurrent disease or distant metastases [59, 125]. It remains unclear if it depends on incomplete excision of benign lesions or radical and curative ablation of malignant mass, respectively.

For these reasons, several other histological techniques are required to improve the accuracy of diagnosing parathyroid carcinoma. Electron microscopy of parathyroid cancer tissue reveals nuclear and mitochondrial alterations and evidence of increased secretory activity, but does not appear to be of value in distinguishing benign from malignant tumors [95, 126–129]. Nuclear diameter appears to be greater and the chromatin is clumped and dispersed through the karyoplasms in parathyroid carcinoma, but this index is not very useful in the individual case [93, 95, 126–129].

Measurement of nuclear DNA content by flow cytometry may be of some value; mean nuclear DNA content is greater, and an aneuploid DNA pattern is more common in parathyroid carcinoma than in adenomas, but it occurs too frequently in parathyroid adenomas to be of great use in differentiating benign from malignant parathyroid lesions [26–28, 130–133].

Studies of the proliferative fractions of parathyroid tumors have revealed higher values in carcinomas than in adenomas. Immunohistochemistry for the cell cycle marker Ki67 has been used; a count above 5% may suggest carcinoma [133, 134], but the overlap of values in equivocal cases has limited the role of this approach [135].

Immunohistochemical staining of Rb protein has been suggested to differentiate benign from malignant parathyroid tumors, since it has been reported to be commonly absent in parathyroid carcinomas while present in adenomas [78, 136], although controversial results have been also reported [137].

An additional approach has involved the use of antibodies to p27, which encodes a cyclin-dependent kinase inhibitor. Carcinomas have a threefold decrease in p27 expression respect of parathyroid adenomas [138]; however, these findings are difficult to be used in single cases because the diagnostic predictive value is often inadequate.

More recently, immunohistochemical evaluation of parafibromin (the product of the HRPT2 gene) has been used to diagnose parathyroid malignancy. Loss of parafibromin may suggest the definitive diagnosis with a sensitivity of 68–96% and a specificity of 99% [21, 25]; however, this protein is also absent in adenomas in HPT-JT patients [17, 51, 52, 59, 67, 68]. Furthermore, normal parafibromin expression has been reported in 80% of metastatic unequivocal parathyroid carcinomas in a series of patients with chronic renal failure [139]. This finding suggests that genetic events other than HRPT2 mutations may be of significance in the genesis of different subsets of parathyroid malignancies [23, 24, 139]. Recently, also the adenomatous polyposis coli (APC, that has an established role in colorectal cancer and play key roles in various fields such as cell migration, adhesion, apoptosis, chromosome segregation) and the protein gene product 9.5 (PGP9.5, encoded by ubiquitin carboxyl-terminal esterase L1) have shown a promising role in the diagnosis of parathyroid carcinoma. In fact, the loss of APC expression and the increased expression of PGP9.5 may be strongly predictive of parathyroid malignancy, especially when associated to the loss of parafibromin expression [22, 140].

Prognosis

The prognosis of parathyroid carcinoma is quite variable, although it usually has a slow, indolent but progressive course because of the rather low malignant potential. In fact, more than 80% of cases are described as "well differentiated" by pathologists [2].

The series of patients with parathyroid carcinoma of the National Cancer Data Base [2] reported a cumulative 5-year and 10-year survival of 86% and 49%, respectively. Other series have reported 5-year survival from 40% to 90% [141]. The most common causes of death are complications of hypercalcemia (renal failure, cardiac arrhythmias, pancreatitis) rather than tumor burden [1, 4, 6–10, 86, 107, 109]. The tumor tends to invade the surrounding structures and to spread to regional lymph nodes (30% of cases). In spite of radical excision, it tends to recur locally at the operative site; recurrence rates from 30% to 80% have been reported [15]. Most recurrences will manifest in the first 3 years [1, 10, 51], but recurrences as late as 20 years have been reported [10, 28]; thus, a prolonged follow-up is required if a parathyroid carcinoma is suspected. It is difficult to predict such a variable aggressiveness; a younger age and preoperative higher calcium levels have been reported as risk factors for early recurrence [1]. Once the disease has recurred, the chances of cure are remote. However, aggressive resection of residual disease and metastasectomy may improve the survival [1–10]. Tumor cells also disseminate hematogenously, and distant metastases occur in lungs (40%), liver (10%), and bones, although very few patients (<5%) have the involvement of regional lymph nodes or distant sites (<2%) at initial presentation [6, 10].

The most important factor affecting prognosis is the completeness of tumor resection [8, 9, 27]. Patients undergoing complete en bloc tumor resection can have survival rates as high as 90% at 5 years and 67% at 10 years [141]. Negative prognostic factors include lymph-node metastases at the time of diagnosis, distant metastases, and incomplete excision [31]; moreover, patients treated initially with simple parathyroidectomy have a worse prognosis, although in some series, tumor size and lymph-node involvement are not prognostic predictive factors [2].

There is no agreed prognostic staging system for parathyroid cancer. A TNM staging system has been proposed by Shaha [142]. Recently, Talat and Schulte have proposed in a meta-analysis of 330 cases a simpler prognostic staging system recognizing low-risk (according to the presence of capsular and soft tissue invasion) and high-risk patterns (according to the presence of vascular invasion and/or lymph node or distant metastases or invasion of vital organs), similarly to other neuroendocrine tumors [32]. This categorization may identify a 3.5-fold increased risk for recurrence and 4.9-fold for death in high-risk patients [32].

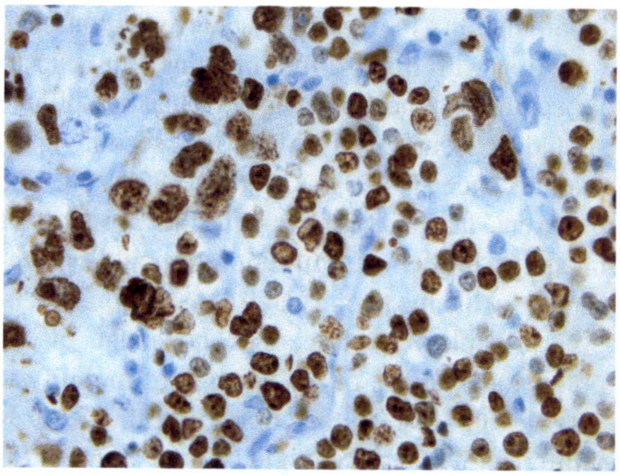

Fig. 8.13 Photomicrograph of a histological section of parathyroid carcinoma. High ki67 labeling index (courtesy of Gianmaria Pennelli, Department of Pathology, University of Padua, Italy)

Aneuploidy appears to be associated with a poorer prognosis [26–28, 123, 129, 143]; higher proliferation rates (Ki67) (see Fig. 8.13) within parathyroid carcinomas predict more aggressive behavior [2, 139, 144].

Surgical Treatment (Please Refer to Chapter on *Surgical Management of Parathyroid Diseases* for Further Discussion)

The single most effective treatment of parathyroid carcinoma is surgery [6, 7, 31, 33, 76, 81, 114, 143]. The gold standard therapy is an "en bloc" resection of the primary lesion at the time of initial operation [6, 7, 31, 37, 76, 145]. This approach consists of parathyroidectomy with the excision of the adjacent ipsilateral thyroid lobe in continuity with the tumor, with minimal manipulation, in order to achieve a complete resection with disease-free margins. Any capsular rupture of the tumor and neoplastic spillage should be accurately avoided, since seeding leads to recurrence [1, 7, 31, 37, 76, 81, 82, 146]. The recurrent laryngeal nerve—in the absence of unequivocal sign of infiltration—should be preserved by the mean of a careful dissection, whenever possible; therefore, the knowledge of the preoperative status of the vocal cord mobility is very useful [15]. To the contrary, if the nerve is infiltrated, its sacrifice might be necessary [7, 15, 30, 33, 37, 82, 108].

Intraoperative assay of quick PTH may confirm the complete removal of all hyperfunctioning parathyroid tissue and possibly it may help to determine the extent of surgery [37, 81]; in fact, it may predict the persistence of the disease suggesting wider excision or prolonged exploration, but does not prevent from late recurrences [147].

More extended procedures have been also proposed, consisting in the removal of the tumor in addition to the surrounding soft tissues, ipsilateral thyroid hemithyroidectomy, skeletonization of trachea, excision of the strap muscles and of the recurrent laryngeal nerve [76]. However, the main criticism to such systematic extensive excisions is related to the possibility of misdiagnosing lesions [15] with the risk of an overtreatment of a parathyroid adenoma. In fact, unfortunately, the definitive diagnosis of parathyroid cancer is hardly available pre- or intraoperatively; subsequently, the morbidity related to systematic aggressive approaches could be unacceptable in case of diagnostic errors, for example, benign lesions with degenerative changes simulating malignancy. However, it should be underlined that—to the contrary—another possible risk is the undertreatment of a true parathyroid cancer; it could be preferable to have a high index of suspicion for parathyroid carcinoma when these features are present than to miss the opportunity for surgical cure by failing to consider it in the differential diagnosis.

Therapeutic cervical lymph-node dissection is usually recommended in case of evident nodal metastases [7, 15, 76, 82, 146]; the mediastinal dissection, along with central compartment dissection, may be required for extension of soft tissue disease through the thoracic inlet [33].

The role of prophylactic nodal dissection is still controversial. Most authors have reported that nodal metastases are exceedingly rare [1, 26–28, 30, 76], and prophylactic neck dissection does not improve the prognosis but may increase the morbidity (recurrent laryngeal nerve palsy and postoperative hypocalcemia) [27, 76, 143].

Recently, others have suggested a systematic clearance of the central compartment (corresponding to level VI) with prophylactic removal of all soft tissues and lymph nodes [3, 32, 33, 145], because nodal metastases might be found in up to 41% of patients undergoing systematic nodal dissection; microscopic nodal involvement may be the source of local recurrences; thus, nodal dissection might improve the cure rate [145].The prophylactic clearance of the lateral compartment in the absence of demonstrable involvement is not recommended, given that jugular lymph-node metastases seem to be uncommon and this procedure does not lead to therapeutic benefits [15, 33, 91, 145].

Effective surgery is usually followed by severe hypocalcemia due to "hungry bone syndrome," requiring adequate calcium and vitamin D replacement and close monitoring of calcium and PTH levels.

When the diagnosis of parathyroid cancer is made in the early postoperative period on the basis of histology, as usually occurs, the management plan becomes more complex and the benefits of further radical operations remain controversial. If the serum calcium and PTH levels are normal, most tend to follow the patient without attempts to immediate reoperations, given that the first surgery could have been curative [5, 30, 148]. Further explorations of the neck have been proposed in case of persistent hypercalcemia [6, 7, 10], following adequate preoperative imaging study to localize the disease as accurately as possible [108, 109].

In spite of every efforts, most patients experience recurrent disease after initial surgery [7, 10, 108]. Reoperation, in these cases, can be considered a good palliation [1, 6, 10, 27, 31, 37, 109, 146]. Appropriate localization studies should be performed in all patients before repeated surgery and, if noninvasive imaging approaches are negative, selective venous sampling for PTH measurement may be an useful tool [6, 7, 108]. Recurrences in the neck and in the mediastinum, including the regional lymph node and all involved structures, should be excised with margins as wide as possible [6, 7, 10]. Multiple reoperations may be required, since they offer a valuable palliative option, although surgical morbidity should be considered [108, 109]. Distant metastases should also be excised [5, 15, 109, 149], although resection is rarely curative, but may result in a period of normocalcemia from months to years. Moreover, also palliative debulking may facilitate the medical management of hypercalcemia [6, 109].

Finally, although surgery remains the mainstay of management in these cases, the availability of new drugs (calcimimetics) is opening new perspectives for the treatment of patients with intractable hypercalcemia [148].

Medical and Adjuvant Treatments

Patients with parathyroid carcinoma generally die from metabolic complications of uncontrollable hypercalcemia rather than from tumor burden; subsequently, serious measures should be taken to reduce serum calcium values. Whenever possible, severe hypercalcemia should be rectified before surgical treatment, because surgery should not be done on an emergency basis but rather once the patient's calcium values have been stabilized by nonsurgical approach [33]. Furthermore, the treatment of hypercalcemia is particularly important in the patients with recurrent or metastatic parathyroid cancer or not suitable for surgical treatment.

At initial presentation, severe hypercalcemia should be treated with urgent restoration of fluid volume through intravenous access along with the administration of diuretics, biphosphonates, and calcimimetic agents. Patients with severe hypercalcemia are significantly dehydrated because of nephrogenic diabetes insipidus and associated nausea and vomiting; an aggressive hydration (200–300 cm^3/h of normal saline) is necessary as initial treatment; loop diuretics, as furosemide, are given to increase renal calcium excretion. Biphosphonates, such as clodronate, etidronate, pamidronate, zolendronate (a class of drugs that inhibit osteoclast-mediated bone resorption by incorporation into the bone matrix) are effective but they lose efficacy over time [7, 10, 26, 33, 37, 82, 143, 150]. The bisphosphonates are poorly absorbed when given orally, therefore, intravenous administration is required. Pamidronate, infused in doses of 30–90 mg/day over 2–4 h, has been effective in lowering serum calcium levels in patients affected by parathyroid cancer, at least transiently; responses last for 1–3 weeks and the treatment can be repeated [26, 82, 143, 150]. Zolendronate has been reported to be more effective at lowering serum calcium levels in patients with hypercalcemia associated with malignancy and can be infused more quickly (4 mg intravenously over 15 min) [8, 82, 151, 152]. However, possible complications of bisphosphonates are represented by avascular necrosis of the jaw and the acute renal failure following rapid intravenous administration in patients with decreased renal function [153]. Furthermore, the effectiveness of these drugs typically decreases over time [82]. When patients are unresponsive to intravenous biphosphonates, mithramycin (an antibiotic found to have calcium lowering properties) has been indicated as a second-line drug for life-threatening hypercalcemia. It is administered intravenously at a dose of 25 μg/kg over 4–8 h and may be repeated at daily intervals for up to 7 days until the serum calcium returns into an acceptable range [10]. However, also this drug is toxic and not very effective, since complete normalization of the calcium values is rarely achieved [7, 10, 15].

Calcitonin and corticosteroids can also be used. Calcitonin inhibits osteoclastic bone resorption and facilitates renal excretion of calcium; it is administered through subcutaneous or intramuscular access at a dose of 3–6 IU/kg and has a rapid onset of action (12–24 h). However, serum calcium levels only show a modest reduction and rapidly return to pretreatment values within 48 h.

Corticosteroids may be used to lower the serum calcium levels increasing the urinary excretion of calcium and decreasing intestinal calcium absorption. However, they have a slow onset of action and may cause side effects such as immunosuppression, hyperglycemia, and cushingoid symptoms. The combination of calcitonin and hydrocortisone may be useful when patients are afflicted by renal failure [82]. Amifostine, a chemoprotective agent that acts by inhibiting PTH secretion, is effective in controlling hypercalcemia but its use is limited because of severe toxicity [10]. Also gallium nitrate is effective to inhibit bone resorption by preventing dissolution of hydroxyapatite crystal but is extremely nephrotoxic [154].

Most part of these treatments has been supplanted by more recent agents; cinacalcet is an effective drug for medical therapy of PTH-related hypercalcemia [82, 155]. Cinacalcet is a calcimimetic acting as an allosteric modulator of calcium-sensing receptors that are responsible for the regulation of PTH secretion. It binds to the calcium receptors on the surface of parathyroid cells and increases the receptor sensitivity to extracellular calcium and subsequently reduces the serum PTH and calcium levels [7, 8, 15, 33, 82, 155, 156]. Cinacalcet is administrated orally (30–60 mg) once daily and is well tolerated [82]; nausea and vomiting are the most common adverse events. Patients with the highest calcium levels have showed the greater reduction, although, it is not usually accompanied by a similar fall in PTH values. There is no evidence that cinacalcet will modify the course of parathyroid cancer; therefore, it cannot replace surgical intervention in case of resectable disease, but in patients with widely metastatic disease or with renal insufficiency this drug can potentially alleviate the consequences of hypercalcemia and represents an important option [6, 15, 33, 155–157].

Finally, octreotide, the somatostatin analog, has been reported to inhibit PTH secretion [158]. Recent reports have demonstrated palliative effects from the use of indium-labeled octreotide therapy for metastatic neuroendocrine tumors; the radiometabolic treatment might represent a therapeutical option in patients with metastatic carcinoma in the future [158].

In the recent years, also antiparathyroid immunotherapy is reported as an useful treatment in patients with refractory hypercalcemia from metastatic disease [7]. A rapid decline of PTH and serum calcium levels, improvement in clinical condition, decrease of the size of lung metastases, without relevant adverse effects have been reported after immunization by a mixture of human and bovine PTH peptides [159]. Dendritic cell immunotherapy has also been used to induce a T-cell immune response [160, 161]. Recently, a monoclonal antibody to PTH has been used also for the treatment of parathyroid carcinoma [162].

Concerning radiotherapy and chemotherapy in parathyroid cancer, all data are derived from case reports [86, 163, 164]. No controlled trials have been carried out, because of the rarity of the disease.

Traditionally, radiotherapy is not considered an effective treatment, either as a single technique or in addition to surgery [31]. A single case of long-term (10 years) apparent cure in a patient with neoplastic invasion of trachea has been reported [86]. In the recent years, the Mayo Clinic and MD Anderson Cancer Center groups have proposed a possible role as adjuvant treatment following surgery, since lower recurrence and longer disease-free have been reported, independently from the type of operation and the disease stage [81, 91, 165]. Unfortunately, these conclusions have been carried out from very small series, and need to be confirmed by further studies. Currently, the best practice seems to be approaching each patient individually in a multidisciplinary fashion.

Also the results of chemotherapy are generally disappointing. Several regimens have been attempted (nitrogen mustard, vincristine, cyclophosphamide, and actinomycin D, and adriamycinaloneorincombinationwithcyclophosphamide and 5-fluorouracil), but none of them has proved to be effective [86, 108, 110]. Currently, there is no role for chemotherapy in the management of patients with parathyroid carcinoma.

References

1. Iacobone M, Lumachi F, Favia G. Up-to-date on parathyroid carcinoma. Analysis of an experience of 19 cases. J Surg Oncol. 2004;88:223–9.
2. Hundahl SA, Fleming ID, Fremgen AM, Menck HR. Two hundred eighty-six cases of parathyroid carcinoma treated in the U. S. between 1985-1995: a National Cancer Data Base Report. The American College of Surgeons Commission on Cancer and the American Cancer Society. Cancer. 1999;86:538–44.
3. Fujimoto Y, Obara T, Ito Y, Kanazawa K, Aiyoshi Y, Nobori M. Surgical treatment of ten cases of parathyroid carcinoma: importance of an initial en bloc tumor resection. World J Surg. 1984;8:392–400.
4. Fujimoto Y, Obara T, Ito Y, Kodama T, Nobori M, Ebihara S. Localization and resection of metastatic parathyroid carcinoma. World J Surg. 1986;10:539–47.
5. Fujimoto Y, Obara T. How to recognize and treat parathyroid carcinoma. Surg Clin North Am. 1987;67:343–57.
6. Marcocci C, Cetani F, Rubin MR, Silverberg SJ, Pinchera A, Bilezikian JP. Parathyroid carcinoma. J Bone Miner Res. 2008;23:1869–80.
7. Rawat N, Khetan N, Williams DW, Baxter JN. Parathyroid carcinoma. Br J Surg. 2005;92:1345–53.
8. Pasieka J, Khalil M. Parathyroid carcinoma. In: Oertli D, Udelsman R, editors. Surgery of the Thyroid and Parathyroid Glands. Berlin: Springer-Verlag; 2007;26:311–25.
9. Marcocci C, Cetani F, Bilezikian JP. Parathryoid Carcinoma. In: Hubbard JGH, Inabnet WB, Lo CY, editors. Endocrine surgery: principles and practice. Springer-Verlag London Limited; 2009;23:321–33.
10. Shane E. Parathyroid carcinoma. J Clin Endocrinol Metab. 2001;86:485–93.
11. Sainton P, Millot J. Degeneration maligne d'un adenome parathyroidienne eosinophile au cours d'une maladie de von Recklinghausen. Ann Anat Pathol. 1933;10:813–4.
12. De Quervain F. Parastruma maligna aberrata. Deutsche Zeitschr Chir. 1904;100:334–52.
13. Delellis RA. Challenging lesions in the differential diagnosis of endocrine tumors. Parathyroid carcinoma. Endocr Pathol. 2008;19:221–5.
14. Johnson SJ. Changing clinicopathological practice in parathyroid disease. Histopathology. 2010;56: 835–51.
15. Givi B, Shah JP. Parathyroid carcinoma. Clin Oncol (R Coll Radiol). 2010;22:498–507.
16. Carpten JD, Robbins CM, Villablanca A, Forsberg L, Presciuttini S, Bailey-Wilson J, Simonds WF, Gillanders EM, Kennedy AM, Chen JD, Agarwal SK, Sood R, Jones MP, Moses TY, Haven C, Petillo D, Leotlela PD, Harding B, Cameron D, Pannett AA, Hoog A, Heath 3rd H, James-Newton LA, Robinson B, Zarbo RJ, Cavaco BM, Wassif W, Perrier ND, Rosen IB, Kristoffersson U, Turnpenny PD, Farnebo LO, Besser GM, Jackson CE, Morreau H, Trent JM, Thakker RV, Marx SJ, Teh BT, Larsson C, Hobbs MR. HRPT2, encoding parafibromin, is mutated in hyperparathyroidism-jaw tumor syndrome. Nat Genet. 2002;32:676–80.
17. Cetani F, Ambrogini E, Viacava P, Pardi E, Fanelli G, Naccarato AG, Borsari S, Lemmi M, Berti P, Miccoli P, Pinchera A, Marcocci C. Should parafibromin staining replace HRTP2 gene analysis as an additional tool for histologic diagnosis of parathyroid carcinoma? Eur J Endocrinol. 2007;156: 547–54.
18. Cetani F, Pardi E, Ambrogini E, Viacava P, Borsari S, Lemmi M, Cianferotti L, Miccoli P, Pinchera A, Arnold A, Marcocci C. Different somatic alterations of the HRPT2 gene in a patient with recurrent sporadic primary hyperparathyroidism carrying an HRPT2 germline mutation. Endocr Relat Cancer. 2007;14:493–9.
19. Howell VM, Haven CJ, Kahnoski K, Khoo SK, Petillo D, Chen J, Fleuren GJ, Robinson BG, Delbridge LW, Philips J, Nelson AE, Krause U, Hammje K, Dralle H, Hoang-Vu C, Haven CJ, Howell VM, Eilers PH, Dunne R, Takahashi M, van Puijenbroek M, Furge K, Kievit J, Tan MH, Fleuren GJ, Robinson BG, Delbridge LW, Philips J, Nelson AE, Krause U, Chen Q, Kaji H, Nomura R, Sowa H, Yamauchi M, Tsukamoto T, Yamaguchi T, Kobayashi A, Sugimoto T, Chihara K. Trial to predict malignancy of affected parathyroid glands in primary hyperparathyroidism. Endocr J. 2003;50:527–34.
20. Howell VM, Gill A, Clarkson A, Nelson AE, Dunne R, Delbridge LW, Robinson BG, Teh BT, Gimm O, Marsh DJ. Accuracy of combined protein gene product 9. 5 and parafibromin markers for immunohistochemical diagnosis of parathyroid carcinoma. J Clin Endocrinol Metab. 2009;94:434–41.
21. Juhlin CC, Villablanca A, Sandelin K, Haglund F, Nordenström J, Forsberg L, Bränström R, Obara T, Arnold A, Larsson C, Höög A. Parafibromin immunoreactivity: its use as an additional diagnostic marker for parathyroid tumor classification. Endocr Relat Cancer. 2007;14:501–12.
22. Juhlin CC, Nilsson IL, Johansson K, Haglund F, Villablanca A, Höög A, Larsson C. Parafibromin and APC as screening markers for malignant potential in atypical parathyroid adenomas. Endocr Pathol. 2010;21:166–77.
23. Mangray S, Kurek KC, Sabo E, DeLellis RA. Immunohistochemical expression of parafibromin is of limited value in distinguishing parathyroid carcinoma from adenoma. Mod Pathol. 2008;21:108.
24. Mangray S, DeLellis RA. Parafibromin as tool for the diagnosis of parathyroid tumors. Adv Anat Pathol. 2008;15:179.
25. Tan MH, Morrison C, Wang P, Yang X, Haven CJ, Zhang C, Zhao P, Tretiakova MS, Korpi-Hyovalti E, Burgess JR, Soo KC, Cheah WK, Cao B, Resau J, Morreau H, Teh BT. Loss of parafibromin immunoreactivity is a distinguishing feature of parathyroid carcinoma. Clin Cancer Res. 2004;10:6629–37.

26. Sandelin K, Thompson NW, Bondeson L. Metastatic parathyroid carcinoma: dilemmas in management. Surgery. 1991;110:978–88.
27. Sandelin K, Auer G, Bondeson L, Grimelius L, Farnebo LO. Prognostic factors in parathyroid cancer: a review of 95 cases. World J Surg. 1992; 16:724–31.
28. Sandelin K, Tullgren O, Farnebo LO. Clinical course of metastatic parathyroid cancer. World J Surg. 1994;18:594–8.
29. Ruda JM, Hollenbeak CS, Stack Jr BC. A systematic review of the diagnosis and treatment of primary hyperparathyroidism from 1995 to 2003. Otolaryngol Head Neck Surg. 2005;132:359–72.
30. Ippolito G, Palazzo FF, Sebag F, De Micco C, Henry JF. Intraoperative diagnosis and treatment of parathyroid cancer and atypical parathyroid adenoma. Br J Surg. 2007;94:566–70.
31. Koea JB, Shaw JH. Parathyroid cancer: biology and management. Surg Oncol. 1999;8:155–65.
32. Talat N, Schulte KM. Clinical presentation, staging and long-term evolution of parathyroid cancer. Ann Surg Oncol. 2010;17:2156–74.
33. Owen RP, Silver CE, Pellitteri PK, Shaha AR, Devaney KO, Werner JA, Rinaldo A, Ferlito A. Parathyroid carcinoma: a review. Head Neck. 2010;33(3):429–36.
34. Hamill J, Maoate K, Beasley SW, Corbett R, Evans J. Familial parathyroid carcinoma in a child. J Paediatr Child Health. 2002;38:314–7.
35. Simonds WF, James-Newton LA, Agarwal SK, Yang B, Skarulis MC, Hendy GN, Marx SJ. Familial isolated hyperparathyroidism: clinical and genetic characteristics of 36 kindreds. Medicine (Baltimore). 2002;81:1–26.
36. Lumachi F, Ermani M, Marino F, Iacobone M, Baldessin M, Cappuzzo G, Zanella S, Favia G. PCNA-LII, Ki-67 immunostaining, p53 activity and histopathological variables in predicting the clinical outcome in patients with parathyroid carcinoma. Anticancer Res. 2006;26:1305–8.
37. Mittendorf EA, McHenry CR. Parathyroid carcinoma. J Surg Oncol. 2005;89:136–42.
38. Rasmuson T, Damber L, Johansson L, Johansson R, Larsson LG. Increased incidence of parathyroid adenomas following X-ray treatment of benign diseases in the cervical spine in adult patients. Clin Endocrinol. 2002;57:731–4.
39. Ireland J, Fleming S, Levison D, Cattell W, Baker L. Parathyroid carcinoma associated with chronic renal failure and previous radiotherapy to the neck. J Clin Pathol. 1985;38:1114–8.
40. Christmas TJ, Chapple CR, Noble JG, Milroy EJ, Cowie AG. Hyperparathyroidism after neck irradiation. Br J Surg. 1988;75:873–4.
41. Cohen J, Gierlowski TC, Schneider AB. A prospective study of hyperparathyroidism in individuals exposed to radiation in childhood. JAMA. 1990; 264:581–4.
42. Schneider AB, Gierlowski TC, Shore-Freedman E, Stovall M, Ron E, Lubin J. Dose–response relationships for radiation-induced hyperparathyroidism. J Clin Endocrinol Metab. 1995;80:254–7.
43. Miki H, Sumitomo M, Inoue H, Kita S, Monden Y. Parathyroid carcinoma in patients with chronic renal failure on maintenance hemodialysis. Surgery. 1996;120:897–901.
44. Berland Y, Olmer M, Lebreuil G, Grisoli J. Parathyroid carcinoma, adenoma and hyperplasia in a case of chronic renal insufficiency on dialysis. Clin Nephrol. 1982;18:154–8.
45. Boyle NH, Ogg CS, Hartley RB, Owen WJ. Parathyroid carcinoma secondary to prolonged hyperplasia in chronic renal failure and celiac disease. Eur J Surg Oncol. 1999;25:100–3.
46. Yoshimoto K, Endo H, Tsuyuguchi M, Tanaka C, Kimura T, Iwahana H, Kato G, Sano T, Itakura T. Familial isolated primary hyperparathyroidism with parathyroid carcinomas: clinical and molecular features. Clin Endocrinol. 1998;48:67–72.
47. Dinnen J, Greenwood R, Jone J, Walker D, Williams E. Parathyroid carcinoma in familial hyperparathyroidism. J Clin Pathol. 1977;30:966–75.
48. Wassif WS, Moniz CF, Friedman E, Wong S, Weber G, Nordenskjold M, Peters TJ, Larsson C. Familial isolated hyperparathyroidism: a distinct genetic entity with an increased risk of parathyroid cancer. J Clin Endocrinol Metab. 1993;77:1485–9.
49. Streeten EA, Weinstein LS, Norton JA, Mulvihill JJ, White BJ, Friedman E, Jaffe G, Brandi ML, Stewart K, Zimering MB, Spiegel AM, Aurbach GD, Marx SJ. Studies in a kindred with parathyroid carcinoma. J Clin Endocrinol Metab. 1992;75:362–6.
50. Marx SJ, Simonds WF, Agarwal SK, Burns AL, Weinstein LS, Cochran C, Skarulis MC, Spiegel AM, Libutti SK, Alexander Jr HR, Chen CC, Chang R, Chandrasekharappa SC, Collins FS. Hyperparathyroidism in hereditary syndromes: special expressions and special managements. J Bone Miner Res. 2002;17:37–43.
51. Masi G, Barzon L, Iacobone M, Viel G, Porzionato A, Macchi V, De Caro R, Favia G, Palù G. Clinical, genetic, and histopathologic investigation of CDC73-related familial hyperparathyroidism. Endocr Relat Cancer. 2008;15:1115–26.
52. Iacobone M, Masi G, Barzon L, Porzionato A, Macchi V, Ciarleglio FA, Palù G, De Caro R, Viel G, Favia G. Hyperparathyroidism-jaw tumor syndrome: a report of three large kindred. Langenbecks Arch Surg. 2009;394:817–25.
53. Haven CJ, van Puijenbroek M, Tan MH, Teh BT, Fleuren GJ, van Wezel T, Morreau H. Identification of MEN1 and HRPT2 somatic mutations in paraffin-embedded (sporadic) parathyroid carcinomas. Clin Endocrinol. 2007;67:370–6.
54. Porzionato A, Macchi V, Barzon L, Masi G, Iacobone M, Parenti A, Palù G, De Caro R. Immunohisto-

chemical assessment of parafibromin in mouse and human tissues. J Anat. 2006;209:817–27.
55. Hampsey M, Reinberg D. Tails of intrigue: phosphorylation of RNA polymerase II mediates histone methylation. Cell. 2003;113:429–32.
56. Rozenblatt-Rosen O, Hughes CM, Nannepaga SJ, Shanmugam KS, Copeland TD, Guszczynski T, Resau JH, Meyerson M. The parafibromin tumor suppressor protein is part of a human Paf1 complex. Mol Cell Biol. 2005;25:612–20.
57. Yart A, Gstaiger M, Wirbelauer C, Pecnik M, Anastasiou D, Hess D, Krek W. The HRPT2 tumor suppressor gene product parafibromin associates with human PAF1 and RNA polymerase II. Mol Cell Biol. 2005;25:5052–60.
58. Ma H, Marsh DJ. Identification of a functional bipartite nuclear localization signal in the tumor suppressor parafibromin. Oncogene. 2005;24:6241–8.
59. Juhlin C, Larsson C, Yakoleva T, Leibiger I, Leibiger B, Alimov A, Weber G, Höög A, Villablanca A. Loss of parafibromin expression in a subset of parathyroid adenomas. Endocr Relat Cancer. 2006;13:509–23.
60. Zhang C, Kong D, Tan MH, Pappas Jr DL, Wang PF, Chen J, Farber L, Zhang N, Koo HM, Weinreich M, Williams BO, Teh BT. Parafibromin inhibits cancer cell growth and causes G1 phase arrest. Biochem Biophys Res Commun. 2006;350:17–24.
61. Chaudhary K, Deb S, Moniaux N, Ponnusamy MP, Batra SK. Human RNA polymerase II-associated factor complex: dysregulation in cancer. Oncogene. 2007;26:7499–507.
62. Lin L, Czapiga M, Nini L, Zhang JH, Simonds WF. Nuclear localization of the parafibromin tumor suppressor protein implicated in the hyperparathyroidism-jaw tumor syndrome enhances its proapoptotic function. Mol Cancer Res. 2007;5:183–93.
63. Bradley KJ, Bowl MR, Williams SE, Ahmad BN, Partridge CJ, Patmanidi AL, Kennedy AM, Loh NY, Thakker RV. Parafibromin is a nuclear protein with a functional monopartite nuclear localization signal. Oncogene. 2007;26:1213–21.
64 Sharretts JM, Simonds WF. Clinical and molecular genetics of parathyroid neoplasms. Best Pract Res Clin Endocrinol Metab. 2010;24:491–502.
65. Woodard GE, Lin L, Zhang JH, Agarwal SK, Marx SJ, Simonds WF. Parafibromin, product of the hyperparathyroidism-jaw tumor syndrome gene HRPT2, regulates cyclin D1/PRAD1 expression. Oncogene. 2005;24:1272–6.
66. Villablanca A, Calender A, Forsberg L, Höög A, Cheng JD, Petillo D, Bauters C, Kahnoski K, Ebeling T, Salmela P, Richardson AL, Delbridge L, Meyrier A, Proye C, Carpten JD, Teh BT, Robinson BG, Larsson C. Germline and de novo mutations in the HRPT2 tumour suppressor gene in familial isolated hyperparathyroidism (FIHP). J Med Genet. 2004;41:32.
67. Gill AJ, Clarkson A, Gimm O, Keil J, Dralle H, Howell VM, Marsh DJ. Loss of nuclear expression of parafibromin distinguishes parathyroid carcinomas and hyperparathyroidism-jaw tumor (HPT-JT) syndrome-related adenomas from sporadic parathyroid adenomas and hyperplasias. Am J Surg Pathol. 2006;30:1140–9.
68. Iacobone M, Barzon L, Porzionato A, Masi G, Macchi V, Marino F, Viel G, Favia G. Parafibromin expression, single-gland involvement, and limited parathyroidectomy in familial isolated hyperparathyroidism. Surgery. 2007;142:984–91.
69. Shattuck TM, Valimaki S, Obara T, Gaz RD, Clark OH, Shoback D, Wierman ME, Tojo K, Robbins CM, Carpten JD, Farnebo LO, Larsson C, Arnold A. Somatic and germ-line mutations of the HRPT2 gene in sporadic parathyroid carcinoma. N Engl Med. 2003;349:1722–9.
70. Cetani F, Pardi E, Borsari S, Vacava P, Dipollina G, Cianferotti L, Ambrogini E, Gazzero E, Colussi G, Berti P, Miccoli P, Pinchera A, Marcocci C. Genetic analyses of the HRPT2 gene in primary hyperparathyroidism: germline and somatic mutations in familial and sporadic parathyroid tumors. J Clin Endocrinol Metab. 2004;89:5583–91.
71. Hewitt KM, Sharma PK, Samowitz W, Hobbs M. Aberrant methylation of the HRPT2 gene in parathyroid carcinoma. Ann Otol Rhinol Laryngol. 2007;116:928–33.
72. Krebs LJ, Shattuck TM, Arnold A. HRPT2 mutational analysis of typical sporadic parathyroid adenomas. J Clin Endocrinol Metab. 2005;90:5015–7.
73. Senior K. Vital gene linked to parathyroid carcinoma. Lancet Oncol. 2003;4:713.
74. Agha A, Carpenter R, Bhattacharya S, Edmonson SJ, Carlsen E, Monson JP. Parathyroid carcinoma in multiple endocrine neoplasia type 1 (MEN1) syndrome: two case reports of an unrecognized entity. J Endocrinol Invest. 2007;30:145–9.
75. Dionisi S, Minisola S, Pepe J, De Geronimo S, Paglia F, Memeo L, Fitzpatrick LA. Concurrent parathyroid adenomas and carcinoma in the setting of multiple endocrine neoplasia type 1: presentation as hypercalcemic crisis. Mayo Clin Proc. 2002;77:866–9.
76. Enomoto K, Uchino S, Ito A, Watanabe S, Shibuya H, Enomoto Y, Noguchi S. The surgical strategy and the molecular analysis of patients with parathyroid cancer. World J Surg. 2010;34:2604–10.
77. Jenkins PJ, Satta MA, Simmgen M, Drake WM, Williamson C, Lowe DG, Britton K, Chew SL, Thakker RV, Besser GM. Metastatic parathyroid carcinoma in the MEN2A syndrome. Clin Endocrinol. 1997;47:747–51.
78. Cryns VL, Thor A, Xu HJ, Hu SX, Wierman ME, Vickery Jr AL, Benedict WF, Arnold A. Loss of the retinoblastoma tumor-suppressor gene in parathyroid carcinoma. N Engl J Med. 1994;330:757–61.
79. Dotzenrath C, Teh BT, Farnebo F, Cupisti K, Svensson A, Toell A, Goretzki P, Larsson C. Allelic loss of the retinoblastoma tumor suppressor gene: a marker for aggressive parathyroid tumors? J Clin Endocrinol Metab. 1996;81:3194–6.

80. Pearce SH, Trump D, Wooding C, Sheppard MN, Clayton RN, Thakker RV. Loss of heterozygosity studies at the retinoblastoma and breast cancer susceptibility (BRCA2) loci in pituitary, parathyroid, pancreatic and carcinoid tumours. Clin Endocrinol. 1996;45:195–200.
81. Clayman GL, Gonzalez HE, El-Naggar A, Vassilopoulou-Sellin R. Parathyroid carcinoma: evaluation and interdisciplinary management. Cancer. 2004;100:900–5.
82. Rodgers SE, Perrier ND. Parathyroid carcinoma. Curr Opin Oncol. 2006;18:16–22.
83. Venkitaraman AR. Chromosome stability, DNA recombination and the BRCA2 tumour suppressor. Curr Opin Cell Biol. 2001;13:338–43.
84. Mallya SM, Arnold A. Cyclin D1 in parathyroid disease. Front Biosci. 2000;5:367–71.
85. Rao SR, Shaha AR, Singh B, Rinaldo A, Ferlito A. Management of cancer of the parathyroid. Acta Otolaryngol. 2002;122:448–52.
86. Wynne AG, van Heerden J, Carney JA, Fitzpatrick LA. Parathyroid carcinoma: clinical and pathologic features in 43 patients. Medicine. 1992;71:197–205.
87. Heath 3rd H, Hodgson SF, Kennedy MA. Primary hyperparathyroidism: incidence, morbidity, and potential economic impact in a community. N Engl J Med. 1980;302:189–93.
88. Silverberg SJ, Shane E, de la Cruz L, Dempster DW, Feldman F, Seldin D, Jacobs TP, Siris ES, Cafferty M, Parisien MV. Skeletal disease in primary hyperparathyroidism. J Bone Miner Res. 1989;4:283–91.
89. Silverberg SJ, Shane E, Jacobs TP, Siris ES, Gartenberg F, Seldin D, Clemens TL, Bilezikian JP. Nephrolithiasis and bone involvement in primary hyperparathyroidism. Am J Med. 1990;89:327–34.
90. Wilkins BJ, Lewis Jr JS. Non-functional parathyroid carcinoma: a review of the literature and report of a case requiring extensive surgery. Head Neck Pathol. 2009;3:140–9.
91. Busaidy NL, Jimenez C, Habra MA, Schultz PN, El-Naggar AK, Clayman GL, Asper JA, Diaz Jr EM, Evans DB, Gagel RF, Garden A, Hoff AO, Lee JE, Morrison WH, Rosenthal DI, Sherman SI, Sturgis EM, Waguespack SG, Weber RS, Wirfel K, Vassilopoulou-Sellin R. Parathyroid carcinoma: a 22-year experience. Head Neck. 2004;26:716–26.
92. Anderson BJ, Samaan NA, Vassilopoulou-Sellin R, Ordonez NG, Hickey RC. Parathyroid carcinoma: features and difficulties in diagnosis and management. Surgery. 1983;94:906–15.
93. Schantz A, Castleman B. Parathyroid carcinoma. A study of 70 cases. Cancer. 1973;31:600–5.
94. Levin K, Galante M, Clark O. Parathyroid carcinoma versus parathyroid adenoma in patients with profound hypercalcemia. Surgery. 1987;101:647–60.
95. Smith J, Coombs R. Histological diagnosis of carcinoma of the parathyroid gland. J Clin Pathol. 1984;37:1370–8.
96. Kung B, Winokur R, Cognetti D, O'Hara B, Rosen D. Parathyroid carcinoma: a rare cause of primary hyperparathyroidism. Ear Nose Throat J. 2009;88:10–3.
97. Okamoto T, Iihara M, Obara T, Tsukada T. Parathyroid carcinoma: etiology, diagnosis, and treatment. World J Surg. 2009;33:2343–54.
98. Cheah WK, Rauff A, Lee KO, Tan W. Parathyroid carcinoma: a case series. Ann Acad Med Singapore. 2005;34:443–6.
99. Caron N, Sturgeon C, Clark OH. Persistent and recurrent hyperparathyroidism. Curr Treat Options Oncol. 2004;5:335–45.
100. Robert JH, Trombetti A, Garcia A, Pache JC, Herrmann F, Spiliopoulos A, Rizzoli R. Primary hyperparathyroidism: can parathyroid carcinoma be anticipated on clinical and biochemical grounds? Report of nine cases and review of the literature. Ann Surg Oncol. 2005;12:526–32.
101. Caron P, Maiza JC, Renaud C, Cormier C, Barres BH, Souberbielle JC. High third generation/second generation PTH ratio in a patient with parathyroid carcinoma: clinical utility of third generation / second generation PTH ratio in patients with primary hyperparathyroidism. Clin Endocrinol. 2009;70:533–8.
102. Rubin MR, Silverberg SJ, D'Amour P, Brossard JH, Rousseau L, Sliney Jr J, Cantor T, Bilezikian JP. An Nterminal molecular form of parathyroid hormone (PTH) distinct from hPTH(1-84) is overproduced in parathyroid carcinoma. Clin Chem. 2007;53:1470–6.
103. Rubin MR, Bilezikian JP, Birken S, Silverberg SJ. Human chorionic gonadotropin measurements in parathyroid carcinoma. Eur J Endocrinol. 2008;159:469–74.
104. Spinelli C, Bonadio AG, Berti P, Materazzi G, Miccoli P. Cutaneous spreading of parathyroid carcinoma after fine needle aspiration cytology. J Endocrinol Invest. 2000;23:255–7.
105. Alwaheeb S, Rambaldini G, Boerner S, Coiré C, Fiser J, Asa SL. Worrisome histologic alterations following fine-needle aspiration of the parathyroid. J Clin Pathol. 2006;59:1094–6.
106. Norman J, Politz D, Browarsky I. Diagnostic aspiration of parathyroid adenomas causes severe fibrosis complicating surgery and final histopathologic diagnosis. Thyroid. 2007;17:1251–5.
107. Thompson SD, Prichard AJ. The management of parathyroid carcinoma. Curr Opin Otolaryngol Head Neck Surg. 2004;12:93–7.
108. Kebebew E, Arici C, Duh QY, Clark OH. Localization and reoperation results for persistent and recurrent parathyroid carcinoma. Arch Surg. 2001;136:878–85.
109. Iacobone M, Ruffolo C, Lumachi F, Favia G. Results of iterative surgery for persistent and recurrent parathyroid carcinoma. Langenbecks Arch Surg. 2005;390:385–90.
110. Kettle AG, O'Doherty MJ. Parathyroid imaging: how good is it and how should it be done? Semin Nucl Med. 2006;36:206–11.
111. Castellani M, Reschini E, Longari V, Paracchi A, Corbetta S, Marotta G, Gerundini P. Role of Tc-99 m sestamibi scintigraphy in the diagnosis and surgical

decision making process in primary hyperparathyroid disease. Clin Nucl Med. 2001;26:139–44.
112. Weber AL, Randolph G, Aksoy FG. The thyroid and parathyroid glands. CT and MR imaging and correlation with pathology and clinical findings. Radiol Clin N Am. 2000;38:1105–29.
113. Kemps B, van Ufford HQ, Creyghton W, de Haas M, Baarslag HJ, Rinkes IB, de Klerk J. Brown tumors simulating metastases on FDG PET in a patient with parathyroid carcinoma. Eur J Nucl Med Mol Imag. 2008;35:850.
114. Pasieka JL. Parathyroid carcinoma. Operative Tech Gen Surg. 1999;1:71–84.
115. Chang Y-J, Mittal V, Remine S, Manyam H, Sabir M, Richardson T, Young S. Correlation between clinical and histological findings in parathyroid tumours suspicious for carcinoma. Am Surg. 2006;72:419–26.
116. Harach HR. The parathyroid. In: Lloyd RV, editor. Endocrine pathology: differential diagnosis and molecular advances. Totowa, NJ: Humana Press; 2004. p. 109–22.
117. Snover D, Foucar K. Mitotic activity in benign thyroid diseases. Am J Clin Pathol. 1981;75:345–7.
118. Bondeson L, Grimeluis L, DeLellis RA, Lloyd R, Akerstrom G, Larsson C, Arnold A, Eng C, Shane E, Bilezikian JP. Parathyroid carcinoma. In: DeLellis RA, Lloyd RV, Heitz PN, Eng C, editors. Pathology and genetics of tumours of endocrine organs (WHO classification). Lyon: IARC; 2004. p. 224–7.
119. Chiofalo MG, Scognamiglio F, Losito S, Lastoria S, Marone U, Pezzullo L. Huge parathyroid carcinoma: clinical considerations and literature review. World J Surg Oncol. 2005;3:39–45.
120. Temmim L, Sinowatz F, Hussein WI, Al-Sanea O, El-Khodary H. Intrathyroidal parathyroid carcinoma: a case report with clinical and histological findings. Diagn Pathol. 2008;3:46–51.
121. Delellis RA. Tumours of the parathyroid gland. Washington, DC: Armed Forces Institute of Pathology; 1993.
122. Reddick RL, Costa J, Marx SJ. Parathyroid hyperplasia and parathyromatosis. Lancet. 1977;1:549.
123. Levin K, Chew K, Ljung B, Mayall B, Siperstein A, Clark O. Deoxyribonucleic acid flow cytometry helps identify parathyroid carcinomas. J Clin Endocrinol Metab. 1988;67:779–84.
124. Guiter GE, DeLellis RA. Risk of recurrence or metastasis in atypical parathyroid adenoma. Mod Pathol. 2000;15:115.
125. Cavaco BM, Guerra L, Bradley KJ, Carvalho D, Harding B, Oliveira A, Santos MA, Sobrinho LG, Thakker RV, Leite V. Hyperparathyroidism-jaw tumor syndrome in Roma families from Portugal is due to a founder mutation of the HRPT2 gene. J Med Genet. 2004;89:1747–52.
126. De la Garza S, De la Garza E, Batres F. Functional parathyroid carcinoma: cytology, histology and ultrastructure of a case. Diag Cytopathol. 1985;1:232.
127. Holck S, Pedersen N. Carcinoma of the parathyroid gland. A light and electron microscopic study. Acta Pathol Microbiol Scand. 1981;89:297–302.
128. Jacobi J, Lloyd H, Smith J. Nuclear diameter in parathyroid carcinomas. J Clin Pathol. 1986;39:1353–4.
129. Lloyd H, Jacobi J, Cooke R. Nuclear diameter in parathyroid adenomas. J Clin Pathol. 1979;32:1278–81.
130. Obara T, Okamoto T, Kanbe M, Iihara M. Functioning parathyroid carcinoma: clinicopathologic features and rational treatment. Sem Surg Oncol. 1997;13:134–41.
131. Mallette LE. DNA quantization in the study of parathyroid lesions. A review. Am J Clin Pathol. 1992;98:305–11.
132. Lumachi F, Ermani M, Marino F, Poletti A, Basso SM, Iacobone M, Favia G. Relationship of AgNOR counts and nuclear DNA content to survival in patients with parathyroid carcinoma. Endocr Relat Cancer. 2004;11:563–9.
133. Dedeurwaerdere F, Van Damme B. Histopathology of the parathyroid glands. Acta Otorhinolaryngol Belg. 2001;55:95–101.
134. Stojadinovic A, Hoos A, Nissan A, Dudas ME, Cordon-Cardo C, Shaha AR, Brennan MF, Singh B, Ghossein RA. Parathyroid neoplasms: clinical, histological, and tissue microarray-based molecular analysis. Hum Pathol. 2003;34:54–64.
135. Abbona GC, Papotti M, Gasparri G, Bussolati G. Proliferative activity in parathyroid tumors as detected by KI-67 immunostaining. Hum Pathol. 1995;26:135–8.
136. Subramaniam P, Wilkinson S, Shepherd JJ. Inactivation of retinoblastoma gene in malignant parathyroid growths: a candidate genetic trigger? Aust NZ J Surg. 1995;65:714–6.
137. Farnebo F, Auer G, Farnebo LO, Teh BT, Twigg S, Aspenblad U, Thompson NW, Grimelius L, Larsson C, Sandelin K. Evaluation of retinoblastoma and Ki-67 immunostaining as diagnostic markers of benign and malignant parathyroid disease. World J Surg. 1999;23:68–74.
138. Erickson LA, Jin L, Wollan P, Thompson GB, van Heerden LA, Lloyd RV. Parathyroid hyperplasia, adenomas and carcinoma: differential expression of p27kip1 protein. Am J Surg Pathol. 1999;23:288–95.
139. TominagaY TT, Matsuoka S, Uno N, Sato T, Shimabukuro S, Goto N, Nagasaka T, Uchida K. Expression of parafibromin in distant metastatic parathyroid tumors in patients with advanced secondary hyperparathyroidism due to chronic kidney disease. World J Surg. 2008;32:815–21.
140. Juhlin CC, Haglund F, Villablanca A, Forsberg L, Sandelin K, Bränström R, Larsson C, Höög A. Loss of expression for the Wnt pathway components adenomatous polyposis coli and glycogen synthase kinase 3-beta in parathyroid carcinomas. Int J Oncol. 2009;34:481–92.
141. Kleinpeter KP, Lovato JF, Clark PB, Wooldridge T, Norman ES, Bergman S, Perrier ND. Is parathyroid carcinoma indeed a lethal disease? Ann Surg Oncol. 2005;12:260–6.
142. Shaha AR, Shah JP. Parathyroid carcinoma: a diagnostic and therapeutic challenge. Cancer. 1999;86: 378–80.

143. Obara T, Fujimoto Y. Diagnosis and treatment of patients with parathyroid carcinoma: an update and review. World J Surg. 1991;15:738–44.
144. Kameyama K, Takami H, Umemura S, Osamura YR, Wada N, Sugino K, Mimura T, Ito K. PCNA and Ki67 as prognostic markers in human parathyroid carcinomas. Ann Surg Oncol. 2000;7:301–4.
145. Schulte KM, Talat N, Miell J, Moniz C, Sinha P, Diaz-Cano S. Lymph node involvement and surgical approach in parathyroid cancer. World J Surg. 2010;34:2611–20.
146. Kebebew E. Parathyroid carcinoma. Curr Treat Options Oncol. 2001;2:347–54.
147. Solorzano CC, Carneiro-Pla DM, Lew JI, Rodgers SE, Montano R, Irvin 3rd GL. Intra-operative parathyroid hormone monitoring in patients with parathyroid cancer. Ann Surg Oncol. 2007;14:3216–22.
148. O'Neill CJ, Chan C, Symons J, Learoyd DL, Sidhu SB, Delbridge LW, Gill A, Sywak MS. Parathyroid carcinoma encountered after minimally invasive focused parathyroidectomy may not require further radical surgery. World J Surg. 2010;35(1):147–53.
149. Koyano H, Shishiba Y, Shimizu T, Suzuki N, Nakazawa H, Tachibana S, Murata H, Furui S. Successful treatment by surgical removal of bone metastasis producing PTH: new approach to the management of metastatic parathyroid carcinoma. Intern Med. 1994;33:697–702.
150. De Papp AE, Kinder B, LiVolsi V, Gupta SM, Stewart AF. Parathyroid carcinoma arising from parathyroid hyperplasia: autoinfarction following intravenous treatment with pamidronate. Am J Med. 1994;97:399–400.
151. Hurtado J, Esbrit P. Treatment of malignant hypercalcaemia. Expert Opin Pharmacother. 2002;3:521–7.
152. Major P, Lortholary A, Hon J, Abdi E, Mills G, Menssen HD, Yunus F, Bell R, Body J, Quebe-Fehling E, Seaman J. Zoledronic acid is superior to pamidronate in the treatment of hypercalcemia of malignancy: a pooled analysis of two randomized, controlled clinical trials. J Clin Oncol. 2001;19:558–67.
153. Lugassy G. Safety and convenience of a 15-minute infusion of zoledronic acid: not so safe. Oncologist. 2005;10:309–10.
154. Hughes TE, Hansen LA. Gallium nitrate. Ann Pharmacother. 1992;26:354–62.
155. Silverberg SJ, Rubin MR, Faiman C, Peacock M, Shoback DM, Smallridge RC, Schwanauer LE, Olson KA, Klassen P, Bilezikian JP. Cinacalcet hydrochloride reduces the serum calcium concentration in inoperable parathyroid carcinoma. J Clin Endocrinol Metab. 2007;92:3803–8.
156. Nemeth EF, SteffeyME HLG, Hung BC, Van Wagenen BC, DelMar EG, Balandrin MF. Calcimimetics with potent and selective activity on the parathyroid calcium receptor. Proc Natl Acad Sci USA. 1998;95:4040–5.
157. Collins MT, Skarulis MC, Bilezikian JP, Silverberg SJ, Spiegel AM, Marx SJ. Treatment of hypercalcemia secondary to parathyroid carcinoma with a novel calcimimetic agent. J Clin Endocrinol Metab. 1998;93:1083–8.
158. Pasieka JL, McEwan A, Rorstad O. The palliative role of 131I MIBG and 111In-octreotide in patients with metastatic parathyroid carcinoma. J Clin Endocrinol Metab. 2004;89:3413–20.
159. Betea D, Bradwell AR, Harvey TC, Mead GP, Schmidt-Gayk H, Ghaye B, Daly AF, Beckers A. Hormonal and biochemical normalization and tumor shrinkage induced by anti-parathyroid hormone immunotherapy in a in a patient with metastatic parathyroid carcinoma. J Clin Endocrinol Metab. 2004;89:3413–20.
160. Schott M, Feldkamp J, Schattenberg D, Krueger T, Dotzenrath C, Seissler J, Scherbaum WA. Induction of cellular immunity in a parathyroid carcinoma treated with tumor lysate-pulsed dendritic cells. Eur J Endocrinol. 2000;142:300–6.
161. Bradwell AR, Harvey TC. Control of hypercalcaemia of parathyroid carcinoma by immunisation. Lancet. 1999;353:370–3.
162. Shoback DM, Arends RH, Roskos L, Shetty S, Wyres M, Huang S, Raienbell GM. Treatment of parathyroid carcinoma with ABX10241, a monoclonal antibody to parathyroid hormone. J Bone Miner Res. 2004;17:SA498.
163. Calandra DB, Chejfec G, Foy BK, Lawrence AM, Paloyan E. Parathyroid carcinoma: biochemical and pathologic response to DTIC. Surgery. 1984;96:1132–7.
164. Bukowski RM, Sheeler L, Cunningham J, Esselstyn C. Successful combination chemotherapy for metastatic parathyroid carcinoma. Arch Intern Med. 1984;144:399–400.
165. Munson ND, Foote RL, Northcutt RC, Tiegs RD, Fitzpatrick LA, Grant CS, van Heerden JA, Thompson GB, Lloyd RV. Parathyroid carcinoma: is there a role for adjuvant radiation therapy? Cancer. 2003;98:2378–84.

9 Biochemistry, Physiology, and Pathophysiology of Parathyroid Hormone-Related Peptide

Bandana Chakravarti, Shailendra K. Dhar Dwivedi, Ambrish Mithal, and Naibedya Chattopadhyay

Abstract

Parathyroid hormone-related peptide (PTHrP) was originally discovered as a systemic humoral factor released by tumor cells that were responsible for humoral hypercalcemia of malignancy. Parathyroid hormone (PTH) and PTHrP are distinct polypeptides having sequence similarity at short N-terminal region. Nascent PTHrP isoforms undergo posttranslational endoproteolytic cleavage and generates three translational products: mature N-terminal, mid-region, and C-terminal secretory forms of PTHrP, each of them having their own physiologic functions and probably their own receptors. Both PTH (1–34) and PTHrP (1–36) bind to the type 1 PTH receptor. This chapter describes various aspects of PTHrP biochemistry, physiology, and pathophysiology. PTHrP plays an important role as a regulator of cell growth, differentiation, and cell death. PTHrP has been shown to regulate branching morphogenesis of mammary gland, fetus-directed transport of maternal calcium across the placental membrane, vascular smooth muscle relaxation and chondrocyte growth and differentiation, and as a regulator of pancreatic beta cell growth and functions. On the pathophysiological side, PTHrP is produced by virtually all tumor types that metastasize to bone such as breast cancer, prostate cancer, lung cancer, and hematological malignancy. The complex regulation of PTHrP gene promoter is beginning to be understood in the context of activation of certain signaling pathways involved in the growth and progression of specific neoplasms. In addition, factors that modulate the entire PTHrP transcriptional unit, as well as the stability of the mRNA, are being

B. Chakravarti, MSc (✉) • S.K.D. Dwivedi, MSc
• N. Chattopadhyay, PhD
Department of Endocrinology, Central Drug Research Institute, Lucknow, Uttar Pradesh, India
e-mail: vandanaks@gmail.com; n_chattopadhyay@cdri.res.in

A. Mithal, MD, DM
Department of Endocrinology and Diabetes, Medanta, The Medicity, Gurgaon, Haryana, India

A.A. Licata and E.V. Lerma (eds.), *Diseases of the Parathyroid Glands*,
DOI 10.1007/978-1-4419-5550-0_9, © Springer Science+Business Media, LLC 2012

elucidated. Finally, strategies to antagonize PTHrP signaling hold therapeutic promise to limit the osteolytic potential of tumors which metastasize to bone.

Keywords
Parathyroid hormone-related peptide • Humoral hypercalcemia syndrome • Posttranslational • Endoproteolytic cleavage • Parathyroid hormone • Osteolytic • Hypercalcemia • Hypophosphatemia • Bone resorption • Nephrogenous cAMP • Proximal nephron • Type I PTH receptor • PTHrP gene • Chromosome 12p11 • PTH gene • Chromosome 11p15 • Preprohormone • Osteoblasts • c-fos protein • Phopholipase C • Inositol triphosphate • Diacylglycerol • Mitogen-activated protein kinase • Physiology • Autocrine • Paracrine • Morphogenesis • Differentiation • Pregnancy • Placental • Trophoblast • Lactating • Estradiol • Mesenchymal cells • Keratinocytes • BMP4 signaling • Cartilage • Growth plate • Chrondrocyte • Endochrondral ossification • Jansen's metaphyseal chrondrodysplasia • Blomstrand osteochondroplasia • Eiken syndrome • Indian hedgehog feedback loop • Canonical BMP pathway • Cardiovascular system • Vascular smooth muscle cell • Dibutyryl cAMP • Forskolin • Platelet-derived growth factor • Myocyte • Chronotropic effect • Pancreatic islets • Hyperinsulinemia • Uncoupling • Histomorphometry • Breast cancer • Immunoreactivity • PTHrP isoforms • Transforming growth factor beta • Calcium-sensing receptor • Connective tissue growth factor • Prostate cancer • Interleukin 1 • Interleukin 6 • Multiple myeloma • Lung cancer • Squamous cell • Adenocarcinoma • Small cell cancer • Renal cancer • Ectopic PTH • Neuroendocrine tumor • Medullary thyroid cancer • 1,25 Dihydroxy vitamin D3 • Vitamin D response element • Retinoid-X-receptor • Glucocorticoids • Leydig cell tumors • Tamoxifen • Medroxyprogesterone

Introduction

It was recognized for many years that hypercalcemia, hypophosphatemia, and increased bone resorption in patients were associated with a variety of solid malignancies. In 1941, Fuller Albright advanced the hypothesis that parathyroid hormone (PTH) is ectopically produced by certain tumor types. However, the altered biochemical profiles observed in malignancies were associated with suppressed, rather than elevated, circulating levels of PTH, ruling out ectopic production of PTH as the disease etiology. Surprisingly, despite suppressed PTH levels in serum, such patients exhibited elevated excretion of nephrogenous cAMP, whose production was determined by PTH receptor activation in the proximal nephron. Pursuing these clues eventually led to the discovery of parathyroid hormone-related peptide (PTHrP), when it was simultaneously purified from human lung cancer [1], breast cancer [2], and renal cell carcinoma [3] by several independent groups and cloned shortly thereafter [4]. Subsequently, it was understood that elevated levels of PTHrP secreted by these tumors produced a humoral syndrome resembling primary hyperparathyroidism (1^0HPT). It also became apparent that the mechanism of action of PTHrP involved its ability to activate the type I PTH receptor (PTHR1), presumably due to similarity in the structures of PTH and PTHrP. Although

PTHrP was discovered as tumor-derived factor, intense research for little over two decades has also established a number of physiological roles of PTHrP both during development and adult life. This chapter aims to explain in detail the biochemistry, physiology, and pathophysiological aspects of PTHrP.

Biochemical Features of PTHrP

PTH and PTHrP are distinct polypeptides having 15% overall sequence homology between them [5, 6]. While PTH is a key regulator of systemic calcium homeostasis, PTHrP was originally discovered as a systemic humoral factor that is released by tumor cells that caused humoral hypercalcemia of malignancy (HHM) [4, 7–9]. In humans, PTHrP gene is located on chromosome 12p11, whereas the gene encoding PTH is in an analogous region on chromosome 11p15. The human PTHrP gene is much larger and more complex than the PTH gene, spanning 15 kb of genomic DNA and having nine exons [10]. The 5′-end of the PTHrP gene contains transcriptional regulation sites consisting of three distinct promoters identified as P1, P2, and P3, respectively [11–15]. Exons 1, 2, 3, and 4 encode the 5′-untranslated regions in the mature PTHrP mRNA; exon 5 encodes for the "prepro" region of the protein; and the exon 6 product contributes to the majority of the coding region. The 3′-end of the gene contains three exons (7, 8, and 9) that may be alternatively spliced to encode carboxyl termini of three distinct mature PTHrP-protein isoforms that are 139, 141, and 173 amino acids in length [4, 12, 16, 17]. In addition, nascent PTHrP isoforms undergo posttranslational processing by members of the prohormone convertase family to at least three fragments: N-terminal PTHrP(1–36), exhibiting PTH-like properties; a mid-region PTHrP(38–94); and a C-terminal PTHrP(107–139)[18]. The midregion domain of PTHrP contains a bipartite nuclear localization sequence (NLS) [residues 61–94 that reside at the junction of the proximal two thirds and distal one third of the molecule] and this sequence allows nuclear import of PTHrP and binding to RNA similar to the NLS in viral and mammalian transcription factors [19]. Subsequent studies revealed that phosphorylation of PTHrP at Thr85 by the cyclin-dependent kinases p33cdk2 and p34cdc2 regulates the nuclear import of PTHrP with the participation of the saturable transport receptor importin-β [20]. The C-terminal domain, also called osteostatin, is able to inhibit bone resorption and, thereby, antagonizes the action of the N-terminal domain of PTHrP [21].

Signaling Aspects of PTHrP

PTHrP shares 70% sequence homology with PTH over the first 13 amino acids at the N terminus, which allows PTHrP to bind to and activate the same PTH receptor (PTHR1) to which PTH binds [22, 23]. PTHR1 is abundantly expressed in osteoblasts in bone and renal tubular cells in kidney; however, low levels of expression of PTHR1 is reported in almost every tissue/cell type studied [24]. While the source of PTH is the parathyroid glands, PTHrP expression was found to be ubiquitous. PTHR1 is a Class II GPCR and is encoded by a multiexonic gene with potential for alternate splicing and promoter usage that was characterized in human, rat, and mouse [25]. In humans, the PTHR1 gene is located on chromosome 3 and the gene involved in its synthesis has a total of 14 exons. The biologically active NH_2-terminal region of PTH (1–34) and PTHrP (1–34) interacts with the J-domain, the functional portion of PTHR1 that contains the 7 TM domains and the connecting loops [26, 27] The C terminal of PTH and PTHrP binds to the extracellular N-domain of PTHR1 promoting association of the NH_2 terminal of the ligand to J-domain [27].

The PTHR1 couples to G_s, G_i, $G_{q/11}$, and $G_{12/13}$ proteins, which subsequently regulate intracellular effectors such as adenylate cyclase, phospholipases, and mitogen-activated protein kinases (MAPK) [28–32]. Activation of Gs pathway following ligand binding to PTHR1 elicits adenylate cyclase (AC) cascade leading to the activation of protein kinase A (PKA) and phosphorylation of the cyclic AMP response element binding (CREB) protein [33–36]. Downstream from this, CREB

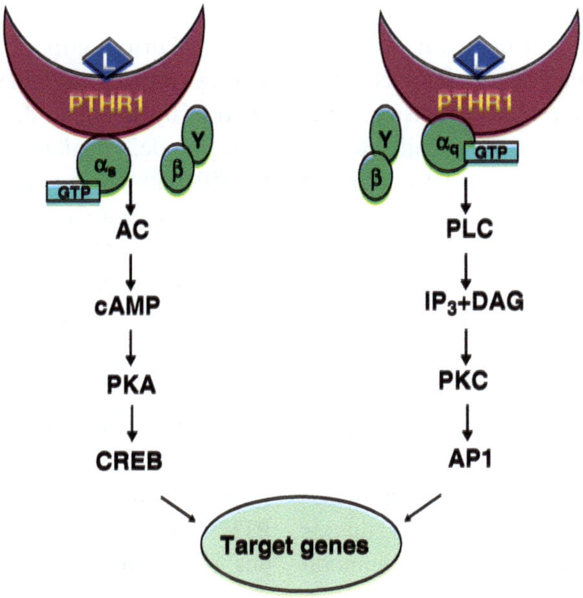

Fig. 9.1 Schematic diagram to illustrate major signaling events that are elicited by PTHrP via the activation of PTHR1. *Left side* shows activation of G_s pathway following ligand binding to PTH1R triggering adenylate cyclase (AC) cascade leading to the activation of PKA, phosphorylation of the CREB and activation of target genes. *Right side* shows activation of Gq pathway following ligand binding to PTH1R and stimulation of phospholipase C (PLC) cascade. Stimulation of the PLC signaling cascade leads to the accumulation of inositol trisphosphate (IP_3) and diacylglycerol (DAG). DAG activates protein kinase C (PKC) pathway and IP_3 induces rise in cytosolic Ca^{2+} via the activation of PLC pathway, and subsequent activation of various genomic effects through transcription factors (c-fos, c-jun, and AP1) regulated by the calcium and PKC

binds to the cAMP response element (CRE) in the promoter region of target genes including the c-fos and induces its expression [37]. Reports from various in vitro and in vivo studies have suggested that c-fos is a key mediator of PTH and PTHrP actions in development [38]. The FOS protein is a member of the AP-1 transcription factor that binds to the promoter region of various target genes [39]. The AP-1 protein is a heterogeneous transcription factor composed of a dimer of Jun (c-Jun, JunB, and JunD) and Fos (c-Fos, FosB, Fra-1, and Fra-2) family members [40]. All the FOS family members are upregulated in response to PTH and PTHrP, but only the JunB member of the JUN family is upregulated [41]. The Jun and Fos family members interact through leucine zipper motifs and bind DNA through a basic region [42]. There are wide array of genes important in bone and hematopoiesis that have AP-1 sites in their promoters and hence could be targets of PTHrP action in the bone microenvironment [43].

Activation of G_q pathway following ligand binding to PTHR1 stimulates phospholipase C (PLC) cascade [34]. Stimulation of the PLC signaling cascade leads to the accumulation of inositol trisphosphate (IP_3) and diacylglycerol (DAG). Protein kinase C (PKC) may be activated in response to DAG and IP_3-stimulated increased cytosolic calcium generated via PLC, resulting in subsequent activation of various genomic effects through transcription factors regulated by the calcium and PKC. Activation of both PKA and PLC pathways then trigger distinct as well as overlapping members of MAPK that finally culminate in transcription of PTH/PTHrP target genes (Fig. 9.1). Although ligand-induced PTHR1 activation could trigger both PKA and PLC pathways, however, agonist efficacy and potency profiles observed in assays of the PLC/PKC pathway were generally lower than those of the AC/PKA pathway [44]. In other words, activation of PLC pathway requires higher ligand concentration than PKA pathway. Since PTH concentrations in plasma are in subnanomolar range, locally produced PTHrP at higher concentrations such as in the developing growth plate [26] is a physiologically relevant scenario for the activation of PLC pathway via the PTHR1. At present, the non-adenylyl cyclase-mediated pathways appear more complex than the AC/PKA pathway and may involve multiple phospholipase isoforms (e.g., PLD and PLC), and be sensitive to variations in cell type, receptor density, and receptor species derivation (28, 103, 104). Signaling of the PTHR1 is also modified by scaffolding proteins such as the Na+/H+ exchanger regulatory factor (NHERF) 1 and 2 through PDZ1 and PDZ2 domains [45, 46].

Like many other GPCRs, PTHR1 goes through cyclical receptor activation, desensitization, and internalization [47]. After ligand binding, PTHR1 is endocytosed and then either recycled to the cell membrane or targeted for degradation. G protein-coupled receptor kinases (GRK) upon phosphorylation by the ligand binding prepares PTHR1 for arrestin binding that contributes to the desentization of both Gs and Gq-mediated PTHR1 signaling [48].

Physiological Roles of PTHrP

Normal individuals do not have detectable circulating levels of PTHrP, suggesting that under physiological condition PTHrP acts as a local regulator in the tissues where it is produced [49]. The extensive distribution of the PTH/PTHrP receptor in nonclassical PTH target tissues (outside bone and kidney) further supports autocrine/paracrine mode of action of PTHrP [20]. By these mechanisms, PTHrP has been shown to regulate chondrocyte growth and differentiation, branching morphogenesis of mammary gland, vascular smooth muscle relaxation, and fetus-directed transport of maternal calcium across the placental membrane [50]. Table 9.1 summarizes various physiological functions of PTHrP.

Table 9.1 Normal physiological functions of PTHrP in different organ systems

Organ	Role of PTHrP	References
Pregnancy and lactation	Midregion of PTHrP interacts with a yet unidentified receptor to maintain maternofetal calcium transport. Regulate trophoblast differentiation and placenta formation. PTHrP act as a calciotropic hormone during lactation.	[57] [58] [59] [60]
Mammary gland	PTHrP and the PTH1R are required for normal mammary gland development. PTHrP interact with BMP signaling and initiates ductal branching and morphogenesis.	[64] [66] [69]
Cartilage	Important autocrine/paracrine factor for chondrocyte metabolism. PTHrP-Ihh feedback loop regulates chondrocytes proliferation and differentiation. The Ihh/PTHrP pathway acts cooperatively with canonical BMP pathway.	[82] [83] [87]
Cardiovascular system	PTHrP is expressed in blood vessels from a variety of vascular beds. On smooth muscle cells, PTH and PTHrP reduce the influence of extracellular calcium, through cAMP-dependent mechanisms. PTHrP production is stimulated by vasoconstrictor agents such as angiotensin II, by mechanical stretching of arterial smooth muscle. PTHrP in the control of vascular tone by acting as a potent vasodilator and hypotensive factor. PTHrP is an inhibitor of vascular smooth muscle cell (VSMC) proliferation. PTHrP, but not PTH, was found to exert positive inotropic effects.	[88] [95] [97, 98] [96] [100] [107]
Pancreatic islets	Normal islets express PTHR1 and PTHrP induces intracellular calcium response in these cells. RIP-PTHrP mice displayed islet cell hyperplasia, significant hypoglycemia.	[108, 110] [111]

Role of PTHrP in Pregnancy and Lactation

During pregnancy, more than 20 g of calcium is transported from the maternal to fetal site through the placenta [51, 52]. Free and rapid transplacental Ca^{2+} transport occurs in which PTH and 1,25(OH)-vitamin D make relatively minor contributions. This active transport of Ca^{2+} across placenta is stimulated by locally (amniotic epithelial cells and trophoblasts) produced PTHrP (1–141) and the midmolecule fragment of PTHrP (67–86), but not by PTHrP (1–34), suggesting that PTHrP stimulates receptor/s distinct from PTHR1. PTHrP derived from the fetal parathyroids is also critical for the maintenance of the active placental calcium gradient, as demonstrated in thyroparathyroidectomy experiments in fetal lambs [53, 54] and decapitation studies on fetal rats [55]. In another model in which cervical dislocation was made in fetal rats to create parathyroidectomy, PTH(1–34) failed to have an effect on placental calcium transport [55, 56]. In addition to the well-studied effect of PTHrP in maternofetal calcium transport, PTHrP appears to play important role in trophoblast differentiation and placenta formation via its differentiation inducing effect on trophoblast giant cells [57–59]. Further, role of PTHrP in early placental function and fetal growth during midgestation has been demonstrated in rats.

Lactating breast is another major site of production of PTHrP and lactation appears to be the only physiological state in which PTHrP acts as a hormone [60]. Increased circulating PTHrP during lactation is coupled with low estradiol resulting in dramatic increase in maternal bone turnover allowing large movements of calcium from maternal skeleton to milk. As a result, lactating women frequently have postpartum osteoporosis and mild hypercalcemia, which is usually self-limiting and resolves gradually after weaning. In mouse, the mammary gland has been shown to become a calcium-"sensing" organ during lactation by robustly upregulating the expression of calcium-sensing receptor (CaSR), a GPCR [61]. CaSR resides in the basolateral side of the luminal epithelial cells of the mammary ducts, and CaSR activation decreases PTHrP secretion [62]. In this respect, the lactating breast resembles the parathyroid gland and appears to act to provide an optimal level of calcium for transport into milk.

Role of PTHrP in Mammary Gland Development

Both PTHrP and the PTHR1 are required for normal mammary gland development. In the absence of PTHrP or its receptor in mice, loss of PTHR1 function in humans results in the absence of mammary gland [63–66]. Mammary epithelial cells express PTHrP as early as the placode stage and the PTHR1 is expressed on immature mesenchymal cells located beneath the embryonic epidermis. During bud formation, PTHrP from the epithelium communicates with the surrounding mesenchyme that leads to the formation of the specialized dense mammary mesenchyme [67]. In response to PTHrP, these mesenchymal cells carry the mammary fate of the epithelial cells, induce the overlying epidermis to form the nipple sheath, and initiate ductal branching and morphogenesis. Disruption of PTHrP signaling causes differentiation of mammary epithelial cells into skin, resulting in the absence of nipple formation and interruption of morphogenesis. Conversely, overexpression of PTHrP in basal keratinocytes using the keratin 14 promoter in mice leads to the conversion of the ventral dermis into condensed mammary mesenchyme with nipple-like characteristics and the suppression of hair follicle development [68]. Regulation of ductal morphogenesis is critically dependent on BMP4-BMPR1a (BMP) signaling in variety of tissues including salivary glands, lung, kidneys, ureter, and prostate. In the embryonic mammary mesenchyme, PTHrP interacts with BMP signaling and initiates ductal morphogenesis [63]. PTHrP released from the bud epithelial cells upregulates the expression of BMPR1a on the mesenchymal cells which facilitates BMP4 signaling, the net effect of which appears to be reduced formation of hair follicles around the primary mammary duct and induction of ductal branching morphogenesis [69].

Role of PTHrP in Cartilage Development

The cartilage growth plate is a highly specialized skeletal structure, essential for bone growth and development. Exact coordination of growth plate chondrocyte proliferation is necessary for normal endochondral bone development and growth. During limb development, a cartilaginous template is formed from mesenchymal condensations that perform the skeletal elements [70]. Subsequent longitudinal bone growth is dependent upon the process of endochondral ossification whereby chondrocytes sequentially proliferate and differentiate. Chondrocyte differentiation is marked by profound physical and biochemical changes, including a 5–10-fold increase in volume and expression of alkaline phosphatase and type X collagen [71, 72]. The process of chondrocyte differentiation culminates in calcification of the matrix and cellular apoptosis [73, 74]. The calcified matrix subsequently serves as the template for primary bone formation.

PTHrP and its receptor are the major players in the dynamics of the growth plate, where transition from pristine cartilage to advancing bone takes place. The crucial role of PTHrP in skeletal development has recently been emphasized by gene deletion experiments in mice and by a natural mutation in humans. PTHrP-*null* mice exhibit skeletal deformities that are due to a decrease in proliferation and the accelerated differentiation of chondrocytes in the developing skeleton [75, 76]. As a result, these mice die prematurely due to small and inappropriately mineralized rib cage. In contrast, mice overexpressing PTHrP exhibit delay in chondrocyte terminal differentiation [77]. At the other end of the spectrum, striking skeletal deformities are observed in Jansen's metaphyseal chondrodysplasia, a human form of shortlimbed dwarfism with delayed endochondral maturation [78] due to ligand-independent constitutively activating mutation of PTHR1. In contrast to Jansen's metaphyseal chondrodysplasia, inactivating mutations in PTHR1 cause Blomstrand lethal osteochondrodysplasia (BOCD) [79]. This rare dysplasia is characterized by advanced skeletal maturation and premature ossification of the skeleton [80]. The phenotype of BOCD closely resembles the malformations reported in PTHR1-*null* mice [79]. In addition, recessive mutations have been described in Eiken syndrome where truncation mutation in the C-terminal tail of the PTHR1gene is responsible for this syndrome. Eiken syndrome is a rare familial skeletal dysplasia characterized by multiple epiphyseal dysplasia with extremely retarded ossification, principally of the epiphyses, pelvis, hands and feet, as well as by abnormal modeling of the bones in hands and feet, abnormal persistence of cartilage in the pelvis and mild growth retardation [81].

Each end of a long bone has a growth zone that is comprised of chondrocytes that move through a sequence of differentiation program (round–flat–prehypertrophic–hypertrophic) that is regulated by the PTHrP-Indian hedgehog (Ihh) feedback loop [82]. The physiological balance between these two factors regulates chondrocytes proliferation and differentiation [83]. It should be noted, that the perichondrial cells produce PTHrP, but PTHR1 is expressed particularly in the prehypertrophic cells and the lower proliferating zone, suggesting paracrine mode of action of PTHrP [18]. By this mechanism, PTHrP acts on chondrocytes to keep the chondrocytes proliferating and to delay the differentiation of the chondrocytes into prehypertrophic and hypertrophic chondrocytes [84, 85]. After chondrocytes stop proliferating, they then produce the secreted factor, Ihh. Ihh synthesis begins throughout mesenchymal condensation, increases during cartilage formation and later decreases [86]. Loss of Ihh leads to premature hypertrophy, growth plate disorganization, and reduced population of osteoblasts at endochondral sites. Ihh acts to increase the synthesis of PTHrP, to accelerate the differentiation of round proliferative chondrocytes into flat proliferating chondrocytes, to increase the rate of proliferation of adjacent chondrocytes, and to direct perichondrial cells to differentiate into osteoblasts. By stimulating the differentiation of the flat proliferating chondrocytes that form columns that extend in the longitudinal axis of long bones, Ihh acts to reinforce the asymmetry of bone growth in the long bones. Interestingly, this action of Ihh is not required during intramembranous bone formation in the skull [84]. The Ihh/PTHrP pathway acts cooperatively with canonical BMP pathway involving the functionally redundant receptor Smads 1 and 5, which in turn can directly activate the Ihh promoter [87].

Role of PTHrP in Cardiovascular System

PTHrP is expressed in blood vessels from a variety of vascular beds, including rat aorta, vena cava, kidney microvessels, and arterial and venous supplies of the mammary gland. The expression of PTHrP in the blood vessels has been localized in the smooth muscle cells and endothelial cells [88, 89]. Exogenous application of synthetic PTHrP peptides exert relaxant activity on both conductance and resistance vessels from different species [90, 91]. On smooth muscle cells, PTH and PTHrP reduce the influence of extracellular calcium, through cAMP-dependent mechanisms [92–94]. These inhibitory effects on voltage-dependent L-type calcium channels of smooth muscle cells cause vasorelaxation [95, 96]. Cultured arterial vascular smooth muscle cells (VSMCs) express both PTHrP and PTHR1. In addition, PTHrP production by cultured VSMCs is stimulated by vasoconstrictor agents such as angiotensin II [97], by mechanical stretching of arterial smooth muscle [98], and by the induction of hypertension with mineralocorticoids, suggesting the presence of a short feedback loop through which the local vasorelaxant actions of PTHrP function to counter pressor (excitation/contraction coupling) activity of angiotensin II and other vasoconstrictor agents [99, 100]. In addition, targeted overexpression of either PTHrP or PTHR1 in vascular smooth muscle of transgenic mice leads to arterial hypotension, probably through sustained activation of the receptor by endogenous ligand [101]. Collectively, these reports support a role for PTHrP in the control of vascular tone by acting as a potent vasodilator and hypotensive factor.

PTHrP is an inhibitor of VSMC proliferation, and that PTHrP acts in smooth muscle via the cell surface PTH/PTHrP receptor. The aortic VSMC proliferation rate in the PTHrP null mouse is markedly lower than that in aortic VSMC from wild-type mouse [102]. The antimitogenic effect requires N-terminal portion of PTHrP and could be mimicked by dibutyryl cAMP or forskolin, suggesting requirement of PKA pathway. The downstream events involved in the antimitogenic effect include induction of cyclin-dependent kinase inhibitor (p27kip1), with consequent inhibition of retinoblastoma (Rb) phosphorylation, which result in G1 cell cycle arrest. PTHrP also inhibits platelet-derived growth factor (PDGF)-directed proliferation and migration of VSMC [18]. The effects of PTHrP on VSMC proliferation and migration in vitro are likely to be relevant to conditions under which these VSMC functions are affected in vivo, for example, during the development of cardiovascular system [18]. In this regard, NLS composed of multibasic amino acids in the 88–106 region of PTHrP was found to promote proliferation of VSMC [103]. These set of reports suggest that nuclear-targeted PTHrP may participate in the normal proliferation and development of the arterial wall in embryonic life [104]. As PTHrP is upregulated in the media and neointima of angioplastied and diseased arteries and local delivery of PTHrP devoid of NLS to the arterial wall at the time of angioplasty might prevent neointimal hyperplasia, the NLS-deleted form, may have therapeutic benefit in disorders associated with arterial smooth muscle cell proliferation, migration, and matrix secretion [104].

PTHrP, but not PTH, was found to exert positive inotropic effects on the heart by virtue of its influence on coronary flow and heart rate, but not by any direct effect on contractile elements in the heart [105]. PTHrP is released from coronary endothelium under hypoxia and energy-depleting conditions, which then results in positive contractile and positive lusitropic effect on adult ventricular cardiomyocytes thus suggesting that PTHrP influences vascular and contractile function of the heart during an early phase of reperfusion [106]. PTHrP is also produced in the cardiac myocyte and its release is stimulated by mechanical forces like stretch [107]. PTHrP has positive chronotropic effect in heart by influencing conductance properties of pacemaker cells of heart [107].

Role of PTHrP in Pancreatic Islets

Pancreatic islets produce PTHrP under normal circumstances as well as in adenoma and carcinoma. Normal islets express PTHR1 and PTHrP induces intracellular calcium response in these cells. The effect of PTHrP in pancreatic cells was studied in a transgenic mouse having PTHrP fused in rat insulin promoter (RIP-PTHrP) [108, 109]. These mice displayed islet cell hyperplasia, significant hypoglycemia under both fasting and nonfasting conditions, as well as inappropriate hyperinsulinemia. The increase in beta cell mass in these mice was not due to increased rate of proliferation [109] but appeared to be due to reduced apoptosis [110]. Insulin expression was shown to be upregulated both at the messenger RNA and protein level in whole pancreas of RIP-PTHrP mice [111]. These findings suggest that PTHrP may be useful as gene therapeutic strategies for increasing beta cell mass and function. Specifically, PTHrP could prove to be valuable in improving islet transplant survival in type 1 diabetes. This area merits further study.

Pathophysiological Role of PTHrP

Hypercalcemia is as a state in which serum calcium concentrations are greater than 12 mg/dl, corrected for serum albumin concentration [112, 113]. As already described, PTHrP is undetectable in serum of normal human being except during pregnancy and lactation [114]. Generally, hypercalcemia associated with increased serum PTHrP in lactating women is mild and reversible after weaning. However, the incidence of increased plasma concentrations of PTHrP is high in patients with solid tumors. One estimate is that approximately 80% of hypercalcemic patients with solid tumors have detectable or elevated circulating PTHrP levels [2, 115, 116]. In addition to mediating hypercalcemia, PTHrP promotes osteolytic bone metastasis, regulating growth of cancer cells and acting as survival factor for cancer cells [49, 117–120]. Despite similarities between the syndromes of HHM and primary hyperparathyroidism (1^0HPT) and the similar biological actions of PTHrP and PTH respectively, unexplained differences between these syndromes have been observed. First, patients with PTHrP-mediated HHM have low 1,25 $(OH)_2$ vitamin D_3 levels compared with patients with 1^0HPT, when both hormones stimulate 1α-hydroxylase activity [113, 121]. Secondly, while both syndromes have marked increases in osteoclastic bone resorption, many patients with HHM do not have the physiologically coupled increase in osteoblastic activity that is observed in the setting of 1^0HPT. Studies using either serum markers of bone turnover [122] or quantitative bone histomorphometry [123] have demonstrated uncoupling of bone resorption from bone formation in HHM patients. Finally, unlike the metabolic acidosis observed in patients with 1^0HPT, HHM patients often have a metabolic alkalosis apparent from a low plasma chloride and high plasma bicarbonate concentration. Some explanations exist for the discrepancies between HHM and 1^0HPT, such as the pulsatile secretion of PTH versus the apparent continuous secretion of PTHrP, circulating levels of biologically active PTHrP fragment [124] and, suppression of bone formation and 1α-hydroxylase activity by other tumor-derived factors. However, further elucidation for the differences between HHM and 1^0HPT is required.

PTHrP and Breast Cancer

The association of hypercalcemia with women in breast cancer is strong and is presented with extensive osteolytic lesions [49]. PTHrP expression by primary breast cancer is more commonly associated with the development of bone metastasis and hypercalcemia [116]. Reports from several studies indicate expression of PTHrP in tumor cells of approximately 60% of the invasive tumors [125–128]. Further, by immunohistochemistry PTHrP was localized in 92% of breast cancer metastases in bone but only 17% of metastases in nonbone sites, suggesting high affinity for PTHrP expressing tumors to bone [43, 128–130]. A recent study showed immunoreactive PTHrP in 68% of early breast cancer samples compared with 100% of bone metastases [131]. Expression of immunoreactive PTHrP is generally considered to be inversely correlated with tumor stage and extent of nodal involvement at the time of diagnosis although contrary report of PTHrP as an indicator of improved prognosis of breast cancer is available [132]. Use of different antibodies against PTHrP (whole peptide versus 1–34) could explain differing results among studies. In addition, a prospective clinical study has shown that PTHrP expression by primary breast cancer cells correlates with decreased metastasis to bone, suggesting different roles for this factor at primary and metastatic sites [133, 134].

When differential expression of PTHrP isoforms was studied in different stages of breast cancer, the levels of the 1–139 isoform mRNA was found to be much higher in the tumors of patients who later developed metastases than in those of patients who developed no metastases [135]. This isoform was also more abundant in breast cancer patients who developed bone metastases than in those of patients who developed metastases in soft tissues. By contrast, the levels of the 1–141 isoform mRNA in these three groups of tumors were similar. These findings suggest that 1-139 isoform of PTHrP could be specifically involved in metastases of breast tumors to bone [136].

Growth of metastatic cancer in bone is dependent on the interaction of tumor cells with the resident cells of the bone microenvironment [137]. Production of PTHrP by the cancer cell in the bone microenvironment stimulates the cells of the osteoblast lineage which express PTHR1. Activation of PTHR1 potently stimulates production of a potent osteoclastogenic cytokine, RANK-ligand by osteoblasts [20]. This sets in motion the natural bone resorptive process that lead to the formation of active bone-resorbing osteoclast. As a result of osteoclast-mediated destruction of the mineral and protein components of bone, growth factors stored in matrix are released. These factors stimulate survival and proliferation of cancer cells at sites of bone metastasis, which becomes a fertile environment for further growth of the tumor cells. Thus a vicious cycle results where bone resorption, initially stimulated by the metastatic cancer cells, then results in increased tumor growth and further destruction of bone [10].

One of the most abundant growth factors in bone matrix is TGFβ. TGFβ has been demonstrated to enhance metastasis and bone destruction via PTHrP in human ER negative breast cancer cells [138, 139]. However, TGFβ also stimulates the production of other osteolytic factors including interleukin-11 and VEGF by breast cancer cells [140, 141]. It is interesting that the effect of TGFβ on tumor cells to stimulate PTHrP may result in adverse effects only when tumor cells are localized in bone rather than in soft tissue sites [139]. In addition to TGFβ, high levels of extracellular Ca^{2+} are produced at the metastatic sites of the tumor due to bone resorptive action. CaSR expressed in human breast cancer cells has been shown to be stimulated by elevated extracellular Ca^{2+} and pharmacological agonists of CaSR resulting in increased synthesis and secretion of PTHrP [142, 143]. Furthermore, high extracellular Ca^{2+} has been shown to synergize the action of TGFβ in stimulating PTHrP release by human breast cancer cells, suggesting a cooperative of Ca^{2+} and TGFβ in generating a vicious cycle of tumor-induced bone resorption, begetting further bone resorption in the setting of skeletal metastases of breast cancers (Fig. 9.2) [20]. Any chemotherapeutic measure directed at suppressing the vicious cycle could be effective for interrupting malignant progression in bone. In this regard, blocking PTHrP action could be valuable therapy for tumor bone metastasis. It is intriguing that activating the CaSR in primary mammary epithelial cells suppresses PTHrP secretion which is opposite to the stimulatory effect of CaSR on PTHrP secretion in breast cancer cells. The opposite effect of extracellular calcium on PTHrP secretion in normal versus transformed breast cells is the result of opposing effects on AC activity associated with alternative G-protein usage as the CaSR couples to $G_{\alpha i}$ while in MCF-7 cells it couples to $G_{\alpha s}$ [144].

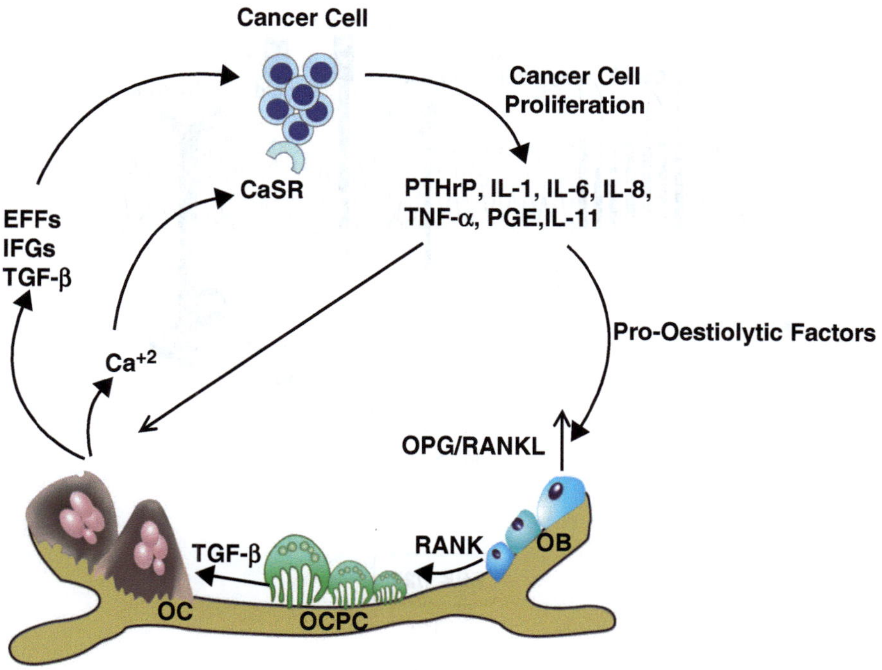

Fig. 9.2 PTHrP and the vicious cycle of bone metastasis. Tumor cells secrete PTHrP, IL-1, IL-6, IL-8, IL-11, TNFα, and PGE which stimulates bone resorption via RANKL expression in osteoblastic cells. Bone resorption results in release of growth factors including TGFβ, EGF, IGF, and calcium from the extracellular matrix. Calcium and growth factors both feedback to tumor cells to enhance PTHrP production. This unique interaction amplifies favorable signals for tumor localization to bone. *IL* interleukin, *TNF* tumor necrosis factor, *RANKL* receptor activator of nuclear factor kappa B ligand, *TGF* transforming growth factor, *EGF* epidermal growth factor, *IGF* insulin-like growth factor, OC-osteoclast, OB-osteoblast, OCPC-osteoclast progenitor cells

Connective tissue growth factor (CCN2) is a mediator of local angiogenesis induced by breast cancer. CCN2 was found to localize with TGFβ and PTHrP in breast cancer cells metastasized to bone. PTHrP was found to increase CCN2 levels via the PKC and PKA pathways [133]. Neutralizing CCN2 by a neutralizing antibody inhibited the extent of osteolytic metastasis of ER-negative human tumor cells [145]. In addition, CCN2 inhibited osteoclastogenesis. Together, these findings suggest that PTHrP also mediates metastasis and osteolysis via CCN2.

PTHrP and Prostate Cancer

In the prostate gland, the physiological role of PTHrP is unknown. However, evidence that there is higher PTHrP expression in prostatic dysplasia (prostate intraepithelial neoplasia) than in normal prostate epithelium and higher PTHrP expression in prostate carcinoma than in benign prostatic hyperplasia suggests that PTHrP participates in the pathophysiology of prostate cancer [146–149]. PTHrP has been shown to promote growth of androgen receptor-negative human prostate cancer cells, PC-3, which expresses functional PTHR1. Also, the level of PTHrP expression is higher in prostate cancer than in normal prostate tissue and that PC-3 cells secrete a significantly higher amount of PTHrP (1–34) than do the androgen receptor positive, LNCaP prostate cancer cell line [150]. Since PTHrP levels in PC-3 was also found to be higher in than DU 145, another androgen receptor negative prostate cancer cells, it thus appears unlikely that PTHrP levels determine aggressiveness of hormone insensitive forms of prostate cancer [151].

Both PTHrP and PTHR1 are expressed in primary prostate cancers as well as in bone metastases [152]. In addition, PTHrP seems to influence cell adhesion by enhancing the synthesis of several

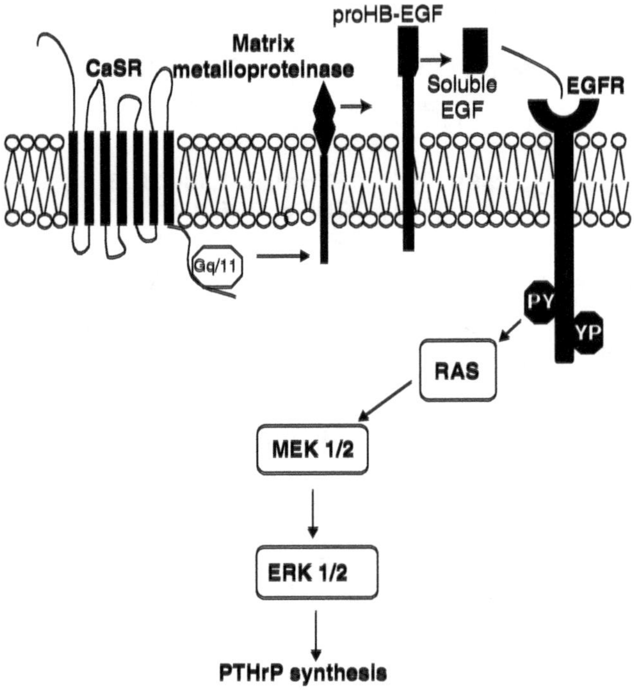

Fig. 9.3 Schematic diagram showing transactivation of EGF receptor (EGFR) by the CaSR and downstream activation of MAP kinases. CaSR can activate one or more matrix metalloproteinases (MMPs), which then cleave proheparin-bound (HB)-EGF to release soluble HB-EGF. HB-EGF then binds to EGFR, and the activated EGFR becomes autophosphorylated. This, in turn, activates the Ras/Raf/MEK pathway, finally resulting in increased PTHrP synthesis and secretion

extracellular matrix proteins and some integrin subunits that would facilitate tumor invasiveness and skeletal metastases through paracrine–autocrine and probably intracrine mechanisms [43]. Elevated Ca2+ by activating the CaSR has been shown to stimulate PTHrP secretion from PC-3 cells [153]. In addition, as in breast cancer cells, in PC-3 cells also, high Ca2+, presumably via the CaSR, accentuates the stimulatory action of TGFb on PTHrP secretion, suggesting that CaSR could "inappropriately" synergize actions of other promalignant cytokines in the progression of prostate cancer [20]. The mechanism underlying CaSR-mediated PTHrP secretion in prostate cancer cells has been shown to be transactivation of epidermal growth factor (EGF) receptor (EGFR) by the CaSR [154–158]. A major regulatory pathway present in a variety of cancer types, including prostate, uses the EGFR [159]. Transactivation of EGFR by the CaSR triggers the activation of ERK1/2, which appears to be the effector MAPK arm of CaSR-stimulated PTHrP secretion by PC-3 cells [160]. At the molecular level, the transactivation of EGFR by CaSR is mediated by matrix metalloproteinase (MMP) as broad spectrum inhibitor of MMP produced a decrease in ERK1/2 activation by the CaSR activation [157, 161]. This scheme to action of CaSR in stimulating PTHrP secretion is consistent with previous reports of convergence of GPCR signals on the receptor tyrosine kinases (RTKs), particularly the EGFR. Transactivation of EGFRs by GPCRs have been shown to occur via the activation of MMPs, which then cleave proheparin-bound (HB)-EGF, thereby releasing HB-EGF to activate EGFR (Fig. 9.3) [160, 162].

PTHrP and Hematological Malignancies

Hematological malignancies may be associated with osteolytic bone destruction and with hypercalcemia

[163]. PTHrP has been demonstrated to be an important pathogenic factor in the development of hypercalcemia in some patients with hematologic malignancies. Expression of PTHrP gene has been extensively studied in adult T-cell leukemia/lymphoma, a malignancy associated with human T-cell leukemia virus type 1 (HTLV-1) infection. This malignancy is frequently associated with the HHM syndrome [164, 165]. Transcript of PTHrP has been demonstrated in the cultures of HTLV-1-infected T cells, and immunohistochemical staining detected PTHrP in neoplastic lymph nodes [164]. In addition, approximately 30% of all patients with multiple myeloma exhibit hypercalcemia. Hypercalcemia is also reported in both non-Hodgkin's and Hodgkin's lymphoma [166]. In a clinical study of 76 patients with various hematological malignancies, 50% of the 14 hypercalcemic patients had significant increases in plasma PTHrP concentrations [167]. Of these, five had non-Hodgkin's lymphoma, one had Hodgkin's disease, and one had multiple myeloma [167]. The serum 1,25-(OH)2D3 concentrations, when measured, were low in the hypercalcemic non-Hodgkin's lymphoma patients who had increased plasma PTHrP concentrations, a characteristic of HHM-induced hypercalcemia as opposed to 1^0HPT [49]. These observations indicate that PTHrP-mediated hypercalcemia not only occurs in association with solid tumors with or without skeletal metastases, but can also occur in association with hematological malignancies [163, 166]. However, it should be noted that myeloma cells produce various other osteoclast activating cytokines including tumor necrosis factor b, interleukin-1b and IL-6, in addition to PTHrP [168–170]. Therefore, it seems likely that PTHrP is another cytokine contributing to the hypercalcemia and the skeletal complications of this disease. It is possible that PTHrP has a role as local mediator of increased bone resorption in multiple myeloma, and that at times produced in excess to reach the circulation and engender an endocrine effect. Such a process could contribute to both osteoporosis and hypercalcemia in multiple myeloma [164].

PTHrP and Lung Cancer

PTHrP expression is frequently observed in all major lung cancer cell types [171]. An estimated 50% or more of human lung tumors express PTHrP [171–173]. The expression of PTHrP appears to be more common in squamous cell carcinoma and less common in adenocarcinoma compared with other lung cancer types [173, 174]. Hypercalcemia occurs most typically with squamous cell carcinoma of the lung despite the fact that adenocarcinoma and small-cell carcinoma frequently metastasize to the bone [43, 164]. Increased expression of PTHrP in lung cancer patients is also reflected in systemic circulation and urine [174]. One report provided strong evidence to support that lung cancer cells might acquire the ability to produce more PTHrP with the progression of malignancy [175].

PTHrP and Renal Carcinoma

PTHrP expression is very common in renal cell carcinoma [176]. However, there appears to be no correlation between the levels of immunoreactive PTHrP and the patient's serum calcium level [177]. Also, there is lack of consensus on the greater PTHrP expression in renal carcinoma of granule cells type versus clear cell type. According to one study, PTHrP was detectable in sera of 15% of 243 renal carcinoma patients but serum PTHrP did not correlate with tumor stage [178]. Patients with PTHrP exhibited a trend of hypercalcemia.

Ectopic Sources of PTH in Malignancies?

Although HHM syndromes are mostly associated with elevated plasma PTHrP, currently there are at least eight convincing case reports of patients with cancers having elevated PTH in plasma. These cases include small cell carcinomas of the lung (two cases), squamous carcinoma of the lung, thymoma, undifferentiated neuroendocrine tumor, clear cell adenocarcinoma of the ovary, thyroid papillary carcinoma, and medullary thyroid carcinoma. In case of small cell carcinomas of the lung, it was a postmortem autopsy description of small cell lung cancer expressing PTH mRNA, high plasma PTH, and histologically normal parathyroids [179]. The second and most thoroughly studied case was that of a 74-year-old woman with severe hypercalcemia and elevated PTH. Initial evaluation failed to demonstrate any cancer. Neck exploration revealed normal parathyroid glands, however, surgical ablation of 3½ glands failed to abate hypercalcemia. Repeat evaluation revealed right ovarian mass characteristic of ovarian adenocarcinoma, which upon resection resulted in rapid decline in PTH levels and hypercalcemia. Southern blot analysis of tumor cells revealed clonal rearrangements upstream of one copy of PTH gene, which either abolished a silencer in this region or was an enhancer of PTH gene. In another recent case report [180] with fatal, decompensated hyperparathyroidism caused by ectopic production of PTH by a metastatic neuroendocrine tumor of the pancreas no such gene rearrangements were found. Instead, the tumor showed transactivation of the PTH gene due to hypomethylation of the PTH promoter. In the recently reported Japanese patient with a medullary thyroid cancer producing PTH, there was no apparent association between PTH expression and GCM2 gene expression, despite coexpression of the two genes [181].

It is clearly documented that most patients with malignancy-associated hypercalcemia have suppressed plasma PTH concentrations. It should be emphasized that the most likely cause of hypercalcemia in the setting of malignancy that is associated with a normal or increased serum PTH concentration is coexisting primary hyperparathyroidism. However, these cases demonstrate that authentic ectopic hyperparathyroidism does occur and may be misdiagnosed as primary hyperparathyroidism. Unless the offending malignant neoplasm is obvious at initial evaluation, such confusion may lead to unsuccessful parathyroidectomy.

Regulation of PTHrP Gene

TGFβ is one of the most abundant growth factors stored in bone and is released in its active form during osteoclastic resorption of bone [139]. TGFβ was originally reported to stimulate PTHrP gene expression in squamous cell carcinoma cell lines and in the MDA-MB-231 cell lines [10, 182, 183]. In MDA-MB-231 line, activation of PTHrP gene expression by TGFb was mediated exclusively by upregulating the level of PTHrP promoter P3-derived RNA that was dependent on smad3/Ets1 (a proto-oncoprotein belonging to Ets family of transcription factor) synergism. *Ras*-MAPK pathway has been shown to regulate PTHrP secretion in H-500, rat Leydig tumor cell line (copiously producing PTHrP to elicit hypercalcemia in male rats) [184–186]. Both Erk and JNK effector arms that are downstream of *Ras*-MAPK pathway are activated leading to increased expression of PTHrP gene in H-500 cells [10, 127]. Recently, studies in human keratinocytes revealed that EGFR-mediated activation of PTHrP expression was critically dependent on Ets binding site (EBS) for full *Ras*-Erk-mediated activation of the P3 promoter by EGFR signaling [187–189]. Therefore, *Ras*-MAPK represents a major routing pathway in the stimulation of PTHrP gene expression by various growth factors/cytokines (Fig. 9.4a).

The P1 promoter of PTHrP is regulated by cAMP responsive element (CRE) when studied in human lung carcinoma cell line (BEN), suggesting that P1 may be primary responsive promoter to the cAMP/PKA/CREB pathway (Fig. 9.4b) [190]. Although PTHrP P2 promoter appears to be expressed in a wide variety of cell lines and tumors, paucity of data makes it difficult to say if this promoter makes a substantial contribution to PTHrP gene expression in physiological or pathological circumstances [10, 184].

1,25 D3 and its various normocalcemic derivatives have been proposed as potential therapeutic agents that could reduce hypercalcemia induced by excessive PTHrP expression as well

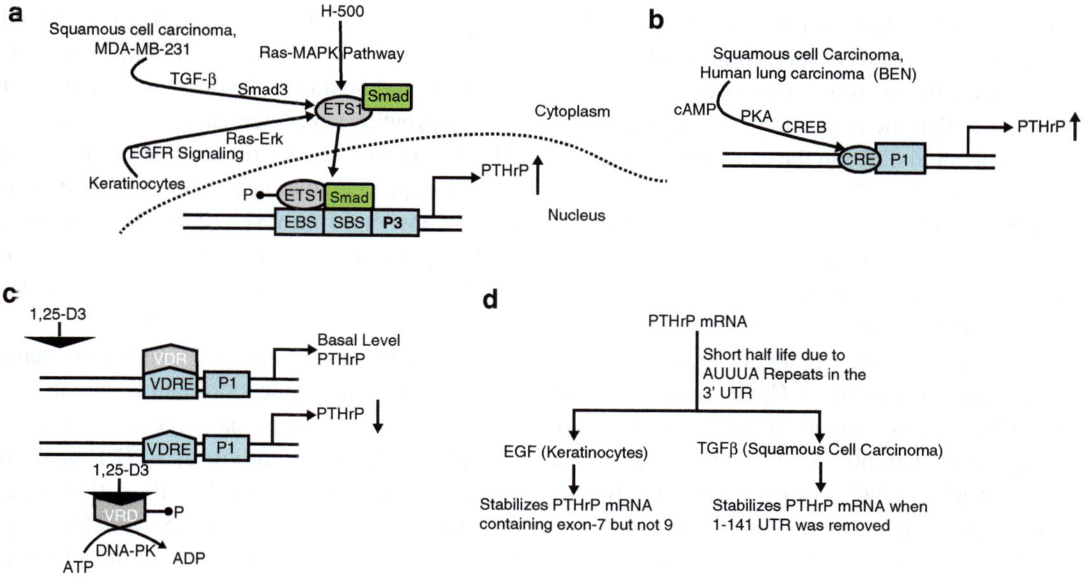

Fig. 9.4 Schematic representations of the regulation of PTHrP gene. (**a**) Transcription factors and coactivators proposed to mediate PTHrP transcription in different cancer model through P3 promoter. All pathways appear to converge on the ETS proteins that interact with the PTHrP-P3 core promoter. In MDA-MB-231 cells, activation of P3 promoter is mediated by TGFβ pathway, in rat Leydig tumor cell line (H-500) by Ras-MAPK pathway, and in keratinocytes through EGFR signaling pathway. (**b**) Activation of P1 promoter: P1 is one of the primary responsive promoter to the cAMP/PKA/CREB pathway in the Human lung carcinoma cell line (BEN). (**c**) Regulation by vitamin D: in the absence of vitamin D3, VDR remains bound to VDRE maintaining basal activity of P1 promoter, while in the presence of the hormone, VDR gets phosphorylated by DNA-dependent protein kinase resulting its dissociation from the VDRE from the region upstream of P1 leading to repression of gene expression from this promoter. (**d**) Mechanisms regulating stabilization of PTHrP mRNA: in keratinocytes PTHrP mRNA lacking exon 9 and containing exon 7 is stabilized, while in case of squamous cell carcinoma PTHrP mRNA lacking 1-141 untranslated region (UTR) is stabilized

as its production by breast and prostate cancers that have metastasized to the bone. The inhibitory effect of these compounds on the expression of PTHrP gene has been reported in a variety of human cancer cells, including prostate cancer, pancreatic cancer, *Ras*-transformed keratinocytes, several human squamous cell carcinomas, and HTLV-1 transformed cells [191–198]. 1,25 D3 represses transcription of PTHrP gene at both basal and stimulated (by growth factor/cytokines) conditions, and resembles the 1,25-(OH)2D3-mediated repression of PTH gene transcription in the parathyroid gland that serves as a feedback loop to control calcium homeostasis [195, 196, 199]. The ability to repress PTHrP gene expression in diverse groups of human cancer cells suggests that this sterol can repress all three promoters. The human PTHrP gene has an unusual vitamin D-responsive element (VDRE) located 517–546 [−3,849 to −3,840] bp upstream of P1 that is homologous to a similar inhibitory response element found in the upstream region of the human PTH gene [196]. Unlike the classical VDRE regulation where vitamin D/VDR recruits the retinoid-X-receptor (RXR) to form a functionally active heterodimer at the VDRE present in the promoters of genes activated by the hormone, the negative regulation of human PTH and PTHrP gene expression by vitamin D does not involve RXR [200]. Instead, unliganded VDR remains bound to the chromatinized VDRE to maintain basal level of expression of PTH or PTHrP gene, and upon ligand binding, VDR undergoes phosphorylation by a DNA-dependent protein kinase resulting its dissociation from the VDRE from the region upstream of P1 leading to repression of gene expression from this promoter (Fig. 9.4c) [201]. However, there are reports showing that vitamin D failed to repress PTHrP gene expression in primary cultures of prostate epithelial cells and skin keratinocytes, raising the possibility that the regulation of PTHrP gene by the sterol could differ in the cancer and nontransformed cells [202, 203].

DNA methylation is an important epigenetic factor that influences gene expression [204]. Studies with a panel of renal carcinoma cells revealed that methylation of residues upstream of the CpG island may negatively regulate PTHrP gene expression [205]. A CpG island is defined as a DNA region ranging from 500 bp to 5 kb, having more than 60% G+C content, and with a ratio of CpG to GpC of at least 0.6 [206]. In normal tissues, CpG islands are mostly unmethylated, whereas methylation of cytosine residues in CpG dinucleotides is frequently observed in cancer and is associated with gene silencing. In the lung squamous cell carcinoma cell line, BEN, extensive methylation was observed in the intron upstream of the CpG island (overlapping those in the region studied in the renal carcinoma) but did not prevent expression of any of the three PTHrP promoters [205]. Barring these conflicting data little is known about how methylation influences PTHrP gene expression in normal cells and cancers derived from specific cell types.

Although the transcription rate of PTHrP is high, yet the steady-state levels of PTHrP transcripts are low because of rapid mRNA turnover similar to that observed in early response genes, such as *c-fos*, GM-CSF, and IL-2[194, 199, 207]. All three PTHrP isoforms contain multiple copies of an AUUUA instability motif, which is responsible for the short half-life of the isoforms. Among the three isoforms of PTHrP, 1–141 mRNA had the shortest half-life (approximately 30 min) and 1–173 mRNA had the longest with a half-life of up to several hours [208]. EGF and TGFb have been shown to increase the half life of PTHrP mRNA in human immortalized keratinocytes (HaCaT) and squamous carcinoma cell lines, respectively [209]. EGF increased stabilization of PTHrP mRNA containing exon 7 (PTHrP 139), but not 9 (PTHrP 141) in keratinocytes [209]. TGFb dramatically increased the stability of PTHrP transcript in squamous carcinoma cells when the PTHrP 1-141 UTR was removed (Fig. 9.4d) [182]. The later effect of mRNA stabilization could be due to the decreased binding of various proteins to *cis* element present within the PTHrP terminal coding region that are involved in transcript degradation [210]. The likely reasons of the rapid turnover of PTHrP transcript could be due to AU-rich instability elements in the 3′ UTR and altered protein binding to *cis* elements in the coding region [211, 212].

P1 and P2 promoters of PTHrP gene have numerous potential glucocorticoid response elements. Glucocorticoids have been shown to potently inhibit transcription of PTHrP gene in squamous carcinoma cells, Leydig cell tumors, and thyroid carcinoma cells [194, 213–216]. However, glucocorticoids failed to reduce PTHrP levels in animals with hypercalcemia [217, 218]. Thus, glucocorticoids have no in vivo application in limiting hypercalcemia. The precise relationship between sex steroid and PTHrP is difficult to evaluate in endocrine cancers based on the conflicting nature of literature. Estradiol, tamoxifen, and hydroxyl-tamoxifen produced a twofold stimulation of PTHrP mRNA expression and secretion in ER-positive MCF-7 cells [219]. However, freshly isolated breast cancer cells treated with estradiol had no effect on PTHrP mRNA expression, but medroxyprogesterone repressed transcript levels [220]. Testosterone activated PTHrP gene expression in LNCaP cells, an androgen receptor (AR)-positive human prostate cancer cell line [221]. In contrast, androgens have been reported to induce downregulation of PTHrP mRNA expression in PC-3 cells (an AR negative human prostate cancer cell line). It is possible that the influence of sex hormones on PTHrP expression may be dependent on specific oncogenic events that give rise to individual breast or prostate cancers.

Conclusion

This chapter sought to cover the biological and pathophysiological roles of PTHrP. With three functional isoforms, PTHrP functions as a polyhormone. By virtue of its 70% sequence homology with PTH over the first 13 amino acids at the N terminus, PTHrP binds with a GPCR, PTHR1 (common PTH/PTHrP receptor). However, unlike PTH, PTHrP synthesis is not regulated by serum calcium, and circulating levels of PTHrP are very low in healthy adults. PTH/PTHrP binding to PTHR1 stimulates both intracellular cAMP and IP3 through Gsα and Gαq, respectively and subsequent activation of PKA or PKC pathway. Since its discovery in little over two decades, the role of PTHrP has been explored in almost all of the mammalian physiological systems both during developmental and adult life. PTHrP is produced in a wide variety of normal adult and fetal tissues, including cartilage, heart, kidney, hair follicles, placenta, breast, lungs, and other epithelial cells, thus suggesting regulation of biological functions by PTHrP other than those linked to the regulation of mineral ion metabolism. Indeed, PTHrP has established roles during development through its prominent action in endochondral bone growth, mammary gland development and tooth eruption. In the cardiovascular system, PTHrP plays homeostatic and hemodynamic functions. In pancreas, PTHrP increases beta cell mass with attendant increase in insulin production. Burgeoning data emerging from the studies on the effects and mechanism of action of PTHrP reveal PTHrP to be a multifunctional peptide that can be simultaneously secreted and targeted to nucleus, and acts via the endocrine, autocrine, paracrine, and intracrine modes. The importance of PTHrP in normal development has been substantiated by studies that have shown dramatic developmental abnormalities in mice genetically modified to either overexpress or not express PTHrP.

In addition to its physiological roles, PTHrP is considered to be a major mediator of hypercalcemia, a very common metabolic complication of malignant disease. Hypercalcemia is not distributed evenly throughout the cancer population. Primary tumors of the breast, lung, kidney, head and neck, and ovary have a higher incidence of hypercalcemia than other cancers. PTHrP-mediated hypercalcemia not only occurs with solid tumors with or without skeletal metastases but also in hematological malignancies. PTHrP has been particularly implicated as a deleterious factor of malignancy causing metastatic lesions; however, its expression with regard to cancer outcomes in patients has been controversial. Additional studies are necessary to precisely define correlations of PTHrP and tumor progression in humans. Strategies to antagonize PTHrP signaling hold therapeutic promise to limit the osteolytic potential of tumors which metastasize to bone.

Acknowledgment Generous funding from the Ministry of Health and Family Welfare, Government of India, is acknowledged.

References

1. Moseley JM, et al. Parathyroid hormone-related protein purified from a human lung cancer cell line. Proc Natl Acad Sci USA. 1987;84(14):5048–52.
2. Burtis WJ, et al. Immunochemical characterization of circulating parathyroid hormone-related protein in patients with humoral hypercalcemia of cancer. N Engl J Med. 1990;322(16):1106–12.
3. Strewler GJ, et al. Parathyroid hormonelike protein from human renal carcinoma cells. Structural and functional homology with parathyroid hormone. J Clin Invest. 1987;80(6):1803–7.
4. Suva LJ, et al. A parathyroid hormone-related protein implicated in malignant hypercalcemia: cloning and expression. Science. 1987;237(4817):893–6.
5. Usdin TB, Gruber C, Bonner TI. Identification and functional expression of a receptor selectively recognizing parathyroid hormone, the PTH2 receptor. J Biol Chem. 1995;270(26):15455–8.
6. Schluter KD. PTH and PTHrP: similar structures but different functions. News Physiol Sci. 1999;14:243–9.
7. Wysolmerski JJ, Broadus AE. Hypercalcemia of malignancy: the central role of parathyroid hormone-related protein. Annu Rev Med. 1994;45:189–200.
8. Lam MH, et al. PTHrP and cell division: expression and localization of PTHrP in a keratinocyte cell line (HaCaT) during the cell cycle. J Cell Physiol. 1997;173(3):433–46.
9. Grill V, Rankin W, Martin TJ. Parathyroid hormone-related protein (PTHrP) and hypercalcaemia. Eur J Cancer. 1998;34(2):222–9.
10. Richard V, Rosol TJ, Foley J. PTHrP gene expression in cancer: do all paths lead to Ets? Crit Rev Eukaryot Gene Expr. 2005;15(2):115–32.
11. Mangin M, et al. Two distinct tumor-derived, parathyroid hormone-like peptides result from alternative ribonucleic acid splicing. Mol Endocrinol. 1988;2(11):1049–55.
12. Mangin M, et al. Isolation and characterization of the human parathyroid hormone-like peptide gene. Proc Natl Acad Sci USA. 1989;86(7):2408–12.

13. Suva LJ, et al. Structure of the 5′ flanking region of the gene encoding human parathyroid-hormone-related protein (PTHrP). Gene. 1989;77(1):95–105.
14. Yasuda T, et al. Characterization of the human parathyroid hormone-like peptide gene. Functional and evolutionary aspects. J Biol Chem. 1989;264(13):7720–5.
15. Vasavada RC, et al. Identification and characterization of a GC-rich promoter of the human parathyroid hormone-related peptide gene. Mol Endocrinol. 1993;7(2):273–82.
16. Mangin M, et al. Identification of a cDNA encoding a parathyroid hormone-like peptide from a human tumor associated with humoral hypercalcemia of malignancy. Proc Natl Acad Sci USA. 1988;85(2):597–601.
17. Gillespie MT, Martin TJ. The parathyroid hormone-related protein gene and its expression. Mol Cell Endocrinol. 1994;100(1–2):143–7.
18. Clemens TL, et al. Parathyroid hormone-related protein and its receptors: nuclear functions and roles in the renal and cardiovascular systems, the placental trophoblasts and the pancreatic islets. Br J Pharmacol. 2001;134(6):1113–36.
19. Kumari R, Robertson JF, Watson SA. Nuclear targeting of a midregion PTHrP fragment is necessary for stimulating growth in breast cancer cells. Int J Cancer. 2006;119(1):49–59.
20. Chattopadhyay N. Effects of calcium-sensing receptor on the secretion of parathyroid hormone-related peptide and its impact on humoral hypercalcemia of malignancy. Am J Physiol Endocrinol Metab. 2006; 290(5):E761–70.
21. Lozano D, et al. Osteostatin-loaded bioceramics stimulate osteoblastic growth and differentiation. Acta Biomater. 2010;6(3):797–803.
22. Gardella TJ, Juppner H. Interaction of PTH and PTHrP with their receptors. Rev Endocr Metab Disord. 2000;1(4):317–29.
23. Lanske B, et al. The parathyroid hormone (PTH)/PTH-related peptide receptor mediates actions of both ligands in murine bone. Endocrinology. 1998; 139(12):5194–204.
24. Kronenberg HM, et al. Functional analysis of the PTH/PTHrP network of ligands and receptors. Recent Prog Horm Res. 1998;53:283–301. discussion 301–3.
25. Bettoun JD, et al. Developmental upregulation of human parathyroid hormone (PTH)/PTH-related peptide receptor gene expression from conserved and human-specific promoters. J Clin Invest. 1998;102(5):958–67.
26. Datta NS, Abou-Samra AB. PTH and PTHrP signaling in osteoblasts. Cell Signal. 2009;21(8):1245–54.
27. Hoare SR, Gardella TJ, Usdin TB. Evaluating the signal transduction mechanism of the parathyroid hormone 1 receptor. Effect of receptor-G-protein interaction on the ligand binding mechanism and receptor conformation. J Biol Chem. 2001;276(11):7741–53.
28. Huang Z, et al. The N-terminal region of the third intracellular loop of the parathyroid hormone (PTH)/PTH-related peptide receptor is critical for coupling to cAMP and inositol phosphate/Ca2+ signal transduction pathways. J Biol Chem. 1996;271(52):33382–9.
29. Iida-Klein A, et al. Mutations in the second cytoplasmic loop of the rat parathyroid hormone (PTH)/PTH-related protein receptor result in selective loss of PTH-stimulated phospholipase C activity. J Biol Chem. 1997;272(11):6882–9.
30. Singh AT, et al. G alpha12/G alpha13 subunits of heterotrimeric G proteins mediate parathyroid hormone activation of phospholipase D in UMR-106 osteoblastic cells. Endocrinology. 2005;146(5): 2171–5.
31. Syme CA, Friedman PA, Bisello A. Parathyroid hormone receptor trafficking contributes to the activation of extracellular signal-regulated kinases but is not required for regulation of cAMP signaling. J Biol Chem. 2005;280(12):11281–8.
32. Gensure RC, Gardella TJ, Juppner H. Parathyroid hormone and parathyroid hormone-related peptide, and their receptors. Biochem Biophys Res Commun. 2005;328(3):666–78.
33. Romero G, et al. Parathyroid hormone receptor directly interacts with dishevelled to regulate beta-Catenin signaling and osteoclastogenesis. J Biol Chem. 2010;285(19):14756–63.
34. Abou-Samra AB, et al. Expression cloning of a common receptor for parathyroid hormone and parathyroid hormone-related peptide from rat osteoblast-like cells: a single receptor stimulates intracellular accumulation of both cAMP and inositol trisphosphates and increases intracellular free calcium. Proc Natl Acad Sci USA. 1992;89(7):2732–6.
35. Mahon MJ, Shimada M. Calmodulin interacts with the cytoplasmic tails of the parathyroid hormone 1 receptor and a sub-set of class b G-protein coupled receptors. FEBS Lett. 2005;579(3):803–7.
36. Mahon MJ, et al. A docking site for G protein betagamma subunits on the parathyroid hormone 1 receptor supports signaling through multiple pathways. Mol Endocrinol. 2006;20(1):136–46.
37. Cui TX, Kwok R, Schwartz J. Cooperative regulation of endogenous cAMP-response element binding protein and CCAAT/enhancer-binding protein beta in GH-stimulated c-fos expression. J Endocrinol. 2008;196(1):89–100.
38. Demiralp B, et al. Anabolic actions of parathyroid hormone during bone growth are dependent on c-fos. Endocrinology. 2002;143(10):4038–47.
39. Rauscher 3rd FJ, et al. Common DNA binding site for Fos protein complexes and transcription factor AP-1. Cell. 1988;52(3):471–80.
40. Kaminska B, et al. Modulation of the composition of AP-1 complex and its impact on transcriptional activity. Acta Neurobiol Exp (Wars). 2000;60(3):395–402.
41. Berry JE, et al. JunB as a downstream mediator of PTHrP actions in cementoblasts. J Bone Miner Res. 2006;21(2):246–57.
42. Abate C, Luk D, Curran T. Transcriptional regulation by Fos and Jun in vitro: interaction among multiple activator and regulatory domains. Mol Cell Biol. 1991;11(7):3624–32.
43. Liao J, McCauley LK. Skeletal metastasis: established and emerging roles of parathyroid hormone

related protein (PTHrP). Cancer Metastasis Rev. 2006;25(4):559–71.
44. Bringhurst FR, et al. Cloned, stably expressed parathyroid hormone (PTH)/PTH-related peptide receptors activate multiple messenger signals and biological responses in LLC-PK1 kidney cells. Endocrinology. 1993;132(5):2090–8.
45. Wang B, et al. NHERF1 regulates parathyroid hormone receptor membrane retention without affecting recycling. J Biol Chem. 2007;282(50):36214–22.
46. Bhattacharya S, et al. A conformational switch in the scaffolding protein NHERF1 controls autoinhibition and complex formation. J Biol Chem. 2010;285(13): 9981–94.
47. Wang B, et al. NHERF1 regulates parathyroid hormone receptor desensitization: interference with beta-arrestin binding. Mol Pharmacol. 2009;75(5): 1189–97.
48. Miedlich SU, Abou-Samra AB. Eliminating phosphorylation sites of the parathyroid hormone receptor type 1 differentially affects stimulation of phospholipase C and receptor internalization. Am J Physiol Endocrinol Metab. 2008;295(3): E665–71.
49. Clines GA, Guise TA. Hypercalcaemia of malignancy and basic research on mechanisms responsible for osteolytic and osteoblastic metastasis to bone. Endocr Relat Cancer. 2005;12(3):549–83.
50. Garrett JE, et al. Calcitonin-secreting cells of the thyroid express an extracellular calcium receptor gene. Endocrinology. 1995;136(11):5202–11.
51. Kovacs CS, Kronenberg HM. Maternal-fetal calcium and bone metabolism during pregnancy, puerperium, and lactation. Endocr Rev. 1997;18(6): 832–72.
52. Care AD. The placental transfer of calcium. J Dev Physiol. 1991;15(5):253–7.
53. Care AD, et al. Stimulation of ovine placental transport of calcium and magnesium by mid-molecule fragments of human parathyroid hormone-related protein. Exp Physiol. 1990;75(4):605–8.
54. Rodda CP, et al. Evidence for a novel parathyroid hormone-related protein in fetal lamb parathyroid glands and sheep placenta: comparisons with a similar protein implicated in humoral hypercalcaemia of malignancy. J Endocrinol. 1988;117(2):261–71.
55. Robinson NR, et al. Fetal control of calcium transport across the rat placenta. Pediatr Res. 1989;26(2): 109–15.
56. Shaw AJ, et al. Effects of two synthetic parathyroid hormone-related protein fragments on maternofetal transfer of calcium and magnesium and release of cyclic AMP by the in-situ perfused rat placenta. J Endocrinol. 1991;129(3):399–404.
57. Bond H, et al. Increased maternofetal calcium flux in parathyroid hormone-related protein-null mice. J Physiol. 2008;586(7):2015–25.
58. El-Hashash AH, Esbrit P, Kimber SJ. PTHrP promotes murine secondary trophoblast giant cell differentiation through induction of endocycle, upregulation of giant-cell-promoting transcription factors and suppression of other trophoblast cell types. Differentiation. 2005;73(4):154–74.
59. Wlodek ME, et al. PTH/PTHrP receptor and mid-molecule PTHrP regulation of intrauterine PTHrP: PTH/PTHrP receptor antagonism increases SHR fetal weight. Placenta. 2004;25(1):53–61.
60. Martin TJ, Moseley JM, Williams ED. Parathyroid hormone-related protein: hormone and cytokine. J Endocrinol. 1997;154(Suppl):S23–37.
61. VanHouten JN. Calcium sensing by the mammary gland. J Mammary Gland Biol Neoplasia. 2005;10(2): 129–39.
62. VanHouten J, et al. The calcium-sensing receptor regulates mammary gland parathyroid hormone-related protein production and calcium transport. J Clin Invest. 2004;113(4):598–608.
63. Hens JR, et al. BMP4 and PTHrP interact to stimulate ductal outgrowth during embryonic mammary development and to inhibit hair follicle induction. Development. 2007;134(6):1221–30.
64. Wysolmerski JJ, et al. Rescue of the parathyroid hormone-related protein knockout mouse demonstrates that parathyroid hormone-related protein is essential for mammary gland development. Development. 1998;125(7):1285–94.
65. Dunbar ME, et al. Stromal cells are critical targets in the regulation of mammary ductal morphogenesis by parathyroid hormone-related protein. Dev Biol. 1998;203(1):75–89.
66. Foley J, et al. PTHrP regulates epidermal differentiation in adult mice. J Invest Dermatol. 1998; 111(6):1122–8.
67. Dunbar ME, et al. Parathyroid hormone-related protein signaling is necessary for sexual dimorphism during embryonic mammary development. Development. 1999;126(16):3485–93.
68. Foley J, et al. Parathyroid hormone-related protein maintains mammary epithelial fate and triggers nipple skin differentiation during embryonic breast development. Development. 2001;128(4):513–25.
69. Hens J, et al. Analysis of gene expression in PTHrP–/– mammary buds supports a role for BMP signaling and MMP2 in the initiation of ductal morphogenesis. Dev Dyn. 2009;238(11):2713–24.
70. Wright E, et al. The Sry-related gene Sox9 is expressed during chondrogenesis in mouse embryos. Nat Genet. 1995;9(1):15–20.
71. Buckwalter JA, et al. Morphometric analysis of chondrocyte hypertrophy. J Bone Joint Surg Am. 1986;68(2):243–55.
72. Linsenmayer TF, et al. Collagen types IX and X in the developing chick tibiotarsus: analyses of mRNAs and proteins. Development. 1991;111(1):191–6.
73. Gibson GJ, Kohler WJ, Schaffler MB. Chondrocyte apoptosis in endochondral ossification of chick sterna. Dev Dyn. 1995;203(4):468–76.
74. Lewinson D, Silbermann M. Chondroclasts and endothelial cells collaborate in the process of cartilage resorption. Anat Rec. 1992;233(4):504–14.
75. Amizuka N, et al. Parathyroid hormone-related peptide-depleted mice show abnormal epiphyseal

cartilage development and altered endochondral bone formation. J Cell Biol. 1994;126(6):1611–23.
76. Karaplis AC, et al. Lethal skeletal dysplasia from targeted disruption of the parathyroid hormone-related peptide gene. Genes Dev. 1994;8(3):277–89.
77. Weir EC, et al. Targeted overexpression of parathyroid hormone-related peptide in chondrocytes causes chondrodysplasia and delayed endochondral bone formation. Proc Natl Acad Sci USA. 1996;93(19): 10240–5.
78. Holthusen W, Holt JF, Stoeckenius M. The skull in metaphyseal chondrodysplasia type Jansen. Pediatr Radiol. 1975;3(3):137–44.
79. Hoogendam J, et al. Novel mutations in the parathyroid hormone (PTH)/PTH-related peptide receptor type 1 causing Blomstrand osteochondrodysplasia types I and II. J Clin Endocrinol Metab. 2007;92(3): 1088–95.
80. Baldridge D, et al. Signaling pathways in human skeletal dysplasias. Annu Rev Genomics Hum Genet. 2010;11:189–217.
81. Duchatelet S, et al. Recessive mutations in PTHR1 cause contrasting skeletal dysplasias in Eiken and Blomstrand syndromes. Hum Mol Genet. 2005; 14(1):1–5.
82. Chen X, et al. Regulation of articular chondrocyte proliferation and differentiation by indian hedgehog and parathyroid hormone-related protein in mice. Arthritis Rheum. 2008;58(12):3788–97.
83. Labrador JP, et al. The collagen receptor DDR2 regulates proliferation and its elimination leads to dwarfism. EMBO Rep. 2001;2(5):446–52.
84. Kronenberg HM. PTHrP and skeletal development. Ann N Y Acad Sci. 2006;1068:1–13.
85. Kronenberg HM, Chung U. The parathyroid hormone-related protein and Indian hedgehog feedback loop in the growth plate. Novartis Found Symp. 2001;232:144–52. discussion 152-7.
86. Kronenberg HM. Developmental regulation of the growth plate. Nature. 2003;423(6937):332–6.
87. Pogue R, Lyons K. BMP signaling in the cartilage growth plate. Curr Top Dev Biol. 2006;76:1–48.
88. Rian E, et al. Parathyroid hormone-related protein is produced by cultured endothelial cells: a possible role in angiogenesis. Biochem Biophys Res Commun. 1994;198(2):740–7.
89. Ishikawa M, et al. Immunocytochemical detection of parathyroid hormone-related protein in vascular endothelial cells. Biochem Biophys Res Commun. 1994;199(2):547–51.
90. Maeda S, et al. Targeted overexpression of parathyroid hormone-related protein (PTHrP) to vascular smooth muscle in transgenic mice lowers blood pressure and alters vascular contractility. Endocrinology. 1999; 140(4):1815–25.
91. Mok LL, et al. Parathyroid hormone as a smooth muscle relaxant. Endocr Rev. 1989;10(4):420–36.
92. Hongo T, et al. Abundant expression of parathyroid hormone-related protein in primary rat aortic smooth muscle cells accompanies serum-induced proliferation. J Clin Invest. 1991;88(6):1841–7.
93. Okano K, et al. Parathyroid hormone (PTH)/PTH-related protein (PTHrP) receptor and its messenger ribonucleic acid in rat aortic vascular smooth muscle cells and UMR osteoblast-like cells: cell-specific regulation by angiotensin-II and PTHrP. Endocrinology. 1994;135(3):1093–9.
94. Kawashima H. Parathyroid hormone causes a transient rise in intracellular ionized calcium in vascular smooth muscle cells. Biochem Biophys Res Commun. 1990;166(2):709–14.
95. Wang R, et al. The effects of parathyroid hormone on L-type voltage-dependent calcium channel currents in vascular smooth muscle cells and ventricular myocytes are mediated by a cyclic AMP dependent mechanism. FEBS Lett. 1991;282(2):331–4.
96. Pang PK, et al. Hypotensive action of parathyroid hormone preparations on rats and dogs. Proc Natl Acad Sci USA. 1980;77(1):675–8.
97. Pirola CJ, et al. Angiotensin II regulates parathyroid hormone-related protein expression in cultured rat aortic smooth muscle cells through transcriptional and post-transcriptional mechanisms. J Biol Chem. 1993;268(3):1987–94.
98. Pirola CJ, et al. Mechanical stimuli induce vascular parathyroid hormone-related protein gene expression in vivo and in vitro. Endocrinology. 1994;134(5): 2230–6.
99. Massfelder T, Helwig JJ, Stewart AF. Parathyroid hormone-related protein as a cardiovascular regulatory peptide. Endocrinology. 1996;137(8):3151–3.
100. Massfelder T, et al. Opposing mitogenic and anti-mitogenic actions of parathyroid hormone-related protein in vascular smooth muscle cells: a critical role for nuclear targeting. Proc Natl Acad Sci USA. 1997;94(25):13630–5.
101. Fritsch S, et al. Intravenous delivery of PTH/PTHrP type 1 receptor cDNA to rats decreases heart rate, blood pressure, renal tone, renin angiotensin system, and stress-induced cardiovascular responses. J Am Soc Nephrol. 2004;15(10):2588–600.
102. Song GJ, Fiaschi-Taesch N, Bisello A. Endogenous parathyroid hormone-related protein regulates the expression of PTH type 1 receptor and proliferation of vascular smooth muscle cells. Mol Endocrinol. 2009;23(10):1681–90.
103. Henderson JE, et al. Nucleolar localization of parathyroid hormone-related peptide enhances survival of chondrocytes under conditions that promote apoptotic cell death. Mol Cell Biol. 1995;15(8):4064–75.
104. Fiaschi-Taesch N, et al. Parathyroid-hormone-related protein as a regulator of pRb and the cell cycle in arterial smooth muscle. Circulation. 2004;110(2): 177–85.
105. Brutsaert DL. Cardiac endothelial-myocardial signaling: its role in cardiac growth, contractile performance, and rhythmicity. Physiol Rev. 2003;83(1): 59–115.

106. Schluter K, et al. Expression, release, and biological activity of parathyroid hormone-related peptide from coronary endothelial cells. Circ Res. 2000;86(9): 946–51.
107. Hara M, et al. Positive chronotropic actions of parathyroid hormone and parathyroid hormone-related peptide are associated with increases in the current, I(f), and the slope of the pacemaker potential. Circulation. 1997;96(10):3704–9.
108. Vasavada RC, et al. Overexpression of parathyroid hormone-related protein in the pancreatic islets of transgenic mice causes islet hyperplasia, hyperinsulinemia, and hypoglycemia. J Biol Chem. 1996;271(2):1200–8.
109. Porter SE, et al. Progressive pancreatic islet hyperplasia in the islet-targeted, parathyroid hormone-related protein-overexpressing mouse. Endocrinology. 1998;139(9):3743–51.
110. Vasavada RC, et al. Targeted expression of placental lactogen in the beta cells of transgenic mice results in beta cell proliferation, islet mass augmentation, and hypoglycemia. J Biol Chem. 2000;275(20): 15399–406.
111. Garcia-Ocana A, et al. Using beta-cell growth factors to enhance human pancreatic Islet transplantation. J Clin Endocrinol Metab. 2001;86(3):984–8.
112. Chattopadhyay N, Brown EM. Role of calcium-sensing receptor in mineral ion metabolism and inherited disorders of calcium-sensing. Mol Genet Metab. 2006;89(3):189–202.
113. Horwitz MJ, et al. Direct comparison of sustained infusion of human parathyroid hormone-related protein-(1-36) [hPTHrP-(1-36)] versus hPTH-(1-34) on serum calcium, plasma 1,25-dihydroxyvitamin D concentrations, and fractional calcium excretion in healthy human volunteers. J Clin Endocrinol Metab. 2003;88(4):1603–9.
114. Mather KJ, Chik CL, Corenblum B. Maintenance of serum calcium by parathyroid hormone-related peptide during lactation in a hypoparathyroid patient. J Clin Endocrinol Metab. 1999;84(2):424–7.
115. Goltzman D. Studies on the mechanisms of the skeletal anabolic action of endogenous and exogenous parathyroid hormone. Arch Biochem Biophys. 2008;473(2):218–24.
116. Guise TA, Mundy GR. Cancer and bone. Endocr Rev. 1998;19(1):18–54.
117. Martin TJ. Manipulating the environment of cancer cells in bone: a novel therapeutic approach. J Clin Invest. 2002;110(10):1399–401.
118. Luparello C, et al. Transforming growth factor-beta 1, beta 2, and beta 3, urokinase and parathyroid hormone-related peptide expression in 8701-BC breast cancer cells and clones. Differentiation. 1993;55(1): 73–80.
119. Li H, et al. Effect of endogenously produced parathyroid hormone-related peptide on growth of a human hepatoma cell line (Hep G2). Endocrinology. 1996;137(6):2367–74.
120. Chen HL, et al. Parathyroid hormone and parathyroid hormone-related protein exert both pro- and anti-apoptotic effects in mesenchymal cells. J Biol Chem. 2002;277(22):19374–81.
121. Schilling T, et al. Parathyroid hormone-related protein (PTHrP) does not regulate 1,25-dihydroxyvitamin D serum levels in hypercalcemia of malignancy. J Clin Endocrinol Metab. 1993;76(3):801–3.
122. Nakashima M, et al. Expression of parathyroid hormone (PTH)-related peptide (PTHrP) and PTH/PTHrP receptor in giant cell tumour of tendon sheath. J Pathol. 1996;180(1):80–4.
123. Philbrick WM, et al. Defining the roles of parathyroid hormone-related protein in normal physiology. Physiol Rev. 1996;76(1):127–73.
124. Plawner LL, et al. Cell type-specific secretion of parathyroid hormone-related protein via the regulated versus the constitutive secretory pathway. J Biol Chem. 1995;270(23):14078–84.
125. Aklilu F, et al. Increased PTHRP production by a tyrosine kinase oncogene, Tpr-Met: role of the Ras signaling pathway. Am J Physiol. 1996;271(2 Pt 1): E277–83.
126. Aklilu F, et al. Induction of parathyroid hormone-related peptide by the Ras oncogene: role of Ras farnesylation inhibitors as potential therapeutic agents for hypercalcemia of malignancy. Cancer Res. 1997;57(20):4517–22.
127. Aklilu F, et al. Role of mitogen-activated protein kinases in the induction of parathyroid hormone-related peptide. Cancer Res. 2000;60(6):1753–60.
128. Southby J, et al. Immunohistochemical localization of parathyroid hormone-related protein in human breast cancer. Cancer Res. 1990;50(23):7710–6.
129. Vargas SJ, et al. Localization of parathyroid hormone-related protein mRNA expression in breast cancer and metastatic lesions by in situ hybridization. J Bone Miner Res. 1992;7(8):971–9.
130. Powell GJ, et al. Localization of parathyroid hormone-related protein in breast cancer metastases: increased incidence in bone compared with other sites. Cancer Res. 1991;51(11):3059–61.
131. Linforth R, et al. Coexpression of parathyroid hormone related protein and its receptor in early breast cancer predicts poor patient survival. Clin Cancer Res. 2002;8(10):3172–7.
132. Liapis H, et al. Expression of parathyroidlike protein in normal, proliferative, and neoplastic human breast tissues. Am J Pathol. 1993;143(4):1169–78.
133. Shimo T, et al. Pathogenic role of connective tissue growth factor (CTGF/CCN2) in osteolytic metastasis of breast cancer. J Bone Miner Res. 2006;21(7): 1045–59.
134. Henderson M, et al. Parathyroid hormone-related protein production by breast cancers, improved survival, and reduced bone metastases. J Natl Cancer Inst. 2001;93(3):234–7.
135. Richard V, et al. Quantitative evaluation of alternative promoter usage and 3′ splice variants for parathyroid

hormone-related protein by real-time reverse transcription-PCR. Clin Chem. 2003;49(8):1398–402.
136. Bouizar Z, Spyratos F, De vernejoul MC. The parathyroid hormone-related protein (PTHrP) gene: use of downstream TATA promotor and PTHrP 1-139 coding pathways in primary breast cancers vary with the occurrence of bone metastasis. J Bone Miner Res. 1999;14(3):406–14.
137. Yoneda T, Hiraga T. Crosstalk between cancer cells and bone microenvironment in bone metastasis. Biochem Biophys Res Commun. 2005;328(3):679–87.
138. Cailleau R, et al. Breast tumor cell lines from pleural effusions. J Natl Cancer Inst. 1974;53(3):661–74.
139. Yin JJ, et al. TGF-beta signaling blockade inhibits PTHrP secretion by breast cancer cells and bone metastases development. J Clin Invest. 1999;103(2): 197–206.
140. Guise TA. Breaking down bone: new insight into site-specific mechanisms of breast cancer osteolysis mediated by metalloproteinases. Genes Dev. 2009;23(18):2117–23.
141. Dunn LK, et al. Hypoxia and TGF-beta drive breast cancer bone metastases through parallel signaling pathways in tumor cells and the bone microenvironment. PLoS One. 2009;4(9):e6896.
142. Sanders JL, et al. Extracellular calcium-sensing receptor expression and its potential role in regulating parathyroid hormone-related peptide secretion in human breast cancer cell lines. Endocrinology. 2000;141(12):4357–64.
143. Buchs N, et al. Calcium stimulates parathyroid hormone-related protein production in Leydig tumor cells through a putative cation-sensing mechanism. Eur J Endocrinol. 2000;142(5):500–5.
144. Mamillapalli R, et al. Switching of G-protein usage by the calcium-sensing receptor reverses its effect on parathyroid hormone-related protein secretion in normal versus malignant breast cells. J Biol Chem. 2008;283(36):24435–47.
145. Leask A, Abraham DJ. All in the CCN family: essential matricellular signaling modulators emerge from the bunker. J Cell Sci. 2006;119(Pt 23):4803–10.
146. Brown JE, Neville-Webbe H, Coleman RE. The role of bisphosphonates in breast and prostate cancers. Endocr Relat Cancer. 2004;11(2):207–24.
147. Iwamura M, et al. Immunohistochemical localization of parathyroid hormone-related protein in prostatic intraepithelial neoplasia. Hum Pathol. 1995;26(7):797–801.
148. Dougherty KM, et al. Parathyroid hormone-related protein as a growth regulator of prostate carcinoma. Cancer Res. 1999;59(23):6015–22.
149. Keller DL. Prostate cancer prevention (August 2009). Cleve Clin J Med. 2009;76(11):630. author reply 630.
150. Pizzi H, et al. Androgen regulation of parathyroid hormone-related peptide production in human prostate cancer cells. Endocrinology. 2003;144(3):858–67.
151. Deftos LJ, et al. Direct evidence that PTHrP expression promotes prostate cancer progression in bone. Biochem Biophys Res Commun. 2005;327(2): 468–72.
152. Liao J, et al. Tumor expressed PTHrP facilitates prostate cancer-induced osteoblastic lesions. Int J Cancer. 2008;123(10):2267–78.
153. Sanders JL, et al. Ca(2+)-sensing receptor expression and PTHrP secretion in PC-3 human prostate cancer cells. Am J Physiol Endocrinol Metab. 2001;281(6):E1267–74.
154. Wetzker R, Bohmer FD. Transactivation joins multiple tracks to the ERK/MAPK cascade. Nat Rev Mol Cell Biol. 2003;4(8):651–7.
155. Fischer OM, et al. EGFR signal transactivation in cancer cells. Biochem Soc Trans. 2003;31(Pt 6): 1203–8.
156. Luttrell LM, Daaka Y, Lefkowitz RJ. Regulation of tyrosine kinase cascades by G-protein-coupled receptors. Curr Opin Cell Biol. 1999;11(2):177–83.
157. Prenzel N, et al. EGF receptor transactivation by G-protein-coupled receptors requires metalloproteinase cleavage of proHB-EGF. Nature. 1999; 402(6764):884–8.
158. Schafer B, Gschwind A, Ullrich A. Multiple G-protein-coupled receptor signals converge on the epidermal growth factor receptor to promote migration and invasion. Oncogene. 2004;23(4):991–9.
159. Kingsley LA, et al. Molecular biology of bone metastasis. Mol Cancer Ther. 2007;6(10):2609–17.
160. Yano S, et al. Calcium-sensing receptor activation stimulates parathyroid hormone-related protein secretion in prostate cancer cells: role of epidermal growth factor receptor transactivation. Bone. 2004;35(3):664–72.
161. Yan Y, Shirakabe K, Werb Z. The metalloprotease Kuzbanian (ADAM10) mediates the transactivation of EGF receptor by G protein-coupled receptors. J Cell Biol. 2002;158(2):221–6.
162. MacLeod RJ, et al. Extracellular calcium-sensing receptor transactivates the epidermal growth factor receptor by a triple-membrane-spanning signaling mechanism. Biochem Biophys Res Commun. 2004;320(2):455–60.
163. Sargent JT, Smith OP. Haematological emergencies managing hypercalcaemia in adults and children with haematological disorders. Br J Haematol. 2010;149(4):465–77.
164. Grill V, Martin TJ. Hypercalcemia of malignancy. Rev Endocr Metab Disord. 2000;1(4):253–63.
165. Fukumoto S, et al. Clinical evaluation of calcium metabolism in adult T-cell leukemia/lymphoma. Arch Intern Med. 1988;148(4):921–5.
166. Seymour JF, Gagel RF. Calcitriol: the major humoral mediator of hypercalcemia in Hodgkin's disease and non-Hodgkin's lymphomas. Blood. 1993;82(5): 1383–94.
167. Kremer R, et al. Parathyroid-hormone-related peptide in hematologic malignancies. Am J Med. 1996;100(4):406–11.
168. Roodman GD. Biology of osteoclast activation in cancer. J Clin Oncol. 2001;19(15):3562–71.

169. Roodman GD. Mechanisms of bone metastasis. N Engl J Med. 2004;350(16):1655–64.
170. Michigami T, et al. Cell–cell contact between marrow stromal cells and myeloma cells via VCAM-1 and alpha(4)beta(1)-integrin enhances production of osteoclast-stimulating activity. Blood. 2000;96(5):1953–60.
171. Brandt DW, et al. All major lung cancer cell types produce parathyroid hormone-like protein: heterogeneity assessed by high performance liquid chromatography. Endocrinology. 1991;129(5):2466–70.
172. Kitazawa S, et al. Immunohistologic evaluation of parathyroid hormone-related protein in human lung cancer and normal tissue with newly developed monoclonal antibody. Cancer. 1991;67(4):984–9.
173. Davidson LA, et al. Lung tumours immunoreactive for parathyroid hormone related peptide: analysis of serum calcium levels and tumour type. J Pathol. 1996;178(4):398–401.
174. Nishigaki Y, et al. Increased serum and urinary levels of a parathyroid hormone-related protein COOH terminus in non-small cell lung cancer patients. Clin Cancer Res. 1999;5(6):1473–81.
175. Hidaka N, Nishimura M, Nagao K. Establishment of two human small cell lung cancer cell lines: the evidence of accelerated production of parathyroid hormone-related protein with tumor progression. Cancer Lett. 1998;125(1–2):149–55.
176. Iwamura M, et al. Parathyroid hormone-related protein is an independent prognostic factor for renal cell carcinoma. Cancer. 1999;86(6):1028–34.
177. Gotoh A, et al. Common expression of parathyroid hormone-related protein and no correlation of calcium level in renal cell carcinomas. Cancer. 1993;71(9):2803–6.
178. Papworth K, et al. Parathyroid hormone-related protein and serum calcium in patients with renal cell carcinoma. Tumour Biol. 2005;26(4):201–6.
179. Yoshimoto K, et al. Ectopic production of parathyroid hormone by small cell lung cancer in a patient with hypercalcemia. J Clin Endocrinol Metab. 1989;68(5):976–81.
180. VanHouten JN, et al. Hypercalcemia of malignancy due to ectopic transactivation of the parathyroid hormone gene. J Clin Endocrinol Metab. 2006;91(2):580–3.
181. Demura M, et al. Ectopic production of parathyroid hormone in a patient with sporadic medullary thyroid cancer. Endocr J. 2010;57(2):161–70.
182. Sellers RS, Capen CC, Rosol TJ. Messenger RNA stability of parathyroid hormone-related protein regulated by transforming growth factor-beta1. Mol Cell Endocrinol. 2002;188(1–2):37–46.
183. Lindemann RK, et al. Transforming growth factor beta regulates parathyroid hormone-related protein expression in MDA-MB-231 breast cancer cells through a novel Smad/Ets synergism. J Biol Chem. 2001;276(49):46661–70.
184 Richard V, et al. Transcriptional regulation of parathyroid hormone-related protein promoter P3 by ETS-1 in adult T-cell leukemia/lymphoma. Leukemia. 2005;19(7):1175–83.
185. Lindemann RK, Nordheim A, Dittmer J. Interfering with TGFbeta-induced Smad3 nuclear accumulation differentially affects TGFbeta-dependent gene expression. Mol Cancer. 2003;2:20.
186. Cataisson C, et al. Ets-1 activates parathyroid hormone-related protein gene expression in tumorigenic breast epithelial cells. Mol Cell Endocrinol. 2003;204(1–2):155–68.
187. Lorch G, et al. Inhibition of epidermal growth factor receptor signalling reduces hypercalcaemia induced by human lung squamous-cell carcinoma in athymic mice. Br J Cancer. 2007;97(2):183–93.
188. Gilmore JL, et al. Amphiregulin-EGFR signaling regulates PTHrP gene expression in breast cancer cells. Breast Cancer Res Treat. 2008;110(3):493–505.
189. Cho YM, et al. Regulation of parathyroid hormone-related protein gene expression by epidermal growth factor-family ligands in primary human keratinocytes. J Endocrinol. 2004;181(1):179–90.
190. Chilco PJ, Leopold V, Zajac JD. Differential regulation of the parathyroid hormone-related protein gene P1 and P3 promoters by cAMP. Mol Cell Endocrinol. 1998;138(1–2):173–84.
191. Tovar Sepulveda VA, Falzon M. Prostate cancer cell type-specific regulation of the human PTHrP gene via a negative VDRE. Mol Cell Endocrinol. 2003;204(1–2):51–64.
192. Abe M, et al. Inhibitory effects of 1,25-dihydroxyvitamin D3 and 9-cis-retinoic acid on parathyroid hormone-related protein expression by oral cancer cells (HSC-3). J Endocrinol. 1998;156(2):349–57.
193. Falzon M, Zong J. The noncalcemic vitamin D analogs EB1089 and 22-oxacalcitriol suppress serum-induced parathyroid hormone-related peptide gene expression in a lung cancer cell line. Endocrinology. 1998;139(3):1046–53.
194. Ikeda K, et al. Expression of transcripts encoding a parathyroid hormone-related peptide in abnormal human parathyroid tissues. J Clin Endocrinol Metab. 1989;69(6):1240–8.
195. Henderson J, et al. Dysregulation of parathyroid hormone-like peptide expression and secretion in a keratinocyte model of tumor progression. Cancer Res. 1991;51(24):6521–8.
196. Nishishita T, et al. A negative vitamin D response DNA element in the human parathyroid hormone-related peptide gene binds to vitamin D receptor along with Ku antigen to mediate negative gene regulation by vitamin D. J Biol Chem. 1998;273(18):10901–7.
197. Endo K, et al. Evidence for the uptake of a vitamin D analogue (OCT) by a human carcinoma and its effect of suppressing the transcription of parathyroid hormone-related peptide gene in vivo. J Biol Chem. 1994;269(51):32693–9.
198. Michigami T, et al. Conflicting actions of parathyroid hormone-related protein and serum calcium as

regulators of 25-hydroxyvitamin D(3)-1 alpha-hydroxylase expression in a nude rat model of humoral hypercalcemia of malignancy. J Endocrinol. 2001;171(2):249–57.
199. Ikeda K, et al. Transcriptional regulation of the parathyroid hormone-related peptide gene by glucocorticoids and vitamin D in a human C-cell line. J Biol Chem. 1989;264(27):15743–6.
200. Haussler MR, et al. New understanding of the molecular mechanism of receptor-mediated genomic actions of the vitamin D hormone. Bone. 1995;17 (2 Suppl):33S–8S.
201. Okazaki T, et al. Vitamin D-dependent recruitment of DNA-PK to the chromatinized negative vitamin D response element in the PTHrP gene is required for gene repression by vitamin D. Biochem Biophys Res Commun. 2003;304(4):632–7.
202. Kremer R, et al. Regulation of parathyroid hormone-like peptide in cultured normal human keratinocytes. Effect of growth factors and 1,25 dihydroxyvitamin D3 on gene expression and secretion. J Clin Invest. 1991;87(3):884–93.
203. Cramer SD, et al. Parathyroid hormone-related protein (PTHrP) is an epidermal growth factor-regulated secretory product of human prostatic epithelial cells. Prostate. 1996;29(1):20–9.
204. Jones PA, Baylin SB. The fundamental role of epigenetic events in cancer. Nat Rev Genet. 2002;3(6): 415–28.
205. Holt EH, et al. Region-specific methylation of the parathyroid hormone-related peptide gene determines its expression in human renal carcinoma cell lines. J Biol Chem. 1993;268(27):20639–45.
206. Merlo A, et al. 5′ CpG island methylation is associated with transcriptional silencing of the tumour suppressor p16/CDKN2/MTS1 in human cancers. Nat Med. 1995;1(7):686–92.
207. Ikeda K, et al. Regulation of parathyroid hormone-related peptide gene expression by cycloheximide. J Biol Chem. 1990;265(10):5398–402.
208. Southby J, et al. Cell-specific and regulator-induced promoter usage and messenger ribonucleic acid splicing for parathyroid hormone-related protein. Endocrinology. 1996;137(4):1349–57.
209. Heath JK, et al. Epidermal growth factor-stimulated parathyroid hormone-related protein expression involves increased gene transcription and mRNA stability. Biochem J. 1995;307(Pt 1):159–67.
210. Bevilacqua A, et al. Post-transcriptional regulation of gene expression by degradation of messenger RNAs. J Cell Physiol. 2003;195(3):356–72.
211. Wilson GM, et al. Structural remodeling of an A + U-rich RNA element by cation or AUF1 binding. J Biol Chem. 2001;276(42):38400–9.
212. Chen CY, et al. AU binding proteins recruit the exosome to degrade ARE-containing mRNAs. Cell. 2001;107(4):451–64.
213. Merryman JI, et al. Regulation of parathyroid hormone-related protein production by a squamous carcinoma cell line in vitro. Lab Invest. 1993;69(3):347–54.
214. Glatz JA, et al. Dexamethasone regulation of parathyroid hormone-related protein (PTHrP) expression in a squamous cancer cell line. Mol Cell Endocrinol. 1994;101(1–2):295–306.
215. Kasono K, et al. Effects of glucocorticoids and calcitonin on parathyroid hormone-related protein (PTHrP) gene expression and PTHrP release in human cancer cells causing humoral hypercalcemia. Jpn J Cancer Res. 1991;82(9):1008–14.
216. Liu B, Goltzman D, Rabbani SA. Regulation of parathyroid hormone-related peptide production in vitro by the rat hypercalcemic Leydig cell tumor H-500. Endocrinology. 1993;132(4):1658–64.
217. Schilling T, et al. Glucocorticoids decrease the production of parathyroid hormone-related protein in vitro but not in vivo in the Walker carcinosarcoma 256 rat model. Bone. 1996;18(4):315–9.
218. Cohen-Solal ME, et al. 1,25 Dihydroxyvitamin D and dexamethasone decrease in vivo Walker carcinoma growth, but not parathyroid hormone related protein secretion. Horm Metab Res. 1995;27(9):403–7.
219. Funk JL, Wei H. Regulation of parathyroid hormone-related protein expression in MCF-7 breast carcinoma cells by estrogen and antiestrogens. Biochem Biophys Res Commun. 1998;251(3):849–54.
220. Sugimoto T, et al. Suppression of parathyroid hormone-related protein messenger RNA expression by medroxyprogesterone acetate in breast cancer tissues. Breast Cancer Res Treat. 1999;56(1):11–23.
221. Asadi F, et al. Effect of parathyroid hormone related protein, and dihydrotestosterone on proliferation and ornithine decarboxylase mRNA in human prostate cancer cell lines. Int Urol Nephrol. 2001;33(3): 417–22.

Ectopic Parathyroid Glands

10

Jean-François Henry and Maurizio Iacobone

Abstract

Parathyroid glands in major ectopic locations are rare but may present a considerable challenge to the endocrinologist, the radiologist, and the surgeon. The prevalence of parathyroid ectopias is unclear and is probably underestimated by failure to search for and identify these ectopic glands when they are normal. In most cases, an ectopic parathyroid gland is identified because it is hyperfunctioning and sought for in a patient presenting with hyperparathyroidism. Nowadays, most ectopic hyperfunctional parathyroid glands can be identified prior to surgery by imaging studies or during surgery. A thorough knowledge of the anatomy and an understanding of the embryonic development of the parathyroid glands are the keys to successful localization and successful resection.

Keywords

Parathyroid ectopias • Hyperparathyroidism • Cryopreservation • Autotransplantation • Selective venous sampling • Hyperfunctional

Introduction

The prevalence of parathyroid ectopias is unclear and is probably underestimated by failure to search for and identify these ectopic glands when they are normal. In most cases, an ectopic parathyroid gland is identified because it is hyperfunctioning and sought for in a patient presenting with hyperparathyroidism (HPT). In addition, few organs have such variable locations as parathyroid glands, and, therefore, the boundaries of the usual territory of orthotopic parathyroid glands are difficult to establish. This explains that the incidence of parathyroid ectopias ranges from 4 to 22% in the literature depending on whether one considers that a gland is located in its usual territory or not. Even if major parathyroid ectopias account for less than 10%, they remain a challenge to the clinician.

J.-F. Henry, MD, FRCS (✉)
Department of Endocrine Surgery, University Hospital La Timone, 264, Rue St. Pierre, Marseille 13385, France
e-mail: JeanFrancois.HENRY@ap-hm.fr

M. Iacobone, MD, FEBS
Endocrine Surgery Unit, Department of Surgical, Oncological and Gastroenterological Sciences, University of Padua, Via Giustiniani 2, Padua 35128, Italy
e-mail: maurizio.iacobone@unipd.it

A.A. Licata and E.V. Lerma (eds.), *Diseases of the Parathyroid Glands*,
DOI 10.1007/978-1-4419-5550-0_10, © Springer Science+Business Media, LLC 2012

Normal Locations of Parathyroid Glands

The normal or orthotopic location of parathyroid glands can be determined from knowledge of their embryonic development. The parathyroid glands arise from the endoderm of the third and fourth branchial pouches. Differentiation of the parathyroid tissue takes place in the embryo at the 8–10-mm stage.

The inferior parathyroid glands arise from the dorsal part of the third branchial pouches. They are numbered PIII to recall their origin. The thymus arises from the ventral portion of the same pouch. This common origin justifies labeling PIII as the "thymic" parathyroids or parathymus complex.

The superior parathyroid glands arise from the dorsal part of the fourth branchial pouches and are therefore numbered PIV. The incorporation of the fifth pouch with the fourth pouch leads to the formation of the "caudal pharyngeal complex," which includes not only PIV but the ultimobranchial bodies or lateral thyroids and a ventral diverticulum.

At the 13–14-mm stage, the PIII and the PIV migrate together with the thymus and ultimobranchial bodies, respectively. The PIII-thymus complex separates from the pharyngeal wall and moves towards the caudal and median region. Because of the extension of the cervical spine and the descent of the heart and great vessels, the thymus, and with it the PIII, is drawn towards the superior mediastinum. At the 20-mm stage, the cephalic regression of the thymus brings about its separation from the PIII, which is thus abandoned at the level of the anterior or posterolateral region of the inferior poles of the thyroid lobes, or at the level of the thyrothymic ligaments, vestigial structures indicative of their former connections.

The PIV follow the thyroid migration of the ultimobranchial bodies, which travel towards the lateral part of the main median thyroid rudiment. Their descent in the neck is thus relatively limited. They remain in contact with the posterior part of the middle third of the thyroid lobes.

The short course of embryologic migration of PIV explains why they remain relatively stable in their topography when they are not pathologic. Thus, in 85% of cases they are grouped at the posterior aspect of the thyroid lobes, in an area of 2 cm diameter, the center of which is situated about 1 cm above the crossing of the inferior thyroid artery and the recurrent nerve [1] (Fig. 10.1).

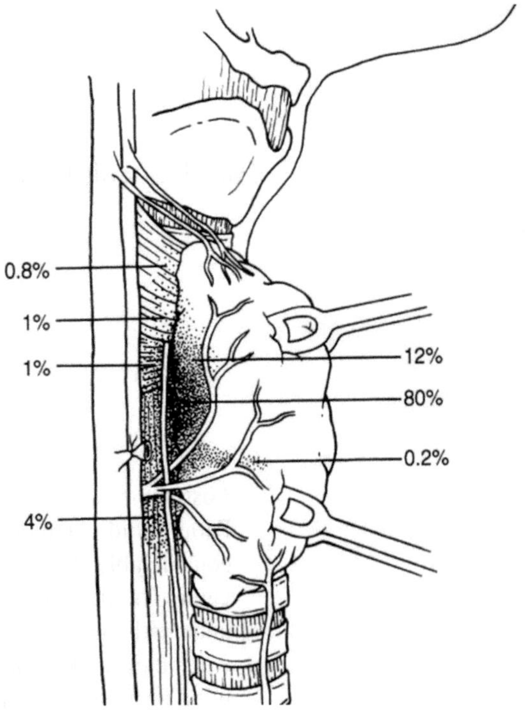

Fig. 10.1 Location of superior parathyroid glands (P IV). The numbers represent the percentages of glands found at different locations in an autopsy study of 503 cases. Modified from Akerstrom G, Malmaeus J, and Bergstrom R. Surgical anatomy of human parathyroid glands. Surgery 1984; 95:14–21

On the contrary, the territory of the normal PIII is much more extensive. In 61% of cases, they are situated at the level of the inferior poles of the thyroid lobes, on the posterior, lateral, or anterior aspects. In 26% of cases, they are situated in the thyrothymic ligaments or in the upper, cervical portion of the thymus. More rarely, in 7% of cases, they are situated higher up, at the level of the middle third of the posterior aspect of the thyroid lobes, and may then be confused with PIV [1] (Fig. 10.2). The other sites are not amenable to classification [1–3].

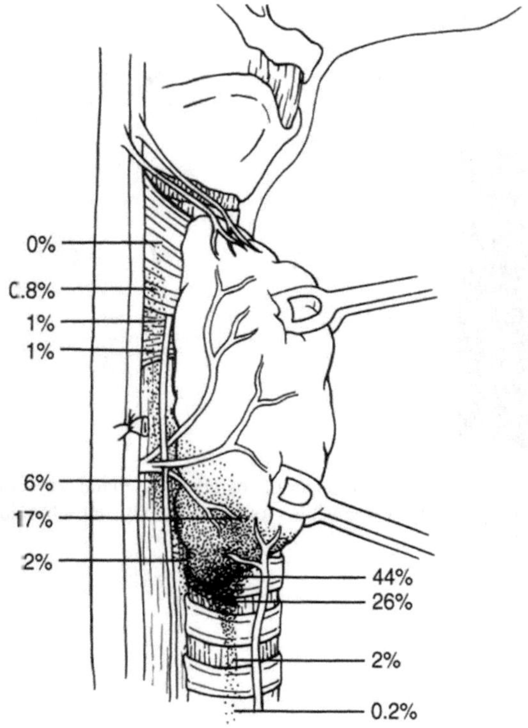

Fig. 10.2 Location of inferior parathyroid glands (P III). The numbers represent the percentages of glands found at different locations in an autopsy study of 503 cases. Modified from Akerstrom G, Malmaeus J, and Bergstrom R. Surgical anatomy of human parathyroid glands. Surgery 1984; 95:14–21

Mechanisms of Parathyroid Ectopias

Parathyroid ectopias may be congenital or acquired. A thorough knowledge of the embryonic development of the parathyroid glands is the key to understanding congenital ectopias. A thorough knowledge of the anatomy is the key to understanding acquired ectopias.

Congenital ectopias may be caused by abnormal embryological migration of one of the four glands. This abnormal embryological migration, whether deficient or excessive, may be responsible for more or less ectopic locations.

The other mechanism of congenital ectopias is related to supernumerary glands. Parathyroid glands derive from embryologic mesenchyme, which is also responsible for the development of the pharynx and its associated cartilagenous, muscular, neural, and vascular stuctures. Supernumerary glands develop from accessory parathyroid debris arising from fragmentation of the pharyngotracheal duct when the pharyngeal pouches separate from the pharynx. Therefore, it is not surprising that parathyroid fragments can be found in these adjacent structures.

Apart from the congenital ectopias, the surgeon must be familiar with the existence of acquired ectopias due to tumoral glands, since a tumoral parathyroid may migrate under the influence of gravity. This migration is favored by ascending movements of the larynx and pharynx during swallowing and by a suction phenomenon due to the negative intrathoracic pressure. A tumoral gland may then leave its proper site and acquire a progressively ectopic site. These migrations depend on the initial topography of the gland before it becomes tumoral.

Congenital Ectopias due to Anomalies of Embryological Migration

Because the area of dispersal of the PIV is limited by their short migratory course, congenital ectopias of PIV are rarely major ectopias. On the contrary, as the embryologic descent of the thymus extends from the angle of the mandible to the pericardium, anomalies of migration of the parathymus, whether excessive or defective, can result in major ectopias of PIII.

Congenital ectopias of PIV are rarely major ectopias. In 12–13% of cases, the glands are on the posterior aspect of the superior pole of the thyroid lobe in a latero-cricoid, latero-pharyngeal, or intercrico-thyroid position, exceptionally, in less than 1% of cases, above the upper pole of the lobe. In 1–4% of cases, they are frankly posterior, behind the pharynx or esophagus [1]. All these locations are probably due to a deficient migration. Conversely, an excessive migration of a PIV is probably responsible for its strictly intrathyroid localization (Fig. 10.3). A PIV may become included within the thyroid at the time of fusion of the ultimobranchial bodies

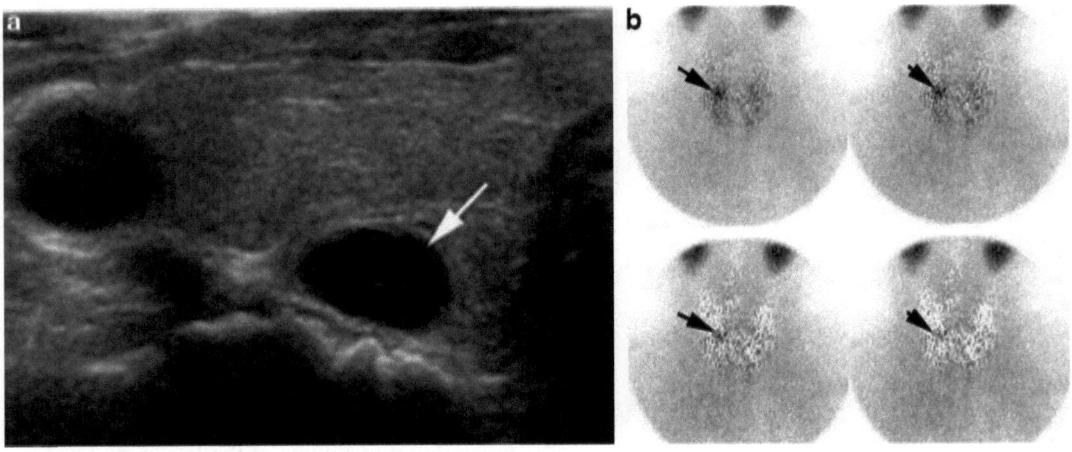

Fig. 10.3 Transverse ultrasound image (**a**) and 99mTc-sestamibi scintigraphy image (**b**) of an intrathyroid parathyroid adenoma. An excessive congenital migration of the right superior parathyroid gland (P IV) is probably responsible for this strictly intrathyroid location

with the median thyroid rudiment [4]. However, not all intrathyroid parathyroid glands are PIV, and undeniable cases of a normal or pathologic PIII included in the lower poles of the thyroid lobes have been reported [5–8]. The embryological explanation proposed for PIV cannot be applied to the PIII, which do not arise from the fourth branchial pouches. The incidence of intrathyroidal parathyroid glands found at autopsy is very low, 0–1.3% [1–3]. The incidence of intrathyroidal adenomas at a first cervical exploration is significantly higher, ranging from 1.4 to 3.2% [6]. In reoperative parathyroid surgery for persistent or recurrent primary hyperparathyroidism (PHPT), this incidence has been reported up to 27.2% [6]. Overall, the incidence of intrathyroid ectopias which seem to involve both PIII and PIV should be estimated between 0.5 and 4%.

Inferior parathyroid glands or PIII descend with the thymus during embryological development. Therefore, deficient migration of the parathymus complex is responsible for high ectopia in the neck and excessive migration is responsible for low ectopia in the anterosuperior mediastinum (Fig. 10.4).

PIII in high cervical ectopia, or undescended PIII, are located on the cranial side of the upper pole of the thyroid lobe (Fig. 10.5). Their prevalence is unclear, but it is probably underestimated by failure to search for and identify these ectopic glands when they are normal. On the basis of autopsy studies of normal subjects as well as description of locations of parathyroid glands found during exploration for PHPT, the incidence

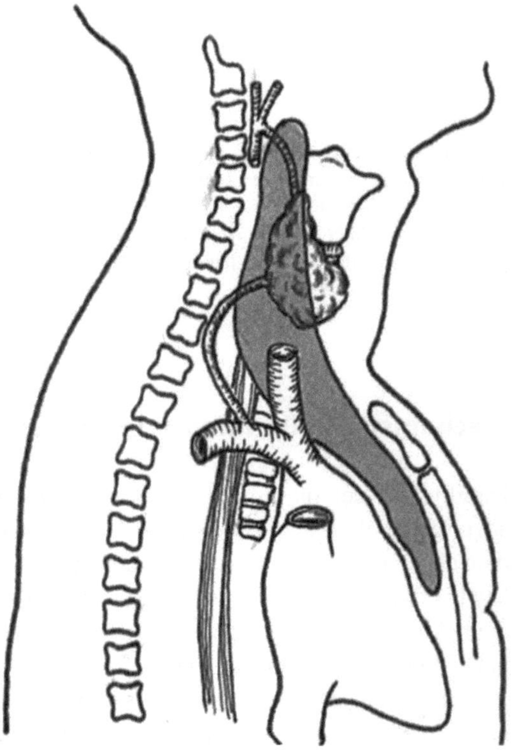

Fig. 10.4 The embryonic migration of the inferior parathyroid gland (P III)-thymus complex results in an extensive area of dispersal of the P III from the angle of the mandible to the pericardium

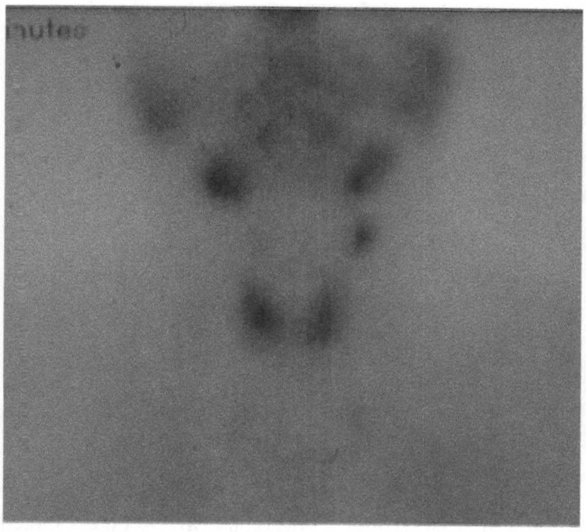

Fig. 10.5 Undescended abnormal left inferior (P III) parathyroid gland identified on 99mTc-sestamibi scintigraphy. At surgery, this gland was found on the antero-medial side of the carotid sheath and was associated with a small amount of thymic tissue. A defect of congenital migration of the parathymus complex was responsible for this high ectopia in the neck

of undescended parathyroid glands would seem to be quite low, less than 1% [3, 9]. Undescended parathyroid adenomas comprise a small, but significant proportion of abnormal glands in patients undergoing reoperations for PHPT. In prominent published series of reoperations for persistent or recurrent HPT the incidence of undescended parathyroid adenomas is up to 7–8% [9–11]. All the factors capable of impeding or arresting the descent of the parathymus result in a deficient migration along the carotid sheath, from the angle of the mandible to the lower pole of the thyroid lobe. Undescended parathyroid glands are located adjacent to the carotid sheath on its antero-medial side with a small amount of associated thymic tissue and parathymic fat. It has been suggested that, in some patients, undescended glands are superior parathyroid glands [12]. These glands are not associated with thymic tissue and are probably PIV lodged in a high position, at the level of the superior thyroid pedicle.

If the PIII are not abandoned by the thymus at the level of the inferior pole of the thyroid, then they are dragged down into the anterior mediastinum to a varying degree, resulting in an ectopic mediastinal location (Fig. 10.6). They are then usually within the thymus, or at the posterior aspect of its capsule, more or less in contact with the great mediastinal vessels. Most of the ectopic PIII, which descend below the level of innominate vein and aortic arch, develop an ectopic arterial blood supply. Generally this is derived from the internal mammary artery. Occasionally the blood supply may come from a thymic artery or a direct branch from the aorta. These low ectopias due to excessive embryologic migration in the anterosuperior mediastinum are observed in 4–5% of cases [3, 8, 13].

Supernumerary Parathyroid Glands and Other Congenital Ectopias

Supernumerary parathyroid glands arise from rests of normal parathyroid tissue when the pharyngeal pouches separate from the pharynx. The incidence of supernumerary glands is far from negligible, since Akerstöm [1] found one or more in 13% of cases in a series of 503 autopsies. This author counted as many as 11 parathyroid glands or fragments of gland in one subject [1]. The continuous growth stimulation in both primary and secondary parathyroid hyperplasia may stimulate the rudiments of parathyroid glands to grow, and many of them may thus appear as proper supernumerary glands. They may be hidden in the perithyroid fatty tissue, usually close to the main gland. They are located most often at the level of the lower poles of the thyroid lobes, in the thyrothymic region and in the thymus itself, but they may also be situated in major ectopic positions. Akerström [1] distinguishes between accessory parathyroid glands containing parathyroid fragments weighing less than 5 mg, usually found very close to the main glands and true supernumerary glands weighing more than 5 mg (average weight of 24 mg) situated apart from the other main glands. These true supernumerary parathyroids are then revealed by tumoral formations developing from them and are responsible for the HPT syndrome. Supernumerary hyperfunctional parathyroid glands have been documented in the pharyngeal structures of the neck [14], within the carotid sheath [1–3, 15], lateral to the jugulocarotid axis [16], in the middle mediastinum, at the level of the aorto-pulmonary

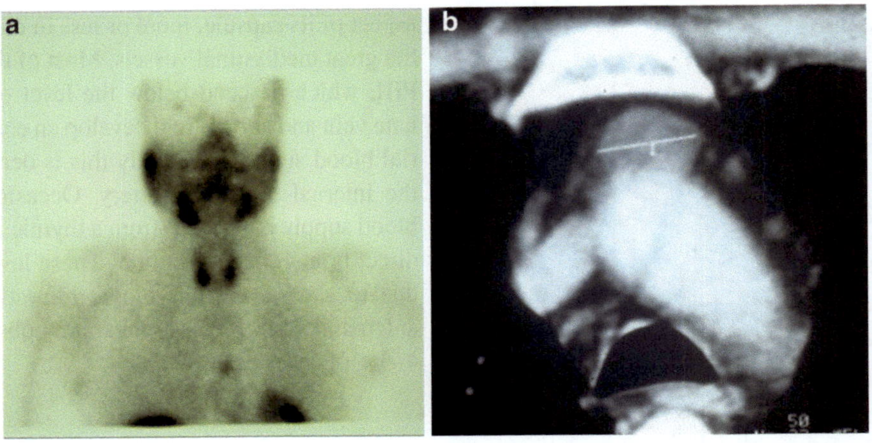

Fig. 10.6 Ectopic mediastinal parathyroid adenoma identified on 99mTc-sestamibi scintigraphy (**a**) and on computed tomography (**b**)

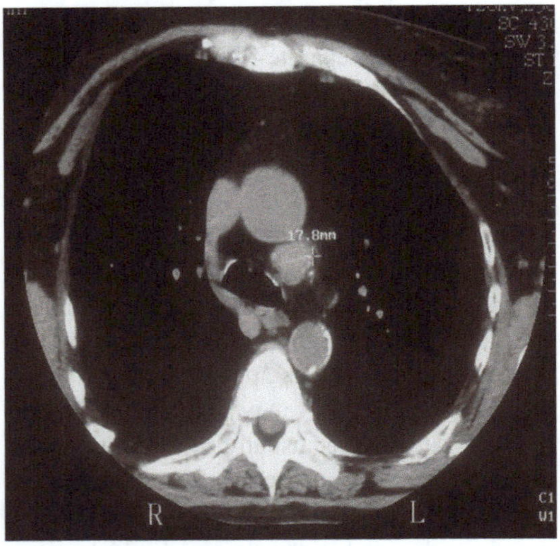

Fig. 10.7 Computed tomography image of a supernumerary ectopic abnormal parathyroid gland located in the aorto-pulmonary window. This patient was reoperated on for persistent hyperparathyroidism. At initial surgery, four normal glands were identified in the neck

window [17], or in association with the vagus nerve [18–21]. The migration of a PIII or a PIV seems very improbable in such cases. The embryologic hypotheses rather suggest a precocious fragmentation of parathyroid tissue and more precisely of the PIV.

Several hypotheses have been proposed to explain the location of parathyroid glands in the aorto-pulmonary window (Fig. 10.7). Based on the observation of Gilmour [15], who noted that PIV is in contact with pericardium in the 3-mm embryo, and those of Frazer [22], who reported that the fourth branchial pouch surrounds the aortic arch on the left side, some parathyroid fragments could separate from the main gland and remain attached to the pericardium. Another hypothesis is in favor of the fragmentation of the PIV. In the 7.5–11-mm embryo, PIV develops close to the sixth branchial artery. If separation of PIV occurs at this stage, some parathyroid fragments would be present near the origin of the future right pulmonary artery, and indeed adenomas located in the aorto-pulmonary window are often found just above or behind the right pulmonary artery and it is often necessary to open the pericardium or to divide the arterial ligament to excise them [17].

Parathyroid tissue and parathyroid adenomas within the vagus nerve have also been described [18–21] (Fig. 10.8). Intravagal parathyroid tissue has been documented in autopsy reports with a frequency rate up to 6% [18]. This leads us to introduce a new concept: the paravagal complex. The vagus nerve is the nerve of the musculature of the fourth and sixth arches. The musculature of the fourth arch is supplied by the superior laryngeal branch of the vagus nerve, and that of the sixth arch by the inferior laryngeal branch or recurrent branch of the vagus nerve. Therefore, the fourth pharyngeal arch is flanked on either

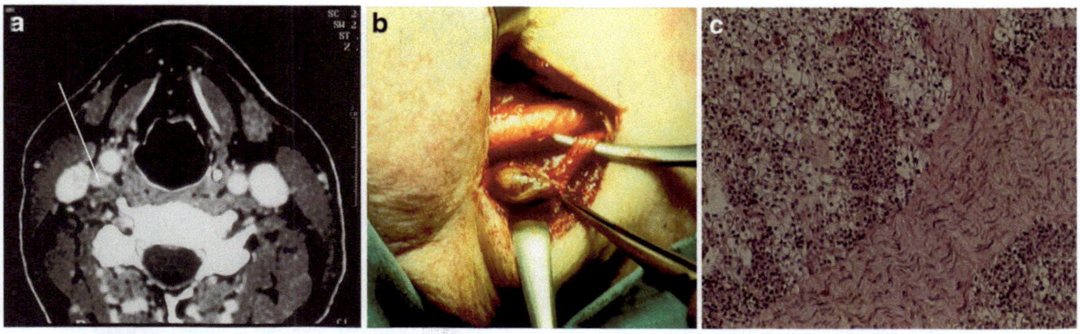

Fig. 10.8 Computed tomography image of a supernumerary abnormal parathyroid gland within the right vagus nerve (**a**) Intraoperative view (**b**) in this case, enucleation of the parathyroid gland from the nerve was not possible and a cephalic portion of the nerve was resected. Microscopic examination shows collection of chief cells within the vagus (**c**)

side by the third and fourth pouches, and the sixth pharyngeal arch is in close contact with the fourth pouch. The close spatial relationship that exists during embryologic development between the sixth arch and the fourth pouch may explain the presence of intravagal parathyroid tissue or the presence of parathyroid tissue in close contact with the vagus nerve and more precisely with the fibers of the inferior laryngeal branch. In our own experience, in 3,478 patients who have undergone parathyroidectomy for HPT, hyperfunctional parathyroid glands within or in close contact with the vagus nerve were only observed at the level of its cervical portion or at the level of its supero mediastinal portion, but never lower than where the inferior laryngeal nerve recurs; that is: on the right side at the level of the right subclavian artery, and on the left side in the aorto-pulmonary window. The concept of the paravagus complex is an additional hypothesis in favor of the fragmentation of the PIV and could explain the location of some parathyroid adenomas in the aorto-pulmonary window.

Acquired Ectopias

As the glands become larger and heavier because of adenomatous or hyperplastic change, they are more likely to shift downward into tissue planes that offer least resistance. This mechanism of migration is more often observed with PIV than with PIII of which the descent appears quite limited, probably because the adjacent anatomic structures are less favorable to gravity-induced displacement.

The PIV, which are relatively constant in their orthotopic site, always migrate in the same direction: posteriorly and towards the posterosuperior mediastinum. They travel against the prevertebral plane, along which they may glide more or less downward. During this course they usually pass behind the trunk of the inferior thyroid artery and remain in very close contact with the esophagus. Whereas 1–4% of the normal P IV is in para—or retroesophageal positions, 40% of the adenomas they develop are found in posterior locations. Usually the tumoral glands are found at the level of the inferior lobes of the thyroid just above the trunk of the inferior thyroid artery. Sometimes, the adenoma is straddled or actually embraced by the artery. In other cases the adenoma is frankly mediastinal, either very posterior, beside or behind the esophagus, or in the tracheoesophageal angle (Fig. 10.9). The lower a PIV, the more posterior it is. In all cases these tumoral glands, even if situated very low down in the posterior mediastinum, retain a cervical blood supply arising from the thyroid system, the origin of their pedicle indicating their initial site. The cervical origin of this vascularisation explains why they can be easily excised through a cervical approach without risk of hemorrhage.

Acquired ectopias of P III are less frequent and more debatable. In practice, the sites of tumoral glands arising from P III are much the same as those of normal glands. Migration occurs towards the anterosuperior mediastinum, the

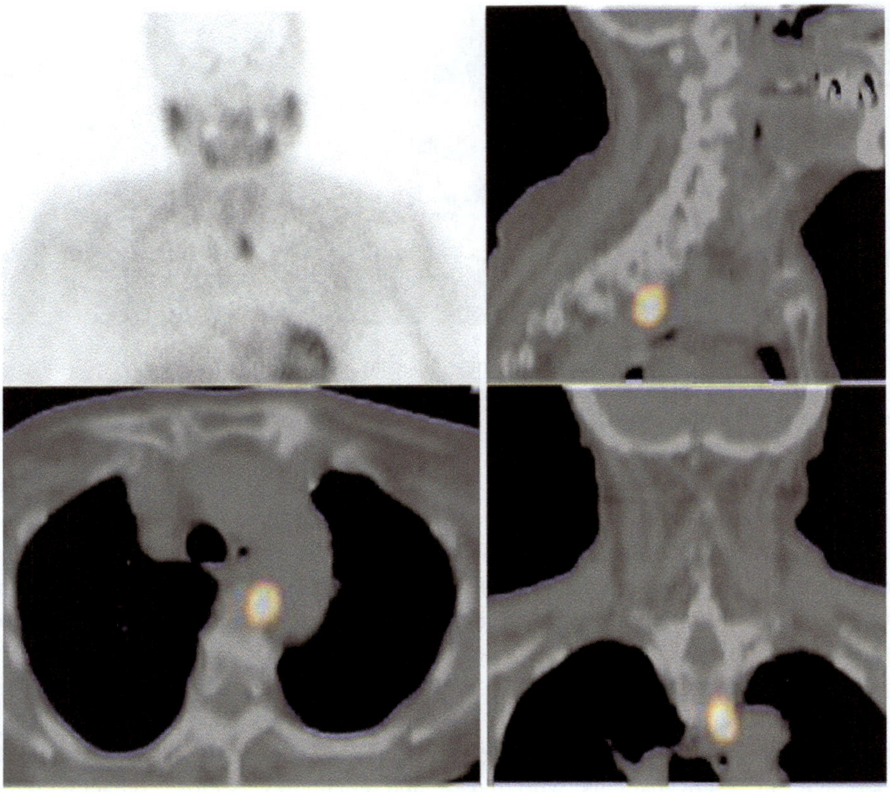

Fig. 10.9 99mTc-sestamibi scintigraphy images of a left superior parathyroid adenoma which has migrated towards the posterosuperior mediastinum by gravity. Planar image finds a left parathyroid adenoma. SPECT images (sagittal, axial, and coronal imaging planes) help in the diagnosis of left paraesophageal location

tumoral gland following the pathway traced by the thyrothymic ligament and the thymus. Nevertheless, this descent is usually limited. More rarely, if the pathologic gland was initially located at the posterolateral part of the lower pole of the thyroid lobe, its hypertrophy may lead to its descent into the posterosuperior mediastinum to acquire a paraesophageal position. But in these cases, unlike the adenomas developed from PIV, the vascular pedicle does not cross the trunk of the inferior thyroid artery.

Surgeons must keep in mind that acquired ectopias may also be due to previous neck surgery: thyroidectomy or unsuccessful parathyroid exploration. In these cases anatomical structures linking the parathyroids to the thyroid are accidentally divided during the initial operation and consequently parathyroids tend to more or less migrate, and acquire sometimes an ectopic site, even when they are not enlarged. Acquired ectopias due to previous surgery are often observed with PIII when they are initially located along the thyrothymic axis; once the thyrothymic ligament has been divided the PIII is dragged down into the superior and anterior mediastinum by the thymus.

Thus, one may distinguish grossly between (Table 10.1):

1. Congenital ectopias, due to abnormal embryologic migration, whether deficient or excessive, and related essentially to PIII,
2. Congenital ectopias due to the development of accessory parathyroid fragments arising from the pharyngotracheal duct when the pharyngeal pouches separate from the pharynx, and related essentially to supernumerary glands, and
3. Acquired ectopias, due to migration affected by gravity, secondary to tumoral pathology, and essentially related to PIV.

Table 10.1 Sites, mechanisms and frequency of major ectopias of hyperfunctional parathyroid glands

Site	Parathyroid	Mechanism	Frequency (%)
Undescended in the neck	P III	Congenital Defect of migration	1
Anterior mediastinum	P III	Congenital Excess of migration	5
Middle mediastinum Aorto-pulmonary window	P V	Congenital Fragmentation and migration	0.25
Posterior mediastinum	P IV	Acquired Migration by gravity	5
Intrathyroid	 P IV P III	Congenital Excess of migration (Unclear)	1.4–3.2

Management of Patients with Ectopic Hyperfunctional Parathyroid Glands

When to Suspect an Ectopic Hyperfunctional Parathyroid Gland?

Not all blind surgical parathyroid explorations are due to a missed ectopic parathyroid adenoma. The diagnosis of PHPT, and particularly in case of suspicion of persistent disease, must be confirmed before any reoperation. It has been estimated that 2–10% of surgical failures may be attributed to an incorrect diagnosis! Today, the diagnosis of PHT can be made with nearly 100% confidence by documenting an increased serum PTH level in a patient with an increased ionized or total calcium. Therefore, all other causes of hypercalcemia and all other causes of PTH elevation must be eliminated [23–25]. A few patients have been documented as having nonparathyroid tumors that produce pure PTH [26].

Not all parathyroid adenomas missed at initial surgery are in ectopic location. In most cases persistent PHPT is due to technical errors during the first operation. It has been estimated that 2/3 of the previously missed abnormal glands are found in their normal site at reoperation.

In case of persistent HPT, an ectopia must be particularly suspected when the previous operation has been performed by an experienced surgeon. The more expert the initial operator, the more probable the ectopia of the missed adenoma. An ectopic mediatinal location must be particularly suspected when four normal glands have been identified in the neck.

An ectopia must be also suspected in patients with virulent forms of HPT such as renal HPT or HPT associated with multiple endocrine neoplasia type I, and more particularly in case of recurrent disease. The continuous growth stimulation in both primary and secondary parathyroid hyperplasia may stimulate the rudiments of parathyroid glands to grow, and many of them may thus appear as proper supernumerary glands. This is observed as well after subtotal resection as after total parathyroidectomy associated with immediate partial transplantation.

Localization of Ectopic Hyperfunctional Parathyroid Glands

For many years bilateral cervical exploration with identification of four glands remained the gold standard in parathyroid surgery, and routine preoperative imaging for initial surgery was considered unnecessary and not cost effective. Indeed, when performed by an experienced endocrine surgeon, the success rate of this procedure was reported to be 95–98% [27]. The failure rate, in most cases related with ectopic glands, not in the neck but located deeply in the mediastinum and virtually inaccessible from the cervical route, was considered too low to justify systematic preoperative imaging. In addition, only invasive localization procedures (angiography and selective venous sampling) were available. Therefore, localization of ectopic parathyroid glands was limited to reoperative cases.

Today, the development and the reported efficacy of non-invasive localization tests have tempted many endocrinologists and many surgeons to order non-invasive techniques on patients undergoing first-time parathyroidectomy. Moreover, more than half the surgeons performing parathyroid surgery now consider that bilateral parathyroid exploration is no longer the only option in patients with HPT. In patients presenting with sporadic PHPT, a focused approach can be proposed when preoperative localization studies are clearly in favor of a solitary adenoma. This explains that today many ectopic hyperfunctional parathyroid glands are identified, more or less incidentally, before initial surgery.

For initial bilateral parathyroid exploration, numerous benefits of successful localization of ectopic parathyroid glands have been reported. Proper localization directs and limits surgical exploration and therefore may reduce surgical failure rate, complication rates and operative time [28]. On the other hand, one should keep in mind that the success of parathyroid operation is above all based on the experience of the surgeon, on a thorough knowledge of the anatomy and on an understanding of the embryological evolution of the glands. The failure rate of an initial cervical exploration performed by an experienced parathyroid surgeon does not exceed 5%. Without any preoperative localization, the experienced parathyroid surgeon is still one of the most sensitive, specific, and cost effective "tool" to identify an ectopic parathyroid gland in the neck or in the mediastinum. Therefore, before initial bilateral cervical exploration, it remains questionable whether the routine use of localization studies is justified and financially sustainable in all cases of PHPT [29].

The clinician must also keep in mind that a negative neck examination does not automatically mean that the adenoma is in an ectopic mediastinal site. Ultrasonography (US) has been shown to have sensitivity and a specificity of 70–85% and 90–95%, respectively [30, 31]. Nevertheless, US sensitivity is highly dependent on the size of the parathyroid gland. US can identify 95% of adenomas that weigh in excess of 1000 mg but fewer than 50% of adenomas weighing less than 200 mg. Other common causes of false-negative US examinations include adenomas associated with multinodular goiter, adenomas obscured by the acoustic shadow of the trachea such as adenomas in the tracheoesophageal groove, or by the acoustic shadow of bone such as adenomas behind the clavicles or sternum. Reported sensitivities of parathyroid scintigraphy for detecting adenomas range from 70 to 100%, mainly depending on gland weights and PTH values [30–32]. False-negative results are attributed to small parathyroid lesions, cystic adenomas after necrosis or cystic degeneration and hyperplastic glands in cases of sporadic or familial multiglandular diseases.

Only an inexpensive, highly sensitive, and highly specific and non-invasive test should be considered for initial surgery [30, 31]. Many authors use routinely US and/or sestamibi scan and consider that other tests are not indicated, even when US and sestamibi are negative.

The problem is different in case of persistent or recurrent HPT. Nearly all authors consider that ultrasonography and sestamibi scan should be performed routinely and are first line in the work-up for any persistent or recurrent HPT [31]. Single-photon emission tomography (SPECT) which provides simultaneous 3D information can be helpful for more precise localization of adenomas in both neck and mediastinum [31–36]. The use of SPECT-CT fusion images is particularly helpful for localizing ectopic glands in the mediastinum [37]. Four-dimensional computed tomography (4D-CT), when available, can be preferred [38].

When US and sestamibi scan are in favor of an ectopic hyperfunctional gland in the neck, there is no need for an additional localization test

When sestamibi scan is in favor of an ectopic mediastinal location, CT or MRI is mandatory to confirm the location and to give additional anatomic information. CT scan and MRI are also indicated in patients in whom both ultrasonography and sestamibi scan have failed and especially when the missing abnormal gland is strongly suspected to be located in the mediastinum. In the mediastinum, (18F)-2-fluorodesoxyglucose-Positron emission tomography (FDG-PET) or 11C-methionine PET have also been proposed [31, 39, 40].

In case of suspicion of an ectopic gland, the surgeon must be aware that the main risk of imaging techniques is a false-positive result. Overall, false-positive results of US vary from 15 to 20%. With sestamibi scan, potential false-positive findings are related to thyroid carcinomas, thymomas, and metastatic or inflammatory lymph nodes. For this reason, in some cases, and more particularly when an ectopic mediastinal site is suspected, additional functional invasive tests may be indicated. In the neck, the diagnosis can be confirmed or rejected by US-directed fine-needle aspiration for parathyroid hormone which is highly sensitive and specific [41, 42]. This test is particularly useful when an intrathyroid parathyroid adenoma is suspected as these adenomas have an ultrasonographic appearance indistinguishable from that of hypoechoic thyroid nodules. PTH determination is more helpful than cytological examination because the sample may be insufficient and because differentiating between parathyroid and thyroid tissue may be difficult.

Invasive procedures, including selective venous sampling (SVS) for PTH as well as selective angiography eventually associated with SVS and QPTH, should be performed only if noninvasive procedures are inconclusive [31, 43–46]. SVS for PTH is a very sensitive test which depends on gland function rather than gland size. The samples must be taken as selectively as possible from the smallest venous branches as to offer a precise gradient map as a guide to the surgeon. At least a twofold gradient of PTH level is required for the diagnosis result to be significant. In the published reports, sensitivity and specificity of the SVS range from 63 to 94.7% and 86 to 100%, respectively [31, 43–46]. Proper parathyroid angiography includes examination of the thyrocervical trunks for glands in lower cervical sites, the carotid arteries and superior thyroid arteries for upper cervical sites, and internal mammary arteries for thymic and mediastinal sites. Parathyroid adenomas appear highly vascularized with an ovoid or round blush. Limit size is 4 mm. Sensitivity approaches 60% [47]. False positives are due to thyroid nodules and enlarged lymph nodes. This is an additional argument to associate angiography with SVS and QPTH. As SVS, parathyroid angiography is a difficult and expensive technique with potentially serious complications.

Finally, one can estimate that when used together, imaging techniques correctly identify ectopic abnormal glands in nearly 95% of cases [31, 48–53].

Indications for Surgery

Once the diagnosis has been confirmed or reconfirmed, the indications for initial operation or reoperation must be discussed. Not every patient needs to be routinely operated on. This is even more true in case of mediastinal location or in case of persistent or recurrent HPT. The risks of doing so, even in the most expert hands, should be assessed and balanced against those of leaving the patient with PHPT. An asymptomatic HPT in an elderly patient may not justify an invasive thoracic operation to excise an ectopic mediastinal adenoma. This may be even more true in case of persistent or recurrent disease. In reoperative surgery, the recurrent nerve paralysis rate and the hypoparathyroidism rate have been reported up to 10% and 35% respectively [53]. Definitive hypoparathyroidism can be a worse disease than mild asymptomatic persistent or recurrent PHPT.

In patients with persistent disease, early reoperations are rarely required. The decision to reoperate should never be made hastily, and with the use of biphosphonates or calcimimetics, acute HPT is no longer life-threatening. When indicated, surgical revision in the first few weeks or months should be avoided because the operation site is still very much affected by inflammatory scarring which considerably hampers dissection. This delay will also allow the surgeon to assemble all the information required for analysis of the case history.

In patients who are not operative or reoperative candidates, one should consider alternative therapeutic modalities versus follow-up of hypercalcemia. FNA can be combined with alcohol ablation of the hyperfunctioning gland, but persistent or recurrent HPT is likely and the procedure has to be repeated [54]. In addition, inferior laryngeal nerve injury has been reported. This nonoperative procedure requires an expert radiologist.

In selected cases, it is possible to do an angiographic embolization of the localized adenoma [55]. This technique is only indicated for poor-risk surgical patients with persistent HPT related with mediastinal parathyroid adenoma.

Initial Surgery for Ectopic Hyperfunctional Parathyroid Glands

The surgical strategy depends on the location of the ectopic gland and its accessibility from a cervical route.

In case of high ectopia in the neck, the surgeon can perform a limited approach, directly focused on the site of the ectopic gland. The exploration of the other glands is not mandatory but the use of intraoperative QPTH assay, to confirm the radicality of the excision, is strongly recommended [56]. This targeted parathyroidectomy must be reserved for patients with sporadic HPT and without suspicion of multiglandular disease on preoperative imaging studies. It is not indicated in patients with familial disease or in case of secondary HPT.

In all other cases, and when the gland is accessible from a cervical route, the approach is the classic cervicotomy with bilateral exploration. Through this access, the operator can explore orthotopic glands and excise not only ectopic glands located in the neck but also most mediastinal adenomas located in the posterior mediastinum, or in the anterior mediastinum above the aortic arch, and notably those which are intrathymic.

In case of ectopic PIV located in the posterior mediastinum, the surgeon should not hesitate to slip his finger as low as possible along the prevertebral plane to explore the posterosuperior mediastinum. If the adenoma is felt, it is progressively extracted by bringing its pedicle upward by progressive traction. In case of ectopic PIII located in the anterior mediastinum, the surgeon must not hesitate to sit at the head of the patient to get a good look down into the superior mediastinum. While exploration of the posterosuperior mediastinum is digital, that of the anterosuperior mediastinum is visual. The thyrothymic ligament is dissected as far as the upper part of the thymus. Since the space between the manubrium and the trachea is very narrow, the exploration must be made by bringing the thymic lobe upward by gentle progressive traction. This maneuver, which may seem somewhat acrobatic, just requires ligation of some veins and may be performed in complete safety. The thymus may thus be exteriorised over 8–10 cm. The elevated thymic lobe must then be dissected since some adenomas are deeply embedded in its substance.

The possibility of an intrathyroid parathyroid adenoma justifies careful palpation of the thyroid parenchyma. Intraoperative ultrasonography may be helpful here. Most of these so-called intrathyroid adenomas are more or less deeply embedded in a crevice of the thyroid parenchyma. Some other adenomas are hidden just under the thyroid capsule and are revealed by a localized discoloration of the surface of the thyroid capsule which darkens progressively during the dissection. Simple incision of the thyroid capsule then allows their dislodgment from their thyroid resting place. True intrathyroidal parathyroid adenomas require thyroid incision. A plane of cleavage always exists between the thyroid and the parathyroid and so, these adenomas can be excised by enucleation. Thyroid excision is the last available procedure. One should be reluctant to perform a blind thyroid lobectomy. Nevertheless, when suspicion remains high but incision has failed to locate the lesion, thyroid lobectomy on the appropriate side is clearly indicated, with unremitting care not to devascularize the normal ipsilateral parathyroid gland.

Initial mediastinal approaches are indicated in the 1–2% of ectopic mediastinal adenomas which are virtually inaccessible from the cervical route. Only adenomas located deep in the anterior mediastinum or in the middle mediastinum require a thoracic approach. The appropriate approach will be dependent upon careful consideration of localizing studies and the depth of the lesion in the mediastinum. Precise localization can allow a less invasive approach than sternal split: anterior extrapleural mini-thoracotomy or left thoracoscopy may be preferable to partial or total sternotomy. In case of initial mediastinal approach, the exploration of the orthotopic cervical glands is not mandatory but the use of intraoperative QPTH assay is strongly recommended.

Reoperation for Ectopic Hyperfunctional Parathyroid Glands

Most often, reoperations for ectopic persistent adenomas are performed after a delay of 4–6 months. Nevertheless, in patients initially operated on without any localization studies, a sestamibi scan may be performed the day after unsuccessful surgery, and if the localization of the missed adenoma is unequivocal, very early reoperation can be proposed. When the ectopic gland is accessible from the same cervical route, reoperation must be performed within 24–72 h to avoid inflammatory tissue. When an ectopic mediastinal location is suspected, sestamibi scan must be associated with CT scan or MRI and a clear topographic diagnosis must be established by convergence of their results. Mediastinal explorations using a thoracic access are too invasive to be recommended when results of localization studies are equivocal.

After reoperation for persistent or recurrent HPT the risk of hypoparathyroidism is considerable and the postoperative morbidity confirms this. Prevention of tetany may require temporary continuous intravenous calcium infusion followed by prolonged oral calcium and vitamin D therapy. Before a reoperation the surgeon is not always aware of how many glands have been left in place. He must keep in mind that the ectopic adenoma may be the only parathyroid gland remaining in the patient. Moreover, some glands—whether or not discovered initially—may have been devitalised by successive dissections. This implies at least the possession of the operative record and the histological report from previous operations. A reading of the histological report should specify the number of glands removed or eventually biopsied. The number, site, and nature of excisions should be systematically compared with those mentioned in the operative record. If biopsy has not been done, the identification of the gland is questionable. Therefore, when the different operative records suggest that more than two glands have been removed or devitalized, immediate autotransplantation using a fragment of the discovered ectopic gland may be proposed. This attitude is debatable since the hyperfunctional grafts may interfere with assessment of the results of parathyroidectomy. Transplantation of hyperfunctional tissue can result in recurrent disease in 7–17% of patients. This explains that most surgeons routinely abstain from immediate autotransplantation at the time of the parathyroidectomy, whatever the nature of the lesions and the number of glands previously removed. In this case, cryopreservation should be arranged. Cryopreservation is an essential adjunct to reoperation for ectopic parathyroid glands. On the one hand, it allows the surgeon to forego immediate autotransplantation, and on the other it allows for secondary autografting in the event of persistent hypoparathyroidism. In cases of postoperative hypocalcemia, delayed autotransplantation based on cryopreserved tissue should not be done too soon. Some hypocalcemic patients do not regain normocalcemia until after 6 months. This is the delay that seems necessary before considering delayed autotransplantation. Grafts may fail to function in 6–50% of transplanted tissue, with failure occurring more frequently when using cryopreserved tissue. However, when there is no available facility for cryopreservation, immediate autotransplantation may be done provided the surgeon is certain that previous successive procedures have led to the excision of at least three normal glands, and the ectopic gland found is an adenoma.

Nearly all reoperations for ectopic glands are performed via an access targeted on the gland preoperatively located. The exploration of the other glands is not performed but intraoperative QPTH monitoring is strongly recommended. Intraoperative ultrasound, gamma probe, frozen section, and recurrent laryngeal nerve monitoring may be useful during these reoperations [56].

To avoid the scar field of previous neck operation(s) two different approaches can be used: the posterolateral approach and the thyrothymic approach. The posterolateral approach or "back-door" approach should be considered when the sought for adenoma has been visualized in a posterocervical site or in a posterosuperior mediastinal site. The previous transverse incision is laterally enlarged on the anterior border of the sternocleidomastoid. The approach is behind the muscles and the thyroid, in a zone that is intact or little affected by the previous operation.

The thyrothymic approach or "front-door" approach should be considered when the sought for adenoma has been visualized in an anterosuperior mediastinal site. A transverse skin incision is used along the previous cervical incision. The infrahyoid muscles are divided as low as possible allowing direct access to the thyrothymic ligaments. This maneuver avoids any dissection between the prethyroid muscles and the thyroid capsule.

Ectopic mediastinal adenomas not accessible from a cervical route require a specific thoracic access. Endoscopic minimally invasive thoracic approaches are more and more often used.

Conclusion

Parathyroid glands in major ectopic locations are rare but may present a considerable challenge to the endocrinologist, the radiologist, and the surgeon. Today, most ectopic hyperfunctional parathyroid glands can be identified prior to surgery by imaging studies or during surgery by an expert parathyroid surgeon. A thorough knowledge of the anatomy and an understanding of the embryonic development of the parathyroid glands are the keys to successful localization and successful resection.

References

1. Akerstrom G, Malmaeus J, Bergstrom R. Surgical anatomy of human parathyroid glands. Surgery. 1984;95:14–21.
2. Gilmour JR. The gross anatomy of the parathyroid glands. J Pathol Bact. 1938;46:133–49.
3. Wang CA. The anatomic basis of parathyroid surgery. Ann Surg. 1976;183:271–5.
4. Wang CA. Hyperfunctioning intra-thyroid parathyroid gland: a potential cause of failure in parathyroid surgery. J R Soc Med. 1981;74:49–51.
5. Wheeler MH, Williams ED, Wade JSH. The hyperfunctioning intrathyroïd parathyroid gland: a potential pitfall in parathyroid surgery. World J Surg. 1987;11:110–4.
6. Feliciano DV. Parathyroid pathology in an intrathyroidal position. Am J Surg. 1992;164:496–500.
7. Bahar G, Feinmesser R, Joshua B, et al. Hyperfunctioning intrathyroid parathyroid gland: a potential cause of failure in parathyroidectomy. Surgery. 2006;39:821–6.
8. Thompson NW, Eckhauser FE, Harness JK. The anatomy of primary hyperparathyroidism. Surgery. 1982;92:814–21.
9. Matsuoka S, Tominaga Y, Uno N, et al. Surgical significance of undescended parathyroid gland in renal hyperparathyroidism. Surgery. 2006;139:815–20.
10. Fraker DL, Doppman JL, Shawker TH, et al. Undescended parathyroid adenoma: an important etiology for failed operations for primary hyperparathyroidism. World J Surg. 1990;14:342–8.
11. Edis AJ, Purnell DC, Van Heerden JA. The undescended parathymus: an occasional cause of failed neck exploration for hyperparathyroidism. Ann Surg. 1979;190:64–8.
12. Simeone DM, Sandelin K, Thompson NW. Undescended superior parathyroid gland: a potential cause of failed cervical exploration for hyperparathyroidism. Surgery. 1995;118:949–56.
13. Wang CA, Gaz RD, Moncure AC. Mediastinal parathyroid exploration: a clinical and pathologic study of 47 cases. World J Surg. 1986;10:687–95.
14. Chan TS, Libutti SK, McCart JA, et al. Persistent primary hyperparathyroïdism caused by adenomas identified in pharyngeal or adjacent structures. World J Surg. 2003;27:675–9.
15. Gilmour JR. The embryology of the parathyroid glands, the thymus and certain associated rudiments. J Pathol Bact. 1937;45:507–26.
16. Udekwu AO, Kaplan EL, Wu TC, et al. Ectopic parathyroid adenoma of the lateral triangle of the neck: report of two cases. Surgery. 1987;101:114–8.
17. Arnault V, Beaulieu A, Lifante JC, et al. Multicenter study of 19 aortopulmonary window parathyroid tumors: the challenge of embryologic origin. World J Surg. 2010;34:2211–6.
18. Lack EE, Delay S, Linnoila RL. Ectopic parathyroid tissue within the vagus nerve. Arch Pathol Lab Med. 1988;112:304–30.
19. Reiling RB, Cady B, Clerkin EP. Aberrant parathyroid adenoma within vagus nerve. Lahey Clin Bull. 1972;21:158–62. denoma Nerve.
20. Doppman JL, Shawker TH, Fraker DL, et al. Parathyroid adenoma within the vagus. AJR Am J Roentgenol. 1994;163:943–5.
21. Takimoto T, Okabe Y, Ito M, et al. Intravagal parathyroid adenoma. J Laryngol Otol. 1989;103:704–6.
22. Frazer JE. The nomenclature of diseased states caused by certain vestigial structures in the neck. Br J Surg. 1923;11:131–6.

23. Lundgren E, Rastad J, Ridefelt P. Long-term effects of parathyroid operation on serum calcium and parathyroid hormone values in sporadic primary hyperparathyroidism. Surgery. 1992;112:1123–9.
24. Nordenstrom E, Westerdahl J, Isaksson A. Patients with elevated serum parathyroid hormone levels after parathyroidectomy showing signs of decreased peripheral parathyroid hormone sensitivity. World J Surg. 2003;27:212–5.
25. Marx SI, Stock JL, Attie MF, et al. Familial hypocalciuric hypercalcemia: recognition among patients referred after unsuccessful parathyroid exploration. Ann Intern Med. 1980;92:351–6.
26. Stremler GH, Budayr AA, Clark OH, et al. Production of parathyroid hormone by a malignant nonparathyroid tumor in a hypercalcemic patient. J Clin Endocrinol Metab. 1993;76:1373–6.
27. Van Heerden JA, Grant CS. Surgical treatment of primary hyperparathyroïdism: an institutional perspective. World J Surg. 1991;15:688–98.
28. Wei JP, Burke GJ. Analysis of savings in operative time for primary hyperparathyroidism using localization with technetium 99m sestamibi scan. Am J Surg. 1995;170:488–91.
29. Schell SR, Dudley NE. Clinical outcomes and fiscal consequences of bilateral neck exploration for primary idiopathic hyperparathyroidism without preoperative radionuclide imaging or minimally invasive techniques. Surgery. 2003;133:32–9.
30. Lumachi F, Ermani M, Basso S. Localization of parathyroid tumours in the minimally invasive era: which technique should be chosen? Population-based analysis of 253 patients undergoing parathyroidectomy and factors affecting parathyroid gland detection. Endocr Relat Cancer. 2001;8:63–9.
31. Mihai R, Simon D, Hellman P. Imaging for primary hyperparathyroidism: an evidence-based analysis. Langenbecks Arch Surg. 2009;394:765–84.
32. Taieb D, Hassad R, Sebag F, et al. Tomoscintigraphy improves the determination of the embryologic origin of parathyroid adenomas, especially in apparently inferior glands: imaging features and surgical implications. J Nucl Med Technol. 2007;35:135–9.
33. Moka D, Voth E, Dietlein M, et al. Technetium 99m-MIBI-SPECT: a highly sensitive diagnostic tool for localization of parathyroid adenomas. Surgery. 2000;128:29–35.
34. Civelek AC, Ozalp E, Donovan P, et al. Prospective evaluation of delayed technetium-99m sestamibi SPECT scintigraphy for preoperative localization of primary hyperparathyroidism. Surgery. 2002;131: 149–57.
35. Lorberboym M, Minski I, Macadziob S, et al. Incremental diagnostic value of preoperative 99mTc-MIBI SPECT in patients with a parathyroid adenoma. J Nucl Med. 2003;44:904–8.
36. Gayed IW, Kim EE, Broussard WF, et al. The value of 99mTc-sestamibi SPECT/CT over conventional SPECT in the evaluation of parathyroid adenomas or hyperplasia. J Nucl Med. 2005;46:248–52.
37. Profanter C, Wetscher GJ, Gabriel M, et al. CT-MIBI image fusion: a new preoperative localisation technique for primary, recurrent and persistent hyperparathyroidism. Surgery. 2004;135:157–62.
38. Rodgers SE, Hunter GJ, Hamberg LM, et al. Improved preoperative planning for directed parathyroidectomy with 4-dimensional computed tomography. Surgery. 2006;140:932–40.
39. Neumann DR, Esselstyn CB, Maclntyre WJ, et al. Comparison of FDG-PET and sestamibi-SPECT in primary hyperparathyroidism. J Nucl Med. 1996;37: 1809–15.
40. Cook GJ, Wong JC, Smellie WJ, et al. [11C] Methionine positron emission tomography for patients with persistent or recurrent hyperparathyroidism after surgery. Eur J Endocrinol. 1998;139:195–7.
41. Sacks BA, Pallotta JA, Cole A, et al. Diagnosis of parathyroid adenomas: efficacy of measuring parathormone levels in needle aspirates of cervical masses. AJR Am J Roentgenol. 1994;163:1223–6.
42. MacFarlane MP, Fraker DL, Shawker TH, et al. Use of preoperative fine-needle aspiration in patients undergoing reoperation for primary hyperparathyroidism. Surgery. 1994;116:959–64.
43. Jones JJ, Brunaud L, Dowd CF, et al. Accuracy of selective venous sampling for intact parathyroid hormone in difficult patients with recurrent or persistent hyperparathyroidism. Surgery. 2002;132:944–50.
44. Chaffanjon PC, Voirin D, Vasdev A, et al. Selective venous sampling in recurrent and persistent hyperparathyroidism: indication, technique, and results. World J Surg. 2004;28:958–61.
45. Eloy JA, Mitty H, Genden EM. Preoperative selective venous sampling for nonlocalising parathyroid adenomas. Thyroid. 2006;16:787–90.
46. Reidel MA, Schilling T, Graf S, et al. Localisation of hyperfunctioning parathyroid glands by selective venous sampling in reoperation for primary or secondary hyperparathyroidism. Surgery. 2006;140:907–13.
47. Miller DL. Pre-operative localization and interventional treatment of parathyroid tumors: when and how? World J Surg. 1991;15:706–15.
48. Shen W, Duren M, Morita E, et al. Reoperation for persistent or recurrent hyperparathyroidism. Arch Surg. 1996;131:861–9.
49. Jaskowiak N, Norton JA, Alexander, et al. A prospective trial evaluating a standard approach to reoperation for missed parathyroid adenoma. Ann Surg. 1996;224:308–22.
50. Thompson GB, Grant CS, Perrier ND, et al. Reoperative parathyroid surgery in the era of sestamibi scanning and intraoperative parathyroid hormone monitoring. Arch Surg. 1999;134:699–704.
51. Yen YWF, Wang TS, Doffek KM, et al. Reoperative parathyroidectomy: an algorithm for imaging and monitoring of intraoperative parathyroid hormone levels that results in a successful focused approach. Surgery. 2008;144:611–21.
52. Hessman O, Stalberg P, Sundin A, et al. High success rate of parathyroid reoperation may be achieved with

improved localisation diagnosis. World J Surg. 2008; 32:774–81.
53. Mihai R, Barczynski M, Iacobone M, et al. Surgical strategy for sporadic primary hyperparathyroidism: an evidence-based approach to surgical strategy, patient selection, and reoperation. Langenbecks Arch Surg. 2009;394:785–98.
54. Harman CR, Grant CS, Hay ID, et al. Indications, technique, and efficacy of alcohol injection of enlarged parathyroid glands in patients with primary hyperparathyroidism. Surgery. 1998;124: 1011–9.
55. McIntyre Jr RC, Kumpe DA, Liechty RD. Reexploration and angiographic ablation for hyperparathyroidism. Arch Surg. 1994;129:499–503.
56. Harrison BJ, Triponez F. Intraoperative adjuncts in surgery for primary hyperparathyroidism. Langenbecks Arch Surg. 2009;394:799–809.

Hyperparathyroidism in Multiple Endocrine Neoplasia

11

Syeda S. Zaidi, Vipul T. Lakhani, and James T. Broome

Abstract

Multiple endocrine neoplasia (MEN) describes a group of syndromes characterized by neoplasms in two or more endocrine organs. Neoplasms can be benign, malignant, and in some cases nonsecretory. To date there are seven MEN syndromes, which includes MEN 1, MEN 2, MEN 4, Carney Complex, McCune–Albright syndrome, Von Hippel–Lindau disease, and neurofibromatosis type 1. This chapter focuses on those syndromes in which primary hyperparathyroidism (PHPT) has been described: MEN 1, MEN 2, and MEN 4 [1]. MEN 1 and MEN 2 are neoplastic syndromes which demonstrate an autosomal dominant inheritance pattern. Due to the unique expression, evaluation, and management of PHPT and the associated endocrine neoplasms in these hereditary syndromes, special discussion on these disorders is deserved.

S.S. Zaidi, MD
Department of Endocrinology and Metabolism, Vanderbilt University Hospital, 1215 21st Avenue South, Suite 8015, MCE, South Tower, Nashville, TN 37232-0475, USA

V.T. Lakhani, MD (✉)
Division of Endocrinology, Department of Medicine, Vanderbilt University School of Medicine, 1215 21st Avenue South, Suite 8015, MCE, South Tower, Nashville, TN 37232, USA
e-mail: vipul.t.lakhani@Vanderbilt.Edu

J.T. Broome, MD
Division of Surgical Oncology/Endocrine Surgery, Department of Surgical Sciences, Vanderbilt University, 597 Preston Research Bldg., 2200 Pierce Ave, Nashville, TN 37232, USA

A.A. Licata and E.V. Lerma (eds.), *Diseases of the Parathyroid Glands*,
DOI 10.1007/978-1-4419-5550-0_11, © Springer Science+Business Media, LLC 2012

Keywords
Multiple endocrine neoplasia • Hyperparathyroidism • Insulinoma • Glucagonoma • VIPoma • GHRHoma • Somatostatinoma and nonfunctional neuroendocrine tumors • Vasoactive intestinal peptide • Hypercalcemia • Carcinoid • Hypogonadism • Galactorrhea • Prolactinoma • Zollinger-Ellison syndrome • Necrolytic migratory erythema • Menin • Mutation • RET codon • Pheochromocytoma

Introduction

Multiple endocrine neoplasia (MEN) describes a group of syndromes characterized by neoplasms in two or more endocrine organs. Neoplasms can be benign, malignant, and in some cases nonsecretory. To date there are seven MEN syndromes, which includes MEN 1, MEN 2, MEN 4, Carney Complex, McCune–Albright syndrome, Von Hippel–Lindau disease, and neurofibromatosis type 1. This chapter focuses on those syndromes in which PHPT has been described: MEN 1, MEN 2, and MEN 4 [1]. MEN 1 and MEN 2 are neoplastic syndromes which demonstrate an autosomal dominant inheritance pattern. Due to the unique expression, evaluation, and management of PHPT and the associated endocrine neoplasms in these hereditary syndromes, special discussion on these disorders is deserved.

MEN 1

Epidemiology

MEN 1 (formerly called Wermer syndrome) causes a multiplicity of endocrine neoplasms. The estimated prevalence of MEN 1 is 0.02–0.2/1,000 [2–4]. However, incomplete clinical identification of the syndrome may be frequent and likely renders this an underestimation of true prevalence. For the clinical diagnosis of MEN 1, a patient must display two of the three main MEN 1-related endocrine tumors [5, 6]: parathyroid adenomas, enteropancreatic endocrine tumors, and pituitary tumors. Familial MEN 1 is an autosomal dominant disorder in which one person in the family has MEN 1 plus at least one first-degree relative with one of the three main MEN-related endocrine tumors [7]. PHPT is the most frequent (>90%) and usually the earliest expression of the MEN 1 syndrome [6, 8, 9]. In MEN 1 patients, pancreatic islet cell tumors are present in 30–80% [10] and consist of gastrinomas, insulinomas, glucagonomas, VIPomas, pancreatic polypeptideomas and other nonfunctioning neuroendocrine tumors of the pancreas. Zollinger-Ellison syndrome (i.e., gastrinoma) is one of the more common pancreatic tumors [11]. Other less common functional tumors include GHRHoma and somatostatinoma. Anterior pituitary tumors consisting of prolactinomas, somatotrophinomas, corticotrophinomas, or nonfunctioning adenomas occur in 30% of patients [9]. Thymic (2%), bronchial (2–4%) or intestinal (10%) carcinoids, lipomas (30%), benign adrenal adenomas (20%), pheochromocytomas (<1%), and thyroid follicular adenomas represent other tumors seen in MEN 1 [3, 7, 12–14].

Several MEN 1 variants with unique expressions have been described. The prolactinoma or Burin variant of MEN 1 combines PHPT (90%) with an unusually high penetrance of prolactinoma (35–65%) and low penetrance of gastrinoma (3–11%) [3, 15, 16]. Carcinoid tumors are also seen more commonly in few the families with this variant [3]. Insulinoma variant of familial MEN 1 has also been reported in some families [17]. In contrast to MEN 2, the genotype–phenotype correlation in MEN 1 families is more heterogeneous.

Hyperparathyroidism in MEN 1

PHPT is the most common endocrinopathy in MEN 1 [3, 14], reaching 90% penetrance by age 35 years [18] and nearly 100% by age 50 years [2, 6, 7, 12, 19, 20]. Rare MEN 1 mutation carriers do not express hyperparathyroidism throughout their life span [3]. Although hyperparathyroidism is the most common presenting endocrinopathy, it may go undiagnosed for years [21]. Parathyroid hyperfunction in this syndrome is virtually always expressed as hyperplasia of all parathyroid glands over the lifetime of the patient with an increased incidence of supernumerary glands (up to 20%) [22, 23]. These supernumerary glands often occur in ectopic locations (e.g., intrathyroidal, intrathymic, or soft tissues of the anterior mediastinum) [8, 18]. Parathyroid hyperplasia can be diffuse, nodular, or asymmetric [24, 25]. It is difficult to establish if a visually normal gland is pathologic or not. The likelihood of finding normal weight glands decreases as the age of the patient increases [14]. For these reasons, the surgical management is distinct and will be reviewed in detail later.

Clinical Presentation

Clinical Presentation of Hyperparathyroidism in MEN 1

PHPT in MEN 1 has an earlier age of onset with cases as early as age 5 having been reported [3, 26]. The average age of onset is 25 years in MEN 1, as compared to 55 years in sporadic hyperparathyroidism [8]. Hyperparathyroidism in MEN 1 exhibits an equal female to male ratio [3, 7, 10], as opposed to sporadic hyperparathyroidism which has ~3:1 female to male ratio. The peak incidence of symptoms in women with MEN 1 is during the third decade of life, whereas the peak incidence in men is during the fourth decade [7, 14]. The symptoms of PHPT are those related to hypercalcemia such as fatigue, polydipsia, polyuria, myalgia, arthralgia, and abdominal pain. Interestingly, only 20–30% of patients with MEN 1 have symptoms [8, 19]. Since calcium serves as a secretagogue for gastrin secretion, uncontrolled hypercalcemia can exacerbate the symptoms of Zollinger-Ellison syndrome, a major cause of morbidity in these patients [27]. Nephrolithiasis, which may be asymptomatic, is found in up to 50% of cases, while osteitis fibrosa cystica is diagnosed in up to 25%. MEN 1-related hyperparathyroidism often occurs at a younger age when bone growth is at its peak, increasing the risk of osteopenia. By the third decade of life, osteopenia affects more than 40% of MEN 1 patients with hyperparathyroidism [28]. Even mild or asymptomatic hypercalcemia can be associated with reduced bone mineral density [28]. If left untreated, this can lead to osteoporosis and increased risk of fracture. Neuropsychiatric manifestations of hyperparathyroidism may affect the MEN 1 patient who is otherwise thought to be asymptomatic. Hyperparathyroidism is believed to affect sleep, cognition, mood, and overall quality of life (Table 11.1).

Clinical Presentation of Other MEN 1-Related Tumors

Gastrinomas are the most common enteropancreatic tumors in MEN 1 and cause abdominal pain, reflux, and diarrhea. Untreated, overproduction of acid can lead to multiple gastrointestinal ulcers in atypical locations and in extreme cases, perforation. Other rare enteropancreatic tumors include insulinoma, glucagonoma, VIPoma, GHRHoma, somatostatinoma, and nonfunctional neuroendocrine tumors. Hypoglycemia is seen in patients with insulinomas. Glucagonoma can cause rash (necrolytic migratory erythema), weight loss, glucose intolerance, and anemia. Vasoactive intestinal

Table 11.1 Expression of primary hyperparathyroidism by syndrome

Feature	Sporadic hyperparathyroidism	MEN 1	MEN 2A
Inheritance	None	Autosomal dominant	Autosomal dominant
Average age of onset	55 years	25 years	>30 years
F:M ratio	3:1	1:1	1:1
Multiplicity	Single ~80% of cases	Multiple	Can be multiple
Other common tumors	None	Pancreatic tumors Pituitary tumors	Medullary thyroid cancer Pheochromocytoma

peptide secreted in VIPoma can cause severe watery diarrhea, hypokalemia, and hypochlorhydria.

The most common pituitary tumor in MEN 1 is a prolactinoma which can present with galactorrhea and hypogonadism. Other rare growth hormone or ACTH-producing tumors can present with acromegaly or Cushing's syndrome, respectively. Nonfunctioning pituitary tumors may present with bitemporal hemianopsia or be found incidentally on imaging.

Carcinoid tumors in MEN 1 typically occur in the thymus, bronchus, stomach, pancreas, or duodenum. They rarely secrete serotonin. They are typically discovered incidentally on imaging, after surgery or when they have widely metastasized.

Laboratory Evaluation

Laboratory Tests for the Diagnosis of Hyperparathyroidism

Diagnosis of hyperparathyroidism is confirmed by finding an elevated albumin-adjusted serum calcium or ionized calcium and inappropriately normal or high concentrations of PTH in the circulation. Other laboratory tests that can be helpful to rule out other conditions are serum phosphate, alkaline phosphatase, 25 OH vitamin D, 24-h urine calcium, and creatinine. It is important that these tests are done in the same blood drawn to ensure clinically relevant results. In patients who have undergone initial total parathyroidectomy with forearm autograft, it is essential to draw levels from the opposite arm if monitoring for recurrence to avoid spuriously elevated PTH levels.

Laboratory Tests for the Diagnosis of Other MEN 1-Related Tumors

Full discussion regarding the laboratory diagnosis of other endocrine tumors associated with MEN 1 is beyond the scope of this chapter. What follows is a cursory look at the basics of the diagnostic workup. Gastrinomas are diagnosed based on elevated fasting serum gastrin levels as well as increased basal gastric acid. When measuring serum gastrin levels it is important that patient is not on acid suppressing medications which can alter the test results. Insulinoma is diagnosed based on performing a 72-h fast which demonstrates inappropriately elevated insulin, proinsulin, and C-peptide levels during hypoglycemia. The diagnosis of VIPoma is based on an elevated serum VIP level and large fasting stool volumes. Elevated glucagon levels and glucose intolerance characterize glucagonomas.

Prolactinomas are diagnosed based on elevated prolactin levels. Acromegaly is diagnosed by demonstrating unsuppressed growth hormone secretion in the setting of glucose loading. Testing of excess cortisol secretion is generally performed with 24-h urine collection for free cortisol. Other commonly used testing for this syndrome includes midnight salivary cortisol testing and 1 mg dexamethasone suppression testing.

Diagnosis

Genetics

MEN 1 is caused by a germline mutation in the *MEN 1* gene [4, 29]. This is a tumor suppressor gene located on chromosome 11 encoding a protein called menin [1, 8, 10]. Approximately 85% of patients with MEN 1 have identifiable mutations in the *MEN 1* gene [30]. Inactivation of the *MEN 1* gene is believed to play a role in parathyroid hyperplasia. Menin is required for transforming growth factor (TGF) beta to inhibit parathyroid cell proliferation [31]. More than 1,100 different germline mutations in *MEN 1* have been reported with no consistent genotype–phenotype correlation [21, 32]. As such the utility of genetic testing is limited for several reasons. The phenotypic expression of the disease is highly variable between individual families sharing the same mutation and even within families with the same mutation. Therefore, prophylactic therapy targeted at the parathyroid, pituitary, or pancreas is not feasible. Therapy is indicated when or if a particular endocrinopathy or nonfunctional tumor arises. The identification of a patient with MEN 1, however, is useful as it guides further evaluation and management. For example, the choice of operative procedure is different if treating

PHPT in sporadic disease as opposed to disease in the setting of MEN 1. Additionally, screening and appropriate management of comorbid endocrinopathies is unique to MEN 1.

Indications for Genetic Testing in MEN 1 and Genetic Counseling

Cancer can be prevented or cured by prophylactic or early treatment in MEN 2 but not in MEN 1. Therefore, genetic testing and genetic counseling have different roles in these two disorders, but in either case genetic counseling should be offered to all patients being considered for genetic testing [1]. Identification of MEN 1 in patients with familial [33] or apparent sporadic hyperparathyroidism helps to guide the management of the disease and to plan the most appropriate operative procedure [4]. The diagnosis of MEN 1 in a patient carries important implications for other family members since MEN 1 is autosomal dominant. First-degree relatives have a 50% risk of inheriting the genetic mutation. Genetic testing is suggested in all young patients <40 years with multiglandular hyperparathyroidism [34], though routine MEN 1 analysis in all patients with hyperparathyroidism is not recommended.

Screening

At this time, there is no consistent genotype–phenotype correlation to direct surveillance for specific tumors in MEN 1. Extensive past medical and family history should be obtained for the identification of previously unrecognized carriers [30]. Detailed family history regarding any family member with nephrolithiasis, high calcium levels, neck surgery, ulcer disease, pancreatic cancer, brain tumor, and infertility should be obtained [4]. Screening for MEN 1 in patients involves detection of tumors by clinical presentation, biochemical testing, and radiologic investigations. Several suggested screening regimens have been proposed for highly likely or genetically confirmed MEN 1 patients. It is suggested [7] that screening is started as early as 5 years for insulinoma and pituitary adenoma with annual serum fasting glucose, insulin levels and prolactin and IGF-1, respectively. Pituitary MRI is also recommended every 3 years. For parathyroid adenoma and hyperparathyroidism, screening begins at age 8 with annual serum calcium and PTH. When the patient reaches age 20, annual serum gastrin levels, gastric acid output, secretin-stimulated gastrin are recommended to screen for gastrinoma. Also at this age, other enteropancreatic tumors are screened for with annual chromogranin-A, glucagon, and proinsulin. CT or MRI of the chest and abdomen is also utilized every 3 years for carcinoid and enteropancreatic tumors. Carcinoids are typically diagnosed on imaging. The biochemical and radiological testing and frequency should be modified based on the specific clinical situation of each patient.

Differential Diagnosis

Diseases in which hyperparathyroidism and hypercalcemia can be seen are hyperparathyroidism-jaw tumor syndrome, familial hypocalciuric hypercalcemia (FHH), neonatal severe hyperparathyroidism, familial hypercalcemia with hypercalciuria, and familial isolated hyperparathyroidism [5, 35].

Imaging Studies

Imaging Studies for Hyperparathyroidism

In patients with sporadic hyperparathyroidism, in which single adenomas are the cause of disease in >80% of cases, the use of preoperative imaging can significantly change the operation performed. But in known MEN 1 patients, the use of extensive preoperative imaging is unlikely to alter the surgical procedure, since bilateral central compartment exploration along with transcervical thymectomy should be performed in all patients. Ultrasound is helpful in evaluating concurrent thyroid pathology and is the preferred preoperative imaging modality.

Localization tests are essential in patients being considered for reoperation for recurrent or persistent hyperparathyroidism to identify the site(s) of disease [12]. Reoperative surgery in the central neck has increased rates of complications specifically with regard to injury to the recurrent laryngeal or external branch of the superior laryngeal nerve. This increased risk makes preoperative localization crucial to minimizing unnecessary dissection and complications. Combination of technetium-99 m sestamibi scintigraphy and ultrasound performed by well-trained operators with up-to-date instruments appear to be the best diagnostic tools for the pre-operative localization of diseased parathyroid glands [36]. Sestamibi scanning detects more than 90% of parathyroid adenomas in patients who have not had surgery but this technique images only about 60% of enlarged glands in multigland parathyroid disease [12, 37]. This technique and contrast-enhanced computed tomographic (CT) imaging have the advantage of being able to identify parathyroid glands in ectopic locations [18, 38, 39]. MIBI subtraction scintigraphy can detect more than 90% of parathyroid adenomas in ectopic locations [40]. Studies have shown that 4D-CT provides significantly greater sensitivity than ultrasonography and sestamibi scans for localization of parathyroid adenomas [41, 42]. Positron emission tomography (PET) with 11 C-methionine has also been successfully used to identify hyperplastic parathyroid glands in patients with primary or secondary hyperparathyroidism. Cost–benefit analyses of these more expensive techniques have not been conducted. Two concordant studies are highly recommended prior to reoperation [18]. Sestamibi and ultrasound are usually the first tests with CT, selective venous sampling, and arteriography [12] reserved for failure of the first two tests. Venous sampling provides not only information about multiple sites of residual parathyroid tissue but also the functional status of parathyroid autografts. It is limited, however, by its lack of anatomic detail giving surgeons only "regions" of increased activity rather than the specific anatomic locations delineated by CT scans or ultrasound.

Imaging Studies for Other MEN 1-Related Tumors

CT scan of the chest, abdomen, and pelvis is useful for the localization of enteropancreatic tumors and carcinoid tumors. Pituitary MRI is the imaging modality of choice for the localization of pituitary tumors.

Treatment

MEN syndromes tend to present with more severe hyperparathyroidism, and assessment of all four glands at initial operation is mandatory. Surgery is the treatment of choice in hyperparathyroidism associated with MEN 1 [43], however, timing for parathyroidectomy remains controversial. Some believe that parathyroidectomy should be delayed since surgery is more complicated than sporadic hyperparathyroidism with slightly higher risks of either persistent or recurrent hyperparathyroidism or postoperative hypoparathyroidism. Others believe that early surgical intervention should be done to prevent complications related to hyperparathyroidism. These complications include decline in bone mineral density, risk of nephrolithiasis, worsening of kidney function, pancreatitis, and worsening of symptoms in patients with gastrinoma [7, 9]. Even mild and asymptomatic hypercalcemia can be associated with reduced bone mineral density. If osteopenia is advanced, it may not be possible to achieve age appropriate bone mineral density in this population, however, successful parathyroidectomy does improve bone mineral density in the majority of patients. Recurrent hyperparathyroidism is more common after parathyroidectomy in MEN 1, further complicating the decision of when to recommend surgery. Given these multiple complexities, collaboration between the endocrinologist and the experienced surgeon is imperative in delivering the most appropriate care for these patients.

Initial Surgery for Hyperparathyroidism

(Please refer to Chap. 20 for further discussion)

Parathyroidectomy should be performed by a skilled surgeon, knowledgeable in the treatment of hyperparathyroidism due to multiple gland hyperplasia and experienced in the identification of ectopic glands. The initial surgery should be extensive, and it is important to identify all diseased parathyroid glands [20]. Confirmation of parathyroid tissue should be obtained from pathology or PTH washings at the time of surgery to minimize the chance of inaccurate identification of the glands. The main goal of surgery is to maintain lifelong eucalcemia while preventing permanent hypocalcemia or recurrent hyperparathyroidism [7]. The indications for surgical intervention for hyperparathyroidism in MEN 1 are similar to those in sporadic PHPT [44]. The criteria usually include significant hypercalcemia (serum calcium >1 mg/dl above the upper limit of normal), nephrolithiasis, osteoporosis, age <50, worsening renal function (creatinine clearance <60 ml/min), or symptomatic gastrinoma [4, 45]. Because surgery is the most effective strategy for preserving bone density in patients with hyperparathyroidism [46], bone density evaluation should play an important role in planning the timing of parathyroid surgery in MEN 1 patients with asymptomatic hyperparathyroidism. Uncontrolled hypercalcemia may exacerbate gastrointestinal symptoms in patients who have co-existent gastrinoma, since calcium acts as a secretagogue for gastrin secretion [27]. For this reason, it is often beneficial to treat the patient's hyperparathyroidism prior to the decision to operate on a patient's gastrinoma.

Total and Subtotal Parathyroidectomy

Since multiple gland hyperplasia is characteristic of MEN 1, four-gland parathyroidectomy with autotransplantation of parathyroid tissue or subtotal parathyroidectomy with removal of 3.5 gland and leaving a parathyroid remnant is recommended [7, 8, 12, 18, 21, 23, 25, 47, 48]. Both approaches should be combined with efforts to exclude supernumerary glands and ectopic parathyroid tissue by including bilateral central neck exploration, resection of fatty tissue from the central neck compartment, and transcervical thymectomy in all patients [5, 47]. The thymus may contain a parathyroid adenoma or potential carcinoid tumor. After total parathyroidectomy, ten to twenty 1-mm pieces of parathyroid tissue are transplanted into individual pockets created in the brachioradialis muscle of the nondominant forearm [47]. Placement in the forearm allows easier, less invasive reoperation should hyperplasia of the autograft become problematic later. For subtotal parathyroidectomy, it is suggested that the largest three of the four parathyroid glands be removed along with transcervical thymectomy. The parathyroid gland of the smallest size is typically left in situ and trimmed to a near-normal size [18] (of no more than 60 mg [47]) to maintain eucalcemia [5]. If the gland to be left in situ is not greater than two times normal size, then it is left undisturbed. The residual parathyroid tissue is marked with a nonabsorbable suture and/or a metallic clip which can be used to attach the gland to the thyroid capsule away from the recurrent laryngeal nerve thereby facilitating reoperative surgery [47]. Great care is taken when performing partial parathyroid resection so as not to seed the local region with hyperplastic cells, resulting in inadvertent parathyroid autografting (parathyromatosis) within the operative bed, sternocleidomastoid muscle, sternothyroid muscle, or wall of the esophagus.

Intraoperative PTH assay may be of some utility in determining the adequacy of or need for subtotal resection of the parathyroid remnant gland. The accuracy of intraoperative PTH for testing residual parathyroid function during surgery in the setting of multiglandular disease is still controversial [49]. Following parathyroidectomy for nonfamilial PHPT, a decrease in the plasma PTH level of >50% from the highest baseline levels indicates an adequate resection of parathyroid tissue [38]. However, significant false-positive rates in patients with MEN 1 have been reported using this cutoff [8, 50]. It has been suggested that more stringent criteria should be applied, such as an 80% reduction in PTH prior to accepting adequate excision of parathyroid tissue in MEN 1 [8, 50, 51]. No specific recommendations are available for the use of this assay because of the limited clinical experience. At this time, the most important surgical adjunct is an experienced surgeon doing a complete initial exploration and resection based on sound clinical judgment and an understanding of the pathophysiology of the syndrome (Table 11.2).

Table 11.2 Comparison of surgical techniques in the management of hyperparathyroidism in MEN 1

	Total parathyroidectomy	Subtotal parathyroidectomy
Number of parathyroid glands removed	4	3.5
Parathyroid gland left in situ	No	Yes ~ 60 mg
Cryopreservation or autotransplantation	Yes	No
Bilateral central neck exploration	Yes	Yes
Transcervical thymectomy	Yes	Yes
Surgery	Initial or reoperative	Initial
Persistent or recurrent hyperparathyroidism	3–30%	14–38%
Postoperative hypoparathyroidism	33%	0–24%

While the initial surgery should be extensive, the surgeon must bear in mind that permanent hypoparathyroidism can often be more difficult to control than mild hyperparathyroidism. Subtotal parathyroidectomy is preferred by some surgeons over total parathyroidectomy to avoid permanent hypoparathyroidism after the initial cervical operation [52].

Hypo and Hyperparathyroidism After the Surgery

Persistent hyperparathyroidism is seen in 14–38% of cases after subtotal parathyroidectomy [20]. Autograft hyperfunction after total parathyroidectomy can result in hypercalcemia in 3–30% of cases [18, 53]. Despite the potential for recurrent hyperparathyroidism, parathyroid autografts are the only way to avoid permanent hypoparathyroidism after a total parathyroidectomy.

The incidence of hypoparathyroidism after the parathyroid surgery is relatively high at 10–25% [20, 22, 54]. Permanent hypocalcemia is seen in 0–24% cases after subtotal parathyroidectomy [5, 25, 55] and approximately one third of patients undergoing total parathyroidectomy with forearm autografting [18, 20, 52]. Hypoparathyroidism is due to ischemic necrosis of parathyroid remnants or grafts or inadequate volumes of viable tissue remaining to support calcium homeostasis. To deal with this high prevalence of postoperative hypoparathyroidism, cryopreservation of parathyroid tissue should be performed whenever facilities are available. Delayed autografting of cryopreserved parathyroid tissue is done for persistent hypocalcaemia, although success rates are highly variable and decrease over time as the tissue is stored.

Reoperative Parathyroid Surgery

There is high rate of recurrent hyperparathyroidism (38–50%) 10 years after initial surgery, depending on the experience of the surgeon. This results in the need for reoperation in many patients with MEN 1 [10, 18, 20, 22, 25, 52, 54, 56]. In comparison, only 2–5% of patients develop recurrence in sporadic PHPT at 10–15 years. Recurrent hyperparathyroidism is more common when diagnosis of MEN 1 is not known at the time of initial surgery and less extensive surgery is performed. The indications of reoperation are similar to the indications for initial neck exploration. In patients requiring reoperation for hyperparathyroidism, surgical cure and long-term control of hypercalcemia are more difficult and less successful than at the time of primary operation [25]. Despite the increased risk of permanent hypocalcemia, it is recommended [5] to perform total parathyroidectomy with autotransplantation in patients requiring reoperation for recurrent hypercalcemia because of the high rate of failure with a lesser procedure [21]. Given the higher rate of overall complications in reoperative neck surgery as well as decreased cure rates, extensive imaging is recommended prior to repeat surgical exploration (see discussion above). Recurrent disease may be caused by the hyperfunctioning parathyroid remnant after subtotal parathyroidectomy, ectopic parathyroid glands in the neck or mediastinum, parathyromatosis from disruption of the gland(s)

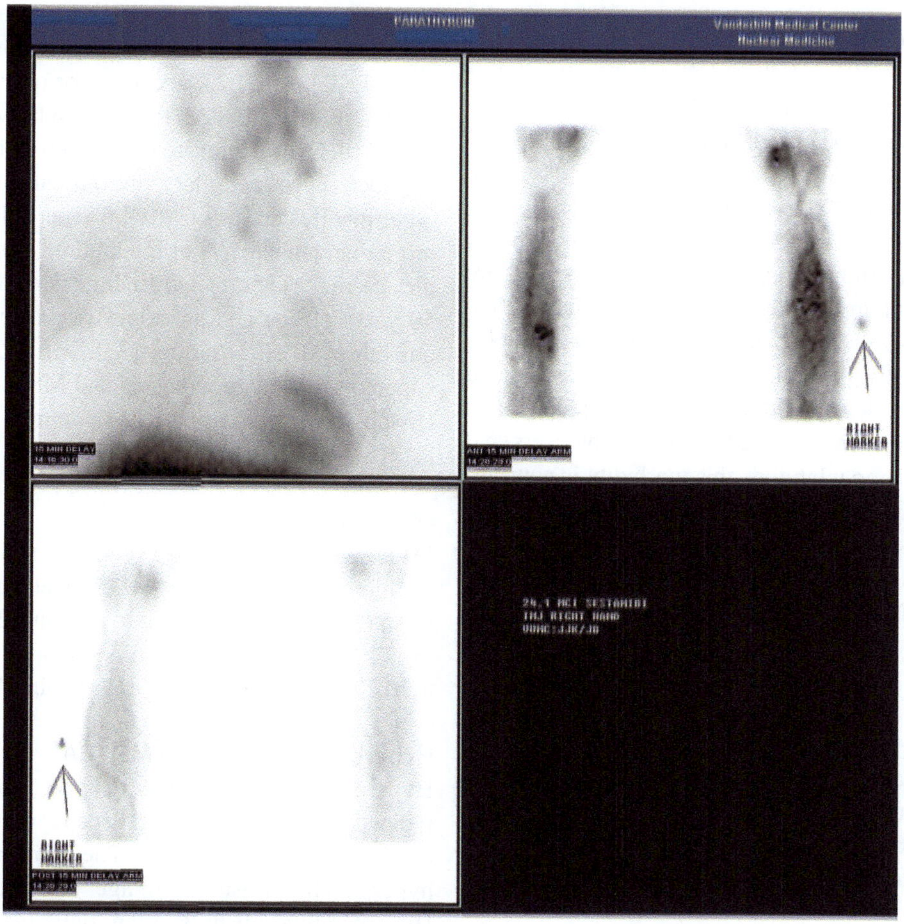

Fig. 11.1 Technetium-99 m Sestamibi scan of a patient with MEN 1 hyperparathyroidism. Patient has already undergone attempted four-gland excision with re-implantation into the left forearm. Anterior images of the forearm demonstrate uptake within the patient's known parathyroid autografts in addition to persistent uptake within the anterior neck

during initial surgery, from a hyperfunctioning forearm graft after total parathyroidectomy or from any combination of the above (Fig. 11.1) [5, 21, 57]. The goal of reoperative surgery is to render the patient eucalcemic for as long as possible while avoiding hypoparathyroidism and permanent dependence of oral supplements to maintain adequate calcium homeostasis.

Medical Management

For those high risk and complicated patients in whom surgery is not an appropriate option, medical management can be considered [43]. Estrogen therapy has shown some modest reduction in serum calcium levels with increased bone density [58]. Also, bisphosphonates have been shown to increase bone mass in patients with PHPT [59, 60]. However, estrogen therapy and bisphosphonates do not address the elevated PTH level [60]. Calcimimetic agents have proven effective in the treatment of patients with hypercalcemia from various causes and will likely play a role in the management of patients with MEN 1 who develop persistent or recurrent hypercalcemia following surgery [61]. Calcimimetic agents normalize serum calcium levels and lower serum levels of PTH [61, 62] but do not significantly affect either bone turnover or BMD [60]. In addition to the medical management of recurrent hypercalcemia, percutaneous alcohol ablation of localized parathyroid glands may have some role in amelioration of symptoms [63].

Prognosis

Patients with MEN 1 have decreased life expectancy, with 50% probability of death by age 50 [14]. One third of deaths in MEN 1 cases are caused by MEN 1 associated malignancies [14, 64, 65] with pancreatic neuroendocrine tumors being the most common cause [14, 64]. Gastrinomas are malignant in 18–60% of cases and have often metastasized before they are detected [27, 66]. Historically, gastrinomas caused excessive acid secretion, leading to perforation, bleeding, and obstruction. With the advent of H2 blockers and proton pump inhibitors, this morbidity is now significantly less [64]. PHPT in MEN 1 almost never progresses to parathyroid carcinoma [5].

Unlike medullary thyroid cancer in MEN 2, the MEN 1-related cancers have no effective prevention (except prophylactic thymectomy for thymic carcinoid). This is mainly because, in MEN 1, the principal cancer host organs (parathyroid, pancreas, pituitary, duodenum, and lungs) are difficult to screen for early tumor occurrences and as yet do not have any effective, low risk prophylactic intervention. Lifelong surveillance as summarized above is important in the continuing care of these patients.

MEN 2

Epidemiology

MEN 2 is characterized by neoplasia involving the thyroid gland (specifically the C cells), the adrenal medulla, the parathyroid glands, or mucosal neuromas [67]. MEN 2 exhibits a high penetrance for medullary thyroid carcinoma (MTC) with greater than 90% of MEN 2 carriers eventually showing evidence for MTC (either from a biopsy proven thyroid nodule or from biochemical testing) [68, 69]. MEN 2 has an estimated prevalence of 2.5 per 100,000 in the general population [5, 70]. MEN 2 has several variants: MEN 2A, familial medullary thyroid cancer (FMTC), MEN 2A with cutaneous lichen amyloidosis, MEN 2A with Hirschsprung's disease and MEN 2B. All MEN 2 variants are caused by germline mutations in the *RET* proto-oncogene [10, 71, 72]. MEN 2A accounts for over 75% of MEN 2 [72], MEN 2B for 5%, and FMTC for 15% [10]. FMTC refers to those families in which members have medullary thyroid cancer but no other manifestations of MEN 2. There should be more than ten carriers in the kindred with multiple carriers or affected members older than 50 years of age and an extensive history ruling out other MEN 2 tumors [73]. MEN 2A with cutaneous lichen amyloidosis and MEN 2A with Hirschsprung's disease are less common variants [5, 10].

MEN 2A

MEN 2A (formerly Sipple syndrome) consists of medullary thyroid cancer (90%), pheochromocytoma (50%), and hyperparathyroidism (20–30%) [5, 7]. Hyperparathyroidism is a feature specific to MEN 2A patients and is not seen in MEN 2B.

Hyperparathyroidism in MEN 2A

Hyperparathyroidism in MEN 2A patients is typically seen after the third decade with median age at 38 years [8, 71]. The penetrance of hyperparathyroidism is age related [71]. Hyperparathyroidism is seen only in 20–30% patients with MEN 2A and is usually asymptomatic or milder than in MEN 1 [74]. PHPT can be one-gland hyperplasia (in 27–48% cases) or multiglandular disease (in 48% cases) [8, 75]. Ectopic (in 43% cases) or supernumerary glands (in 8.6 % cases) are also reported [8, 75]. In 75–80% of patients, the diagnosis of hyperparathyroidism occurs synchronously with the diagnosis of medullary thyroid cancer or pheochromocytoma. In the remainder, PHPT can be detected years after total thyroidectomy performed for MTC [7, 74]. Only 15–25% of the patients develop clinical signs of their disease. In some kindreds, hyperparathyroidism occurs more frequently than others, although it has been noticed that hyperparathyroidism may not occur in those gene carriers who have undergone thyroidectomy at early age [73]. RET codon 634 mutations (in particular, cysteine to arginine amino acid substitution) have been found to be strongly predictive of para-

Table 11.3 Phenotype–genotype correlation in MEN 2A

Hyperparathyroidism	634, 630 most common
Pheochromocytoma	634, 918 up to 50% of patients 609, 611, 618, 620 up to 20% of patients 791, 804 rare
Medullary thyroid cancer	All RET codon mutations are associated with MTC. RET mutations 918, 883 have the most aggressive disease

thyroid involvement [21, 71]. In fact, RET codon 634 mutations have been reported in 73–85% of MEN 2A families with parathyroid disease [71, 74]. PHPT is less common with mutations in codons 609, 611, 618, 620, and 791 but has been reported (Table 11.3).

MEN 2B

MEN 2B is the most aggressive of the MEN 2 variants [7]. MEN 2B consists of medullary thyroid cancer (100%), pheochromocytoma (50%), plus marfanoid habitus, and mucosal and intestinal ganglioneuromatosis [7]. PHPT is not a feature of MEN 2B, though occult parathyroid hyperplasia without hypercalcemia may be recognized by careful microscopic analysis [76].

Clinical Presentation

MEN 2A

Clinical Presentation of Hyperparathyroidism in MEN 2A

Hyperparathyroidism in these patients is usually asymptomatic and milder than that in MEN 1 [74], with some patients showing normal circulating PTH values even if pathologically enlarged parathyroid glands are found at the time of thyroid surgery for MTC [8]. Signs and symptoms of hyperparathyroidism are the same as mentioned above.

Clinical Presentation of Other MEN 2A-Related Tumors

MTC occurs in >90% of MEN 2A patients and generally presents as a neck mass or thyroid nodule.

Pheochromocytoma can occur in 50% of MEN 2A patients and half of them are bilateral. Palpitations, jitteriness, hypertension, headaches, and diaphoresis are seen in these patients. Pheochromocytoma rarely can cause hypercalcemia due to production of parathyroid hormone-related protein (PTHrp) [73].

Cutaneous lichen amyloidosis is a unilateral or bilateral pruritic skin lesion seen on the upper back in some families with MEN 2A [73]. It is typically seen with RET 634 mutation.

MEN 2B

Parathyroid disease does not occur in MEN 2B.

Laboratory Evaluation

Laboratory Tests for the Diagnosis of Hyperparathyroidism

Blood work to diagnose hyperparathyroidism in MEN 2A is identical to the laboratory evaluation done for the diagnosis of hyperparathyroidism in MEN 1.

Laboratory Tests for the Diagnosis of Other MEN 2-Related Tumors

Historically, pentagastrin-stimulated calcitonin levels were checked in screening and diagnosing the disease preoperatively. With the identification of the *RET* proto-oncogene, pentagastrin stimulation has become less necessary. All patients with positive RET mutation should undergo thyroidectomy and the timing is based on the codon mutation [77]. Measurement of plasma calcitonin, which is secreted by the C cells of the thyroid, is especially useful after thyroidectomy since detectable levels indicate the presence of persistent or recurrent MTC, even though it may not be clinically evident [7]. Carcinoembryonic antigen (CEA) is also secreted by the C cells and is a useful tumor marker, though it is not specific to MTC [10, 73].

Pheochromocytoma should be ruled out in all MEN 2 patients prior to any surgical procedure. Poor outcomes are seen in patients with undiagnosed pheochromocytoma who are taken to the operating room for surgical interventions on other tumors. Complications include hypertensive crisis, myocardial infarction, or cerebrovascular accident. Diagnosis of pheochromocytoma is made biochemically and imaging is done for localization purposes. Resting plasma-free metanephrines and normetanephrines are checked for the diagnosis. Other testing includes 24-h urine collections for free catecholamines and metanephrines. It is essential to remember that many common medications can affect the test results and should be avoided or withheld when a patient is being tested. A full discussion of pheochromocytoma evaluation and management is beyond the scope of this chapter.

Diagnosis

Genetics

MEN 2 results from germline mutations in the *Rearranged during Transfection (RET)* proto-oncogene. This gene is located in the centromeric region of chromosome 10 [1, 73, 78]. It encodes for a tyrosine kinase receptor [8]. *RET* mutations can be identified in approximately 97% of patients with MEN 2 [74]. To date just over 50 different missense mutations have been identified which are associated with MEN 2 [78]. It is estimated that up to 7% of patients [7] with apparently sporadic MTC actually harbor germline *RET* mutations. Therefore, all patients with medullary thyroid cancer should be tested for the common *RET* mutations. Each variant of MEN 2 results from a different *RET* gene mutation, with a strong genotype–phenotype correlation [70, 78]. Approximately 85% of patients with MEN 2A and hyperparathyroidism have codon 634 mutation and the remainder have mutations of codon 609, 611, 618, 620, and 630 [70]. MEN 2A with cutaneous lichen amyloidosis is also specifically associated with a mutation at codon 634. More than 95% of MEN 2B patients have mutations in codon 918 and rarely in codon 883 [70] (Table 11.3).

Indications for Genetic Testing in MEN 2 and Genetic Counseling

In contrast to MEN 1, timely diagnosis of MEN 2 plays a major role in decreasing mortality by medullary thyroid cancer. Since medullary thyroid cancer is the most common cause of death in these patients, it is important to identify patients with MEN 2 before medullary thyroid cancer can metastasize. If germline *RET* mutation is identified in the family, genetic counseling and *RET* mutation analysis should be offered to all first-degree relatives [78]. It is also essential to identify pheochromocytoma in these patients before they are taken to the operating room for treatment of hyperparathyroidism or medullary thyroid cancer.

Screening

Guidelines [7] suggest that the decision for prophylactic thyroidectomy in MEN 2 should be based predominantly on the result of *RET* mutation testing, rather than on basal or stimulated calcitonin testing [77, 79]. Several unique features of MEN 2 support this recommendation. Early detection and intervention can alter the clinical course of MTC. Prevention or treatment of early MTC by thyroidectomy is well tolerated even by most infants [80]. Abnormal calcitonin tests to dictate thyroidectomy have 5–10% chance of false-positive results [5]. The *RET* genetic testing has a higher rate of true positives and a lower rate of false negatives and false positives than the calcitonin testing [7]. After surgical resection, calcitonin becomes an integral part of screening for recurrence. *RET* germline mutation analysis is recommended for all first-degree relatives of known MEN 2 patients. *RET* germline mutation testing has replaced calcitonin testing as the basis for carrier diagnosis in MEN 2 families. It reveals *RET* mutation in over 95% of MEN 2 index cases [7]. Because there is a stronger genotype–phenotype correlation between specific codon mutation and neoplasm expression, periodic screening for tumors in MEN 2 carriers is based upon the MEN 2 variants, *RET* mutations and by manifestations in the rest of the family. The combination of greater clinical benefit, fewer total causative mutations, more predictable genotype–phenotype correlation and the ability to perform relatively low risk targeted prophylactic thyroidectomy and adrenalectomy, results in a more widespread application of the *RET* germline mutation analysis over the *MEN 1* germline mutation analysis (Table 11.3).

Differential Diagnosis

Differential of hyperparathyroidism is briefly discussed under the MEN 1 section.

Imaging Studies

Imaging Studies for Hyperparathyroidism in MEN 2

Imaging modalities for localization for parathyroid tumors is the same as discussed in the MEN 1 section. Imaging prior to the initial operation is not necessary although paramount to improving success rates in reoperative cases.

Imaging Studies for Other Tumors Related to MEN 2A and MEN 2B

Thyroid ultrasound is done to evaluate for thyroid nodules and lymph node disease.

Once pheochromocytoma is biochemically diagnosed, CT or MRI of the abdomen or MIGB scanning is performed to localize the disease.

Treatment

The overall experience regarding the surgical approach to hyperparathyroidism in MEN 2 is limited. Although hyperparathyroidism in MEN 2 can be due to multiple gland hyperplasia, the rate of four-gland hyperplasia is not as high as MEN 1 and a less radical approach is suggested. Hyperparathyroidism in MEN 2 is less frequently expressed and involves all four parathyroid glands in less than 50% of cases. Hypercalcemia is often milder and recurrent hyperparathyroidism after initial surgery is less frequent than in MEN 1. A conservative approach encompassing identification of all four parathyroid glands with excision reserved for only those visually enlarged glands without transcervical thymectomy is recommended [7, 8, 25, 74]. Subtotal parathyroidectomy is the treatment option for cases with more severe hypercalcemia or hyperplasia evident at the time of four-gland exploration. There is no role at this time for the use of minimally invasive/guided parathyroidectomy techniques in MEN 2.

Rarely a pheochromocytoma can cause hypercalcemia by production of PTHrp [73]. Biochemical analysis should demonstrate elevated calcium, normal (or suppressed) PTH levels with elevated levels of PTHrp in the serum. The surgeon should rule-out a functional pheochromocytoma prior to either thyroidectomy or parathyroidectomy in MEN 2 patients. If a pheochromocytoma is identified, it is treated with premedication and surgical excision prior to parathyroidectomy.

Timing of prophylactic thyroidectomy is dependent on the specific RET mutation and typically is performed before age 6 months in MEN 2B and before age 5 years in MEN 2A [7, 77]. Policies about central lymph node dissection at initial thyroidectomy are controversial and may differ among the MEN 2 variants. During thyroidectomy for patients with MEN 2A, it is important to evaluate the parathyroid glands, because they may be enlarged even though preoperative serum calcium levels are normal [7]. At the present moment, prophylactic parathyroidectomy of morphologically normal parathyroid glands at the time of thyroidectomy for medullary thyroid cancer is not justified [8]; however, parathyroidectomy can be done if the patient is symptomatic or enlarged parathyroid glands are seen at the time of surgery.

Prognosis

All variants of MEN 2 have medullary thyroid cancer, which is the cause of mortality in 15–25% of all cases with MEN 2 [5]. Morbidity is more severe and mortality is earlier in MEN 2B than MEN 2A. The two major comorbid MEN 2B conditions are MTC and intestinal ganglioneuromatosis. MEN 2 variants differ in aggressiveness of MTC with MEN 2B being the most aggressive, followed by MEN 2A, and then by FMTC.

MEN 4

A new MEN syndrome has been identified in animals and humans with phenotypic overlap of both MEN 1 and MEN 2. It consists of bilateral pheochromocytomas, parathyroid adenomas, multifocal thyroid C-cell hyperplasia, paragangliomas, and endocrine pancreatic hyperplasia. Only a few cases have been identified [8]. Germline mutations in the tumor suppressor gene CDKN1B, encoding for cyclin-dependent kinase inhibitor p27 is the cause [81]. Little is known about this newly described syndrome limiting our clinical knowledge of prognosis or treatment options.

References

1. Marx SJ. Molecular genetics of multiple endocrine neoplasia types 1 and 2. Nat Rev Cancer. 2005;5(5):367–75.
2. Brandi ML, Marx SJ, Aurbach GD, Fitzpatrick LA. Familial multiple endocrine neoplasia type I: a new look at pathophysiology. Endocr Rev. 1987;8(4):391–405.
3. Marx S. Multiple Endocrine Neoplasia type 1. The parathyroids: basic and clinical concepts. Academic Press: San Diego; 2001. p. 535–84.
4. Glascock MJ, Carty SE. Multiple endocrine neoplasia type 1: fresh perspective on clinical features and penetrance. Surg Oncol. 2002;11(3):143–50.
5. Malone JP, Srivastava A, Khardori R. Hyperparathyroidism and multiple endocrine neoplasia. Otolaryngol Clin North Am. 2004;37(4):715–36. viii.
6. Marx S. Multiple endocrine neoplasia type 1. In: Vogelstein B, Kinzler KW, editors. Genetics basis of human cancer. 1st ed. New York: McGraw Hill; 1998. p. 489–506.
7. Brandi ML, Gagel RF, Angeli A, Bilezikian JP, Beck-Peccoz P, Bordi C, Conte-Devolx B, Falchetti A, Gheri RG, Libroia A, Lips CJ, Lombardi G, Mannelli M, Pacini F, Ponder BA, Raue F, Skogseid B, Tamburrano G, Thakker RV, Thompson NW, Tomassetti P, Tonelli F, Wells Jr SA, Marx SJ. Guidelines for diagnosis and therapy of MEN type 1 and type 2. J Clin Endocrinol Metab. 2001;86(12):5658–71.
8. Tonelli F, Marcucci T, Giudici F, Falchetti A, Brandi ML. Surgical approach in hereditary hyperparathyroidism. Endocr J. 2009;56(7):827–41.
9. Benson L, Ljunghall S, Akerstrom G, Oberg K. Hyperparathyroidism presenting as the first lesion in multiple endocrine neoplasia type 1. Am J Med. 1987;82(4):731–7.
10. Lakhani VT, You YN, Wells SA. The multiple endocrine neoplasia syndromes. Annu Rev Med. 2007;58:253–65.
11. Alzahrani AS, Al-Khaldi N, Shi Y, Al-Rijjal RA, Zou M, Baitei EY, Amin T. Diagnosis by serendipity: Cushing syndrome attributable to cortisol-producing adrenal adenoma as the initial manifestation of multiple endocrine neoplasia type 1 due to a rare splicing site MEN1 gene mutation. Endocr Pract. 2008;14(5):595–602.
12. Marx S, Spiegel AM, Skarulis MC, Doppman JL, Collins FS, Liotta LA. Multiple endocrine neoplasia type 1: clinical and genetic topics. Ann Intern Med. 1998;129(6):484–94.
13. Thakker RV. Multiple endocrine neoplasia type 1. Endocrinol Metab Clin North Am. 2000;29(3): 541–67.
14. Doherty GM. Multiple endocrine neoplasia type 1. J Surg Oncol. 2005;89(3):143–50.
15. Hershon KS, Kelly WA, Shaw CM, Schwartz R, Bierman EL. Prolactinomas as part of the multiple endocrine neoplastic syndrome type 1. Am J Med. 1983;74(4):713–20.
16. Bear JC, Briones-Urbina R, Fahey JF, Farid NR. Variant multiple endocrine neoplasia I (MEN IBurin): further studies and non-linkage to HLA. Hum Hered. 1985;35(1):15–20.
17. Marx SJ, Spiegel AM, Levine MA, Rizzoli RE, Lasker RD, Santora AC, Downs Jr RW, Aurbach GD. Familial hypocalciuric hypercalcemia: the relation to primary parathyroid hyperplasia. N Engl J Med. 1982;307(7):416–26.
18. Lambert LA, Shapiro SE, Lee JE, Perrier ND, Truong M, Wallace MJ, Hoff AO, Gagel RF, Evans DB. Surgical treatment of hyperparathyroidism in patients with multiple endocrine neoplasia type 1. Arch Surg. 2005;140(4):374–82.
19. Lamers CB, Froeling PG. Clinical significance of hyperparathyroidism in familial multiple endocrine adenomatosis type I (MEA I). Am J Med. 1979;66(3):422–4.
20. Rizzoli R, Green III J, Marx SJ. Primary hyperparathyroidism in familial multiple endocrine neoplasia type I. Long-term follow-up of serum calcium levels after parathyroidectomy. Am J Med. 1985;78(3):467–74.
21. Evans DB, Rich TA, Cote GJ. Surgical management of familial hyperparathyroidism. Ann Surg Oncol. 2007;14(5):1525–7.

22. Hellman P, Skogseid B, Oberg K, Juhlin C, Akerstrom G, Rastad J. Primary and reoperative parathyroid operations in hyperparathyroidism of multiple endocrine neoplasia type 1. Surgery. 1998;124(6):993–9.
23. Tonelli F, Marcucci T, Fratini G, Tommasi MS, Falchetti A, Brandi ML. Is total parathyroidectomy the treatment of choice for hyperparathyroidism in multiple endocrine neoplasia type 1? Ann Surg. 2007;246(6):1075–82.
24. Marx SJ, Menczel J, Campbell G, Aurbach GD, Spiegel AM, Norton JA. Heterogeneous size of the parathyroid glands in familial multiple endocrine neoplasia type 1. Clin Endocrinol (Oxf). 1991;35(6): 521–6.
25. O'Riordain DS, O'Brien T, Grant CS, Weaver A, Gharib H, van Heerden JA. Surgical management of primary hyperparathyroidism in multiple endocrine neoplasia types 1 and 2. Surgery. 1993;114(6):1031–7. discussion 1037–9.
26. Stratakis CA, Schussheim DH, Freedman SM, Keil MF, Pack SD, Agarwal SK, Skarulis MC, Weil RJ, Lubensky IA, Zhuang Z, Oldfield EH, Marx SJ. Pituitary macroadenoma in a 5-year-old: an early expression of multiple endocrine neoplasia type 1. J Clin Endocrinol Metab. 2000;85(12):4776–80.
27. Jensen RT. Management of the Zollinger-Ellison syndrome in patients with multiple endocrine neoplasia type 1. J Intern Med. 1998;243(6):477–88.
28. Burgess JR, David R, Greenaway TM, Parameswaran V, Shepherd JJ. Osteoporosis in multiple endocrine neoplasia type 1: severity, clinical significance, relationship to primary hyperparathyroidism, and response to parathyroidectomy. Arch Surg. 1999;134(10):1119–23.
29. Larsson C, Skogseid B, Oberg K, Nakamura Y, Nordenskjold M. Multiple endocrine neoplasia type 1 gene maps to chromosome 11 and is lost in insulinoma. Nature. 1988;332(6159):85–7.
30. Yip L, Ogilvie JB, Challinor SM, Salata RA, Thull DL, Yim JH, Carty SE. Identification of multiple endocrine neoplasia type 1 in patients with apparent sporadic primary hyperparathyroidism. Surgery. 2008;144(6):1002–6. discussion 1006–7.
31. Davenport C, Agha A. The role of menin in parathyroid tumorigenesis. Adv Exp Med Biol. 2009;668: 79–86.
32. Lemos MC, Thakker RV. Multiple endocrine neoplasia type 1 (MEN1): analysis of 1336 mutations reported in the first decade following identification of the gene. Hum Mutat. 2008;29(1):22–32.
33. Cetani F, Pardi E, Ambrogini E, Lemmi M, Borsari S, Cianferotti L, Vignali E, Viacava P, Berti P, Mariotti S, Pinchera A, Marcocci C. Genetic analyses in familial isolated hyperparathyroidism: implication for clinical assessment and surgical management. Clin Endocrinol (Oxf). 2006;64(2):146–52.
34. Skandarajah A, Barlier A, Morlet-Barlat N, Sebag F, Enjalbert A, Conte-Devolx B, Henry JF. Should routine analysis of the MEN1 gene be performed in all patients with primary hyperparathyroidism under 40 years of age? World J Surg. 2010;34(6):1294–8.
35. DeLellis RA, Mazzaglia P, Mangray S. Primary hyperparathyroidism: a current perspective. Arch Pathol Lab Med. 2008;132(8):1251–62.
36. De Feo ML, Colagrande S, Biagini C, Tonarelli A, Bisi G, Vaggelli L, Borrelli D, Cicchi P, Tonelli F, Amorosi A, Serio M, Brandi ML. Parathyroid glands: combination of (99 m)Tc MIBI scintigraphy and US for demonstration of parathyroid glands and nodules. Radiology. 2000;214(2):393–402.
37. Johnston LB, Carroll MJ, Britton KE, Lowe DG, Shand W, Besser GM, Grossman AB. The accuracy of parathyroid gland localization in primary hyperparathyroidism using sestamibi radionuclide imaging. J Clin Endocrinol Metab. 1996;81(1):346–52.
38. Tonelli F, Spini S, Tommasi M, Gabbrielli G, Amorosi A, Brocchi A, Brandi ML. Intraoperative parathormone measurement in patients with multiple endocrine neoplasia type I syndrome and hyperparathyroidism. World J Surg. 2000;24(5):556–62. discussion 562–53.
39. Weber AL, Randolph G, Aksoy FG. The thyroid and parathyroid glands. CT and MR imaging and correlation with pathology and clinical findings. Radiol Clin North Am. 2000;38(5):1105–29.
40. Doppman JL. Preoperative localization of parathyroid tissue in primary hyperparathyroidism. The parathyroids: basic and clinical concepts. San Diego: Academic Press; 2001. p. 475–86.
41. McHenry CR. Four-dimensional computed tomography permits preoperative planning for directed parathyroidectomy. Surgery. 2006;140(6):942.
42. Rodgers SE, Hunter GJ, Hamberg LM, Schellingerhout D, Doherty DB, Ayers GD, Shapiro SE, Edeiken BS, Truong MT, Evans DB, Lee JE, Perrier ND. Improved preoperative planning for directed parathyroidectomy with 4-dimensional computed tomography. Surgery. 2006;140(6):932–40. discussion 940–31.
43. Bilezikian JP, Khan AA, Potts Jr JT. Guidelines for the management of asymptomatic primary hyperparathyroidism: summary statement from the third international workshop. J Clin Endocrinol Metab. 2009;94(2):335–9.
44. Bilezikian JP, Potts Jr JT, Fuleihan GH, Kleerekoper M, Neer R, Peacock M, Rastad J, Silverberg SJ, Udelsman R, Wells SA. Summary statement from a workshop on asymptomatic primary hyperparathyroidism: a perspective for the 21st century. J Clin Endocrinol Metab. 2002;87(12):5353–61.
45. Silverberg SJ, Lewiecki EM, Mosekilde L, Peacock M, Rubin MR. Presentation of asymptomatic primary hyperparathyroidism: proceedings of the third international workshop. J Clin Endocrinol Metab. 2009;94(2):351–65.
46. Udelsman R, Pasieka JL, Sturgeon C, Young JE, Clark OH. Surgery for asymptomatic primary hyperparathyroidism: proceedings of the third international workshop. J Clin Endocrinol Metab. 2009;94(2):366–72.
47. Hubbard JG, Sebag F, Maweja S, Henry JF. Primary hyperparathyroidism in MEN 1–how radical should surgery be? Langenbecks Arch Surg. 2002;386(8):553–7.

48. Hubbard JG, Sebag F, Maweja S, Henry JF. Subtotal parathyroidectomy as an adequate treatment for primary hyperparathyroidism in multiple endocrine neoplasia type 1. Arch Surg. 2006;141(3):235–9.
49. Pellitteri PK. The role of intraoperative measurement of parathyroid hormone in parathyroid surgery. ORL J Otorhinolaryngol Relat Spec. 2008;70(5):319–30.
50. Clerici T, Brandle M, Lange J, Doherty GM, Gauger PG. Impact of intraoperative parathyroid hormone monitoring on the prediction of multiglandular parathyroid disease. World J Surg. 2004;28(2):187–92.
51. Thompson GB, Grant CS, Perrier ND, Harman R, Hodgson SF, Ilstrup D, van Heerden JA. Reoperative parathyroid surgery in the era of sestamibi scanning and intraoperative parathyroid hormone monitoring. Arch Surg. 1999;134(7):699–704. discussion 704–695.
52. Elaraj DM, Skarulis MC, Libutti SK, Norton JA, Bartlett DL, Pingpank JF, Gibril F, Weinstein LS, Jensen RT, Marx SJ, Alexander HR. Results of initial operation for hyperparathyroidism in patients with multiple endocrine neoplasia type 1. Surgery. 2003;134(6):858–64. discussion 864–5.
53. Demeter JG, De Jong SA, Lawrence AM, Paloyan E. Recurrent hyperparathyroidism due to parathyroid autografts: incidence, presentation, and management. Am Surg. 1993;59(3):178–81.
54. Burgess JR, David R, Parameswaran V, Greenaway TM, Shepherd JJ. The outcome of subtotal parathyroidectomy for the treatment of hyperparathyroidism in multiple endocrine neoplasia type 1. Arch Surg. 1998;133(2):126–9.
55. Goudet P, Cougard P, Verges B, Murat A, Carnaille B, Calender A, Faivre J, Proye C. Hyperparathyroidism in multiple endocrine neoplasia type I: surgical trends and results of a 256-patient series from Groupe D'etude des Neoplasies Endocriniennes Multiples Study Group. World J Surg. 2001;25(7):886–90.
56. Gagel RF. Multiple endocrine neoplasia. Williams textbook of endocronology. 11th ed. Philadelphia, PA: Saunders; 2008. 1705–46.
57. Brandi ML, Aurbach GD, Fitzpatrick LA, Quarto R, Spiegel AM, Bliziotes MM, Norton JA, Doppman JL, Marx SJ. Parathyroid mitogenic activity in plasma from patients with familial multiple endocrine neoplasia type 1. N Engl J Med. 1986;314(20):1287–93.
58. Selby PL, Peacock M. Ethinyl estradiol and norethindrone in the treatment of primary hyperparathyroidism in postmenopausal women. N Engl J Med. 1986;314(23):1481–5.
59. Khan AA, Bilezikian JP, Kung AW, Ahmed MM, Dubois SJ, Ho AY, Schussheim D, Rubin MR, Shaikh AM, Silverberg SJ, Standish TI, Syed Z, Syed ZA. Alendronate in primary hyperparathyroidism: a double-blind, randomized, placebo-controlled trial. J Clin Endocrinol Metab. 2004;89(7):3319–25.
60. Khan A, Grey A, Shoback D. Medical management of asymptomatic primary hyperparathyroidism: proceedings of the third international workshop. J Clin Endocrinol Metab. 2009;94(2):373–81.
61. Silverberg SJ, Bone III HG, Marriott TB, Locker FG, Thys-Jacobs S, Dziem G, Kaatz S, Sanguinetti EL, Bilezikian JP. Short-term inhibition of parathyroid hormone secretion by a calcium-receptor agonist in patients with primary hyperparathyroidism. N Engl J Med. 1997;337(21):1506–10.
62. Shoback DM, Bilezikian JP, Turner SA, McCary LC, Guo MD, Peacock M. The calcimimetic cinacalcet normalizes serum calcium in subjects with primary hyperparathyroidism. J Clin Endocrinol Metab. 2003;88(12):5644–9.
63. Harman CR, Grant CS, Hay ID, Hurley DL, van Heerden JA, Thompson GB, Reading CC, Charboneau JW. Indications, technique, and efficacy of alcohol injection of enlarged parathyroid glands in patients with primary hyperparathyroidism. Surgery. 1998;124(6):1011–9. discussion 1019–20.
64. Doherty GM, Olson JA, Frisella MM, Lairmore TC, Wells Jr SA, Norton JA. Lethality of multiple endocrine neoplasia type I. World J Surg. 1998;22(6):581–6. discussion 586–7.
65. Dean PG, van Heerden JA, Farley DR, Thompson GB, Grant CS, Harmsen WS, Ilstrup DM. Are patients with multiple endocrine neoplasia type I prone to premature death? World J Surg. 2000;24(11):1437–41.
66. Lowney JK, Frisella MM, Lairmore TC, Doherty GM. Pancreatic islet cell tumor metastasis in multiple endocrine neoplasia type 1: correlation with primary tumor size. Surgery. 1998;124(6):1043–8. discussion 1048–9.
67. Gimm O. Multiple endocrine neoplasia type 2. In: DeLellis R, Lloyd R, Heitz P, Eng C, editors. Pathology and genetics of tumors of endocrine organs. 1st ed. Lyon: IARC Press; 2004. p. 211–7.
68. Ponder BA, Ponder MA, Coffey R, Pembrey ME, Gagel RF, Telenius-Berg M, Semple P, Easton DF. Risk estimation and screening in families of patients with medullary thyroid carcinoma. Lancet. 1988; 1(8582):397–401.
69. Easton DF, Ponder MA, Cummings T, Gagel RF, Hansen HH, Reichlin S, Tashjian Jr AH, Telenius-Berg M, Ponder BA. The clinical and screening age-at-onset distribution for the MEN-2 syndrome. Am J Hum Genet. 1989;44(2):208–15.
70. Raue F, Frank-Raue K. Genotype–phenotype relationship in multiple endocrine neoplasia type 2. implications for clinical management. Hormones (Athens). 2009;8(1):23–8.
71. Schuffenecker I, Virally-Monod M, Brohet R, Goldgar D, Conte-Devolx B, Leclerc L, Chabre O, Boneu A, Caron J, Houdent C, Modigliani E, Rohmer V, Schlumberger M, Eng C, Guillausseau PJ, Lenoir GM. Risk and penetrance of primary hyperparathyroidism in multiple endocrine neoplasia type 2A families with mutations at codon 634 of the RET proto-oncogene. Groupe D'etude des Tumeurs a Calcitonine. J Clin Endocrinol Metab. 1998;83(2):487–91.
72. Ponder BA. Multiple endocrine neolasia type 2. The metabolic and molecular bases of inherited disease. New York: McGraw Hill; 2001. 931–42.

73. Gagel RF. Multiple endocrine neoplasia type 2 The parathyroids: basic and clinical concepts. San Diego: Academic press; 2001. 585–600.
74. Kraimps JL, Denizot A, Carnaille B, Henry JF, Proye C, Bacourt F, Sarfati E, Dupond JL, Maes B, Travagli JP, Boneu A, Roger P, Houdent C, Barbier J, Modigliani E. Primary hyperparathyroidism in multiple endocrine neoplasia type IIa: retrospective French multicentric study. Groupe d'Etude des Tumeurs a Calcitonine (GETC, French Calcitonin Tumors Study Group), French Association of Endocrine Surgeons. World J Surg. 1996;20(7):808–12. discussion 812–3.
75. Herfarth KK, Bartsch D, Doherty GM, Wells Jr SA, Lairmore TC. Surgical management of hyperparathyroidism in patients with multiple endocrine neoplasia type 2A. Surgery. 1996;120(6):966–73. discussion 973–4.
76. Carney JA, Roth SI, Heath III H, Sizemore GW, Hayles AB. The parathyroid glands in multiple endocrine neoplasia type 2b. Am J Pathol. 1980;99(2):387–98.
77. Kloos RT, Eng C, Evans DB, Francis GL, Gagel RF, Gharib H, Moley JF, Pacini F, Ringel MD, Schlumberger M, Wells Jr SA. Medullary thyroid cancer: management guidelines of the American Thyroid Association. Thyroid. 2009;19(6):565–612.
78. Raue F, Frank-Raue K. Update multiple endocrine neoplasia type 2. Fam Cancer. 2010;9(3):449–57.
79. Lips CJ. Clinical management of the multiple endocrine neoplasia syndromes: results of a computerized opinion poll at the Sixth International Workshop on Multiple Endocrine Neoplasia and von Hippel-Lindau disease. J Intern Med. 1998;243(6):589–94.
80. Skinner MA, Moley JA, Dilley WG, Owzar K, Debenedetti MK, Wells Jr SA. Prophylactic thyroidectomy in multiple endocrine neoplasia type 2A. N Engl J Med. 2005;353(11):1105–13.
81. Georgitsi M, Raitila A, Karhu A, van der Luijt RB, Aalfs CM, Sane T, Vierimaa O, Makinen MJ, Tuppurainen K, Paschke R, Gimm O, Koch CA, Gundogdu S, Lucassen A, Tischkowitz M, Izatt L, Aylwin S, Bano G, Hodgson S, De Menis E, Launonen V, Vahteristo P, Aaltonen LA. Germline CDKN1B/p27Kip1 mutation in multiple endocrine neoplasia. J Clin Endocrinol Metab. 2007;92(8):3321–5.

Familial Hypocalciuric Hypercalcemia

12

Ogo I. Egbuna and Edward M. Brown

Abstract

Previously referred to as "familial benign hypercalcemia (FBH)," familial hypocalciuric hypercalcemia (FHH) is a benign autosomal dominant disorder of mineral metabolism most often caused by a mutation in the gene encoding the extracellular calcium-sensing receptor (CaSR).

The importance of distinguishing between FHH and the much more common primary hyperparathyroidism (PHPT) has been recognized. In contrast to the benign clinical course of most FHH patients, patients with PHPT can develop a variety of complications, e.g., bone loss, impaired renal function, kidney stone, etc. In terms of management, for those with the complications of PHPT, successful surgical removal of hyperfunctioning parathyroid tissue cures the hypercalcemia and arrests or partially reverses renal and skeletal complications of the disease. On the other hand, in FHH, anything less than total parathyroidectomy is generally accompanied by persistence or prompt recurrence of hypercalcemia. In contrast, in almost all FHH cases, parathyroid surgery is contraindicated, both because of their benign clinical course and by the failure of the usual surgical treatment of PTH-dependent forms of hypercalcemia (e.g., PHPT) to restore normocalcemia in FHH.

Keywords

Parathyroidectomy • Hyperfunctioning • Hypercalcemia • Hypocalciuria • Calcium-sensing receptor • Acquired or autoimmune hypocalciuric hypercalcemia

O.I. Egbuna, MD, MSc, FASN (✉)
Amgen Inc, Bone Therapeutic Area,
1 Amgen Center Drive, Mail Stop 38-B-A,
Room 38 2D-1-2, Thousand Oaks, CA 91320, USA
e-mail: ogo.egbuna@gmail.com

E.M. Brown, MD
Division of Endocrinology, Diabetes and Hypertension,
Brigham and Women's Hospital, EBRC223A,
221 Longwood Ave., Boston, MA 02186, USA

A.A. Licata and E.V. Lerma (eds.), *Diseases of the Parathyroid Glands*,
DOI 10.1007/978-1-4419-5550-0_12,

Introduction

A distinct form of idiopathic "familial benign hypercalcemia" (FBH) was first described by Foley and colleagues in 1972 [1]. Marx and colleagues in a series of papers starting soon afterward, reported many of the metabolic characteristics of this syndrome (hypercalcemia, normal or low serum phosphorus, inappropriately normal or elevated parathyroid hormone (PTH) levels, and relative or absolute hypocalciuria) and applied the more commonly used term—familial hypocalciuric hypercalcemia (FHH) [2–13]. Typically, FHH is a benign autosomal dominant disorder of mineral metabolism *most often* caused by a mutation in the gene encoding the extracellular calcium-sensing receptor (CaSR), a G protein-coupled receptor that resides on the long arm of chromosome 3. The CaSR is an extracellular sensor capable of detecting changes in the blood calcium concentration of only a few percent, and it modulates the functions of parathyroid gland and kidney so as to restore blood calcium to normal. In the parathyroid, it inhibits the secretion of the calcium-elevating hormone, PTH; PTH, in turn, produces net release of calcium from bone, increases renal tubular reabsorption of calcium, and promotes formation of the most active naturally occurring form of vitamin D, 1,25-dihydroxyvitamin D_3 [$1,25(OH)_2D_3$]. In FHH, the parathyroid glands are less sensitive than normal to extracellular calcium. In contrast to the indirect effect of the CaSR on tubular reabsorption of calcium mediated by CaSR-regulated PTH secretion, the CaSR in the kidney directly inhibits renal calcium reabsorption, thereby counteracting the effect of PTH. The phenotype of FHH—mild to moderate, PTH-dependent hypercalcemia accompanied by relative or absolute hypocalciuria—reflects the biochemical impact of loss of one allele of the CaSR in parathyroid and kidney, producing what can be thought of as "resistance" of these two tissues to extracellular calcium.

There is a clear gene dosage effect of loss-of-function mutations of the CaSR: individuals who are heterozygous for these mutations are usually clinically asymptomatic and present as FHH. Homozygotes (or compound heterozygotes), in contrast, owing to their total lack of normally functioning CaSRs, often present at the other end of the clinical spectrum with life-threatening neonatal hypercalcemia requiring urgent parathyroidectomy, a condition called neonatal severe hyperparathyroidism (NSHPT) [14]. With the availability of molecular genetic tests to identify individuals with hypercalcemia that results from inactivating mutations of the CaSR, there has been a progressive blurring of the classical descriptions of FHH and NSHPT and the distinction between them. In addition to the typical presentation of FHH, patients heterozygous for inactivating mutations of the CaSR can present as (1) NSHPT [15]; (2) neonatal hyperparathyroidism (NHPT) [16] that is intermediate in severity between FHH and NSHPT; (3) more severe hypercalcemia in adults than is typically found in FHH [17], or (4) a clinical picture indistinguishable from that of primary hyperparathyroidism (PHPT) [18]. Conversely, not all patients homozygous for inactivating mutations present as life-threatening hyperparathyroidism at birth, but may only be diagnosed serendipitously later in childhood [19] or even as largely asymptomatic adults [20]. Thus, an important focus of this discussion is to discuss the widening clinical spectrum of inactivating mutations of the CaSR, and the resulting impact on the diagnosis and management of the variants of the classical diseases, FHH and NSHPT.

The importance of distinguishing between FHH and the much more common, PTH-dependent hypercalcemic disorder, PHPT, has been recognized for some time [21]. In contrast to the benign clinical course of most FHH patients, patients with PHPT can develop a variety of complications, including bone loss, impaired renal function, kidney stones, and others, which increase in frequency with the duration of the disease [22]. In patients with the complications of PHPT, successful surgical removal of hyperfunctioning parathyroid tissue cures the hypercalcemia and arrests or partially reverses renal and skeletal complications of the disease. In FHH, in contrast, anything less than total parathyroidectomy is generally accompanied by persistence or prompt recurrence of hypercalcemia [4, 18] as the residual parathyroid tissue once again "resets" the serum calcium concentration to the elevated level dictated by the presence of the inactive mutant CaSR. Thus in almost all FHH cases, parathyroid surgery is contraindicated, both because of their benign clinical course and by the failure of the usual surgical treatment of PTH-dependent forms of hypercalcemia (e.g., PHPT) to restore normocalcemia in FHH. Therefore, distinguishing between FHH, NSHPT, and other PTH-dependent forms of hypercalcemia, especially PHPT, will be another important focus of this chapter.

Epidemiology

By virtue of its benign clinical features, relatively little is known of the true prevalence of FHH. However, some increase in apparent prevalence has been reported due to routine biochemical testing of blood chemistries, including calcium, as part of the investigation of other clinical conditions. One study from the West of Scotland estimated a prevalence of about 1 in 78,000 [23]. Most other estimates of the prevalence of FHH are derived from sporadic reports of the syndrome in families in Israel [24], Italy [25–27], France [28–30], Spain [31], Norway [32], Sweden [33, 34], Denmark [35–38], the Netherlands [39–41], Switzerland [42], and Japan [43–46], likely reflecting the quality of care in these countries, but suggesting that FHH is more prevalent than is currently appreciated.

At the present time, there is insufficient data to draw conclusions on racial predisposition, although FHH is relatively rarely reported in African Americans [47]. The prevalence of PHPT is considerably higher (≈10-fold or more) than that of FHH but varies geographically and in different reports [48–53]. Therefore, as described in more detail later, while only a minority of cases of PHPT have biochemical features resembling FHH (e.g., about 10% have relative hypocalciuria), and the absolute number of PHPT cases whose biochemical features could be confused with FHH is comparable to that of the latter.

Pathogenetic Basis of FHH

FHH has since been indexed in the Online Mendelian Inheritance In Man (OMIM®) database (http://www.ncbi.nlm.nih.gov/omim/145980) as MIM #145980 [hypocalciuric hypercalcemia 1 (HHC1)] based on evidence that the phenotype attributed to this condition in many *but not all* cases is caused by a mutation in the gene encoding the calcium-sensing receptor (CaSR). Linkage analysis has shown that the predominant locus of the FHH disease gene (e.g., the CaSR gene) resides on the long arm of chromosome 3 (band q21–24) [54]. However, FHH is not always linked to chromosome 3q. Notably, one family with clinical features similar to FHH showed linkage to the short arm of chromosome 19 (HHC2, 19p13.3, MIM #145981) [55], while two others showed linkage to a site on the long arm of the same chromosome (19q13, HHC3, MIM #600740) [56, 57]. Based on the features of the first family that was shown to be linked to 19q13, this form of the condition (HHC3) was called the *Oklahoma variant* (FBHOk). Patients in this family exhibited hypophosphatemia, a tendency to an age-dependent rise in serum PTH to frankly elevated levels, and the presence of the bone disease, and osteomalacia (defective mineralization of bone) in some family members [56]. In the second family identified with HHC3, however, these features atypical of FHH were less apparent [57]. HHC2 and HHC3 likely represent a minority of the ~30% of FHH cases without an identifiable mutation in the coding region of the CaSR gene. The remaining cases of FHH that are linked to chromosome 3 but do not have an identifiable mutation presumably harbor mutations in regulatory regions of the CaSR gene that control its expression, but this remains to be shown directly.

As many as 213 mutations have been described in the coding region or splice sites of the CaSR gene (188 missense, 17 nonsense, 6 insertion and/or deletion, 1 silent, and 1 splice mutation) in the CaSR mutation database (http://www.casrdb.mcgill.ca) related to FHH, NSHPT (MIM #239200), or autosomal dominant hypoparathyroidism (ADH, MIM #601298) either in families

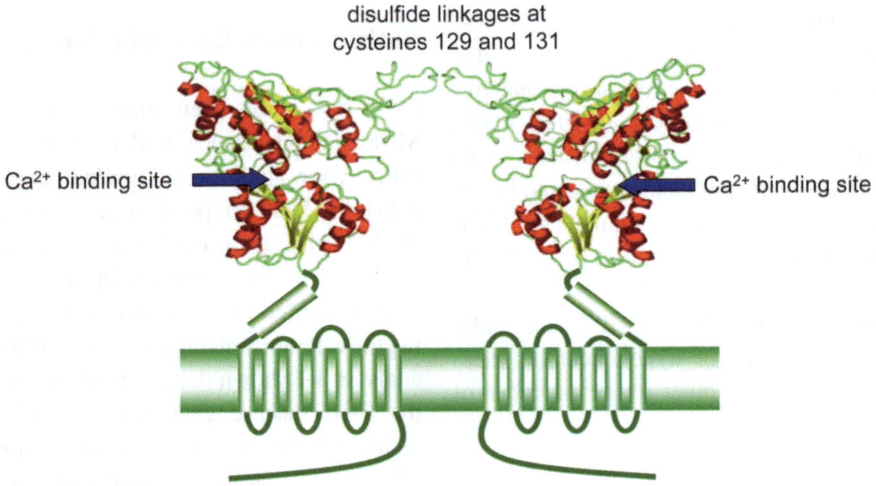

Fig. 12.1 Model of the predicted structure of the dimeric CaSR. Shown are the two extracellular domains (ECDs) of the dimeric CaSR with alpha helices shown in *red* and intermolecular disulfide bonds involving cysteines 129 and 131. The dimeric, Venus flytrap structure of the CaSR enables dominant negative interactions between a normal and a mutant CaSR in a heterodimeric state. A binding site for calcium is indicated in the crevice between the two lobes of each monomeric ECD. The seven-membrane spanning helices as well as the intracellular (IC) tail domains of each CaSR are shown in the *lower part* of the figure. This research was originally published in the Journal of Biological Chemistry. Huang, et al. Identification and dissection of Ca^{2+}-binding Sites in the extracellular domain of Ca^{2+}-sensing receptor. J Biol Chem. 2007;282:19000–10. ©The American Society for Biochemistry and Molecular Biology

or as de novo disease. ADH, in contrast to FHH and NSHPT, is an inherited disorder of calcium metabolism caused by gain-of-function mutations in the CaSR that present most commonly as asymptomatic hypocalcemia/hypoparathyroidism. Over 150 inactivating mutations of the CaSR have been described in association with FHH and/or NSHPT [58, 59]. Most of these mutations are missense mutations, the rest being nonsense, insertion, or deletion/insertion mutations [58–61].

The functional, cell surface form of the CaSR is a dimer (Fig. 12.1), and the two monomers within the dimeric CaSR are linked by disulfide bonds involving cysteine residues 129 and 131 within each monomer [62, 63]. Some mutations, such as nonsense mutations close to the translational start site of the receptor protein [64], likely produce simple haploinsufficiency, similar to that present in mice heterozygous for targeted inactivation of the CASR gene [65]. That is, it is simply the loss of one allele of the CASR gene and the resultant, presumably ~50% reduction in the normal complement of cell surface CaSRs that reduces effective signaling through the receptor in parathyroid and kidney. As a result, a higher than normal level of extracellular calcium is needed to achieve the functional activity of the CaSR present in normocalcemic, otherwise normal individuals. FHH patients with such null mutations may have only mild hypercalcemia [64], as is observed in the heterozygous CaSR knockout mouse.

A number of missense mutations also produce a comparable degree of mild hypercalcemia [16, 17]. In these cases, statistical considerations would suggest that 25% of the receptors in parathyroid and kidney cells are wild-type homodimers, 25% are mutant homodimers, and 50% are mutant-wild type heterodimers. For this complement of receptors to signal equivalently to the 50% complement of normal CaSRs thought to be present with heterozygous null CaSR mutations, the 50% of mutant-wild type heterodimers would need to signal with the same efficiency as the 25% wild-type homodimers. This may imply, therefore, that the mutant receptor in the wild type-mutant heterodimers interferes to some extent with the function of its normal partner (i.e., exerts a dominant negative effect). In fact, more pronounced dominant negative effects of some mutant CaSRs (S137P, R185Q, R227L, R795W, and F881L) have been described in vitro, which can be associated with more pronounced hypercalcemia in vivo than is the norm in FHH [17, 34, 64, 66, 67]. Three cases of de novo NSHPT have been described that were heterozygous for missense mutations located in the extracellular domain of the CaSR, with no mutation found in the parents [15, 68]. One such individual with de novo NSHPT has been reported as heterozygous for a previously described mutation in an FHH family [15]. It is thought that this scenario is most likely to occur with dominant negative mutations. The severity of the disease in these neonates may also be related to the gestation of an affected fetus in a normal mother. Because the fetal parathyroid glands would read the mother's normocalcemia as "hypocalcemia," this would lead to further hyperplasia of the fetal parathyroid glands and hypersecretion of PTH.

As many as 11 single nucleotide polymorphisms (SNPs) have been identified (http://www.casrdb.mcgill.ca/?Topic=CasrMutation&v=new) and at the present time, although SNPs have been identified in families with FHH [57, 69], the base pair change is present in both affected and unaffected persons, and these SNPs do not appear to segregate with known diseases of divalent ion metabolism [14]. The presence of certain SNPs in the general population, however, can be associated with slight but significant alterations in renal calcium handling or in serum calcium concentration within the normal range. For example, the 990 G SNP variant of the CaSR has been reported to influence renal CaSR activation, urinary calcium excretion, and probably the risk for nephrolithiasis [70]. In addition, certain haplotypes of SNPs are associated with alterations in serum calcium concentration within the normal range [71], thereby providing a likely mechanism and contributing to the fact that the normal range for serum calcium concentration, which is about ±10% of its mean value, is several-fold greater than that measured in any given normal individual, which varies by only a few percent (~±1–2%). Nevertheless, the magnitude of the variation in blood calcium resulting from these haplotypes is considerably less than the normal range for calcium, suggesting a role for other factors as well. It is likely, however, that certain haplotypes of SNPs might modify the degree of hypercalcemia present within a given FHH family or in unrelated families with the same mutation [72].

FHH, as the name suggests, is distinct from the later onset form of hypocalciuric hypercalcemia, usually in adult life, that has been termed acquired or autoimmune hypocalciuric hypercalcemia (AHH) [73]. The distinction between the acquired and hereditary forms is important because in occasional cases, glucocorticoids may control the acquired form and parathyroidectomy is rarely necessary for FHH. Kifor and colleagues described a total of four affected individuals in two families with PTH-dependent hypercalcemia, three of whom exhibited hypocalciuria [74]. In contrast, the fourth individual had hypercalciuria, pointing out that the biochemical presentation of this condition can be similar to that of PHPT. Kifor and colleagues, however, were not able to identify mutations in the CASR gene [74], and their other autoimmune manifestations prompted a search for an autoimmune basis for their hypocalciuric hypercalcemia. All four patients, in fact, harbored inactivating anti-CaSR antibodies that mitigated high Ca^{2+}-stimulated activation of PLC and MAPK and stimulated PTH secretion.

A subsequent report from the same group [75] described a 66-year-old hypercalcemic woman with multiple autoimmune manifestations (psoriasis, adult-onset asthma, Coomb's positive hemolytic anemia, rheumatoid arthritis, uveitis, bullous pemphigoid, sclerosing pancreatitis, and autoimmune hypophysitis with hypothyroidism and diabetes insipidus). Her hypercalcemia (as high as 13.4 mg/dl) was accompanied by elevated intact PTH levels (75–175 pg/ml) and hypocalciuria. A diagnosis of PHPT had been made earlier, but a subtotal parathyroidectomy was followed within 3 weeks by recrudescence of her hypercalcemia. Remarkably, her hypercalcemia subsequently resolved during treatment of her bullous pemphigoid with glucocorticoids, and her intact PTH level decreased concomitantly to the upper limit of normal. While hypercalcemic, her serum harbored anti-CaSR antibodies, but there was a substantial drop in their titer during glucocorticoid therapy. As in the earlier four cases of AHH [74], the persistence of PTH-dependent hypercalcemia proves unequivocally that the anti-CaSR antibodies had a clear functional impact on PTH secretion without destroying the patients' parathyroid glands.

Pathophysiology

In FHH, inappropriately normal PTH levels or, in about 20% of cases, frankly elevated values, given the coexistent hypercalcemia, reflect a right-shift in the set-point for calcium-regulated PTH release [76]. This proves, along with the findings in CaSR knockout mice, the physiological importance of the CaSR in maintaining mineral ion homeostasis. The set-point shift likely results from any combination of reduced complement of normal receptors, reduced function of the mutant receptors, or, as noted above, dominant negative actions of the mutant CaSR on the wild-type partner within heterodimers. Elegant studies by Attie and colleagues more than 30 years ago homed in on the ascending limb of the loop of Henle as the "major renal locus of abnormal calcium transport" in this disorder, where hypocalciuria was PTH-independent and persistent despite coexistent hypercalcemia [77]. This alteration in renal calcium handling reflects "resistance" of the kidney to the usual hypercalciuric action of hypercalcemia, and is the equivalent in the kidney of the resistance of PTH secretion by the parathyroid to the normal inhibitory effect of high calcium. Another consequence of the impaired Ca^{2+}-sensing in the kidney is blunting of the usual hypercalcemia-induced reduction in the urinary concentrating mechanism. This observation is consistent with results of experiments in animals describing a role of the CaSR in modulating vasopressin-regulated permeability and membrane transporters in the inner medullary collecting duct [78].

The crucial role of the CaSR in directly regulating renal transport of calcium, even in the absence of PTH, is of relevance in FHH, and the defense against hypercalcemia induced by various means has recently been more carefully delineated in CaSR knockout mouse models [79, 80]. Note that the CaSR also indirectly regulates renal calcium reabsorption by virtue of its regulation of PTH secretion, which, it turn, modulates renal calcium handling. The use of a loop diuretic promotes renal excretion of calcium in hypoparathyroid subjects with FHH [77], and this clinical observation has been reproduced over two decades later by Egbuna, Brown, and colleagues in observations made using CaSR knockout mouse models of disease [81]. All these observations point to the relative roles of inactivation of the CaSR in the parathyroid and kidney and the contribution of thick ascending limb of the nephron in the anomalous renal handling of calcium in FHH.

Clinical Presentation

The syndrome of FHH most commonly has a benign, asymptomatic course, and patients are frequently not diagnosed until a routine measurement of blood calcium concentration done as part of other diagnostic work-up shows an unexpectedly high value, or family screening is carried out due to the birth of a child with NSHPT. Some symptoms that are present in probands of FHH families, such as chondrocalcinosis or pancreatitis, have not, with the likely exception of pancreatitis, been present in other affected family members with frequencies higher than in unaffected members of the same kindred [82]. The lack of the usual symptoms of hypercalcemia in FHH appears to extend to those kindreds with higher serum calcium concentrations than is typical in FHH, e.g., those with dominant negative mutations in the CaSR. This lack of symptoms despite a substantial degree of hypercalcemia (13–14 mg/dl in some families) suggests that the CaSR mediates at least some of the usual symptoms of hypercalcemia.

Recent studies have readdressed the relationship of pancreatitis to FHH. Several kindreds have been described in which there are family members with recurrent pancreatitis [83], perhaps owing to the specific functional properties of the mutated receptors in these families. Of note in this regard, the CaSR is expressed in the pancreatic ducts, where alterations in its function could potentially be associated with pathology [84]. In one study, FHH patients who also harbored mutations in the SPINK1 gene, which predisposes to the development of pancreatitis, appeared at increased risk of pancreatitis [85]. In fact, mutations in the CaSR are now characterized by some investigators as one of six genes conferring an increased risk for pancreatitis [86]. However, it should be kept in mind that the development of pancreatitis in FHH is unusual and, when considered in the context of FHH as a whole, the incidence of this complication may not be in excess of that of the general population [87]. Further studies are needed to define the role of specific CaSR mutations in predisposing to pancreatitis.

The availability of genetic screening for FHH has identified families with a clinical picture indistinguishable from that of PHPT. One such family had overt hypercalciuria in some family members as well as the presence of one or more parathyroid adenomas at the time of parathyroid surgery [34]. Subtotal parathyroidectomy induced long-term remission of the hypercalcemia in affected patients, in contrast to the recurrence or persistence of hypercalcemia in most FHH patients subjected to parathyroid surgery. More recently, inactivating CaSR mutations have been described as a cause of about 15% of kindreds with familial isolated hyperparathyroidism (FIH) [18, 88], with a clinical presentation in several cases indistinguishable from that of PHPT, including the presence of overt hypercalciuria. As is observed in typical FHH, parathyroid surgery in cases of FIH caused by CaSR mutations was followed by persistent or recurrent hypercalcemia in most cases [18].

There are additional examples of the expanding clinical spectrum of inactivating CaSR mutations. As noted earlier, some infants with heterozygous inactivating CaSR mutations can present with NSHPT (see below for typical clinical features in homozygotes) [15] or the milder variant, NHPT [16]. In addition to having hypercalcemia that is more severe than in newborns with typical FHH, patients with NHPT can have symptoms of hypercalcemia, moderate to severe elevations in PTH, and hyperparathyroid bone disease. Following conservative treatment or, in some cases, subtotal parathyroidectomy, such cases can revert to a more classical FHH phenotype, suggesting the existence of in utero factors contributing to the unusually severe phenotype at birth. These may include gestation in a normal mother (see above) or the co-existence of vitamin D deficiency, which can aggravate the degree of hyperparathyroidism [89]. Rare cases have also been described in which a member of an FHH kindred has a substantially higher calcium concentration than other affected family members owing to the development of a presumably coincidental parathyroid adenoma [90]. The serum calcium concentration in all of these clinical variants of heterozygous inactivating CaSR mutations, however, seldom exceed 14–15 mg/dl, in contrast to what is observed with homozygous or compound heterozygous CaSR mutations.

NSHPT more commonly results from genetic conditions in which there are no normal CaSRs (homozygous or compound heterozygous mutations). Affected infants usually present in the neonatal period with severe, symptomatic, PTH-dependent hypercalcemia to levels as high as 7.7 mM in the most severe cases and, with rare exceptions [19], above 15 mg/dl. Such infants can exhibit weakness, hypotonia, and failure to thrive [14]. The bony changes of severe hyperparathyroidism are a prominent part of the clinical presentation and are often complicated by multiple fractures, which, if involving the ribs, can produce a flail chest syndrome. These infants exhibit significantly higher PTH levels than are observed in FHH or NHPT (not infrequently 5–10-fold the upper limit of normal) and can also manifest polyuria and dehydration in addition to their skeletal and constitutional symptoms [7, 91, 92]. In the total absence of normal CaSRs in the parathyroid glands, PTH may be totally nonsuppressible at high calcium concentrations or exhibit some limited suppressibility if the mutant CaSR retains some capacity to signal.

Screening for mutations in the CaSR in a variety of forms of PTH-dependent hypercalcemia, however, has revealed that not all patients with homozygous inactivating mutations of the CaSR present with the syndrome of NSHPT. Rare patients have been described in whom hypercalcemia was only identified serendipitously in adulthood. Remarkably, despite serum calcium concentrations of 15–17 mg/dl, one such patient, who was said to be of somewhat reduced intelligence due to "encephalitis," was seemingly otherwise asymptomatic, with a PTH level at the upper limit of normal, normal renal function, and no apparent bone disease [20]. Mutational analysis revealed that she was homozygous for a Pro39Ala mutation of the CaSR, which exhibited relatively mild functional impairment when studied in vitro. These clinical findings again support an important role of the CaSR in the genesis of at least some of the symptoms of hypercalcemia and, perhaps, some renal complications. A more recent example of relatively mild clinical presentation of homozygous inactivating mutations of the CaSR was a 5-year old male who first presented at age 2 with moderate hypercalcemia (13 mg/dl). Subsequent levels of calcium varied from 11.9 to 13.1 mg/dl with levels of PTH ranging from normal to about twice the upper limit of normal and fractional excretion of calcium that was well below 0.01 (see below for a discussion of renal calcium handling in FHH) [19]. Given the early age of onset of hypercalcemia, mutational screening of the CaSR was performed and revealed the presence of homozygous Q459R mutation within the extracellular domain of the receptor. Interestingly, all individuals in the family who were heterozygous for the mutation were normocalcemic, albeit in the upper part of the normal range (and significantly higher than unaffected family members). Hence, the proband manifested in an autosomal recessive manner. The milder phenotype of these cases of homozygous inactivating CaSR mutations, most likely reflects sufficient residual activity of the mutant CaSR to maintain the serum calcium concentration within a range compatible with life.

In summary, the clinical presentations of heterozygous inactivating mutations of the CaSR include (1) asymptomatic individuals with mild to moderate, lifelong hypercalcemia or even serum calcium concentrations that are consistently below the upper limit of normal (typical FHH), (2) neonatal hyperparathyroidism of sufficient severity to produce overt bone disease (NHPT), (3) NSHPT, (4) a clinical and biochemical presentation indistinguishable from PHPT, and (5) unusually severe hypercalcemia in a member of an FHH kindred with a superimposed parathyroid adenoma. Homozygous or compound heterozygous mutations can produce clinical and biochemical pictures ranging from moderate to dramatic hypercalcemia (NSHPT) (>30 mg/dl) that is life-threatening and in need of urgent medical and/or surgical intervention. The areas of diagnostic overlap are (1) cases of FHH phenotypically indistinguishable from PHPT; (2) infants with NSHPT, which can result from either heterozygous or homozygous mutations; and (3) very mildly affected homozygotes, who might be confused with PHPT or with FHH patients with unusually high serum calcium concentrations. This broad range of phenotypes resulting from heterozygous or homozygous (or compound heterozygous) inactivating mutations of the CaSR are illustrated in Table 12.1.

Table 12.1 Phenotypes associated with inactivating CaSR mutations

Heterozygous mutations
Typical FHH with hypercalcemia ranging from high normal to moderate
FHH with unusually severe hypercalcemia (e.g., dominant negative mutation)
FHH with superimposed parathyroid adenoma
NSHPT (serum calcium generally <15 mg/dl)
NHPT
Familial isolated hypercalcemia
Homozygous or compound heterozygous mutations
NSHPT
Asymptomatic hypercalcemia in children or adults
Autosomal recessive hypercalcemia

Laboratory Evaluation

The serum calcium concentration in FHH typically averages about 10% above the upper limit of normal (i.e., ~11.5 mg/dl), but ranges from the upper half of the normal range [19] to as high as 13–14 mg/dl in some kindreds [17]. These levels encompass the range encountered in patients with PHPT in the modern era. The serum magnesium concentration in FHH is in the upper half of the normal range or is mildly elevated [4], supporting the early hypothesis by Strewler that the CaSR contributes to the setting of extracellular concentrations of not only calcium but also magnesium [93]. Serum magnesium correlates positively with the serum calcium concentration in FHH, in contrast to PHPT, in which there is an inverse relationship between the serum calcium and magnesium concentrations [4]. Serum phosphorus concentration in FHH is usually normal, although commonly in the lower half of the normal range, and, in a minority of cases, frankly low [94]. Despite lifelong hypercalcemia, renal function is preserved in FHH [4, 94] and chronic renal complications of hypercalcemia, such as impaired renal function and nephrocalcinosis, are absent.

Serum intact PTH levels are normal in about 80% of cases [94]; elevated values may be characteristic of specific families, perhaps reflecting the specific functional impact of that family's mutation (e.g., a dominant negative action) [36]. The mean values of serum 25-hydroxyvitamin D_3 and 1,25-dihydroxyvitamin D_3 concentrations are within the normal range [94]. The failure to observe the elevation in serum $1,25(OH)_2D_3$ commonly seen in PHPT may reflect the generally normal PTH level in FHH. Twenty-four-hour urinary calcium excretion, while averaging within the normal range, is distinctly within the lower part of the normal range (e.g., ~110 mg/24 h in FHH vs. a normal range of 80–320 mg/24 h) in a Danish population [94]. The enhanced renal tubular reabsorption of calcium is most easily documented by calculating the ratio of the renal clearance of calcium to that of creatinine [(UCa/PCa) × (PCr/UCr), where UCr is urinary creatinine, PCr is plasma creatinine, UCa is urinary calcium, and PCr is plasma calcium], which is equivalent to the fractional excretion of calcium. Approximately eighty percent of patients with FHH have a calcium to creatinine clearance ratio (CCa/CCr) of <0.01 (e.g., a fractional excretion of less than 1%), while a similar percentage of patients with PHPT have a value higher than this level (for additional discussion, see section on "Differential Diagnosis" below). Another biochemical finding in FHH patients is their capacity to concentrate urine normally, in contrast to patients with PHPT in whom maximal urinary concentration elicited by dehydration is reduced [6]. This observation is consistent with the role of a functional CaSR in attenuating arginine vasopressin-mediated aquaporin-2 expression and water transport in the collecting duct [78, 95]. Bone density is similar to that of age-matched controls, although markers of bone turnover are often mildly elevated [96]. The parathyroid glands of patients with FHH are typically of normal size and histology, but a few studies of FHH patients have reported the presence of single or multiple parathyroid "adenomas" or in some cases mild chief cell proliferation/lipohyperplasia with one or more glands resembling adenomas [34, 97]. Despite the normal appearing parathyroid glands in most patients with FHH, the recurrence of hypercalcemia after anything short of a total parathyroidectomy is also characteristic of FHH.

Imaging Studies

Two kinds of imaging studies important in the management of the more common endocrine disorder that can be confused with FHH, PHPT, are potentially applicable to FHH. These are measurement of bone mineral density (BMD) and parathyroid localization studies, such as sestamibi scans, ultrasound, CT scan, and/or MRI. In patients with PHPT, determination of BMD is important to assess whether a sufficient degree of bone loss has taken place (i.e., >2.5 standard deviations reduction below normal peak BMD in forearm, spine, or hip) to warrant parathyroid surgery [22]. If BMD is sufficiently low in PHPT, or other surgical criteria are met, such as serum calcium concentration >1 mg/dl above the upper limit of normal or estimated glomerular filtration rate is <60 ml/min, and/or age <50, parathyroid localization studies then guide the surgical approach to be taken [22]. For example, unilateral minimally invasive parathyroid (MIP) surgery may be undertaken if only a single enlarged gland is identified.

However, the need for imaging studies in FHH differs from that in PHPT in several important respects. First, as noted above, BMD in FHH is generally equivalent to that in age-matched normal subjects and higher than that in PHPT [82]. Therefore, there is no need to determine BMD in FHH patients unless there are other reasons to suspect excessive bone loss. The benign clinical course and resultant expectant medical follow-up rather than parathyroid surgery in the vast majority of FHH patients likewise obviates the need for parathyroid localization studies in the vast majority of cases. Only in cases of NSHPT or NHPT or in the rare cases of FHH (i.e., with a superimposed parathyroid adenoma) who might be surgical candidates are parathyroid localization studies a consideration. Given that most of these cases will exhibit four-gland parathyroid hyperplasia, however, one might argue that bilateral parathyroid exploration is necessary in any event and localization studies are superfluous.

Differential Diagnoses

The broad differential diagnosis of FHH encompasses the numerous causes of hypercalcemia. As with the investigation of any clinical entity, the correct diagnosis starts with a detailed medical history and physical examination, which may help distinguish FHH from NSHPT, acquired autoimmune hyperparathyroidism, and hypercalcemia due to neoplastic or other disorders (see Table 12.1). The initial laboratory evaluation, however, provides key information. That is, FHH is a PTH-dependent form of hypercalcemia (i.e., PTH, even when normal, is not appropriately suppressed to or below the lower limit of normal by the prevailing hypercalcemia, as occurs in normal individuals) accompanied by inappropriately normal or frankly low renal calcium excretion, implicating the renal contribution to hypercalcemia characteristic of FHH. Thus, the differential diagnosis in FHH can be limited to the various causes of PTH-dependent hypercalcemia, and, more specifically, those accompanied by hypocalciuria. The distinction between FHH and PHPT is particularly important because the management of the two conditions differs in important ways. It is key in this regard to alert not only the proband but also other affected family members that parathyroid surgery is ill-advised in all but the most unusual of circumstances.

Table 12.2 Causes of PTH-dependent hypocalciuric hypercalcemia

FHH
Primary hyperparathyroidism
Hyperparathyroidism associated with
Very low calcium intake
Vitamin D deficiency
Mild renal insufficiency
Drug-induced hypocalciuric hypercalcemia
Lithium therapy
Treatment with thiazide diuretics
Autoimmune hypocalciuric hypercalcemia

What are the other hypocalciuric forms of hypercalcemia that must be differentiated from FHH (Table 12.2)? The most important differential is between FHH and PHPT. Ten to twenty percent of patients with PHPT have a calcium to creatinine clearance ratio (CCa/CCr) of <0.01, while a similar percentage of FHH patients have a value higher than this level. In a recent study [98], the value of CCa/CCr providing the optimal diagnostic separation between FHH and PHPT was 0.0115 (similar to the widely used value of 0.01) [4], which provided 80% sensitivity and 88% specificity. In any patient with PHPT, coexistent factors that can lower the CCa/CCr further are very low calcium intake, vitamin D deficiency (as assessed by a serum level of 25-hydorxyvitamin D), concomitant administration of a thiazide diuretic or lithium, and mild or moderate renal insufficiency (which reduces the filtered load of calcium). Even mild renal insufficiency (e.g., 50% reduction in GFR) can lower calcium excretion substantially. Such contributory factors should be sought by history and laboratory investigation in the evaluation of PTH-dependent hypocalciuric hypercalcemia. The hypercalcemia caused by lithium and thiazide diuretics is in some cases reversible following cessation of the drug. If not, the drugs may have unmasked mild, preexistent PHPT by their hypocalciuric action or directly contributed to the development of PHPT by stimulating parathyroid growth. As noted earlier, a small number of patients have been described with hypocalciuric hypercalcemia owing to inactivating antibodies to the CaSR. The presence of other autoimmune conditions, such as sprue or Hashimoto's thyroiditis, can be an important clue to this diagnosis.

What is the role of genetic testing in the diagnosis or differential diagnosis of patients suspected of having FHH? In many FHH kindreds, the presence of benign, PTH-dependent hypocalciuric hypercalcemia in an autosomal dominant pattern of inheritance in the proband and in two or more additional family members is diagnostic of FHH and genetic testing adds little. In apparently sporadic cases with PTH-dependent hypercalcemia and CCa/CCr <0.01 or patients in the region of overlap between FHH and PHPT (0.01–0.02), the correct diagnosis is usually straightforward using history (including family history and biochemical screening if appropriate), physical examination, and appropriate laboratory evaluation as noted above. In patients in whom the diagnosis remains unclear, mutational analysis of the exons and exon–intron boundaries of the CaSR gene would be appropriate, bearing in mind that in ~30% of patients with linkage of their FHH to chromosome 3, no mutation will be identified. Such genetic testing is offered by several commercial laboratories. Other situations in which genetic testing should be performed are (1) any patient with FIH; (2) any child <10 with PTH-dependent hypocalciuric hypercalcemia, including those with NHPT or NSHPT, as most such patients have inactivating CaSR mutations; (3) a family with hypocalciuric hypercalcemia and recurrent pancreatitis. Any family with FHH and consanguineous marriages should be counseled about the risk of NSHPT.

Treatment

The most important treatment of typical FHH is no specific treatment. Because of the benign clinical course of the disease in the great majority of these patients, no medical intervention is indicated. It is important that patients with typical FHH and his/her affected family members be counseled as to the inadvisability of parathyroid surgery. There is no evidence that the currently recommended levels of calcium and vitamin D supplementation for the population as a whole pose any risk of exacerbating the hypercalcemia in FHH or inducing hypercalciuria, and these patients should be supplemented in the same way as other, unaffected persons of their age and sex. There are specific recommendations for monitoring the clinical status of patients with asymptomatic PHPT who do not initially meet current guidelines for parathyroid surgery [22], e.g., determinations of serum calcium and creatinine yearly and of BMD every 1–2 years. Given their benign clinical course, less frequent monitoring of these parameters in patients with typical FHH, on the order of every 5 years, would likely suffice, although there have been no systematic studies of this issue.

It is in patients with severe or atypical presentations of inactivating mutations of the CaSR that more active intervention may be warranted. The most severe of such cases are NSHPT due to homozygous inactivating CaSR mutations. NSHPT can be a lethal disease, and prompt parathyroidectomy early in life may be life-saving. In some cases, the bisphosphonate, pamidronate has been used as "rescue" therapy to lower serum calcium concentration and stabilize the affected infant's condition [99]. Another potential medical treatment is the use of the calcimimetic, cinacalcet HCl, which, however, in a patient with a homozygous CaSR mutation would only be effective if the receptor had some residual signaling capacity. In patients only discovered to have homozygous inactivating mutations later in childhood, or even as adults, the need for any kind of medical or surgical intervention would need to be made on a case-by-case basis, but might not be easily justified in an asymptomatic patient without renal or skeletal complications of hyperparathyroidism.

Cinacalcet might also be useful as a temporizing measure in infants with NHPT who are heterozygous for inactivating CaSR mutations [100]. Cinacalcet is not FDA approved for treatment of FHH. Such patients can revert spontaneously, or following subtotal parathyroidectomy, to a picture resembling FHH, with healing of bony lesions. Use of the calcimimetic might obviate the need for parathyroid surgery in this setting.

Other atypical presentations in which active medical or surgical intervention might be considered would be FHH presenting as typical PHPT, rather than FHH, or in patients with pancreatitis. In the former setting, frankly elevated levels of PTH and, in some cases, hypercalciuria may lead to the skeletal and renal consequences, respectively, of PHPT. The only recent recognition, however, that FIH can be caused by inactivating mutations of the CaSR and the small number of families reported, has not allowed an extensive experience to date. Furthermore, there appears to be a high risk of persistence or recurrence of hypercalcemia in this setting [18].

Prognosis

As noted above, the prognosis of typical FHH is excellent, and studies to date of a substantial number of such patients in multiple kindreds have not indicated any premature mortality of affected vs. unaffected family members. Atypical forms of FHH, such as those present in families with unusually high serum calcium and/or PTH levels or recurrent pancreatitis, have not been studied with regard to overall prognosis. However, there might be morbidity, or possibly mortality, associated with the more marked hypercalcemia, chronically elevated PTH levels or pancreatitis per se in such patients. In its severest form, NSHPT, particularly that due to homozygous or compound heterozygous mutations in the CaSR, can be lethal. If a child with NSHPT escapes clinical detection, there can be severe neurodevelopmental consequences. Successful surgical treatment, in contrast, can be associated with prolonged survival, although the number of such cases that have been studied is small.

References

1. Foley Jr TP, Harrison HC, Arnaud CD, Harrison HE. Familial benign hypercalcemia. J Pediatr. 1972;81(6):1060–7.
2. Marx SJ. Familial hypocalciuric hypercalcemia. N Engl J Med. 1980;303(14):810–1.
3. Marx SJ. Uncertainties in distinction of typical primary hyperparathyroidism from familial hypocalciuric hypercalcemia. West J Med. 1982;136(2):145–5.
4. Marx SJ, Attie MF, Levine MA, Spiegel AM, Downs Jr RW, Lasker RD. The hypocalciuric or benign variant of familial hypercalcemia: clinical and biochemical features in fifteen kindreds. Medicine (Baltimore). 1981;60(6):397–412.
5. Marx SJ, Attie MF, Spiegel AM, Levine MA, Lasker RD, Fox M. An association between neonatal severe primary hyperparathyroidism and familial hypocalciuric hypercalcemia in three kindreds. N Engl J Med. 1982;306(5):257–64.
6. Marx SJ, Attie MF, Stock JL, Spiegel AM, Levine MA. Maximal urine-concentrating ability: familial hypocalciuric hypercalcemia versus typical primary hyperparathyroidism. J Clin Endocrinol Metab. 1981;52(4):736–40.
7. Marx SJ, Fraser D, Rapoport A. Familial hypocalciuric hypercalcemia. Mild expression of the gene in heterozygotes and severe expression in homozygotes. Am J Med. 1985;78(1):15–22.
8. Marx SJ, Powell D, Shimkin PM, Wells SA, Ketcham AS, McGuigan JE, et al. Familial hyperparathyroidism. Mild hypercalcemia in at least nine members of a kindred. Ann Intern Med. 1973;78(3):371–7.
9. Marx SJ, Spiegel AM, Brown EM, Koehler JO, Gardner DG, Brennan MF, et al. Divalent cation metabolism. Familial hypocalciuric hypercalcemia versus typical primary hyperparathyroidism. Am J Med. 1978;65(2):235–42.
10. Marx SJ, Spiegel AM, Brown EM, Windeck R, Gardner DG, Downs Jr RW, et al. Circulating parathyroid hormone activity: familial hypocalciuric hypercalcemia versus typical primary hyperparathyroidism. J Clin Endocrinol Metab. 1978;47(6):1190–7.
11. Marx SJ, Spiegel AM, Levine MA, Rizzoli RE, Lasker RD, Santora AC, et al. Familial hypocalciuric hypercalcemia: the relation to primary parathyroid hyperplasia. N Engl J Med. 1982;307(7):416–26.
12. Marx SJ, Spiegel AM, Sharp ME, Brown EM, Gardner DG, Downs Jr RW, et al. Adenosine 3′,5′-monophosphate response to parathyroid hormone: familial hypocalciuric hypercalcemia versus typical primary hyperparathyroidism. J Clin Endocrinol Metab. 1980;50(3):546–8.
13. Marx SJ, Stock JL, Attie MF, Downs Jr RW, Gardner DG, Brown EM, et al. Familial hypocalciuric hypercalcemia: recognition among patients referred after unsuccessful parathyroid exploration. Ann Intern Med. 1980;92(3):351–6.
14. Egbuna OI, Brown EM. Hypercalcaemic and hypocalcaemic conditions due to calcium-sensing receptor mutations. Best Pract Res Clin Rheumatol. 2008;22(1):129–48.
15. Bai M, Pearce SH, Kifor O, Trivedi S, Stauffer UG, Thakker RV, et al. In vivo and in vitro characterization of neonatal hyperparathyroidism resulting from a de novo, heterozygous mutation in the

Ca^{2+}-sensing receptor gene: normal maternal calcium homeostasis as a cause of secondary hyperparathyroidism in familial benign hypocalciuric hypercalcemia. J Clin Invest. 1997;99(1):88–96.
16. Pearce SH, Bai M, Quinn SJ, Kifor O, Brown EM, Thakker RV. Functional characterization of calcium-sensing receptor mutations expressed in human embryonic kidney cells. J Clin Invest. 1996;98(8):1860–6.
17. Bai M, Quinn S, Trivedi S, Kifor O, Pearce SH, Pollak MR, et al. Expression and characterization of inactivating and activating mutations in the human Ca^{2+}-sensing receptor. J Biol Chem. 1996;271(32):19537–45.
18. Simonds WF, James-Newton LA, Agarwal SK, Yang B, Skarulis MC, Hendy GN, et al. Familial isolated hyperparathyroidism: clinical and genetic characteristics of 36 kindreds. Medicine (Baltimore). 2002;81(1):1–26.
19. Lietman SA, Tenenbaum-Rakover Y, Jap TS, Yi-Chi W, De-Ming Y, Ding C, et al. A novel loss-of-function mutation, Gln459Arg, of the calcium-sensing receptor gene associated with apparent autosomal recessive inheritance of familial hypocalciuric hypercalcemia. J Clin Endocrinol Metab. 2009;94(11):4372–9.
20. Aida K, Koishi S, Inoue M, Nakazato M, Tawata M, Onaya T. Familial hypocalciuric hypercalcemia associated with mutation in the human Ca^{2+}-sensing receptor gene. J Clin Endocrinol Metab. 1995;80(9):2594–8.
21. Heath III H. Familial benign (hypocalciuric) hypercalcemia. A troublesome mimic of mild primary hyperparathyroidism. Endocrinol Metab Clin North Am. 1989;18(3):723–40.
22. Bilezikian JP, Khan AA, Potts Jr JT. Guidelines for the management of asymptomatic primary hyperparathyroidism: summary statement from the third international workshop. J Clin Endocrinol Metab. 2009;94(2):335–9.
23. Hinnie J, Bell E, McKillop E, Gallacher S. The prevalence of familial hypocalciuric hypercalcemia. Calcif Tissue Int. 2001;68(4):216–8.
24. Liel Y, Arie R, Vered I. Familial hypocalciuric hypercalcemia in Israel: a preliminary report. Calcif Tissue Int. 1997;61(1):36–8.
25. Cetani F, Pardi E, Borsari S, Tonacchera M, Morabito E, Pinchera A, et al. Two Italian kindreds with familial hypocalciuric hypercalcaemia caused by loss-of-function mutations in the calcium-sensing receptor (CaR) gene: functional characterization of a novel CaR missense mutation. Clin Endocrinol (Oxf). 2003;58(2):199–206.
26. Marcocci C, Borsari S, Pardi E, Dipollina G, Giacomelli T, Pinchera A, et al. Familial hypocalciuric hypercalcemia in a woman with metastatic breast cancer: a case report of mistaken identity. J Clin Endocrinol Metab. 2003;88(11):5132–6.
27. Lo Presti R, Caimi G. Familial hypocalciuric hypercalcemia. Minerva Endocrinol. 1986;11(4):245–51.
28. Sereni D, Chevalier P, Cremer GA, Boissonnas A, Dubost C, Laroche C. Familial hypocalciuric hypercalcemia: two case reports (author's transl). Ann Med Interne (Paris). 1982;133(4):281–4.
29. Langhendries JP, Chanoine F, Corvilain J, Fuss M, Van Geertruyden J. Familial hypocalciuric hypercalcemia. A new family. Rev Rhum Mal Osteoartic. 1985;52(11):609–12.
30. Monfort-Gouraud M, Lanza M, Meyer A, Roussel M, Badoual J. A rare cause of hypercalcemia: familial hypocalciuric hypercalcemia. Arch Fr Pediatr. 1993;50(4):335–7.
31. Gomez JM, Jorge S, Soler J, Lucas T. Familial hypocalciuric hypercalcemia. Report of a new family. J Endocrinol Invest. 1982;5(2):125–7.
32. Gjestvang FT, Olsson S, Sundoy A, Schjoth A, Haug E. Familial hypocalciuric hypercalcemia. Tidsskr Nor Laegeforen. 1992;112(4):476–8.
33. Toss G, Arnqvist H, Larsson L, Nilsson O. Familial hypocalciuric hypercalcaemia: a study of four kindreds. J Intern Med. 1989;225(3):201–6.
34. Carling T, Szabo E, Bai M, Ridefelt P, Westin G, Gustavsson P, et al. Familial hypercalcemia and hypercalciuria caused by a novel mutation in the cytoplasmic tail of the calcium receptor. J Clin Endocrinol Metab. 2000;85(5):2042–7.
35. Schwarz P, Larsen NE, Lonborg Friis IM, Lillquist K, Brown EM, Gammeltoft S. Familial hypocalciuric hypercalcemia and neonatal severe hyperparathyroidism associated with mutations in the human Ca^{2+}-sensing receptor gene in three Danish families. Scand J Clin Lab Invest. 2000;60(3):221–7.
36. Nissen PH, Christensen SE, Heickendorff L, Brixen K, Mosekilde L. Molecular genetic analysis of the calcium sensing receptor gene in patients clinically suspected to have familial hypocalciuric hypercalcemia: phenotypic variation and mutation spectrum in a Danish population. J Clin Endocrinol Metab. 2007;92(11):4373–9.
37. Kassem M, Eriksen EF, Mosekilde L. Familial hypercalciuric hypercalcemia. Nord Med. 1991;106(4):107–8. 11.
38. Lillquist K, Illum N, Jacobsen BB, Lockwood K. Primary hyperparathyroidism in infancy associated with familial hypocalciuric hypercalcemia. Acta Paediatr Scand. 1983;72(4):625–9.
39. Timmers HJ, Karperien M, Hamdy NA, de Boer H, Hermus AR. Normalization of serum calcium by cinacalcet in a patient with hypercalcaemia due to a de novo inactivating mutation of the calcium-sensing receptor. J Intern Med. 2006;260(2):177–82.
40. Menko FH, Bijvoet OL, Fronen JL, Sandler LM, Adami S, O'Riordan JL, et al. Familial benign hypercalcaemia. Study of a large family. Q J Med. 1983;52(206):120–40.
41. van Steensel-Moll HA, Drop SL. Hypercalcemia in childhood. A boy with asymptomatic hypocalciuric hypercalcemia. Tijdschr Kindergeneeskd. 1986;54(5):147–50.

42. Steinmann B, Gnehm HE, Rao VH, Kind HP, Prader A. Neonatal severe primary hyperparathyroidism and alkaptonuria in a boy born to related parents with familial hypocalciuric hypercalcemia. Helv Paediatr Acta. 1984;39(2):171–86.
43. Matsuo M, Okita K, Takemine H, Fujita T. Neonatal primary hyperparathyroidism in familial hypocalciuric hypercalcemia. Am J Dis Child. 1982;136(8):728–31.
44. Watanabe N, Yamauchi Y, Matsumoto J, Sakaguchi K, Fukase M, Tsutsumi M, et al. Familial hypocalciuric hypercalcemia with severe neonatal primary hyperparathyroidism (author's transl). Nippon Naika Gakkai Zasshi. 1982;71(4):479–84.
45. Yawata K, Tanabe Y, Yamamoto I, Hirosawa H, Momotsu T, Ito S, et al. Clinical study of two kindreds of familial hypocalciuric hypercalcemia. Nippon Naika Gakkai Zasshi. 1987;76(1):93–9.
46. Fujita T, Watanabe N, Fukase M, Tsutsumi M, Fukami T, Imai Y, et al. Familial hypocalciuric hypercalcemia involving four members of a kindred including a girl with severe neonatal primary hyperparathyroidism. Miner Electrolyte Metab. 1983;9(1):51–4.
47. Mohammed R, Bray MB, Koch CA, Uwaifo GI. Spontaneous rib fractures in a black woman with familial hypocalciuric hypercalcemia. Med Sci Monit. 2008;14(10):CS102–6.
48. Wermers RA, Khosla S, Atkinson EJ, Hodgson SF, O'Fallon WM, Melton III LJ. The rise and fall of primary hyperparathyroidism: a population-based study in Rochester, Minnesota, 1965-1992. Ann Intern Med. 1997;126(6):433–40.
49. Wermers RA, Khosla S, Atkinson EJ, Achenbach SJ, Oberg AL, Grant CS, et al. Incidence of primary hyperparathyroidism in Rochester, Minnesota, 1993-2001: an update on the changing epidemiology of the disease. J Bone Miner Res. 2006;21(1):171–7.
50. Lundgren E, Rastad J, Thrufjell E, Akerstrom G, Ljunghall S. Population-based screening for primary hyperparathyroidism with serum calcium and parathyroid hormone values in menopausal women. Surgery. 1997;121(3):287–94.
51. Jorde R, Bonaa KH, Sundsfjord J. Primary hyperparathyroidism detected in a health screening. The Tromso study. J Clin Epidemiol. 2000;53(11): 1164–9.
52. Sorva A, Valvanne J, Tilvis RS. Serum ionized calcium and the prevalence of primary hyperparathyroidism in age cohorts of 75, 80 and 85 years. J Intern Med. 1992;231(3):309–12.
53. Lindstedt G, Nystrom E, Lundberg PA, Johansson E, Eggertsen R. Screening of an elderly population in primary care for primary hyperparathyroidism. Scand J Prim Health Care. 1992;10(3):192–7.
54. Hauache OM. Extracellular calcium-sensing receptor: structural and functional features and association with diseases. Braz J Med Biol Res. 2001;34(5): 577–84.
55. Heath III H, Jackson CE, Otterud B, Leppert MF. Genetic linkage analysis in familial benign (hypocalciuric) hypercalcemia: evidence for locus heterogeneity. Am J Hum Genet. 1993;53(1):193–200.
56. Lloyd SE, Pannett AA, Dixon PH, Whyte MP, Thakker RV. Localization of familial benign hypercalcemia, Oklahoma variant (FBHOk), to chromosome 19q13. Am J Hum Genet. 1999;64(1):189–95.
57. Nesbit MA, Hannan FM, Graham U, Whyte MP, Morrison PJ, Hunter SJ, et al. Identification of a second kindred with familial hypocalciuric hypercalcemia type 3 (FHH3) narrows localization to a <3.5 megabase pair region on chromosome 19q13.3. J Clin Endocrinol Metab. 2010;95(4):1947–54.
58. Pidasheva S, D'Souza-Li L, Canaff L, Cole DE, Hendy GN. CASRdb: calcium-sensing receptor locus-specific database for mutations causing familial (benign) hypocalciuric hypercalcemia, neonatal severe hyperparathyroidism, and autosomal dominant hypocalcemia. Hum Mutat. 2004;24(2):107–11.
59. Hendy GN, D'Souza-Li L, Yang B, Canaff L, Cole DE. Mutations of the calcium-sensing receptor (CASR) in familial hypocalciuric hypercalcemia, neonatal severe hyperparathyroidism, and autosomal dominant hypocalcemia. Hum Mutat. 2000;16(4): 281–96.
60. Janicic N, Pausova Z, Cole DE, Hendy GN. Insertion of an Alu sequence in the Ca^{2+}-sensing receptor gene in familial hypocalciuric hypercalcemia and neonatal severe hyperparathyroidism. Am J Hum Genet. 1995;56(4):880–6.
61. D'Souza-Li L, Canaff L, Janicic N, Cole DEC, Hendy GN. An acceptor splice site mutation in the calcium-sensing receptor gene in familial hypocalciuric hypercalcemia and neonatal severe hyperparathyroidism. Hum Mutat. 2001;18(5):411–21.
62. Bai M, Trivedi S, Brown EM. Dimerization of the extracellular calcium-sensing receptor (CaR) on the cell surface of CaR-transfected HEK293 cells. J Biol Chem. 1998;273(36):23605–10.
63. Hofer AM, Brown EM. Extracellular calcium sensing and signalling. Nat Rev Mol Cell Biol. 2003;4(7):530–8.
64. Ward BK, Magno AL, Blitvich BJ, Rea AJ, Stuckey BG, Walsh JP, et al. Novel mutations in the calcium-sensing receptor gene associated with biochemical and functional differences in familial hypocalciuric hypercalcaemia. Clin Endocrinol (Oxf). 2006;64(5):580–7.
65. Ho C, Conner DA, Pollak MR, Ladd DJ, Kifor O, Warren HB, et al. A mouse model of human familial hypocalciuric hypercalcemia and neonatal severe hyperparathyroidism. Nat Genet. 1995;11(4):389–94.
66. Brown EM. Editorial: mutant extracellular calcium-sensing receptors and severity of disease. J Clin Endocrinol Metab. 2005;90(2):1246–8.
67. Tfelt-Hansen J, Ferreira A, Yano S, Kanuparthi D, Romero JR, Brown EM, et al. Calcium-sensing receptor activation induces nitric oxide production in H-500 Leydig cancer cells. Am J Physiol Endocrinol Metab. 2005;288(6):E1206–13.
68. Pearce SH, Trump D, Wooding C, Besser GM, Chew SL, Grant DB, et al. Calcium-sensing receptor mutations in familial benign hypercalcemia and neonatal hyperparathyroidism. J Clin Invest. 1995;96(6): 2683–92.

69. Felderbauer P, Klein W, Bulut K, Ansorge N, Dekomien G, Werner I, et al. Mutations in the calcium-sensing receptor: a new genetic risk factor for chronic pancreatitis? Scand J Gastroenterol. 2006; 41(3):343–8.
70. Vezzoli G, Tanini A, Ferrucci L, Soldati L, Bianchin C, Franceschelli F, et al. Influence of calcium-sensing receptor gene on urinary calcium excretion in stone-forming patients. J Am Soc Nephrol. 2002;13(10):2517–23.
71. Scillitani A, Guarnieri V, De Geronimo S, Muscarella LA, Battista C, D'Agruma L, et al. Blood ionized calcium is associated with clustered polymorphisms in the carboxyl-terminal tail of the calcium-sensing receptor. J Clin Endocrinol Metab. 2004;89(11):5634–8.
72. Toke J, Czirjak G, Patocs A, Enyedi B, Gergics P, Csakvary V, et al. Neonatal severe hyperparathyroidism associated with a novel de novo heterozygous R551K inactivating mutation and a heterozygous A986S polymorphism of the calcium-sensing receptor gene. Clin Endocrinol (Oxf). 2007;67(3):385–92.
73. Makita N, Sato J, Manaka K, Shoji Y, Oishi A, Hashimoto M, et al. An acquired hypocalciuric hypercalcemia autoantibody induces allosteric transition among active human Ca-sensing receptor conformations. Proc Natl Acad Sci USA. 2007; 104(13):5443–8.
74. Kifor O, Moore Jr FD, Delaney M, Garber J, Hendy GN, Butters R, et al. A syndrome of hypocalciuric hypercalcemia caused by autoantibodies directed at the calcium-sensing receptor. J Clin Endocrinol Metab. 2003;88(1):60–72.
75. Pallais JC, Kifor O, Chen YB, Slovik D, Brown EM. Acquired hypocalciuric hypercalcemia due to autoantibodies against the calcium-sensing receptor. N Engl J Med. 2004;351(4):362–9.
76. Auwerx J, Demedts M, Bouillon R. Altered parathyroid set point to calcium in familial hypocalciuric hypercalcaemia. Acta Endocrinol (Copenh). 1984;106(2):215–8.
77. Attie MF, Gill Jr JR, Stock JL, Spiegel AM, Downs Jr RW, Levine MA, et al. Urinary calcium excretion in familial hypocalciuric hypercalcemia. Persistence of relative hypocalciuria after induction of hypoparathyroidism. J Clin Invest. 1983;72(2):667–76.
78. Sands JM, Flores FX, Kato A, Baum MA, Brown EM, Ward DT, et al. Vasopressin-elicited water and urea permeabilities are altered in IMCD in hypercalcemic rats. Am J Physiol. 1998;274(5 Pt 2):F978–85.
79. Kantham L, Quinn SJ, Egbuna OI, Baxi K, Butters R, Pang JL, et al. The calcium-sensing receptor (CaSR) defends against hypercalcemia independently of its regulation of parathyroid hormone secretion. Am J Physiol Endocrinol Metab. 2009;297(4):E915–23.
80. Egbuna O, Quinn S, Kantham L, Butters R, Pang J, Pollak M, et al. The full-length calcium-sensing receptor dampens the calcemic response to 1alpha,25(OH)2 vitamin D3 in vivo independently of parathyroid hormone. Am J Physiol Renal Physiol. 2009;297(3):F720–8.
81. Egbuna O, Quinn S, Kantham L, Pang L, Butters R, Pollak M, et al. editors. PTH-dependent and independent roles of the CaSR in renal handling using diuretics in mice in-vivo. Proceedings of the 40th annual meeting of the American Society of Nephrology. San Francisco; 2007.
82. Law Jr WM, Heath III H. Familial benign hypercalcemia (hypocalciuric hypercalcemia). Clinical and pathogenetic studies in 21 families. Ann Intern Med. 1985;102(4):511–9.
83. Pearce SH, Wooding C, Davies M, Tollefsen SE, Whyte MP, Thakker RV. Calcium-sensing receptor mutations in familial hypocalciuric hypercalcaemia with recurrent pancreatitis. Clin Endocrinol (Oxf). 1996;45(6):675–80.
84. Bruce JI, Yang X, Ferguson CJ, Elliott AC, Steward MC, Case RM, et al. Molecular and functional identification of a Ca^{2+} (polyvalent cation)-sensing receptor in rat pancreas. J Biol Chem. 1999; 274(29):20561–8.
85. Felderbauer P, Hoffmann P, Einwachter H, Bulut K, Ansorge N, Schmitz F, et al. A novel mutation of the calcium sensing receptor gene is associated with chronic pancreatitis in a family with heterozygous SPINK1 mutations. BMC Gastroenterol. 2003; 3:34.
86. Whitcomb DC. Genetic aspects of pancreatitis. Annu Rev Med. 2010;61:413–24.
87. Stuckey BG, Gutteridge DH, Kent GN, Reed WD. Familial hypocalciuric hypercalcaemia and pancreatitis: no causal link proven. Aust N Z J Med. 1990;20(5):718–9. 25.
88. Warner J, Epstein M, Sweet A, Singh D, Burgess J, Stranks S, et al. Genetic testing in familial isolated hyperparathyroidism: unexpected results and their implications. J Med Genet. 2004;41(3):155–60.
89. Zajickova K, Vrbikova J, Canaff L, Pawelek PD, Goltzman D, Hendy GN. Identification and functional characterization of a novel mutation in the calcium-sensing receptor gene in familial hypocalciuric hypercalcemia: modulation of clinical severity by vitamin D status. J Clin Endocrinol Metab. 2007;92(7):2616–23.
90. Brachet C, Boros E, Tenoutasse S, Lissens W, Andry G, Martin P, et al. Association of parathyroid adenoma and familial hypocalciuric hypercalcaemia in a teenager. Eur J Endocrinol. 2009;161(1): 207–10.
91. Heath DA. Familial benign hypercalcemia. Trends Endocrinol Metab. 1989;1(1):6–9.
92. Brown EM. Familial hypocalciuric hypercalcemia and other disorders with resistance to extracellular calcium. Endocrinol Metab Clin North Am. 2000;29(3):503–22.
93. Strewler GJ. Familial benign hypocalciuric hypercalcemia—from the clinic to the calcium sensor. West J Med. 1994;160(6):579–80.
94. Christensen SE, Nissen PH, Vestergaard P, Heickendorff L, Rejnmark L, Brixen K, et al. Plasma 25-hydroxyvitamin D, 1,25-dihydroxyvitamin D, and parathyroid hormone in familial hypocalciuric

hypercalcemia and primary hyperparathyroidism. Eur J Endocrinol. 2008;159(6):719–27.
95. Bustamante M, Hasler U, Leroy V, de Seigneux S, Dimitrov M, Mordasini D, et al. Calcium-sensing receptor attenuates AVP-induced aquaporin-2 expression via a calmodulin-dependent mechanism. J Am Soc Nephrol. 2008;19(1):109–16.
96. Law Jr WM, Wahner HW, Heath III H. Bone mineral density and skeletal fractures in familial benign hypercalcemia (hypocalciuric hypercalcemia). Mayo Clin Proc. 1984;59(12):811–5.
97. Burski K, Torjussen B, Paulsen AQ, Boman H, Bollerslev J. Parathyroid adenoma in a subject with familial hypocalciuric hypercalcemia: coincidence or causality? J Clin Endocrinol Metab. 2002;87(3):1015–6.
98. Christensen SE, Nissen PH, Vestergaard P, Heickendorff L, Brixen K, Mosekilde L. Discriminative power of three indices of renal calcium excretion for the distinction between familial hypocalciuric hypercalcaemia and primary hyperparathyroidism: a follow-up study on methods. Clin Endocrinol (Oxf). 2008;69(5):713–20.
99. Waller S, Kurzawinski T, Spitz L, Thakker R, Cranston T, Pearce S, et al. Neonatal severe hyperparathyroidism: genotype/phenotype correlation and the use of pamidronate as rescue therapy. Eur J Pediatr. 2004;163(10):589–94.
100. Alon US, VandeVoorde RG. Beneficial effect of cinacalcet in a child with familial hypocalciuric hypercalcemia. Pediatr Nephrol. 2010;25(9):1747–50.

Hyperparathyroidism–Jaw Tumor Syndrome

13

Andrew C. Calabria and Michael A. Levine

Abstract

Hyperparathyroidism–jaw tumor syndrome (HPT–JT) is an autosomal dominant disorder characterized by the development of parathyroid tumors, ossifying fibromas of the mandible and maxilla, cystic and neoplastic renal abnormalities, and uterine tumors. One of its unique characteristics is its association with a high prevalence of atypical parathyroid adenomas and carcinomas.

HPT–JT is caused by mutations in the HRPT2 gene that reduce expression or function of parafibromin, a nuclear protein that regulates gene expression and inhibits cellular proliferation (Carpten et al., Nat Genet 32(4):676–680, 2002; Yart et al., Mol Cell Biol 25(12):5052–5060, 2005; Zhang et al., Biochem Biophys Res Commun 350(1):17–24, 2006; Woodard et al., Oncogene 24(7):1272–1276, 2005). Prior to recognition of HRPT2, HPT–JT was diagnosed using clinical criteria and was based on the presence of ossifying jaw tumors in a patient with primary hyperparathyroidism (PHPT) who lacked features of other complex syndromes associated with hyperfunctioning parathyroid glands. Patients with HPT–JT also manifest a more aggressive form of PHPT than is typical of sporadic or other genetic forms of PHPT, due in part to the presence of atypical parathyroid tumors and the increased risk of parathyroid carcinoma (Marx, N Engl J Med 343(25):1863–1875, 2000). Moreover, patients

A.C. Calabria, MD
Division of Endocrinology and Diabetes,
The Children' Hospital of Philadelphia,
34th and Civic Center Blvd., 11NW-Ste30, Philadelphia,
PA 19104, USA

M.A. Levine, MD (✉)
Department of Pediatrics, University of Pennsylvania
School of Medicine, Children's Hospital of Philadelphia,
34th and Civic Center Blvd., Philadelphia, PA 19104, USA
e-mail: levinem@chop.edu

A.A. Licata and E.V. Lerma (eds.), *Diseases of the Parathyroid Glands*,
DOI 10.1007/978-1-4419-5550-0_13, © Springer Science+Business Media, LLC 2012

with HPT–JT have asynchronous development of parathyroid tumors, so recurrence of PHPT is common after removal of one or more parathyroid tumors.

Keywords
Hyperparathyroidism • Parafibromin • Atypical parathyroid adenomas • HRPT2 gene

Introduction

Primary hyperparathyroidism (PHPT) is the most common cause of hypercalcemia. In most cases, PHPT is a sporadic disorder that occurs in patients in their fifth or sixth decade of life and occurs as a consequence of a single, benign parathyroid adenoma. Inherited forms of PHPT occur in up to 20% of cases, however, and are usually associated with the presence of multiple parathyroid tumors and an earlier onset of hypercalcemia. These disorders exhibit autosomal dominant modes of transmission, and over the past few years, molecular genetic research has led to the identification of many of the responsible genes. In turn, clinical genetic testing has facilitated molecular diagnosis in presymptomatic relatives of affected subjects, enabled the identification of affected patients who lack a family history of PHPT, and enhanced specification and characterization of distinct genetic forms of inherited PHPT. Patients with genetic forms of PHPT may have isolated hyperparathyroidism, in which only the parathyroid glands are involved, or may have more complex syndromes in which parathyroid tumors are associated with cellular defects in other endocrine and nonendocrine tissues (Table 13.1) [1]. The most unique of these complex syndromes is the hyperparathyroidism–jaw tumor syndrome (HPT–JT), an autosomal dominant disorder with incomplete penetrance that is characterized by the development of parathyroid tumors, ossifying fibromas of the mandible and maxilla, cystic and neoplastic renal abnormalities, and uterine tumors. In contrast to other forms of familial PHPT in which parathyroid tumors are generally benign, HPT–JT is associated with a high prevalence of atypical parathyroid adenomas and carcinomas [2–5].

Table 13.1 Familial forms of primary hyperparathyroidism

Familial forms of primary hyperparathyroidism(PHPT)	Genetic mutation	Chromosomal location	Inheritance	PHPT features	Associated endocrinopathies
HPT–JT	*HRPT2*	1q21.q31	AD	Adenomas (cystic) Carcinomas	Jaw tumors Renal tumors Uterine tumors
MEN-1	*MEN1*	11q13	AD	Hyperplasia	Pituitary tumors Pancreatic tumors
MEN-2A	*RET*	10q11.2	AD	Hyperplasia	Medullary thyroid carcinoma Pheochromocytoma
FIHP	*HRPT2* *MEN1* *CASR* *Unnamed*	1q21.31 11q13 3q13.3-q21 2q14-p13.3	AD	Adenomas/carcinomas Hyperplasia/adenoma Normal/hyperplasia Hyperplasia/adenoma	By definition, isolated to PHPT
FHH	*CASR*	3q13.3-q21	AD	Normal/hyperplasia	None

Adapted from Carling, T. and R. Udelsman, *Parathyroid surgery in familial hyperparathyroid disorders.* J Intern Med, 2005. **257**(1): p. 27–37

HPT–JT is caused by mutations in the *HRPT2* gene that reduce expression or function of parafibromin, a nuclear protein that regulates gene expression and inhibits cellular proliferation [6–9]. Prior to recognition of *HRPT2*, HPT–JT was diagnosed using clinical criteria and was based on the presence of ossifying jaw tumors in a patient with PHPT who lacked features of other complex syndromes associated with hyperfunctioning parathyroid glands. Patients with HPT–JT also manifest a more aggressive form of PHPT than is typical of sporadic or other genetic forms of PHPT, due in part to the presence of atypical parathyroid tumors and the increased risk of parathyroid carcinoma [5]. Moreover, patients with HPT–JT have asynchronous development of parathyroid tumors, so recurrence of PHPT is common after removal of one or more parathyroid tumors. Some patients with HPT–JT will not have jaw tumors or other typical features of the syndrome, which in the absence of molecular genetic testing can lead to diagnostic confusion with other hereditary parathyroid disorders (Table 13.1) [1] or sporadic presentations of PHPT.

Pathophysiology

The pathophysiology of the HPT–JT syndrome is similar to other forms of PHPT. The primary abnormality in parathyroid cells leads to excessive and inappropriate secretion of parathyroid hormone (PTH), which results in hypercalcemia and other features of PHPT. PTH binds to specific heptahelical receptors (PTHR1) that are expressed on the plasma membrane of target cells, particularly renal tubular cells and osteoblasts, and activates adenylyl cyclase to produce the second messenger cyclic AMP. In the kidney, PTH increases calcium reabsorption in the renal distal tubule and reduces reabsorption of phosphate and bicarbonate in the proximal tubule. In addition, PTH induces expression of renal CYP27b, the enzyme that converts 25(OH)D to 1,25(OH)$_2$D (calcitriol), with consequent elevation of serum levels of this fully active, hormonal form of vitamin D. Elevated levels of calcitriol increase absorption of calcium, and to a lesser extent phosphorus, from the gastrointestinal tract, and together with PTH induce expression of RANKL (receptor activator of nuclear factor of kB ligand) in osteoblasts. Elevated RANKL induces differentiation and activity of osteoclasts, which lead to increased bone resorption and bone turnover. These direct and indirect actions of PTH lead to the principal features of PHPT: hypercalcemia, hypophosphatemia, and preferential loss of cortical bone. Skeletal abnormalities range from mild osteopenia to the classical lesions of osteitis fibrosa cystica. Overt skeletal disease is now uncommon, occurring in only 1.4–14% patients at presentation, but osteoporosis with associated fractures is now increasing [10]. Symptoms in PHPT are often vague and patients may also complain of anorexia, nausea, abdominal pain, constipation, and rarely acute pancreatitis. Peptic ulcer disease has been described in multiple endocrine neoplasia type 1 (MEN-1) if PHPT is present, but this has not been described with HPT–JT. Psychiatric symptoms such as fatigue, weakness, somnolence, lethargy, dementia, stupor, and depression have long been associated with PHPT and are likely related to effects of hypercalcemia on the neurologic system. Many of these changes may be subtle and may not be truly appreciated until after parathyroidectomy. Acute hypercalcemic crisis with nephrogenic diabetes insipidus may also develop if serum calcium levels are greater than 12 mg/dL (3 mmol/L). The degree of hypercalcemia determines the amount of calcium in the glomerular filtrate, and although the fractional excretion of calcium may be reduced, the absolute amount of excreted calcium in the urine is increased in most patients and increases the risk of nephrocalcinosis and nephrolithiasis. Today, due to the routine measurement of serum concentrations of calcium, at least 70–80% of patients with PHPT fail to show obvious signs or symptoms of disease, and are identified through the incidental finding of mild hypercalcemia [11].

In most patients with PHPT (80–85%), hyperparathyroidism is limited to a single monoclonal adenoma, which in most cases is related to a specific somatic gene defect. The other three glands are normal. The average adenoma ranges from 1 to 3 cm in size and weighs about 0.5 g, which is significantly larger than a normal parathyroid gland (25–35 mg). Cystic elements in an adenomatous gland may call attention to HPT–JT, which was originally characterized as *cystic parathyroid adenomatosis*. Approximately 15–20% of patients with PHPT have diffuse hyperplasia of all four glands, a broad category that includes hyperplasia, multiple adenomas, and polyclonal hyperfunction. Multiglandular disease is more likely to occur in younger individuals, and is usually associated with germ line mutations that cause MEN-1 and MEN-2A (Table 13.1) [1]. PHPT rarely is due to parathyroid carcinoma (~1%), but its identification should raise suspicions for HPT–JT.

Hyperparathyroidism–Jaw Tumor Syndrome

Clinical Presentation

In 1987, Mallette et al. described a father and three sons who at early ages developed severe hypercalcemia; in each case, a single parathyroid adenoma was found at surgery [12]. Three members of this family developed recurrent hypercalcemia due to development of a second parathyroid adenoma 6–13 years after resection of the initial parathyroid adenoma; the fourth affected individual had developed hypoparathyroidism after the first operation. Review of the pathologic specimens showed that each parathyroid tumor was a cystic adenoma, and unexpectedly, similar cystic changes were also present in the normal parathyroid glands in these patients. In the originally described cohort, urinary calcium excretion was elevated in all four patients, and one individual had nephrolithiasis. Interestingly, three other first-degree relatives of the affected subjects were hypercalcemic, but two were hypocalciuric, which initially suggested a possible link between this syndrome and familial hypocalciuric hypercalcemia (FHH) that was later disproved. Three of four patients in this cohort also underwent resection of ossifying fibromas of the mandible or maxilla. However, unlike the classic brown tumors of the jaw (epulis) that occasionally occur in other forms of PHPT, these jaw tumors did not have the distinctive appearance of brown tumors as they were found to lack osteoclasts. Review of the literature disclosed previously reported cases of familial parathyroid adenomas in association with fibro-osseous jaw tumors [13, 14], suggesting that these individuals had the same syndrome. Further review of the parathyroid histology in these other kindreds also identified the adenomas as cystic [15]. To date, approximately 50 families of HPT–JT have been described. Subsequent analysis of these additional cases has extended the phenotype of HPT–JT to include uterine tumors and cystic and neoplastic renal anomalies and extended the spectrum of parathyroid disease to include not only cystic adenomas but also parathyroid carcinomas.

Natural History of PHPT in HPT–JT Syndrome

The most common, and sometimes the only feature of HPT–JT, is primary hyperparathyroidism, which has a penetrance of about 80–90% [5, 16]. HPT–JT, similar to other genetic forms of PHPT, presents earlier in life than sporadic forms of PHPT. On average, about 80% of individuals with HPT–JT will manifest PHPT by the end of the third decade [5]. The average age of diagnosis for HPT–JT probands is 32 years, but in some patients PHPT may occur as early as the first decade [17]. With the exception of its very early onset, the clinical presentation of PHPT in HPT–JT is otherwise indistinguishable from that of sporadic or other inherited forms of PHPT. Patients with PHPT often develop renal complications, such as nephrolithiasis (17–37%), nephrocalcinosis, and hypercalciuria [11]. Patients with HPT–JT develop additional unique renal anomalies, such as renal cysts, hamartomas, and adult onset Wilms tumor.

In contrast to sporadic PHPT or other hereditable forms of PHPT, there is a relatively high prevalence of parathyroid carcinoma in HPT–JT, as well as atypical adenomas that have a high potential for malignant transformation. Moreover, although all four parathyroid glands are potentially affected in HPT–JT, the development of adenomas is asynchronous, and often only a single parathyroid tumor is present at diagnosis [3]. This asynchronous presentation is unique among the different forms of inherited PHPT, in which development of parathyroid tumors is more likely to be metasynchronous. Removal of the initially affected parathyroid tumor leads to a presumed cure, only to be followed years later by recurrence of PHPT and the need for additional treatment or surgery [3]. As in the original description of HPT–JT, the adenomas may be cystic, either with micro- or macrocysts, which may aid in diagnosis [3]. In addition, there is a significant association of parathyroid carcinoma in HPT–JT syndrome, with 15% of cases presenting with parathyroid carcinoma, compared to an incidence of <1% in other forms of PHPT [17, 18]. Still, while most experts cite a frequency of 15% for parathyroid carcinomas in HPT–JT syndrome, this number is based on a relatively small number of families and may be confounded by ascertainment bias [19]. In general, parathyroid carcinomas are usually larger, firmer, and more easily palpable than benign parathyroid tumors, and are associated with higher serum levels of PTH and serum calcium levels that are often greater than 14 mg/dL (3.5 mmol/L) [20].

Jaw Tumors

In 1958, Jackson et al. reported a unique multigenerational family with hereditary hyperparathyroidism in which four of the five affected members of the first generation had jaw tumors [21]. Three affected members of the third generation developed similar jaw tumors that progressed after surgical correction of hyperparathyroidism. Reinvestigation of this family disclosed that these maxillary and mandibular tumors were histologically distinct from the classical "brown tumors" of hyperparathyroidism. Brown tumors are focal lesions found within the areas of bone resorption. Radiographic evaluation of these tumors reveals well-defined lytic lesions but histologically brown tumors represent a reparative cellular process. Brown tumors consist of foci of hemorrhage, fibrosis, and granulation tissue, and the characteristic brown color is due to hemosiderin deposition. The lesions contain increased numbers of multinucleate giant cells, osteoblasts, and osteoclasts and poorly mineralized woven bone, and often resemble giant cell lesions. Brown tumors are usually slowly growing and locally destructive lesions, and invasion into surrounding structures may cause a variety of symptoms. Patients often develop significant bone pain, and pathologic fractures may occur. When brown tumors occur in the head or neck, they usually involve the mandible, and only rarely affect the maxilla. Most studies have shown that surgical treatment of PHPT and normalization of excessive levels of serum PTH is typically associated with spontaneous regression of the bony lesions, including brown tumors. Nevertheless, local curettage and enucleation of jaw lesions appear necessary in cases where regression of the brown tumor is incomplete or where disfigurement is significant.

By contrast, the jaw tumors in HPT–JT are fibro-osseous lesions that lack giant cells. The jaw tumors are typically fibrous maxillary or mandibular tumors and resemble ossifying fibromas (cemento-ossifying fibromas) (Fig. 13.1) [22]. The ossifying fibromas of HPT–JT are limited to the jaw, whereas the typical brown tumors of hyperparathyroidism occur in the ribs or knees as well as the jaw. Whereas sporadic jaw tumors generally occur in the third and fourth decades of life, jaw tumors in HPT–JT often arise earlier. Jaw tumors occur in 16–50% of patients with HPT–JT [23], and as they are unrelated to parathyroid status it is not surprising that they do not regress after correction of hyperparathyroidism [24]. Similar to the asynchronous development of parathyroid tumors in HPT–JT, jaw tumors may be asynchronous and may even precede the development of hypercalcemia by several decades. Complete surgical removal of jaw tumors is the recommended treatment, but recurrence is possible [25].

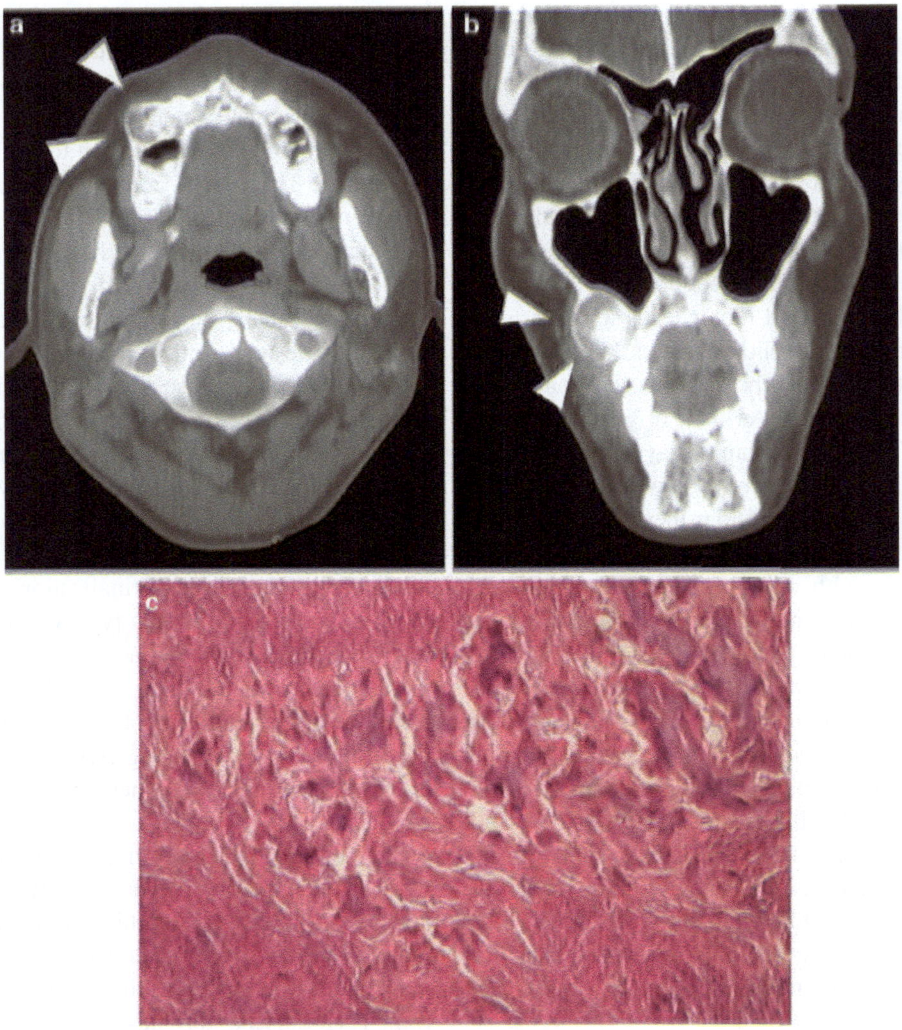

Fig. 13.1 Jaw tumors. Axial (**a**) and coronal (**b**) CT scans showing a well-circumscribed lesion in the right maxilla of an HPT–JT patient, with accompanying histologic evaluation consistent with an ossifying fibroma (**c**) (Reprinted from Int J Oral Maxillofac Surg, 36(4), Yamashita, Y., et al., A case of hyperparathyroidism-jaw tumor syndrome found in the treatment of an ossifying fibroma in the maxillary bone, pp. 365–9, Copyright 2007, with permission from Elsevier)

Kidney Involvement in the HPT–JT Syndrome

The kidney is involved in a limited subset of patients with HPT–JT (~5–15% of cases), raising the possibility that the development of renal cysts and tumors represents a distinct phenotypic variant of HPT–JT [26, 27]. Cystic kidney disease is the most common renal manifestation of this syndrome [26]. The majority of affected HPT–JT patients were discovered to have unsuspected renal involvement by routine ultrasound, but several patients have presented in renal failure [26]. The cysts may range from a few minor cysts to bilateral polycystic lesions that result in renal failure [26]. In addition to renal cysts, some patients often develop rare renal tumors, such as mixed epithelial-stromal tumors and adult Wilms' tumors. The mixed epithelial-stromal tumor, previously reported as a hamartoma, is a very unusual tumor that may be solid or cystic, lacks necrosis, and contains a mesenchymal component with variable spindle cell proliferation [16]. While these tumors demonstrate loss of the wild-type *HRPT2* allele, surgical resection has been curative and malignant behavior (i.e., metastases) has not been noted. Adult Wilms' tumors have been described in multiple HPT–JT families. Wilms' tumors are typically diagnosed in childhood and are usually highly malignant tumors that require surgical resection, chemotherapy, and radiation. The Wilms' tumors in HPT–JT have been identified in patients as old as 53 years but have neither metastasized nor led to death. They are usually bilateral, poorly circumscribed, and of smaller sizes than classical childhood Wilms' tumor, which is an embryonal tumor (e.g., nephroblastoma) that is associated with loss of both copies of the *WT1* tumor suppressor gene. The Wilms tumor of HPT–JT also has distinctive histological features that distinguish it from the childhood Wilms' tumor, such as a low number of mitoses, lack of necrosis and hemorrhages, large mesenchymal components, and the presence of cysts [4]. Papillary renal cell carcinoma and renal cell adenomas have also been described, albeit infrequently, in HPT–JT [28]. These tumors are also likely part of HPT–JT, as both mixed epithelial-stromal tumors and papillary renal cell carcinomas have all shown allelic deletions in the same region on chromosome 1 [4, 28].

Other Features

Characterization of additional, more recently described subjects with HPT–JT has shed new light on the spectrum of endocrinopathies and tumors that can be associated with syndrome. Uterine tumors have been described in association with HPT–JT and may actually be the most common clinical feature in some patients after PHPT, affecting 75% of HPT–JT female patients in some cohorts [19, 23, 29, 30]. In a Japanese family, two women with HPT–JT had unusual multiple small uterine polyps, which were diagnosed as adenomyomatous polyps [31]. It is unclear if these polyps are a variant of adenomyosis or endometriosis or have more aggressive neoplastic potential. Analysis of 33 HPT–JT kindreds revealed that affected women in 13 families suffered from menorrhagia in their second to fourth decades and often required hysterectomy as definitive treatment [30]. Uterine tumors were only diagnosed after surgery and have been linked to reduced fertility in affected women with HPT–JT [30]. Histological analysis of the uterine specimens revealed both benign and malignant tumors, with adenomyosis, adenofibromas, leiomomas, endometrial hyperplasia, and adenosarcomas identified [30]. Uterine myomas have also been described in several families [31]. A large Dutch kindred has also extended the clinical phenotype of HPT–JT syndrome. Thirteen affected members presented with either parathyroid adenoma or carcinoma, but in addition to associated renal anomalies, testicular mixed germ cell tumor with major seminoma component and Hürthle cell thyroid adenoma were also reported [28]. Other conditions, including thyroid carcinoma, thyrotoxicosis, colonic carcinoma, and pituitary cyst, have also been described, but may represent incidental findings. It is unclear whether a predisposition to these less common tumors truly exists.

The HPT–JT Syndrome and Other Forms of Familial PHPT

HPT–JT is one of the several autosomal dominant forms of familial hyperparathyroidism, that include familial isolated hyperparathyroidism (FIHP), MEN-1, multiple endocrine neoplasia type 2A (MEN-2A), and FHH (Table 13.1). In general, inherited forms of PHPT present at an earlier age than sporadic forms and occur with equal frequencies in both sexes. Genetic analyses of these disorders have helped to elucidate some of the underlying molecular mechanisms that may have significant clinical implications (Fig. 13.2) [32]. Multiple small kindreds with two or three affected members with isolated PHPT have received a diagnosis of FIHP. FIHP is a rare autosomal dominant form of PHPT characterized by hypercalcemia, elevated PTH levels, and uni- or multiglandular parathyroid tumors. FIHP is a diagnosis of exclusion and must be distinguished from other familial hypercalcemic

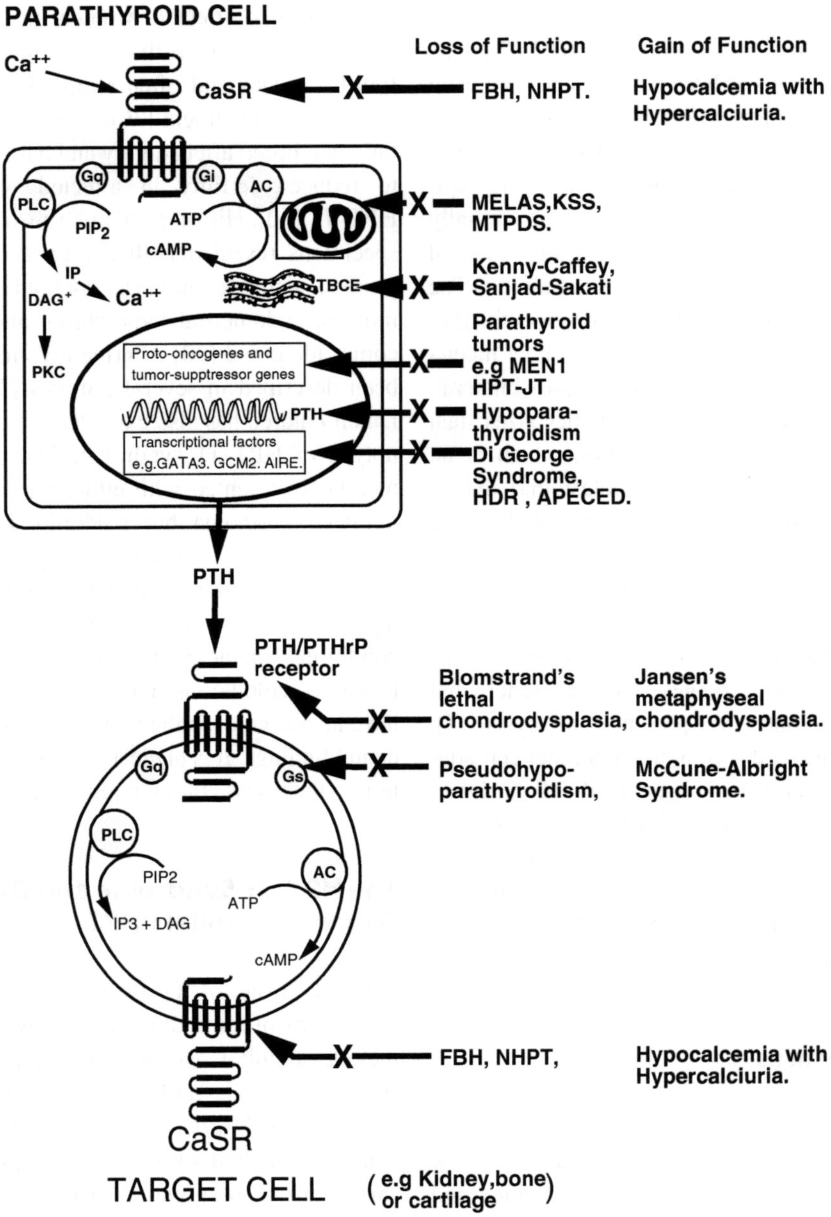

Fig. 13.2 Schematic representation of molecular components of calcium homeostasis. HPT–JT syndrome is caused by a mutation in the *HRPT2* gene and must be differentiated from MEN-1, which is due to inactivating mutations of the tumor suppressor gene *MENIN*; FHH, which is caused by heterozygous loss-of-function mutations of the *CASR* gene encoding the calcium sensing receptor; and FIHP, which has been linked to mutations in *HRPT2*, *MENIN*, and *CASR* in some cases (With kind permission from Springer Science+Business Media: Rev Endocr Metab Disord, Genetics of endocrine and metabolic disorders: Parathyroid, 5(1), 2004, p. 37–51, Thakker, R.V.)

disorders, in particular, FHH, MEN-1, MEN-2A, and HPT–JT (Table 13.1). The genetic locus of FIHP has not yet been disclosed. FHH is a benign autosomal dominant hypercalcemic disorder that is caused by heterozygous loss-of-function mutations of the *CASR* gene encoding the calcium sensing receptor. FHH is characterized by lifelong, nonprogressive hypercalcemia that may be present from birth, inappropriately elevated PTH levels, and hypocalciuria. FHH is related to neonatal severe PHPT, a life-threatening form of severe hypercalcemia that is most commonly due to homozygous loss-of-function mutations in the *CASR* gene. MEN-1 is due to inactivating mutations of the tumor suppressor gene *MENIN*, and the autosomal dominant MEN-1 syndrome is characterized by tumors of the parathyroid, anterior pituitary (most commonly prolactinomas), and endocrine pancreas (most commonly gastrinomas). MEN-1 has near full penetrance, with hyperparathyroidism present at diagnosis in over 90% of cases and invariably associated with multiglandular disease. The presentation of pituitary and pancreatic tumors is generally much later and more variable than hyperparathyroidism in MEN-1. Like MEN-1, MEN-2A is also an autosomal dominant condition, but instead is due to activating mutations of the *RET* proto-oncogene and associated with medullary thyroid cancer, pheochromocytoma, and hyperparathyroidism. PHPT occurs in only 10–15% of patients with MEN-2A, as opposed to MTC, which has nearly 100% penetrance, and pheochromocytoma, which occurs in 50–60% of affected individuals. In contrast to MEN-1, PHPT in MEN-2A is more often caused by uniglandular disease but occasionally presents with multiglandular disease.

HPT–JT may be difficult to distinguish from other forms of familial PHPT, especially when the parathyroid tumors occur in isolation without any evidence of jaw tumors. HPT–JT syndrome is readily differentiated from FHH, as serum calcium levels are elevated in FHH from the neonatal or early infantile period and fractional excretion of calcium is very low (<1%), whereas hypercalcemia in HPT–JT is uncommon in the first decade. The clinical distinction between HPT–JT and MEN-1 in patients who lack other features can be more challenging. Although HPT–JT patients can have multiple parathyroid adenomas, they more commonly will have a single parathyroid adenoma with unusual histology of a parathyroid carcinoma. By contrast, parathyroid disease in patients with MEN-1 is often multiglandular and parathyroid carcinoma does not occur. Long-term follow-up may be required to disclose the development of other lesions in MEN-1, which may explain why some cases of FIHP have been linked to the MEN-1 locus [33]. The distinction between HPT–JT syndrome and FIHP is equally difficult, especially given the incomplete or asynchronous presentation of the additional features associated with HPT–JT. However, this distinction is very important given the higher risk of developing carcinomas in HPT–JT. A personal or family history of parathyroid carcinoma mandates serious consideration of germ line *HRPT2* mutation status in families with FIHP, regardless of whether features associated with HPT–JT are present [34]. An investigation for additional features of HPT–JT, such as jaw tumors, renal, uterine, pancreatic, thyroid, and testicular anomalies, may provide such a distinction and may help identify HPT–JT patients. Specifically, the finding of ossifying fibromas is an important distinguishing feature of HPT–JT from FIHP, and the occurrence of these jaw tumors may occasionally precede the development of hypercalcemia in HPT–JT patients by decades.

Parafibromin and the *HRPT2* Gene

To gain insight into the mechanisms underlying HPT–JT, family linkage studies were undertaken to determine the chromosomal location of the HPT–JT locus. The HPT–JT locus was mapped to chromosome 1q21-q31 and the putative gene designated hyperparathyroidism type 2, *HRPT2*. Positional cloning studies refined the chromosomal map location of *HRPT2*, and a prioritized DNA sequence analysis of the genes located within the critical interval on chromosome 1q31.2 revealed mutations within a gene that encoded a 531 amino acid protein with 17 exons, designated parafibromin or cell division cycle 73 (CDC73) [6]. The mutations identified in HPT–JT patients were found to be scattered through the coding region, with a higher number of mutations in exons 1–2 and 7–8, but none in exons 9–12 and 14–17, and greater than 80% predicting a functional loss through premature truncation [23, 27, 30]. To date, 111 independent CDC73 mutations have been recognized and consist of 68 germ line mutations (>60%), 38 somatic mutations (<35%), and 5 others (<5%) whose origin has not been defined [35]. Of the 111 mutations, 50% were frameshift deletions or insertions, 29% nonsense mutations, 13% missense mutations, 6% splice site mutations, and 2% in-frame deletions or insertions [35]. In another study of HPT–JT kindreds, germ line frameshift and nonsense mutations were the most frequent mutations identified, accounting for 88% of mutations, as opposed to the infrequent finding of germ line missense mutations [23]. No genotype–phenotype correlation has been identified to date [30]. In addition, nonpenetrance has been seen in greater than 30% of mutation carriers, which may have important implications for surveillance considerations [30].

In their original work, Carpten et al. were able to detect *HRPT2* mutations in only 14 of 24 HPT–JT families, most of which had full expression of the syndrome and proven linkage to 1q24-q32 [6, 36]. Mutations in the coding region and splice sites have been identified in more than 80% of the 51 reported HPT–JT families [36]. In the remaining cases, mutations may be present in the promoter or untranslated regions or there may be whole exon or gene deletions that are not detected by PCR-based analysis [36]. Gene silencing through methylation is also a potential mechanism, as is involvement of a second genetic locus [36].

Since the identification of *HRPT2*, germ line *HRPT2* mutations have been found in 7% of FIHP (*HRPT1*) kindreds [6, 17, 23, 27, 30, 34, 37, 38]. In several of these apparent FIHP kindreds, parathyroid carcinomas and atypical adenomas have been identified in individuals carrying a germ line *HRPT2* mutation, again pointing to the tendency for malignant proliferation [6, 30, 34]. Other cases of FIHP had previously been linked to mutations in the MEN-1 gene and *CASR* [39]. In addition, hyperparathyroidism type 3 (*HRPT3*) has also been described, with mapping demonstrating linkage to chromosome 2q14-p13.3 in a FIHP kindred [40]. The remaining cases of FIHP are likely due to as of yet unidentified genes or potentially recently described genes, such as *CDKN1B*, which has been associated with the pathogenesis of sporadic parathyroid adenomas and a rare familial MEN-1-like (MEN-4) disorder but whose role in tumorigenesis remains to be fully elucidated [41]. FIHP may represent a phenotypic variant of different genetic syndromes, such as HPT–JT, MEN-1, and FHH, but with reduced or incomplete penetrance. As such, the clinical diagnosis of FIHP should be considered only provisional, and ultimately the term FIHP may be replaced as more causative genes are recognized.

Parafibromin is thought to function as a tumor suppressor, and consistent with Knudson's two-hit model of inherited cancer, mutations in *HRPT2* generally lead to a truncated or inactive protein. Moreover, germline mutations that inactivate *HRPT2* are present in affected members of HPT–JT kindreds and occur as somatic events in sporadic parathyroid adenomas and carcinomas [6, 24]. In some cases, "two hits" affecting *HRPT2*, either an additional mutation or loss of heterozygosity at the *HRPT2* locus, have been identified in a subset of parathyroid tumors [23, 26, 42–44]. Despite this, immunohistochemical analysis has revealed a loss of parafibromin expression in both parathyroid adenomas and carcinomas but not in normal parathyroid glands in the same subjects [23]. This suggests that the loss of parafibromin immunoreactivity in HPT–JT-related adenomas is a pivotal step in parathyroid tumorigenesis [45]. Still, as parafibromin is only involved in approximately 70% of parathyroid carcinomas and loss of parafibromin immunoreactivity may not be observed in all cases of *HRPT2* mutation, the identification of complementary markers would greatly aid diagnosis [46]. One such candidate marker to loss of parafibromin immunoreactivity is protein gene product 9.5 (PGP9.5), encoded by ubiquitin carboxyl-terminal esterase L1 (*UCHL1*) [46]. Diffuse positive staining for PGP9.5 has been exhibited in parafibromin negative carcinomas and adenomas, as well as parafibromin positive tumors, and may have greater sensitivity with similar specificity to parafibromin negativity as a marker of malignancy [46]. Moreover, these findings were supported by RT-PCR analysis that showed high expression of *UCHL1* in the carcinoma group [46].

The association between other affected tissues in HPT–JT and the *HRPT2* gene has also been explored. Masi et al. compared parafibromin expression in HPT–JT-related uterine polyps to sporadic ones. They noted a loss of parafibromin nuclear staining in both stromal and epithelial components of HPT–JT polyps, supporting a pathogenic role for *HRPT2* mutations in the development of uterine polyps in this syndrome [23]. While linkage to 1q markers was not associated with *HRPT2* in six hereditary Wilms' tumor families [26], additional studies have identified somatic *HRPT2* mutations with sporadic renal tumors, including renal cell carcinoma and Wilms' tumor [47]. Somatic and germ line *HRPT2* mutations have also been identified in sporadic ossifying fibromas and support a potential role for *HRPT2* mutations in the pathogenesis of jaw tumors [48]. The presence of such mutations in the fibromas themselves may explain the lack of clinical improvement in these jaw tumors after parathyroidectomy.

Determination of *HRPT2* mutations is particularly important due to the association with parathyroid carcinoma. Overall, somatic *HRPT2* mutations are present in most sporadic parathyroid carcinomas (20 of 26 cases; 77%) [49–51], and are absent in most sporadic parathyroid adenomas (0–4%). This indicates that *HRPT2* mutations confer a high risk for malignant transformation to carcinoma and may have a direct role in the pathogenesis of parathyroid carcinoma. A recent analysis of the full coding sequence and splice sites of the *HRPT2* gene in 21 parathyroid carcinomas from 15 patients without family history of PHPT revealed that 67% of parathyroid tumors had *HRPT2* mutations, and three patients carried germ line *HRPT2* mutations [51]. The unexpected finding of germ line *HRPT2* mutations in 20–30% of patients with sporadic parathyroid carcinomas suggests that these probands and their relatives may have occult HPT–JT with limited expressivity or a phenotypic variant. Thus, *HRPT2* analysis can provide a sensitive and specific molecular marker for parathyroid carcinoma in tumors with ambiguous or atypical histopathology. This has important clinical implications, as up to 50% of parathyroid tumors that behave in a biologically malignant manner (i.e., recurrence and metastasis) will be considered benign using conventional clinicopathological criteria. Moreover, *HRPT2* analysis facilitates DNA-based testing to identify at-risk relatives of patients with parathyroid cancer who carry germ line *HRPT2* mutations.

The *HRPT2* gene is ubiquitously expressed and evolutionarily conserved. Despite its role as a putative tumor suppressor gene, the function of parafibromin was not initially clear. The C-terminal domain shares 27% sequence identity with the yeast Cdc73 protein, which is a component of the yeast polymerase-associated factor 1 (PAF1) complex, a key transcriptional regulatory complex that interacts directly with RNA polymerase II [7]. Studies in yeast as well as mammalian cells have revealed that parafibromin is a nuclear protein and a mediator of key transcriptional events of histone modification, chromatin remodeling, initiation, and elongation [36]. Studies in *Drosophila* support a role for parafibromin in the regulation of translation, through homologs of the mammalian translational regulatory protein, cytoplasmic polyadenylation element binding protein [52]. Parafibromin has also been recognized to have an activating role as a component of the Wnt signaling pathway [53]. Immunohistochemical and functional studies have demonstrated that *HRPT2* mutations lead to loss of parafibromin expression [42, 45], abnormal localization [54], and abolition of antiproliferative activity [8]. In mammalian cells, parafibromin may have a dual role as an oncoprotein and tumor suppressor, depending on cellular environment, and therefore may have opposing effects in different tissues [36]. Interestingly, loss of HRPT2 expression and parafibromin in mice leads to apoptosis, possibly due to decreased expression of the *Igf1*, *Igf2*, *Hmga1*, and *Hmga2* genes, which are important factors for mammalian growth and adult survival [36, 55]. By contrast, similar loss of HRPT2 expression in human adult parathyroid cells results in tumor development due to increased proliferation. Comparison with the *Men1* knockout mouse provides adjunctive evidence for this divergence of expression. Despite ubiquitous expression, *Men1* knockout mice suggest that loss of a tumor suppressor in susceptible tissues will lead to tumor formation, but will not affect proliferation in nonsusceptible tissues and cells will undergo apoptosis or remain normal [36].

Diagnostic Evaluation

Primary Hyperparathyroidism

The most common clinical presentation of both sporadic and familial forms of PHPT is asymptomatic hypercalcemia. An elevated serum calcium level should be confirmed by repeated measurement of the serum calcium concentration. Measurement of the total serum calcium concentration is generally adequate, but determination of the ionized calcium level may be necessary if serum protein levels and/or acid–base status are abnormal. An ionized calcium level may be more sensitive, as shown in a recent series of patients with PHPT where 12 of 60 subjects had elevated serum ionized calcium levels in the setting of presumed normocalcemia [56]. If possible, previous values for serum calcium levels should be reviewed. The presence of longstanding asymptomatic hypercalcemia raises the possibility of FHH and is also more suggestive of PHPT than nonparathyroid malignancy.

If hypercalcemia is confirmed, PTH levels should be measured using an immunoassay for intact or whole molecule PTH. The diagnosis of PHPT is usually concluded by the combination of an elevated or inappropriately normal serum level of PTH level in a subject with hypercalcemia. Absolute or relative elevations in PTH help to distinguish PHPT from other common causes of hypercalcemia, such as malignancy (Fig. 13.3) [5]. The majority of patients with PHPT have elevated serum levels of PTH, but in some patients the PTH concentration can be within the normal range [57]. These latter cases suggest that not all bioactive PTH can be measured by currently available intact and bioactive assays [57], or that "normal" ranges for serum PTH are not accurate. In suspected cases of PHPT with low-normal PTH levels, it may be helpful to repeat measurement of PTH using assays that detect other epitopes as adenomas may produce a bioactive form of PTH that is not completely measured by the intact or bioactive assays [57]. In addition, the 7–84 PTH peptide makes up roughly 15% of the measured intact assay in normal plasma, whereas the amino-truncated PTH (7–84) may account for at least 30% of the intact assay measurement in PHPT [57]. Conversely, others cases of PHPT may initially present with normocalcemia despite elevated PTH levels, which may represent the earliest manifestation of the disease course of PHPT. In these cases of so-called "incipient" PHPT, elevations of PTH are not associated with frankly elevated levels of serum calcium. In a longitudinal study of 37 patients with normocalcemic PHPT referred to a metabolic bone disease unit, many patients had evidence of classical PHPT, with a history of kidney stones in 14%, fragility fractures in 11%, and osteoporosis in 57% [spine (34%), hip (38%), and/or distal one-third radius (28%)] [58]. Moreover, progressive bone loss was not confined to the distal one-third of the radius, as in classical PHPT, instead occurring at all sites [T scores: spine, -2.00 ± 0.25; hip, -1.84 ± 0.18; distal one-third radius, -1.74 ± 0.22] [58]. Further signs of progressive hyperparathyroidism developed over the duration of the study (median 3 years) in 40% of patients, with 19% developing hypercalcemia [58]. Moreover, the observation that many individuals did not show evidence of hypercalcemia suggests the time course for the development of hypercalcemia in PHPT is highly variable.

Preoperative Imaging

^{99}Tc-labeled sestamibi with single photon emission computerized tomography (SPECT) imaging is the most widely used localization procedure for parathyroid tumors at experienced centers and can help plan the surgical approach in HPT–JT as in other cases of PHPT. However, suspicion for HPT–JT may not arise until the time of surgery, based on operative, histologic, and pathologic findings, or much later, in the event of recurrence

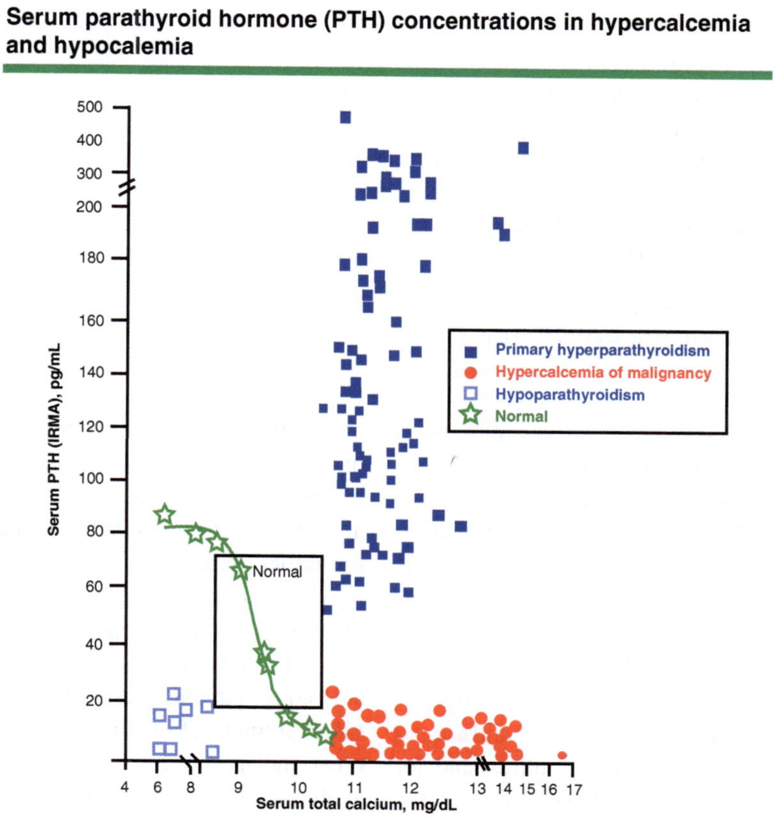

Fig. 13.3 Serum parathyroid hormone (PTH) concentrations (pg/mL) according to serum total calcium concentrations (mg/dL) in various disease states. The normal range is shown in the *white box*. Serum PTH and calcium levels are low in hypoparathyroidism (*open blue squares*) and high in primary hyperparathyroidism (*blue squares*). The serum calcium concentration is high and serum PTH is appropriately low in individuals with hypercalcemia of malignancy (*red circles*). While the diagnosis of a mineral metabolism disorder is usually clear, the PTH levels may overlap with the normal ranges and represent a limitation of the assays available for clinical use today (Reproduced with permission from Fuleihan GE, Silverberg SJ. Diagnosis and differential diagnosis of primary hyperparathyroidism. In: UpToDate, Basow, DS (Ed), UpToDate, Waltham, MA 2011. Copyright © 2011 UpToDate, Inc. For more information visit http://www.uptodate.com)

after initial resection of an isolated adenoma. Overall, the success rate of sestamibi scans is very good, with approximately 85% of parathyroid adenomas identified, but this decreases to about 45% for multiglandular disease [59]. Other modalities such as ultrasound and magnetic resonance imaging (MRI) are less helpful, except in the setting of coexisting thyroid disease and remedial cervical exploration [60]. Invasive localization procedures, such as angiography and venous sampling, are used for patients with recurrent or persistent PHPT [60, 61], and venous sampling in particular has been aided by the introduction of the rapid PTH assay [61].

Additional Diagnostic Testing

Diagnosis of HPT–JT is usually made during the second or third decade of life. Typically, the diagnosis is based on the finding of a single parathyroid adenoma with atypical cystic features and/or parathyroid carcinoma in a patient with jaw tumors. While the finding of carcinoma raises the possibility of HPT–JT, the presentation of a solitary parathyroid adenoma makes it much more difficult to distinguish HPT–JT from other forms of PHPT. Moreover, jaw tumors may be occult, emphasizing the importance of radiological evaluation of the jaw and kidneys in patients with young-onset

Table 13.2 Screening recommendations

Tumor[a]	Test	Frequency[b]
Parathyroid	Serum calcium, parathyroid hormone (PTH)	6 Months
Jaw fibromas	Panoramic jaw X-rays	5 Years
Renal	Renal ultrasound and/or abdominal magnetic resonance imaging (MRI)	5 Years
Uterine	Pelvic ultrasound	Annual

[a]Screening for the most common HPT–JT tumors is listed, but additional tumors, such as thyroid and testicular tumors, have also been reported. When indicated, assessment for these should also be undertaken
[b]Frequency after baseline testing
Adapted from Bradley, K.J., et al., *Uterine tumours are a phenotypic manifestation of the hyperparathyroidism-jaw tumour syndrome.* J Intern Med, 2005. **257**(1): p. 18–26

disease, multiglandular involvement, cystic parathyroid adenomas, and parathyroid carcinoma.

Additional baseline testing in suspected cases of HPT–JT would also be indicated. Pelvic ultrasound may be performed on an annual basis to screen for uterine tumors, which may be more common that originally appreciated [30]. Depending on kindred and any potential known tumors associated with the individual lineage, additional testing, including testicular ultrasound for testicular tumors and thyroid ultrasound for thyroid cancers, can be considered (Table 13.2).

Gene Sequencing and Screening

All patients with young-onset PHPT, multiglandular parathyroid disease, cystic parathyroid adenomas, or positive family history of PHPT should be carefully evaluated for the presence of a germ line gene defect associated with MEN 1, MEN2a, FIHP, FHH, and HPT–JT. The identification of parathyroid carcinoma increases the likelihood of identifying an *HRPT2* mutation. Identification of associated features, such as renal or jaw tumors, which may sometimes precede the identification of PHPT, would also be an indication for gene sequencing for *HRPT2*. Gene sequencing for *HRPT2* as well as other genes that are involved in familial PHPT is available from both several commercial reference laboratories (http://www.ncbi.nlm.nih.gov/sites/GeneTests/?db=GeneTests). The identification of a loss-of-function *HRPT2* mutation in an affected individual has important consequences for ongoing surveillance for additional manifestations of HPT–JT. However, it is equally important to screen at-risk individuals in potential kindreds. Whereas mutation-negative individuals may no longer require close biochemical monitoring, regular surveillance of individuals with a germ line *HRPT2* mutation may allow for earlier detection of hyperparathyroidism, earlier surgical management, and possible prevention or cure of parathyroid carcinoma. DNA testing for *HRPT2* mutations should also be seriously considered for patients presenting with apparent sporadic carcinoma. In addition to sporadic carcinoma, other indications for possible *HRPT2* mutation analysis include young-onset PHPT (less than 35 years of age), sporadic jaw tumors, FIHP (after exclusion of *MEN1* and *CASR*), and parathyroid adenoma, in association with renal cysts or tumors, pancreatic tumors, thyroid tumors, and/or uterine lesions [35].

Screening Recommendations

Semiannual follow-up evaluations have been arbitrarily but appropriately suggested for affected probands with HPT–JT and potentially affected family members. In one such kindred, a 13-year-old boy with parathyroid carcinoma developed a second, albeit more benign, tumor 2 years after the initial malignancy, but his serum calcium and PTH levels were normal 6 months prior to presentation of the second tumor [34]. The rapid progression of PHPT suggests how aggressive this disease can be and reinforces the need for regular and frequent surveillance. Similarly, in the same kindred, an asymptomatic 22-year-old brother developed an aggressive parathyroid tumor that was identified after biochemical monitoring indicated hypercalcemia and an elevated PTH level [34]. This group recommended screening asymptomatic, previously normocalcemic, mutation-positive siblings of the proband using serum calcium and PTH measurements every 6 months [34].

Guidelines for regular surveillance for the development of HPT–JT associated tumors have been suggested but not formally endorsed and will likely continue to evolve [30]. These apply to asymptomatic mutation carriers and first- and second-degree relatives in families without identified germ line *HRPT2* mutations. Monitoring of serum calcium and PTH levels is warranted in such family members, with the goal of early diagnosis and treatment of early parathyroid cancer. If PHPT develops in an at-risk relative, surgery aimed at identifying and examining all parathyroid glands could be advocated, even if a more limited approach might otherwise have been chosen. However, surveillance limited to biochemical monitoring alone would not capture some at-risk individuals. In a family with a germ line mutation of the *HRPT2* gene, discovery of a recurrent atypical adenoma in the normocalcemic proband 12 years after initial resection and the finding of a parathyroid carcinoma in a normocalcemic carrier suggest that adding neck ultrasound to the surveillance may increase sensitivity and lead to earlier detection of potential neoplasms [19]. Given the high worldwide prevalence of vitamin D deficiency, we recommend determination of serum 25-hydroxyvitamin D levels in patients who have elevated serum PTH levels and normal serum calcium concentrations to exclude mild secondary hyperparathyroidism.

The unexpected finding of germline *HRPT2* mutations in patients with apparent sporadic parathyroid carcinoma has forced a reconsideration of the clinical management approach taken not only for affected patients but also for potentially at-risk relatives. On further investigation, these individuals may ultimately have manifestations of HPT–JT or represent a phenotypic variant. When hyperparathyroidism recurs or worsens in such a patient, a new and distinct primary parathyroid tumor should be carefully sought in addition to recurrence or progression of the original neoplasm due to the asynchronous presentation commonly seen in HPT–JT [51]. Surveillance for jaw and renal tumors would also be indicated. As such, genetic testing for *HRPT2* mutations should be offered to all individuals with presumed sporadic parathyroid carcinoma. Moreover, while the identification of a mutation in the coding sequence would be definitive, this would not rule out the existence of a mutation in the noncoding region, a finding that has been recognized in nearly half of families with classic HPT–JT [6]. Relatives of individuals with germline *HRPT2* mutations may also be at risk for the development of parathyroid carcinoma or other findings consistent with HPT–JT if they likewise possess the mutation. While monitoring serum calcium levels on a semiannual basis may be used as a screening test, definitive genetic testing would allow for focused clinical surveillance for family members who carry the mutation. Monitoring of serum calcium levels in *HRPT2*-positive relatives would allow for earlier diagnosis and treatment of parathyroid carcinoma. Similarly, in at-risk individuals, surgery aimed at identifying and examining all parathyroid glands may be advocated. However, as in probands, current technologies will not capture mutations in the noncoding regions, so continued biochemical monitoring may still be considered in those at-risk relatives negative for *HRPT2* mutations.

Treatment

Although surgical intervention remains the primary treatment for patients with specific signs or symptoms of PHPT, most individuals are asymptomatic. The most recent recommendations for management of patients with asymptomatic PHPT are based on the Third International Workshop on the Management of Asymptomatic Primary Hyperparathyroidism, a consensus conference that was convened in 2008 to reassess previous guidelines from 1990 and 2002 workshops in the context of recent advances in our understanding of the natural history of untreated and treated asymptomatic disease [62–64].

The recommendations for surgery in asymptomatic patients with PHPT include the following criteria:

1. Serum calcium concentration that more than 1 mg/dL (>0.25 mmol/L) above the upper limits of normal.
2. Renal stones but not isolated hypercalciuria.
3. GFR less than 60 mL/min 1.73 m^2.
4. Reduction in bone density. Surgery is recommended for peri- or postmenopausal women and men aged 50 and older who have a *T*-score of −2.5 or less at the lumbar spine, femoral neck, total hip, or 33% (one-third) radius. In premenopausal women and in men younger than 50, the *Z*-score of −2.5 or less is recommended as the cut-point below which surgery is advised.
5. The presence of a fragility fracture, which provides clinical evidence of symptomatic low bone density.
6. Age less than 50 years is a guideline for surgery, as evidence supports a greater risk of complications of PHPT in these individuals over time than in those who are older than 50 years.

The 2008 workshop also acknowledged that patients who appeared to have asymptomatic PHPT frequently have significant neurocognitive symptoms that are only appreciated after parathyroidectomy [65]. Moreover, patients with asymptomatic PHPT often have lower bone mineral density and increased fracture rates that may improve with parathyroidectomy [62].

In HPT–JT, like other forms of PHPT, the standard treatment is surgical, but given the relatively small number of cases that have been studied, surgical recommendations continue to evolve. Prophylactic total parathyroidectomy has been suggested in HPT–JT to reduce the risk of parathyroid carcinoma. This approach seems unduly aggressive, however, given the infrequency of parathyroid carcinoma and the difficulties of managing postsurgical hypoparathyroidism.

In cases of sporadic PHPT where imaging studies provide preoperative confirmation of a single parathyroid tumor, and localization is successful, minimally invasive parathyroidectomy (MIP) is emerging as the surgical procedure of choice. MIP offers the potential for curative treatment of a localized tumor with less damage to surrounding tissue, fewer complications and more rapid postoperative recovery [66]. MIP may be considered as an alternative to standard complete cervical exploration with visualization of all four parathyroid glands in patients with HPT–JT when uniglandular uptake is identified on preoperative imaging (e.g., ultrasound examination, 99mTc-sestamibi scanning with concomitant SPECT/CT, CT, and/or MRI) [66]. Because patients with HPT–JT may have additional parathyroid tumors that escape detection by standard imaging techniques, MIP should incorporate intraoperative PTH measurement, and PTH levels should be obtained prior to and 5 and 10 min after tumor resection [66]. As normal parathyroid glands are suppressed by the hypercalcemia, a decline of PTH of greater than 50% after tumor resection is generally considered indicative of a successful operation where no further exploration is required [66]. However, concerns have arisen regarding the reliability of a drop in PTH levels after resection of an adenoma in patients with multiple parathyroid adenomas or multiglandular disease [67], and some have suggested that an 80% reduction in PTH instead be applied [68, 69].

The surgical approach in HPT–JT is further complicated by the increased risk of parathyroid carcinoma. If parathyroid carcinoma is encountered, a more aggressive *en bloc tumor* resection with ipsilateral thyroid lobectomy and resection of adjacent soft tissues has been recommended as definitive treatment [70]. It is important to avoid damaging the tumor, as this could lead to seeding of tumor cells in the local area. Vascular invasion, fibrous, and large size are hallmarks of parathyroid carcinoma. In most series, the median maximal diameter of parathyroid carcinoma is between 3.0 and 3.5 cm compared with approximately 1.5 cm for benign adenomas.

In one report of 12 patients with germ line *HRPT2* mutations (11 adenomas and 1 carcinoma) who underwent limited parathyroidectomy, all but one achieved initial cure, but three required later reoperation due to recurrent disease at 5, 9, and 27 years, respectively [71]. However,

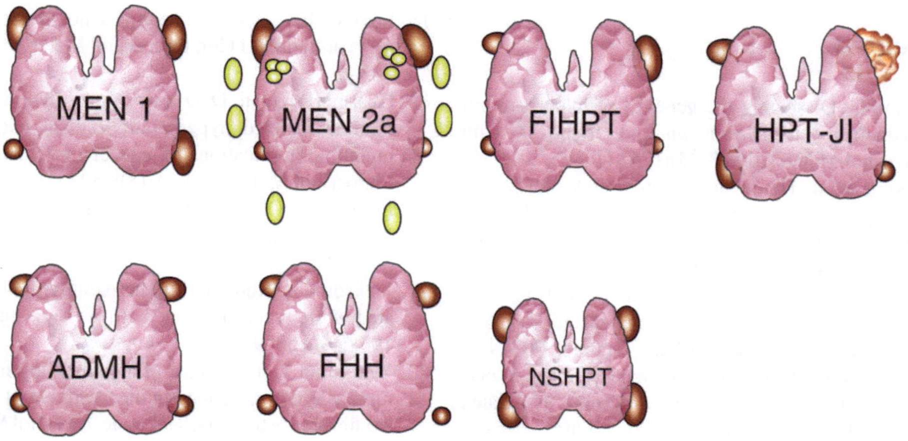

Fig. 13.4 Schematic illustrations of parathyroid abnormalities in familial forms of hyperparathyroidism. Parathyroid tumors in HPT–JT syndrome most commonly present as a single adenoma but may be cystic, and carry a 15% risk of parathyroid carcinoma. By contrast, MEN-1 nearly always has multiglandular involvement, FIHP usually presents with a single adenoma but may also have multiglandular involvement, and FHH exhibits mild hyperplasia. Marked variations exist within each subset (From Carling, T. and R. Udelsman, *Parathyroid surgery in familial hyperparathyroid disorders.* J Intern Med, 2005. **257**(1): p. 27–37)

long-term follow-up of three Brazilian kindreds with germ line *HRPT2* mutations shows that 80% of individuals have either persistence or recurrence of PHPT after focused parathyroidectomy and may support of adoption of a more aggressive initial surgical approach, such as subtotal parathyroidectomy [72]. Still, while no formal consensus exists, neither limited nor subtotal parathyroidectomy is effective for parathyroid carcinoma. By contrast, in other familial forms such as MEN-1, subtotal parathyroidectomy is generally recommended but total parathyroidectomy with heterotopic autotransplantation of resected parathyroid tissue may be considered. A schematic of parathyroid abnormalities in the different familial forms of PHPT is provided in Fig. 13.4 [66].

Conclusion

HPT–JT is a genetic form of PHPT caused by inactivating mutations of the *HRPT2* gene and characterized by parathyroid tumors, jaw tumors, renal and uterine tumors. While the penetrance of PHPT is high, the prevalence of other features is highly variable between kindreds. While only diagnosed in approximately 50 families to date, HPT–JT, unlike other forms of PHPT, is characterized by a high prevalence of atypical adenomas and parathyroid carcinomas. As such, the identification of *HRPT2* mutations in patients has significant clinical implications for screening for related tumors and for screening at-risk asymptomatic relatives for *HRPT2* mutations. As the presentation of the features of HPT–JT may be asynchronous, PHPT may be isolated and it may be difficult to distinguish HPT–JT from other forms of PHPT. Genetic testing for *CASR*, *MEN-1*, and *HRPT2* can help differentiate cases and may even provide a more definitive diagnosis than the provisional diagnosis of FIHP given to some individuals. In HPT–JT, after treatment of an initial parathyroid tumor, additional tumors may occur or the initial tumor may recur, again emphasizing the importance of genetic testing in suspected cases as it may affect surgical management. Identification of *HRPT2* mutations in cases of sporadic parathyroid carcinomas have also provided further justification for genetic testing in these individuals. Screening for jaw tumors, renal tumors, uterine tumors, and other related tumors and endocrinopathies should be pursued on a semiannual basis in affected individuals with HPT–JT and mutation-positive relatives. Treatment for affected cases is surgical.

References

1. Larsson C. Dissecting the genetics of hyperparathyroidism–new clues from an old friend. J Clin Endocrinol Metab. 2000;85(5):1752–4.
2. Szabo J, et al. Hereditary hyperparathyroidism-jaw tumor syndrome: the endocrine tumor gene HRPT2 maps to chromosome 1q21-q31. Am J Hum Genet. 1995;56(4):944–50.
3. Marx SJ, et al. Hyperparathyroidism in hereditary syndromes: special expressions and special managements. J Bone Miner Res. 2002;17 Suppl 2:N37–43.
4. Teh BT, et al. Autosomal dominant primary hyperparathyroidism and jaw tumor syndrome associated with renal hamartomas and cystic kidney disease: linkage to 1q21-q32 and loss of the wild type allele in renal hamartomas. J Clin Endocrinol Metab. 1996;81(12):4204–11.
5. Marx SJ. Hyperparathyroid and hypoparathyroid disorders. N Engl J Med. 2000;343(25):1863–75.
6. Carpten JD, et al. HRPT2, encoding parafibromin, is mutated in hyperparathyroidism-jaw tumor syndrome. Nat Genet. 2002;32(4):676–80.
7. Yart A, et al. The HRPT2 tumor suppressor gene product parafibromin associates with human PAF1 and RNA polymerase II. Mol Cell Biol. 2005;25(12):5052–60.
8. Zhang C, et al. Parafibromin inhibits cancer cell growth and causes G1 phase arrest. Biochem Biophys Res Commun. 2006;350(1):17–24.
9. Woodard GE, et al. Parafibromin, product of the hyperparathyroidism-jaw tumor syndrome gene HRPT2, regulates cyclin D1/PRAD1 expression. Oncogene. 2005;24(7):1272–6.
10. Mazzaglia PJ, et al. The changing presentation of hyperparathyroidism over 3 decades. Arch Surg. 2008;143(3):260–6.
11. Fraser WD. Hyperparathyroidism. Lancet. 2009; 374(9684):145–58.
12. Mallette LE, et al. Familial cystic parathyroid adenomatosis. Ann Intern Med. 1987;107(1):54–60.
13. Heath 3rd H. *Familial benign (hypocalciuric) hypercalcemia.* A troublesome mimic of mild primary hyperparathyroidism. Endocrinol Metab Clin North Am. 1989;18(3):723–40.
14. Jackson CE, Boonstra CE. Hereditary hypercalcemia and parathyroid hyperplasia without definite hyperparathyroidism. J Lab Clin Med. 1966;68:883.
15. Heath III H. The familial benign hypocalciuric hypercalcemia syndromes. In: Raisz L, Bilezikian J, Rodan G, editors. Principles of bone biology. San Diego: Academic; 1996. p. 769–82.
16. Teh BT, et al. A family with isolated hyperparathyroidism segregating a missense MEN1 mutation and showing loss of the wild-type alleles in the parathyroid tumors. Am J Hum Genet. 1998;63(5):1544–9.
17. Simonds WF, et al. Familial isolated hyperparathyroidism: clinical and genetic characteristics of 36 kindreds. Medicine (Baltimore). 2002;81(1):1–26.
18. Streeten EA, et al. Studies in a kindred with parathyroid carcinoma. J Clin Endocrinol Metab. 1992;75(2): 362–6.
19. Guarnieri V, et al. Diagnosis of parathyroid tumors in familial isolated hyperparathyroidism with HRPT2 mutation: implications for cancer surveillance. J Clin Endocrinol Metab. 2006;91(8):2827–32.
20. Fujimoto Y, Obara T. How to recognize and treat parathyroid carcinoma. Surg Clin North Am. 1987;67(2): 343–57.
21. Jackson CE. Hereditary hyperparathyroidism associated with recurrent pancreatitis. Ann Intern Med. 1958;49(4):829–36.
22. Yamashita Y, et al. A case of hyperparathyroidism-jaw tumour syndrome found in the treatment of an ossifying fibroma in the maxillary bone. Int J Oral Maxillofac Surg. 2007;36(4):365–9.
23. Masi G, et al. Clinical, genetic, and histopathologic investigation of CDC73-related familial hyperparathyroidism. Endocr Relat Cancer. 2008;15(4):1115–26.
24. Cavaco BM, et al. The hyperparathyroidism-jaw tumour syndrome in a Portuguese kindred. QJM. 2001;94(4):213–22.
25. Aldred MJ, et al. Dental findings in a family with hyperparathyroidism-jaw tumor syndrome and a novel HRPT2 gene mutation. Oral Surg Oral Med Oral Pathol Oral Radiol Endod. 2006;101(2):212–8.
26. Tan MH, Teh BT. Renal neoplasia in the hyperparathyroidism-jaw tumor syndrome. Curr Mol Med. 2004;4(8):895–7.
27. Bradley KJ, et al. Parafibromin mutations in hereditary hyperparathyroidism syndromes and parathyroid tumours. Clin Endocrinol (Oxf). 2006;64(3):299–306.
28. Haven CJ, et al. A genotypic and histopathological study of a large Dutch kindred with hyperparathyroidism-jaw tumor syndrome. J Clin Endocrinol Metab. 2000;85(4):1449–54.
29. Cavaco BM, et al. Hyperparathyroidism-jaw tumor syndrome in Roma families from Portugal is due to a founder mutation of the HRPT2 gene. J Clin Endocrinol Metab. 2004;89(4):1747–52.
30. Bradley KJ, et al. Uterine tumours are a phenotypic manifestation of the hyperparathyroidism-jaw tumour syndrome. J Intern Med. 2005;257(1):18–26.
31. Fujikawa M, et al. Familial isolated hyperparathyroidism due to multiple adenomas associated with ossifying jaw fibroma and multiple uterine adenomyomatous polyps. Eur J Endocrinol. 1998;138(5): 557–61.
32. Thakker RV. Genetics of endocrine and metabolic disorders: parathyroid. Rev Endocr Metab Disord. 2004;5(1):37–51.
33. Kassem M, et al. Familial isolated primary hyperparathyroidism. Clin Endocrinol (Oxf). 1994;41(4): 415–20.
34. Kelly TG, et al. Surveillance for early detection of aggressive parathyroid disease: carcinoma and atypical adenoma in familial isolated hyperparathyroidism associated with a germline HRPT2 mutation. J Bone Miner Res. 2006;21(10):1666–71.

35. Newey PJ, et al. Cell division cycle protein 73 homolog (CDC73) mutations in the hyperparathyroidism-jaw tumor syndrome (HPT-JT) and parathyroid tumors. Hum Mutat. 2010;31(3):295–307.
36. Newey PJ, Bowl MR, Thakker RV. Parafibromin–functional insights. J Intern Med. 2009;266(1):84–98.
37. Mizusawa N, et al. Genetic analyses in patients with familial isolated hyperparathyroidism and hyperparathyroidism-jaw tumour syndrome. Clin Endocrinol (Oxf). 2006;65(1):9–16.
38. Villablanca A, et al. Germline and de novo mutations in the HRPT2 tumour suppressor gene in familial isolated hyperparathyroidism (FIHP). J Med Genet. 2004;41(3):e32.
39. Hannan FM, et al. Familial isolated primary hyperparathyroidism caused by mutations of the MEN1 gene. Nat Clin Pract Endocrinol Metab. 2008;4(1):53–8.
40. Warner JV, et al. Familial isolated hyperparathyroidism is linked to a 1.7 Mb region on chromosome 2p13.3-14. J Med Genet. 2006;43(3):e12.
41. Costa-Guda J, et al. Somatic mutation and germline sequence abnormalities in CDKN1B, encoding p27Kip1, in sporadic parathyroid adenomas. J Clin Endocrinol Metab. 2011;96(4):E701–6.
42. Gill AJ, et al. Loss of nuclear expression of parafibromin distinguishes parathyroid carcinomas and hyperparathyroidism-jaw tumor (HPT-JT) syndrome-related adenomas from sporadic parathyroid adenomas and hyperplasias. Am J Surg Pathol. 2006;30(9):1140–9.
43. Juhlin C, et al. Loss of parafibromin expression in a subset of parathyroid adenomas. Endocr Relat Cancer. 2006;13(2):509–23.
44. Juhlin CC, et al. Parafibromin immunoreactivity: its use as an additional diagnostic marker for parathyroid tumor classification. Endocr Relat Cancer. 2007;14(2):501–12.
45. Tan MH, et al. Loss of parafibromin immunoreactivity is a distinguishing feature of parathyroid carcinoma. Clin Cancer Res. 2004;10(19):6629–37.
46. Howell VM, et al. Accuracy of combined protein gene product 9.5 and parafibromin markers for immunohistochemical diagnosis of parathyroid carcinoma. J Clin Endocrinol Metab. 2009;94(2):434–41.
47. Zhao J, et al. Sporadic human renal tumors display frequent allelic imbalances and novel mutations of the HRPT2 gene. Oncogene. 2007;26(23):3440–9.
48. Pimenta FJ, et al. HRPT2 gene alterations in ossifying fibroma of the jaws. Oral Oncol. 2006;42(7):735–9.
49. Cetani F, et al. Genetic analyses in familial isolated hyperparathyroidism: implication for clinical assessment and surgical management. Clin Endocrinol (Oxf). 2006;64(2):146–52.
50. Howell VM, et al. HRPT2 mutations are associated with malignancy in sporadic parathyroid tumours. J Med Genet. 2003;40(9):657–63.
51. Shattuck TM, et al. Somatic and germ-line mutations of the HRPT2 gene in sporadic parathyroid carcinoma. N Engl J Med. 2003;349(18):1722–9.
52. Zhang JH, et al. Cytoplasmic polyadenylation element binding protein is a conserved target of tumor suppressor HRPT2/CDC73. Cell Death Differ. 2010;17(10):1551–65.
53. Mosimann C, Hausmann G, Basler K. Parafibromin/Hyrax activates Wnt/Wg target gene transcription by direct association with beta-catenin/Armadillo. Cell. 2006;125(2):327–41.
54. Bradley KJ, et al. Parafibromin is a nuclear protein with a functional monopartite nuclear localization signal. Oncogene. 2007;26(8):1213–21.
55. Wang P, et al. Parafibromin, a component of the human PAF complex, regulates growth factors and is required for embryonic development and survival in adult mice. Mol Cell Biol. 2008;28(9):2930–40.
56. Glendenning P, et al. High prevalence of normal total calcium and intact PTH in 60 patients with proven primary hyperparathyroidism: a challenge to current diagnostic criteria. Aust N Z J Med. 1998;28(2):173–8.
57. Lafferty FW, et al. Primary hyperparathyroidism with a low-normal, atypical serum parathyroid hormone as shown by discordant immunoassay curves. J Clin Endocrinol Metab. 2006;91(10):3826–9.
58. Lowe H, et al. Normocalcemic primary hyperparathyroidism: further characterization of a new clinical phenotype. J Clin Endocrinol Metab. 2007;92(8):3001–5.
59. Civelek AC, et al. Prospective evaluation of delayed technetium-99 m sestamibi SPECT scintigraphy for preoperative localization of primary hyperparathyroidism. Surgery. 2002;131(2):149–57.
60. Alexander Jr HR, et al. Role of preoperative localization and intraoperative localization maneuvers including intraoperative PTH assay determination for patients with persistent or recurrent hyperparathyroidism. J Bone Miner Res. 2002;17 Suppl 2:N133–40.
61. Udelsman R, et al. Rapid parathyroid hormone analysis during venous localization. Ann Surg. 2003;237(5):714–9. discussion 719–21.
62. Bilezikian JP, Khan AA, Potts Jr JT. Guidelines for the management of asymptomatic primary hyperparathyroidism: summary statement from the third international workshop. J Clin Endocrinol Metab. 2009;94(2):335–9.
63. Eastell R, et al. Diagnosis of asymptomatic primary hyperparathyroidism: proceedings of the third international workshop. J Clin Endocrinol Metab. 2009;94(2):340–50.
64. Khan A, Grey A, Shoback D. Medical management of asymptomatic primary hyperparathyroidism: proceedings of the third international workshop. J Clin Endocrinol Metab. 2009;94(2):373–81.
65. Udelsman R, et al. Surgery for asymptomatic primary hyperparathyroidism: proceedings of the third international workshop. J Clin Endocrinol Metab. 2009;94(2):366–72.
66. Carling T, Udelsman R. Parathyroid surgery in familial hyperparathyroid disorders. J Intern Med. 2005;257(1):27–37.

67. Weber CJ, Ritchie JC. Retrospective analysis of sequential changes in serum intact parathyroid hormone levels during conventional parathyroid exploration. Surgery. 1999;126(6):1139–43. discussion 1143–4.
68. Dackiw AP, et al. Relative contributions of technetium Tc 99 m sestamibi scintigraphy, intraoperative gamma probe detection, and the rapid parathyroid hormone assay to the surgical management of hyperparathyroidism. Arch Surg. 2000;135(5):550–5. discussion 555–7.
69. Clerici T, et al. Impact of intraoperative parathyroid hormone monitoring on the prediction of multiglandular parathyroid disease. World J Surg. 2004;28(2):187–92.
70. Carling T, Udelsman R. Parathyroid tumors. Curr Treat Options Oncol. 2003;4(4):319–28.
71. Iacobone M, et al. Parafibromin expression, single-gland involvement, and limited parathyroidectomy in familial isolated hyperparathyroidism. Surgery. 2007;142(6):984–91. discussion 984–91.
72. Sarquis MS, et al. Familial hyperparathyroidism: surgical outcome after 30 years of follow-up in three families with germline HRPT2 mutations. Surgery. 2008;143(5):630–40.

Hypoparathyroidism and Pseudohypoparathyroidism

14

Rajesh V. Thakker

Abstract

This chapter focuses on problems with hypoparathyroidism and pseudohypoparathyroidism, in contrast to previous chapters in which these problems were discussed in children. It provides clinical information on medical history, clinical symptoms and medical management. Up-to-date information is summarized about the genetic abnormalities associated with hypoparathyroid disorders as well as disorders such as pluriglandular autoimmune hypoparathyroidism. Blomstand's disease, mitochondrial disorders associated with hypoparathyroidism, and recessive hypoparathyroid.

Keywords

Hypoparathyroidism • Hypocalcemia • Hyperphosphataemia • DiGeorge syndrome • Autoimmune • Hypomagnesaemia • Pluriglandular disorder • Endocrinopathy • Normal serum calcium • Subcapsular cataract • Papilloedema • 25 Hydroxy vitamin D • 1,25 Dihydroxy vitamin D • Pseudohypoparathyroidism • Tetany • Calcium gluconate • Celiac disease • Persistent hypocalcemia • Cholecalciferol • Ergocalciferol • Alfacalcidiol • Calcitriol • Hypercalciuria • Hypercalcemia • Autosomal disorder • X-linked disorder • Infiltrating metastases • Seizures • PTH gene mutation • Chromosome 11p15 • Autosomal dominant isolated hyperparathyroidism • Autosomal recessive hypoparathyroidism • Calcium receptor • GCMB gene • X-linked recessive hypoparathyroidism • Sox 3 gene • SRY gene • Acquired hypoparathyroidism • Hemochromatosis • Amyloidosis • Sarcoidosis • Thalassemia • Wilson's disease • Neonatal hypoparathyroidism • Kenney Caffey syndrome • Barakat syndrome • Dysmorphic features • Lymphoedema • Deafness • Renal dysplasia • Haploinsufficiency • Mitochondrial disorders • Kearns-Sayre syndrome • MELAS syndrome •

R.V. Thakker, MD, ScD, FRCP, FRCPath, FMedSci (✉)
Nuffield Department of Medicine, University of Oxford,
OCDEM, Churchill Hospital, Oxford,
Oxon OX3 7LJ, UK
e-mail: rajesh.thakker@ndm.ox.ac.uk

A.A. Licata and E.V. Lerma (eds.), *Diseases of the Parathyroid Glands*,
DOI 10.1007/978-1-4419-5550-0_14,

Opthalmoplegia • Pigmentary retinopathy • Cardiomyopathy • Lactic acidosis • Diabetes mellitus • Sensorineural deafness • Trifunctional protein deficiency • Osteosclerosis • Nanophthalmos • Hyperopia • Kirk-Richardson syndrome • Sanjad–Sakati syndrome • Tubulin-specific chaperone • Brachytelephalangy • Blomstrand disease • Chondrodysplasia • Pluriglandular autoimmune hypoparathyroidism • Candidiasis • Hypogonadism • Steatorrhea • Alopecia • Vitiligo • Autoimmune polyglandular candidiasis ectodermal dystrophy • Polyglandular autoimmune type 1 syndrome • Autoantibodies • Addison's disease • Diabetes mellitus type 1 • Inflammasome • Innate immune system • Familial benign hypocalciuric hypercalcemia • Barter syndrome type 5 • Hypokalemic alkalosis • Hyperrenninemia • Hyperaldosteronism • Gain-of-function mutation • Inactivating mutation • Carpopedal spasm • Nephrocalcinosis • Autoimmune acquired hypoparathyroidism • Pseudohypoparathyroidism type 1a and 1b • Pseudopseudohypoparathyroidism • Albright's hereditary osteodystrophy • Dental hypoplasia • Brachydactyly • Adenyl cyclase • Parathyroid hormone-related protein • *GNAS* gene

Introduction

Hypoparathyroidism is characterized by hypocalcaemia and hyperphosphataemia, which are the result of a deficiency in PTH secretion or action (Table 14.1) [1–4]. Hypoparathyroidism may result from agenesis (e.g. the DiGeorge syndrome) or destruction of the parathyroid glands (e.g. following neck surgery, or in autoimmune diseases), from reduced secretion of PTH (e.g. neonatal hypocalcaemia or hypomagnesaemia), or resistance to PTH (which may occur as a primary disorder [e.g. pseudohypoparathyroidism (PHP)], or secondary to hypomagnesaemia) [3, 4]. In addition, hypoparathyroidism may occur as an inherited disorder (Table 14.2) that may either be part of a complex congenital defect (e.g. the DiGeorge syndrome), or as part of a pluriglandular autoimmune disorder, or as a solitary endocrinopathy, which has been referred to as *isolated or idiopathic* hypoparathyroidism (Fig. 14.1) [3, 4].

Table 14.1 Causes of hypoparathyroidism

- Low parathyroid hormone levels (hypoparathyroidism)
  - Parathyroid agensis
    - Isolated or part of complex developmental anomaly (e.g. DiGeorge syndrome)
  - Parathyroid destruction
    - Surgery[a]
    - Radiation
    - Infiltration by metastases or systemic disease (e.g. haemochromatosis, amyloidosis, sarcoidosis, Wilson's disease, thalassaemia)
  - Autoimmune
    - Isolated
    - Polyglandular (type 1)[a]
  - Reduced parathyroid function (that is, parathyroid hormone secretion)
    - Parathyroid hormone gene defects
    - Hypomagnesaemia[a]
    - Neonatal hypocalcaemia (may be associated with maternal hypercalcaemia)
    - Hungry bone disease (post-parathyroidectomy)
    - Calcium-sensing receptor mutations
- High parathyroid hormone levels
  - Parathyroid hormone resistance (e.g. pseudohypoparathyroidism and hypomagnesaemia)

[a]Most common causes

Clinical Features and Investigations

Patients with hypoparathyroidism may be asymptomatic or develop symptoms and signs associated with hypocalcaemia [1, 2]. The clinical presentation of hypocalcaemia ranges from an asymptomatic biochemical abnormality to a severe, life-threatening condition. Normal total serum calcium is 2.15–2.65 mM, and in mild hypocalcaemia (serum calcium 2.00–2.15 mM), patients may be asymptomatic. Those with more

Table 14.2 Inherited forms of hypoparathyroidism and their chromosomal locations

Disease	Inheritance	Gene product	Chromosomal location
Isolated hypoparathyroidism	Autosomal dominant Autosomal recessive X-linked recessive	PTH[a], GCMB PTH[a], GCMB SOX3	11p15, 6p24.2 11p15, 6p24.2 Xq26–27
Hypocalcaemic hypercalciuria	Autosomal dominant	CaSR	3q21.1
Hypoparathyroidism associated with complex congenital syndromes			
DiGeorge type 1 (DGS1)	Autosomal dominant	TBX1	22q11.2
DiGeorge type 2 (DGS2)	Autosomal dominant		10p13–14
HDR	Autosomal dominant	GATA3	10p15
Hypoparathyroidism associated with Kearns–Sayre and MELAS	Maternal	Mitochondrial Genome	
Blomstrand lethal chondrodysplasia	Autosomal recessive	PTH/PTHrPR	3p21.3
Kenney–Caffey, Sanjad–Sakati	Autosomal dominant[b]	TBCE	1q42.3
Barakat	Autosomal recessive[b]	Unknown	?
Lymphoedema	Autosomal recessive	Unknown	?
Nephropathy, nerve deafness	Autosomal dominant[b]	Unknown	?
Nerve deafness without renal dysplasia	Autosomal dominant	Unknown	?
Hypoparathyroidism associated with polyglandular autoimmune syndrome (APECED)	Autosomal recessive	AIRE	21q22.3
Pseudohypoparathyroidism (type Ia)	Autosomal dominant parentally imprinted	GNAS1	20q13.3
Pseudohypoparathyroidism (type Ib)	Autosomal dominant parentally imprinted	GNAS1	20q13.3

HDR hypoparathyrodism, deafness, and renal anomalies, *MELAS* mitochondrial encephalopathy, stroke like episodes and lactic acidosis, ? location not known

[a]Mutations of PTH gene identified only in some families

[b]Most likely inheritance shown

severe (serum calcium less than 1.9 mM) and long-term hypocalcaemia may develop the following: acute symptoms of neuromuscular irritability (Table 14.3), ectopic calcification (e.g. in the basal ganglia, which may be associated with extrapyramidal neurological symptoms), subcapsular cataract, papilloedema, and abnormal dentition. Investigations should be directed at confirming the presence of hypocalcaemia and establishing the cause (Table 14.1). In *hypoparathyroidism*, serum calcium is low, phosphate is high, and PTH is undetectable; renal function and concentrations of the 25-hydroxy and 1,25-dihydroxy metabolites of vitamin D are normal [1, 3]. In PHP these findings are similar to those of hypoparathyroidism except for PTH, which is markedly increased [2, 3].

Management of Acute Hypocalcaemia

The management of acute hypocalcaemia depends on the severity of the hypocalcaemia, the rapidity with which it developed and the degree of neuromuscular irritability (Table 14.3). Treatment should be given to: symptomatic

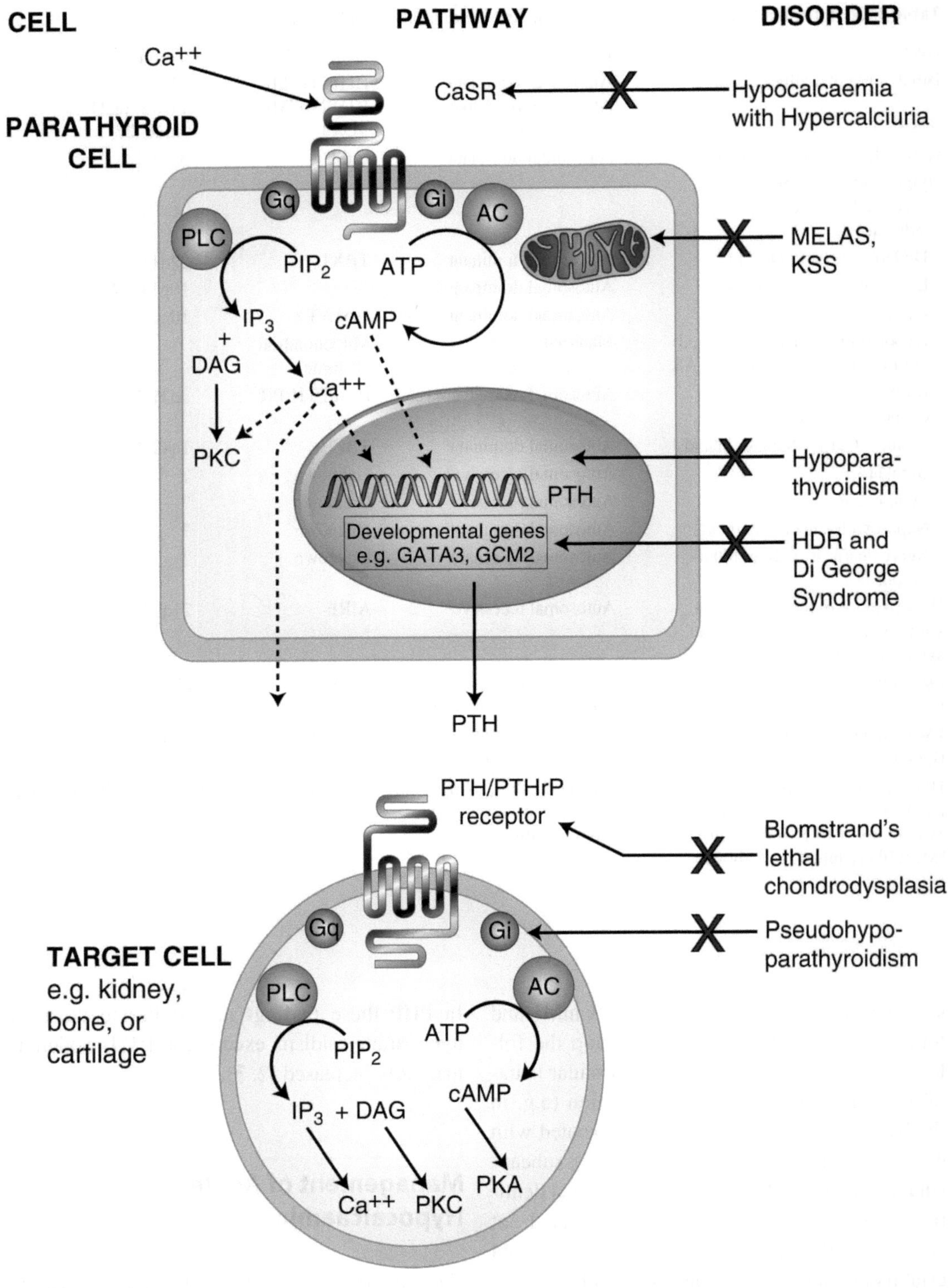

Fig. 14.1 Schematic representation of some of the components involved in calcium homeostasis. Alterations in extracellular calcium are detected by the calcium-sensing receptor (CaSR), which is a 1,078-amino acid G-protein coupled receptor. The PTH/PTHrP receptor is also a G-protein coupled receptor. Thus, Ca^2, PTH, and PTHrP involve G-protein coupled signalling pathways, and interaction with their specific receptors can lead to activation of Gs, Gi, and Gq. Gs stimulates adenylate cyclase (AC) which catalyses the formation of cAMP from ATP.

Table 14.3 Symptoms and signs associated with hypocalcaemia

• Paraesthesia, usually of fingers, toes, and circumoral regions
• Tetany, carpopedal spasm, muscle cramps
• Chvostek's sign[a]
• Trousseau's sign[b]
• Seizures of all types (that is, focal or petit mal, grand mal or syncope)
• Prolonged QT interval on ECG
• Laryngospasm
• Bronchospasm

[a]Chvostek's sign is twitching of the circumoral muscles in response to gentle tapping of the facial nerve just anterior to the ear; it may be present in 10% of normal individuals

[b]Trousseau's sign is carpal spasm elicited by inflation of a blood pressure cuff to 20 mmHg above the patient's systolic blood pressure for 3 min

patients (e.g. with tetany); and asymptomatic patients with a serum calcium of less than 1.90 mM who may be at high risk of developing complications. The preferred treatment for acute symptomatic hypocalcaemia is calcium gluconate, 10 ml 10% *w*/*v* (2.20 mmol of calcium) i.v., diluted in 50 ml of 5% dextrose or 0.9% sodium chloride and given by slow injection (more than 5 min); this can be repeated as required to control symptoms. Serum calcium should be assessed regularly [2, 3]. Continuing hypocalcaemia may be managed acutely by administration of a calcium gluconate infusion; e.g. dilute 10 ampoules of calcium gluconate, 10 ml 10% *w*/*v* (22.0 mmol of calcium), in 1 L of 5% dextrose or 0.9% sodium chloride, start infusion at 50 ml/h and titrate to maintain serum calcium in the low normal range. Generally, 0.30–0.40 mmol/kg of elemental calcium infused over 4–6 h increases serum calcium by 0.5–0.75 mM. If hypocalcaemia is likely to persist, oral vitamin D therapy should also be commenced. It is important to note that, in hypocalcaemic patients who are also hypomagnesaemic, the hypomagnesaemia must be corrected before the hypocalcaemia will resolve. This may occur in the post-parathyroidectomy period or in those with severe intestinal malabsorption, e.g. as in coeliac disease.

Management of Persistent Hypocalcaemia

The two major groups of drugs available for the treatment of hypocalcaemia are supplemental calcium, about 10–20 mmol calcium 6–12 hourly, and vitamin D preparations [3]. Patients with hypoparathyroidism seldom require calcium supplements after the early stages of stabilization on vitamin D. A variety of vitamin D preparations have been used (Table 14.4). These include vitamin D3 (cholecalciferol) or vitamin D2 (ergocalciferol), 25000–100000 U (1.25–5 mg/day); dihydrotachysterol (now seldom used), 0.25–1.25 mg/day; alfacalcidol (1α-hydroxycholecalciferol), 0.25–1.0 μg/day; and calcitriol (1,25-dihydroxycholecalciferol), 0.25–2.0 μg/day. In children, these preparations are prescribed in doses based on body weight. Cholecalciferol and ergocalciferol are the least-expensive preparations, but have the longest durations of action and may result in prolonged toxicity. The other preparations, which do not require renal 1α-hydroxylation, have the advantage of shorter half-lives and thereby minimize the risk of prolonged toxicity. Calcitriol is probably the drug of choice because it is the active metabolite and, unlike alfacalcidol, does not require hepatic 25-hydroxylation. Close monitoring (at about 1–2 weeks intervals) of the patient's serum and urine calcium is required initially, and at 3–6 monthly intervals once stabilization is achieved.

Fig. 14.1 (continued) Gi inhibits AC activity. cAMP stimulates PKA, which phosphorylates cell-specific substrates. Activation of Gq stimulates PLC, which catalyses the hydrolysis of phosphoinositide (PIP_2) to inositol triphosphate (IP_3), which increases intracellular calcium, and diacylglycerol (DAG), which activates PKC. These proximal signals modulate downstream pathways, which result in specific physiological effects. Abnormalities in several genes and encoded proteins in these pathways have been identified in patients with hypoparathyroid disorders (Table 14.1). Adapted from Thakker RV [57]. By permission of Oxford University Press

Table 14.4 Pharmaceutical preparations of vitamin D and active metabolites

	Calciferol[a]	Dihydrotachysterol	Calcifediol	Calcitriol	Alfacalcidiol
Drug	Vitamin D_3 or D_2 • Capsules, 0.25 and 1.25 mg	DHT • Liquid, 0.25 mg/ml	25-Hydroxyvitamin D_3 • Capsules, 20 and 50 μg	$1,25(OH)_2D_3$ • Capsules, 0.25 and 0.5 μg • Injection, 1 μg/ml	$1\alpha(OH)D_3$ • Capsules, 0.25, 0.50 and 1 μg • Liquid, 2 μg/ml • Injection, 2 μg/ml in propylene glycol
Time to maximum effect (week)	4–10	2–4	4–20	0.5–1	0.5–1
Persistence of effect after cessation (week)	6–30	2–8	4–12	0.5–1	0.5–1

[a]Calciferol may contain cholecalciferol or ergocalciferol.

The aim is to avoid hypercalcaemia, hypercalciuria, nephrolithiasis, and renal failure. It should be noted that hypercalciuria may occur in the absence of hypercalcaemia.

Hypoparathyroid Disorders

Isolated Hypoparathyroidism

Isolated hypoparathyroidism may either be *inherited* as an autosomal or X-linked disorder [4], or it may be *acquired* by damage to the parathyroids at surgery, or by infiltrating metastases, or systemic disease (Table 14.1).

Autosomal Hypoparathyroidism

Patients with autosomal forms of hypoparathyroidism may develop hypocalcaemic seizures in the neonatal or infantile periods and require lifelong treatment with oral vitamin D preparations, e.g. calcitriol. These patients may have mutations in the PTH gene, which consists of three exons and is located on chromosome 11p15 [5, 6]. To date, three PTH mutations have been identified [4]. These occurred in one patient with *autosomal dominant isolated hypoparathyroidism* and in two families with *autosomal recessive hypoparathyroidism* [4–6]. However, mutations of the PTH gene have been detected in only a minority of autosomal forms of hypoparathyroidism and this indicates that other genes are likely to be involved (Table 14.2). Two of these are the *CaSR* gene (see below), and the *Gcm2* (*glial cells missing* 2) [7–12]. GCMB (glial cells missing B), which is the human homologue of the Drosphilia gene Gcm, and of the mouse gcm2 gene, is expressed exclusively in the parathyroid glands. Studies of patients with isolated hypoparathyroidism have shown that GCMB mutations are associated with autosomal recessive and dominant forms of hypoparathyroidism [7–11]. Thus, a homozygous intragenic deletion of GCMB has been identified in a patient with autosomal recessive hypoparathyroidism [7], whilst in other families homozygous nonsense and missense mutations has been reported [8, 10]. Heterozygous GCMB mutations, which consist of single nucleotide deletions (c1389deT and c1399delC) that introduce frameshifts and premature truncations and a missense mutation, have been identified in three unrelated families with autosomal dominant hypoparathyroidism [9, 11]. These mutations were shown, by using a GCMB-associated luciferase reporter, to inhibit the action of the wild-type transcription factor, thereby indicating that these GCMB mutants have dominant-negative properties [9, 11].

X-linked Recessive Hypoparathyroidism

X-linked recessive hypoparathyroidism has been reported in two multigenerational kindreds from Missouri, USA [13]. In this disorder only males are affected and they suffer from infantile onset of epilepsy and hypocalcaemia, which is due to an isolated defect in parathyroid gland development [14]. Studies utilizing X-linked polymorphic markers in these families localized the mutant gene to chromosome Xq26-q27 [15], and a molecular deletional–insertion that involves chromosome 2p25 and Xq27 has been identified [16]. This deletion insertion is located approximately 67 kb downstream of SOX3, and hence it is likely to exert a position effect on SOX3 expression. SOX3 belongs to a family of genes encoding high-mobility group (HMG) box transcription factors and is related to SRY, the sex determining gene on the Y chromosome. The location of the deletion-insertion ~67 kb downstream of SOX3 in X-linked recessive hypoparathyroid patients is likely to result in altered SOX3 expression, as SOX3 expression has been reported to be sensitive to position-effects caused by X-chromosome abnormalities [17].

Acquired Forms of Hypoparathyroidism

Hypoparathyroidism may occur after neck *surgery*, *irradiation*, or because of *infiltration by metastases* or *systemic disease*, e.g. haemochromatosis, amyloidosis, sarcoidosis, Wilson's disease, or thalassaemia [2, 3] (Table 14.1). Surgical damage to the parathyroids occurs most commonly after a radical neck dissection, e.g. for laryngeal or oesophageal carcinoma, or a total thyroid resection, or after repeated parathyroidectomies for multi-gland disease, e.g. in multiple endocrine neoplasia type 1 or type 2. Hypocalcaemic symptoms begin 12–24 h postoperatively and may need treatment with oral or intravenous calcium. Parathyroid function often returns, but persistent hypocalcaemia requires treatment with vitamin D preparations [2, 3].

Neonatal hypoparathyroidism resulting in hypocalcaemia may occur in the baby of a mother with hypercalcaemia caused by primary hyperparathyroidism [2, 3]. Maternal hypercalcaemia results in increased calcium delivery to the foetus, and this foetal hypercalcaemia suppresses foetal PTH secretion. Post-partum, the infant's suppressed parathyroids are unable to maintain normocalcaemia. The disorder is usually self-limiting, but occasionally therapy may be required.

Hypoparathyroidism may occur secondary to *severe hypomagnesaemia* (less than 0.40 mM), which may be due to a severe intestinal malabsorption disorder (e.g. Crohn's disease) or a renal tubular disorder [2, 3]. It is associated with hypoparathyroidism because magnesium is required for the release of PTH from the parathyroid gland and also for PTH action via adenyl cyclase. Magnesium chloride, 35–50 mmol i.v. in 1 L of 5% glucose or other isotonic solution given over 12–24 h may be repeatedly required to restore normomagnesaemia.

Complex Syndromes Associated with Hypoparathyroidism

Hypoparathyroidism may occur as part of a complex syndrome which may either be associated with a congenital development anomaly or with an autoimmune syndrome [4]. The congenital developmental anomalies associated with hypoparathyroidism include the DiGeorge, the hypoparathyroidism, deafness and renal anomalies (HDR), the Kenney–Caffey, and the Barakat syndromes and also syndromes associated with either lymphoedema or dysmorphic features and growth failure (Fig. 14.1).

DiGeorge Syndrome

Patients with the DiGeorge syndrome (DGS) typically suffer from hypoparathyroidism, immunodeficiency, congenital heart defects, and deformities of the ear, nose, and mouth [4, 8–20]. The disorder arises from a congenital failure in the development of the derivatives of the third and fourth pharyngeal pouches with resulting absence or hypoplasia of the parathyroids and thymus. Most cases of DGS are sporadic but an autosomal dominant inheritance of DGS has been observed and an association between the syndrome and an unbalanced translocation and deletions involving 22q11.2 have also been reported [18], and this is referred to as DGS type 1 (DGS1). In some patients, deletions of another locus on chromosome 10p have been observed in association with DGS [19] and this is referred to as DGS type 2 (DGS2). Mapping studies of the DGS1 deleted region on chromosome 22q11.2 have defined a 250–3,000-kb critical region [20], which contained approximately 30 genes. Studies of DGS1 patients have reported deletions of several of the genes (e.g. rnex40, nex2.2–nex 3, UDFIL, and TBX1) from the critical region. However, point mutations in DGS1 patients have been detected only in the TBX1 gene [21], and TBX1 is now considered to be the gene causing DGS1 [22]. TBX1 is a DNA-binding transcriptional factor, of the T-Box family, that is known to have an important role in vertebrate and invertebrate organogenesis and pattern formation. The TBX1 gene is deleted in ~96% of all DGS1 patients. Moreover, DNA sequence analysis of unrelated DGS1 patients, who did not have deletions of chromosome 22q11.2, revealed the occurrence of three heterozygous point mutations [21]. One of these mutations resulted in a frameshift with a premature truncation, whilst the other two were missense mutations (Phe148Tyr and Gly310Ser). All of these patients had the complete pharyngeal phenotype but did not have mental retardation or learning difficulties.

Some patients may have a late onset DGS1 and these develop symptomatic hypocalcaemia in childhood or during adolescence with only subtle phenotypic abnormalities [23]. These late-onset DGS1 patients have similar microdeletions in the 22q11 region. It is of interest to note that the age of diagnosis in the families of the three DGS1 patients with inactivating Tbx1 mutations ranged from 7 to 46 years, which is in keeping with late onset DGS1 [21].

Hypoparathyroidism, Deafness, and Renal Anomalies Syndrome

The combined inheritance of hypoparathyroidism, deafness, and renal dysplasia (HDR) as an autosomal dominant trait was reported in one family in 1992 [24]. Patients had asymptomatic hypocalcaemia with undetectable or inappropriately normal serum concentrations of PTH and normal brisk increases in plasma cAMP in response to the infusion of PTH. The patients also had bilateral, symmetrical, sensorineural deafness involving all frequencies. The renal abnormalities consisted mainly of bilateral cysts that compressed the glomeruli and tubules, and lead to renal impairment in some patients. Cytogenetic abnormalities were not detected and abnormalities of the PTH gene were excluded [24]. However, cytogenetic abnormalities involving chromosome 10p14-10pter were identified in two unrelated patients with features that were consistent with HDR. These two patients suffered from hypoparathyroidism, deafness, and growth and mental retardation; one patient also had a solitary dysplastic kidney with vesico-ureteric reflux and a uterus bicornis unicollis, and the other patient, who had a complex reciprocal, insertional translocation of chromosomes 10p and 8q, had cartilaginous exostoses [25]. Neither of these patients had immunodeficiency or heart defects, which are key features of DGS2 (see above), and further studies defined two non-overlapping regions; thus, the DGS2 region was located on 10p13-14 and HDR on 10p14-10pter. Deletion mapping studies in two other HDR patients further defined a critical 200-kb region that contained GATA3 [25], which belongs to a family of zinc-finger transcription factors that are involved in vertebrae embryonic development. DNA sequence analysis in other HDR patients identified mutations that resulted in a haploinsufficiency and loss of GATA3 function [25, 26]. GATA3 has two zinc fingers, and the C-terminal finger (ZnF2) binds DNA, whilst the N-terminal finger (ZnF1) stabilizes this DNA binding and interacts with other zinc-finger proteins, such as the Friends of GATA (FOG) [26]. HDR-associated mutations involving GATA3 ZnF2 or the adjacent basic amino acids were found to result in a loss of DNA binding, whilst those involving ZnF1 either lead to a loss of interaction with FOG2 ZnFs or altered DNA-binding affinity [26]. These findings are consistent with the proposed 3D model of GATA3 ZnF1, which has separate DNA- and protein-binding surfaces [26]. Thus, the HDR-associated GATA3 mutations can be subdivided into two broad classes which depend upon whether they disrupt ZnF1 or ZnF2 and their subsequent effects on interactions with FOG2 and altered DNA binding, respectively. The majority (>75%) of these HDR-associated mutations are predicted to result in truncated forms of the GATA3 protein. Each proband and family will generally have its own unique mutation and there appears to be no correlation with the underlying genetic defect and the phenotypic variation, e.g. the presence or absence of renal dysplasia. Over 90% of patients with two or three of the major clinical features of the HDR syndrome, i.e. hypoparathyroidisim, deafness, or renal abnormalities, have a GATA3 mutation [26]. The remaining 10% of HDR of patients who do not have a GATA3 mutation of the coding region may harbour mutations in the regulatory sequences flanking the GATA3 gene, or else they may represent heterogeneity. The phenotypes of HDR patients with GATA3 mutations appear to be similar to those without GATA3 mutations [26]. It is important to note that HDR patients with GATA3 haploinsufficiency do not have immune deficiency, and this suggests that the immune abnormalities observed in some patients with 10p deletions are most likely to be caused by other genes on 10p. Similarly, the facial dysmorphism, growth, and development delay, commonly seen in patients with larger 10p deletions were absent in the HDR patients with GATA3 mutations, further indicating that these features were likely due to other genes on 10p [25]. These studies of HDR patients indicate an important role for GATA3 in parathyroid development and in the aetiology of hypoparathyroidism.

Mitochondrial Disorders Associated with Hypoparathyroidism

Hypoparathyroidism has been reported to occur in three disorders associated with mitochondrial dysfunction: the Kearns–Sayre syndrome (KSS), the MELAS syndrome, and a mitochondrial trifunctional protein deficiency syndrome. KSS is characterized by progressive external ophthalmoplegia and pigmentary retinopathy before the age of 20 years and is often associated with heart block or cardiomyopathy. The MELAS syndrome consists of a childhood onset of mitochondrial encephalopathy, lactic acidosis, and stroke-like episodes. In addition, varying degrees of proximal myopathy can be seen in both conditions. Both the KSS and MELAS syndromes have been reported to occur with insulin-dependent diabetes mellitus and hypoparathyroidism [27, 28]. A point mutation in the mitochondrial gene tRNA leucine (UUR) has been reported in one patient with the MELAS syndrome who also suffered from hypoparathyroidism and diabetes mellitus [28]. Large deletions, consisting of 6,741 and 6,903 bp and involving more than 38% of the mitochondrial genome, have been reported in other patients who suffered from KSS, hypoparathyroidism, and sensorineural deafness [29]. Rearrangements and duplication of mitochondrial DNA have also been reported in KSS [4]. Mitochondrial trifunctional protein deficiency is a disorder of fatty-acid oxidation that is associated with peripherial neuropathy, pigmentary retinopathy, and acute fatty liver degeneration in pregnant women who carry an affected foetus. Hypoparathyroidism has been observed in one patient with trifunctional protein deficiency [30]. The role of these mitochondrial mutations in the aetiology of hypoparathyroidism remains to be further elucidated.

Kenney–Caffey, Sanjad–Sakati, and Kirk-Richardson Syndromes

Hypoparathyroidism has been reported to occur in over 50% of patients with the Kenney–Caffey syndrome which is associated with short stature, osteosclerosis, and cortical thickening of the long bones, delayed closure of the anterior fontanel, basal ganglia calcification, nanophthalmos, and hyperopia [31]. Parathyroid tissue could not be found in a detailed post-mortem examination of one patient [32] and this suggests that hypoparathyroidism may be due to an embryological defect of parathyroid development. In the Kirk-Richardson and Sanjad–Sakati syndromes, which are similar, hypoparathyroidism is associated with severe growth failure and dysmorphic features [33, 34]. This has been reported in patients of Middle Eastern origin. Consanguinity was noted in the majority of the families, indicating that this syndrome is inherited as an autosomal recessive disorder. Homozygosity and linkage disequilibrium studies located this gene to chromosome 1q42–q43 and molecular genetic investigations have identified that mutations of the tubulin-specific chaperone (TBCE) are associated with the Kenney–Caffey and Sanjad–Sakati syndromes [35]. TBCE encodes one of several chaperone proteins required for the proper folding of α-tubulin subunits and the formation of α-β tubulin heterodimers (Fig. 14.1) [35].

Additional Familial Syndromes

Single familial syndromes in which hypoparathyroidism is a component have been reported (Table 14.2). The inheritance of the disorder in some instances has been established and molecular genetic analysis of the PTH gene has revealed no abnormalities. Thus, an association of hypoparathyroidism, renal insufficiency, and developmental delay has been reported in one Asian family in whom autosomal recessive inheritance of the disorder was established. An analysis of the PTH gene in this family revealed no abnormalities. The occurrence of hypoparathyroidism, nerve deafness, and a steroid-resistant nephrosis leading to renal failure, which has been referred to as the *Barakat syndrome*, has been reported in four brothers from one family, and an association of hypoparathyroidism with congenital lymphoedema, nephropathy, mitral valve prolapse, and brachytelephalangy has been observed in two brothers from another family. Molecular genetic studies have not been reported from these two families.

Blomstrand's Disease

Blomstrand's chondrodysplasia is an autosomal recessive disorder characterized by early lethality, dramatically advanced bone maturation, and accelerated chondrocyte differentiation. Affected infants, who usually have consanguineous unaffected parents, develop pronounced hyperdensity of the entire skeleton with markedly advanced ossification that results in extremely short and poorly modelled long bones. Mutations of the PTH/PTHrP receptor that impair its function are associated with Blomstrand's disease [36]. Thus, it seems likely that affected infants will, in addition to the skeletal defects, also have abnormalities in other organs, which will include secondary hyperplasia of the parathyroid glands, presumably due to hypocalcaemia.

Pluriglandular Autoimmune Hypoparathyroidism

This syndrome comprises of hypoparathyroidism, Addison's disease, candidasis, and two or three of the following: insulin-dependent diabetes mellitus, primary hypogonadism, autoimmune thyroid disease, pernicious anaemia, chronic active hepatitis, steatorrhoea (malabsorption), allopecia (totalis or areata), and vitiligo. The disorder has also been referred to as either the autoimmune polyendocrinopathy-candidiasis-ectodermal dystrophy (APECED) syndrome or the polyglandular autoimmune type 1 syndrome [37]. This disorder has a high incidence in Finland, and a genetic analysis of Finnish families indicated autosomal recessive inheritance of the disorder. In addition, the disorder has been reported to have a high incidence among Iranian Jews, although the occurrence of candidiasis was less common in this population. Linkage studies of Finnish families mapped the APECED gene to chromosome 21q22.3 [38]. Further positional cloning approaches led to the isolation of a novel gene from chromosome 21q22.3. This gene, referred to as AIRE (*a*uto*i*mmune *re*gulator), encodes a 545-amino acid protein that contains motifs suggestive of a transcriptional factor and includes two zinc-finger motifs, a proline-rich region and three LXXLL motifs [39, 40]. Four AIRE1 mutations are commonly found in APECED families, which are the following: Arg257 Stop in Finnish, German, Swiss, British, and Northern Italian families; Arg139 Stop in Sardinian families; Tyr85Cys in Iranian Jewish families; and a 13-bp deletion in exon 8 in British, Dutch, German, and Finnish families [39, 41]. AIRE1 has been shown to regulate the elimination of organ-specific T cells in the thymus, and thus APECED is likely to be caused by a failure of this specialized mechanism for deleting forbidden T cells and establishing immunological tolerance [42]. Patients with APS1 may also develop other autoimmune disorders in association with organ-specific autoantibodies, which are similar to those in patients with non-APS1 forms of the disease. Examples of such autoantibodies and related diseases are GAD6S autoantibodies in Diabetes Mellitus type 1A and 21-dydroxylase autoantibodies in Addison's disease. Patients with APS1 may also develop autoantibodies that react with specific autoantigens that are not found in non-APS1 patients, and examples of this are autoantibodies to type 1 inferferon, which are present in all APS1 patients [43], and to NACHT leucine-rich-repeat-protein 5 (NALP5), which is a parathyroid-specific autoantibody present in 49% of patients with APS1 associated hypoparathyroidism [44]. NALP proteins are essential components of the inflammasone and activate the innate immune system in different inflammatory and autoimmune disorders, such as vitiligo, which involves NALP1, and gout, which involves NALP3 [45]. The precise role of NALP5 in APS1 associated hypoparathyroidism remains to be elucidated.

Calcium-Sensing Receptor Abnormalities

The CaSR, which is located in the plasma membrane of the cell (Fig. 14.1), is at a critical site to enable the cell to recognize changes in extracellular calcium concentration. Thus, an increase in extracellular calcium leads to CaSR activation of the G-protein signalling pathway, which in turn increases the free intracellular calcium concentration and leads to a reduction in transcription of the PTH gene. CaSR mutations that result in a loss of function are associated with familial benign (hypocalciuric) hypercalcaemia (FBH or FHH) [46]. CaSR abnormalities are associated with three hypocalcemic disorders, which are autosomal dominant hypocalcemic hypercalciuria (ADHH), Bartter syndrome type V (i.e. ADHH with a Bartter-like syndrome), and a form of autoimmune hypoparathyroidism (AH) due to CaSR autoantibodies (Table 14.2) [47]. CaSR missense mutations that result in a gain of function (or added sensitivity to extracellular calcium) lead to ADHH [12]. These hypocalcaemic individuals are generally asymptomatic and have serum PTH concentrations that are in the low-normal range, and because of the insensitivities of previous PTH assays in this range, such patients have often been diagnosed to be hypoparathyroid. In addition, such patients may have hypomagnesaemia. Treatment with vitamin D or its active metabolites to correct the hypocalcaemia in these patients may result in marked hypercalciuria, nephrocalcinosis, nephrolithiasis, and renal impairment. Thus, these patients need to be distinguished from those with hypoparathyroidism. Patients with Bartter syndrome type V have the classical features of the syndrome i.e. hypokalemic metabolic alkalosis, hyperreninemia, and hyperaldosteronism [47–49]. In addition, they develop hypocalcaemia, which may be symptomatic and lead to carpopedal spasm, and an elevated fractional excretion of calcium that may be associated with nephrocalcinosis [48, 49]. Such patients have been reported to have heterozygous gain-of-function CaSR mutations, and in vitro functional expression of these mutations has revealed a more severe set-point abnormality for the receptor than that found in patients with ADHH [48, 49]. This suggests that the additional features occurring in Bartter syndrome type V, but not in ADHH, are due to severe gain-of-function mutations of the CaSR.

Autoimmune Acquired Hypoparathyroidism

Twenty percent of patients who had acquired hypoparathyroidism (AH) in association with autoimmune hypothyroidism, were found to have autoantibodies to the extracellular domain of the CaSR [50, 51]. The CaSR autoantibodies did not persist for long; 72% of patients who had AH for less than 5 years had detectable CaSR autoantibodies; whereas only 14% of patients with AH for more than 5 years had such autoantibodies [50]. The majority of the patients who had CaSR autoantibodies were females, a finding that is similar to that found in other auto-antibody mediated diseases. Indeed a few AH patients have also had features of autoimmune polyglandular syndrome type 1 (APS1). These findings establish that the CaSR is an autoantigen in AH [50, 51].

Pseudohypoparathyroidism

Patients with PHP, which may be inherited as an autosomal dominant disorder, are characterized by hypocalcaemia and hyperphosphataemia due to PTH resistance rather than PTH deficiency [1, 4]. Five variants are recognized on the basis of biochemical and somatic features (Table 14.5) and three of these—PHP type Ia (PHPIa), PHP type 1b (PHPIb), and pseudopseudohypoparathyroidism (PPHP)—will be reviewed in further detail. Patients with PHPIa exhibit PTH resistance (hypocalcaemia, hyperphosphataemia, elevated serum PTH, and an absence of an increase in serum and urinary cyclic AMP and urinary phosphate following intravenous human PTH infusion), together with the features of Albright's hereditary osteodystrophy (AHO), which includes short stature, obesity, subcutaneous calcification, mental retardation, round facies, dental hypoplasia, and brachydactyly (i.e. shortening of the metacarpals, particularly the third, fourth, and fifth) [1, 4]. In addition to brachydactyly, other skeletal abnormalities of the long bones and shortening of the metatarsals may also occur. Patients with PHPIb exhibit PTH resistance only and do not have the somatic features of AHO; whilst patients with PPHP exhibit the somatic features of AHO in the absence of PTH resistance [4]. The absence of a normal rise in urinary excretion of cyclic AMP after an infusion of PTH in PHPIa indicated a defect at some site of the PTH receptor–adenyl cyclase system. This receptor system is regulated by at least two G proteins, one of which stimulates (Gsα) and another which inhibits (Giα) the activity of the membrane-bound enzyme that catalyses the formation of the intracellular second messenger cyclic AMP. Interestingly, patients with PHPIa may also show resistance to other hormones, e.g. thyroid-stimulating hormone (TSH), follicle-stimulating hormone (FSH), and luteinizing hormone (LH), that act via G-protein coupled receptors [1, 4].

Table 14.5 Clinical, biochemical, and genetic features of hypoparathyroid and pseudohypoparathyroid disorders

		Pseudohypopara-thyroidism (PHP)				
	Hypoparathyroidism	PHPIa	PPHP	PHPIb	PHPIc	PHPII
AHO manifestations	No	Yes	Yes	No	Yes	No
Serum calcium	↓	↓	N	↓	↓	↓
Serum PO_4	↑	↑	N	↑	↑	↑
Serum PTH	↓	↑	N	↑	↑	↑
Response to PTH						
Urinary cAMP[a] (Chase–Aurbach test)	↑	↓	↑	↓	↓	↑
Urinary PO_4 (Ellsworth–Howard test)	↑	↓	↑	↓	↓	↓
Gsα activity	N	↓	↓	N	N	N
Inheritance	AD/AR/X	AD	AD	AD	AD	Sporadic
Molecular defect	PTH/CaSR/GATA3/ Gcm2/others	GNAS1	GNAS1	?GNAS1	?Adenyl cyclase	?cAMP targets
Other hormonal resistance	No	Yes	No	No	Yes	No

↓ decreased, ↑ increased, *N* normal, *AD* autosomal dominant, *AR* autosomal recessive, *X* X-linked, *AHO* Albright's hereditary osteodystrophy, ? presumed, but not proven
[a]Plasma cAMP responses are similar to those of urinary cAMP

Inactivating mutations of the Gsα gene (referred to as *GNAS1*), which is located on chromosome 20q13.2, have been identified in PHPIa and PPHP patients [52, 53]. However, *GNAS1* mutations do not fully explain the PHPIa or PPHP phenotypes, and studies of PHPIa and PPHP that occurred within the same kindred revealed that the hormonal resistance is parentally imprinted [54]. Thus, PHPIa occurs in a child only when the mutation is inherited from a mother affected with either PHPIa or PPHP; and PPHP occurs in a child only when the mutation is inherited from a father affected with either PHPIa or PPHP. *GNAS1* mutations have not been detected in PHPIb, which has been considered to be due to a defect of the PTH/PTHrP receptor. However, studies of the PTH/PTHrP receptor gene and mRNA in PHPIb patients have not identified mutations [55], and linkage studies in four unrelated kindreds have mapped the PHPIb locus to chromosome 20q13.3, a location that also contains the *GNAS1* gene. In addition, parental imprinting of the genetic defect was observed and this is similar to the findings in kindreds with PHP-type Ia and/or PPHP. Detailed analyses of the GNAS1 gene in PHPIb families have revealed a large 3-kb deletion involving upstream exon(s) referred to as A/B [56]. In affected individuals, the deletion involved the maternal allele, whereas its occurrence on the paternal allele resulted in unaffected healthy carriers [56]. This is consistent with parental imprinting of the GNAS1 abnormality causing PHPIb [57].

Acknowledgements I am grateful: to the Medical Research Council (UK) for support and to Mrs Tracey Walker for typing the manuscript and for expert secretarial assistance.

References

1. Rubin MR, Levine MA. Hypoparathyroidism and pseudohypoparathyroidism. In: Rosen CJ, editor. Primer on the metabolic bone diseases and disorders of mineral metabolism. 7th ed. Washington, DC: American Society of Bone and Mineral Research; 2008. p. 354–61.
2. Shoback D. Hypocalcaemia: definition, etiology, pathogenesis, diagnosis and management. In: Rosen

CJ, editor. Primer on the metabolic bone diseases and disorders of mineral metabolism. 7th ed. Washington, DC: American Society of Bone and Mineral Research; 2008. p. 313–7.
3. Thakker RV. Hypocalcaemic disorders. In: Thakker RV, Wass JAH, editors. Endocrine disorders, medicine. Abingdon, Oxon: The Medicine Group [Journals] Ltd, 25(6):68–70.
4. Thakker RV, Juppner H. Genetic disorders of calcium homeostasis caused by abnormal regulation of parathyroid hormone secretion or responsiveness. In: DeGroot LJ, Jameson JL, editors. Endocrinology. 5th ed. Philadelphia: Elsevier Saunders; 2006. p. 1511–31.
5. Arnold A, Horst SA, Gardella TJ, Baba H, Levine MA, Kronenberg HM. Mutations of the signal peptide encoding region of preproparathyroid hormone gene in isolated hypoparathyroidism. J Clin Invest. 1990;86: 1084–7.
6. Parkinson DB, Thakker RV. A donor splice site mutation in the parathyroid hormone gene is associated with autosomal recessive hypoparathyroidism. Nat Genet. 1992;1:149–52.
7. Ding C, Buckingham B, Levine M. Familial isolated hypoparathyroidism caused by a mutation in the gene for the transcription factor GCMB. J Clin Invest. 2001;108:1215–20.
8. Baumber L, Tufarelli C, Patel S, King P, Johnson CA, Maher ER, Trembath RC. Identification of a novel mutation disrupting the DNA binding activity of GCM2 in autosomal recessive familial isolated hypoparathyroidism. J Med Genet. 2005; 2005(42):443–8.
9. Mannstadt M, Bertrand G, Grandechamp B, Jueppner H, Silve C. Dominant-negative GCMB mutations cause hypoparathyroidism. J Bone Miner Res. 2007;22:S9.
10. Bowl MR, Mirczuk SM, Grigorieva IV, Piret SE, Cranston T, Southam L, Allgrove J, Bahl S, Brain C, Loughlin J, Mughal Z, Ryan F, Shaw N, Thakker YV, Tiosano D, Nesbit MA, Thakker RV. Identification and characterization of novel parathyroid-specific transcription factor glial cells missing homolog B (GCBM) mutations in 8 families with autosomal recessive hypoparathyroidism. Hum Mol Genet. 2010; 19(10):2028–38.
11. Mirczuk SM, Bowl MR, Nesbit MA, Cranston T, Fratter C, Allgrove J, Brain C, Thakker RV. A missense glial cells missing homologue B (GCMB) mutation, Asn502His causes autosomal dominant hypoparathyroidism. J Clin Endocrinol Metab. 2010; 95(7):3512–6.
12. Pearce SH, Williamson C, Kifor O, Bai M, Coulthard MG, Davies M, Lewis-Barned N, McCredie D, Powell H, Kendall-Taylor P, Brown EM, Thakker RV. A familial syndrome of hypocalcaemia with hypocalciuria due to mutations in the calcium-sensing receptor gene. N Engl J Med. 1996;335:1115–22.
13. Whyte MP, Weldon VV. Idiopathic hypoparathyroidism presenting with seizures during infancy: X-linked recessive inheritance in a large Missouri kindred. J Pediatr. 1981;99:608–11.
14. Whyte MP, Kim GS, Kosanovich M. Absence of parathyroid tissue in sex-linked recessive hypoparathyroidism (Letter). J Pediatr. 1986;109:915.
15. Thakker RV, Davies KE, Whyte MP, Wooding C, O'Riordan JLH. Mapping the gene causing X-linked recessive idiopathic hypoparathyroidism to Xq26–Xq27 by linkage studies. J Clin Invest. 1990;6: 40–5.
16. Bowl MR, Nesbit MA, Harding B, Levy E, Jefferson A, Volpi E, Rozzoti K, Lovell-Badge R, Schlessinger D, Whyte M, Thakker RV. An interstitial deletion-insertion involving chromosomes 2p25.3 and Xq27.1, near SOX3, causes X-linked recessive hypoparathyroidism. J Clin Invest. 2005;115:2822–31.
17. Kleinjan DA, van Heyningen V. Long-range control of gene expression: emerging mechanisms and disruption in disease. Am J Hum Genet. 2005;76:8–32.
18. Scambler PJ, Carey AH, Wyse RK, Roach S, Dumanski JP, Nordenskjold M, Williamson R. Microdeletions within 22q11 associated with sporadic and familial DiGeorge syndrome. Genomics. 1991;10: 201–6.
19. Monaco G, Pignata C, Rossi E, et al. DiGeorge anomaly associated with 10p deletion. Am J Med Genet. 1991;39:215–6.
20. Scambler PJ. The 22q11 deletion syndromes. Hum Mol Genet. 2000;9:2421–6.
21. Yagi H, Furutani Y, Hamada H, Sasaki T, Asakawa S, Minoshima S, Ichida F, Joo K, Kimura M, Imamura S, Kamatani N, Momma K, Takao A, Nakazawa M, Shimizu N, Matsuoka R. Role of TBX1 in human del22q11.2 syndrome. Lancet. 2003;362:1366–73.
22. Baldini A. DiGeorge's syndrome: a gene at last. Lancet. 2003;362:1342–3.
23. Sykes KS, Bachrach LK, Siegel-Bartelt J, Ipp M, Kooh SW, Cytrynbaum C. Velocardio-facial syndrome presenting as hypocalcemia in early adolescence. Arch Pediatr Adolesc Med. 1997;151:745–7.
24. Bilous RW, Murty G, Parkinson DB, Thakker RV, Coulthard MG, Burn J, Mathias D, Kendall-Taylor P. Autosomal dominant familial hypoparathyroidism, sensorineural deafness and renal dysplasia. N Engl J Med. 1992;327:1069–84.
25. Van Esch H, Groenen P, Nesbit MA, Schuffenhauer S, Lichtner P, Vanderlinden G, Harding B, Beetz R, Bilous RW, Holdaway I, Shaw NJ, Fryns JP, Van de Ven W, Thakker RV, Devriendt K. GATA3 haploinsufficiency causes human HDR syndrome. Nature. 2000;406:419–22.
26. Ali A, Christie PT, Grigorieva IV, Harding B, Van Esch H, Ahmed SF, Bitner-Glindzicz M, Blind E, Bloch C, Christin P, Clayton P, Gecz J, Gilbert-Dussardier B, Guillen-Navarro E, Hackett A, Halac I, Hendy GN, Lalloo F, Mache CJ, Mughal Z, Ong ACM, Rinat C, Shaw N, Smithson SF, Tolmie J, Weill J, Nesbit MA, Thakker RV. Functional characterisation of GATA3 mutations causing the hypoparathyroidism-deafness-renal (HDR) dysplasia syndrome: insight into mechanisms of DNA binding by the GATA3 transcription factor. Hum Mol Genet. 2007; 16:265–75.

27. Moraes CT, DiMauro S, Zeviani M, Lombes A, Shanske S, Miranda AF, Nakase H, Bonilla E, Werneck LC, Servidei S. Mitochondrial deletions in progressive external ophthalmoplegia and Kearns–Sayre syndrome. N Engl J Med. 1989;320:1293–9.
28. Morten KJ, Cooper JM, Brown GK, Lake BD, Pike D, Poulton J. A new point mutation associated with mitochondrial encephalomyopathy. Hum Mol Genet. 1993;2:2081–7.
29. Isotani H, Fukumoto Y, Kawamura H, Furukawa K, Ohsawa N, Goto Y, Nishino I, Nonaka I. Hypoparathyroidism and insulin-dependent diabetes mellitus in a patient with Kearns–Sayre syndrome harbouring a mitochondrial DNA deletion. Clin Endocrinol. 1996;45:637–41.
30. Dionisi-Vici C, Garavaglia B, Burlina AB, Bertini E, Saponara I, Sabetta G, Taroni F. Hypoparathyroidism in mitochondrial trifunctional protein deficiency. J Pediatr. 1996;129:159–62.
31. Franceschini P, Testa A, Bogetti G, Girardo E, Guala A, Lopez-Bell G, Buzio G, Ferrario E, Piccato E. Kenny-Caffey syndrome in two sibs born to consanguineous parents: evidence for an autosomal recessive variant. Am J Med Genet. 1992;42:112–6.
32. Boynton JR, Pheasant TR, Johnson BL, Levin DB, Streeten BW. Ocular findings in Kenny's syndrome. Arch Ophthalmol (Chicago). 1979;97:896–900.
33 Richardson RJ, Kirk JM. Short stature, mental retardation, and hypoparathyroidism: a new syndrome. Arch Dis Child. 1990;65:1113–7.
34. Sanjad SA, Sakati NA, Abu-Osba YK, Kaddoura R, Milner RD. A new syndrome of congenital hypoparathyroidism, severe growth failure, and dysmorphic features. Arch Dis Child. 1991;66:193–6.
35. Parvari R, Hershkovitz E, Grossman N, Gorodischer R, Loeys B, Zecic A, Mortier G, Gregory S, Sharony R, Kambouris M, Sakati N, Meyer BF, Al Aqeel AI, Al Humaidan AK, Al Zanhrani F, Al Swaid A, Al Othman J, Diaz GA, Weiner R, Khan KT, Gordon R, Gelb BD, HRD/Autosomal Recessive Kenny-Caffey Syndrome Consortium. Mutation of TBCE causes hypoparathyroidism-retardation-dysmorphism and autosomal recessive Kenny-Caffey syndrome. Nat Genet. 2002;32:448–52.
36. Jobert AS, Zhang P, Couvineau A, Bonaventure J, Roume J, Le Merrer M, Silve C. Absence of functional receptors parathyroid hormones and parathyroid hormone-related peptide in Blomstrand chondrodysplasia. J Clin Invest. 1998;102:34–40.
37. Ahonen P, Myllärniemi S, Sipilä I, Perheentupa J. Clinical variation of autoimmune polyendocrinopathy-candidiasis ectodermal dystrophy (APECED) in a series of 68 patients. N Engl J Med. 1990;322: 1829–36.
38. Aaltonen J, Björses P, Sandkuijl L, Perheentupa J, Peltonen L. An autosomal locus causing autoimmune disease: autoimmune polyglandular disease type 1 assigned to chromosome 21. Nat Genet. 1994;8:83–7.
39. Nagamine K, Peterson P, Scott HS, Kudoh J, Minoshima S, Heino M, Krohn KJ, Lalioti MD, Mullis PE, Antonarakis SE, Kawasaki K, Asakawa S, Ito F, Shimizu N. Positional cloning of the APECED gene. Nat Genet. 1997;17:393–8.
40. The Finnish-German APECED consortium. An autoimmune disease, APECED, caused by mutations in a novel gene featuring two PHD-type zinc finger domains. Nat Genet. 1997;17:399–403.
41. Pearce SH, Cheetham T, Imrie H, Vaidya B, Barnes ND, Bilous RW, Carr D, Meeran K, Shaw NJ, Smith CS, Toft AD, Williams G, Kendall-Taylor P. A common and recurrent 13-bp deletion in the autoimmune regulator gene in British kindreds with autoimmune polyendocrinopathy type 1. Am J Hum Genet. 1998;63:1675–84.
42. Liston A, Lesage S, Wilson J, Peltonen L, Goodnow CC. Aire regulates negative selection of organ-specific T cells. Nat Immunol. 2003;4:350–4.
43. Meaager A, Visvalingam K, Peterson P, Moll K, Murumagi A, Krohn K, Eskelin P, Perheentupa J, Husebye E, Kadota Y, Willcox N. Anti-interferon autoantibodies in autoimmune polyendocrinopathy syndrome type 1. PLoS Med. 2006;3:e289.
44. Alimohammadi M, Bjorklund P, Hallgren A, Pontynen N, Szinnai G, Shikama N, Keller MP, Ekwall O, Kinkel SA, Husebye ES, Gustafsson J, Rorsman F, Peltonen L, Betterle C, Perheentupa J, Akerstrom G, Westin G, Scott HS, Hollander GA, Kampe O. Autoimmune polyendocrine syndrome type 1 and NALP5, a parathyroid autoantigen. N Engl J Med. 2008;358:1018–28.
45. Eisenbarth SC, Colegio OR, O'Connor W, Sutterwala FS, Flavell RA. Crucial role for the Nalp3 inflammasome in the immunostimulatory properties of aluminium adjuvants. Nature. 2008;453:1122–6.
46. Pollak MR, Brown EM, Chou YH, Hebert SC, Marx SJ, Steinmann B, Levi T, Seidman CE, Seidman JG. Mutations in the human Ca^{2+}-sensing receptor gene cause familial hypocalciuric hypercalcaemia and neonatal severe hyperparathyroidism. Cell. 1993;75: 1297–303.
47. Thakker RV. Diseases associated with the extracellular calcium-sensing receptor. Cell Calcium. 2004;35: 275–82.
48. Watanabe S, Fukumoto S, Chang H, Takeuchi Y, Hasegawa Y, Okazaki R, Chikatsu N, Fujita T. Association between activating mutations of calcium-sensing receptor and Bartter's syndrome. Lancet. 2002;360:692–4.
49. Vargas-Poussou R, Huang C, Hulin P, Houillier P, Jeunemaitre X, Paillard M, Planelles G, Dechaux M, Miller RT, Antignac C. Functional characterization of a calcium-sensing receptor mutation in severe autosomal dominant hypocalcemia with a Bartter-like syndrome. J Am Soc Nephrol. 2002;13:2259–66.
50. Li Y, Song YH, Rais N, Connor E, Schatz D, Muir A, Maclaren N. Autoantibodies to the extracellular

domain of the calcium sensing receptor in patients with acquired hypoparathyroidism. J Clin Invest. 1996;97:910–4.
51. Kifor O, Moore Jr FD, Delaney M, Garber J, Hendy GN, Butters R, Gao P, Cantor TL, Kifor I, Brown EM, Wysolmerski J. A syndrome of hypocalciuric hypercalcemia caused by autoantibodies directed at the calcium-sensing receptor. J Clin Endocrinol Metab. 2003;88:60–72.
52. Weinstein LS, Gejman PV, Friedman E, et al. Mutations of the Gsα-subunit gene in Albright hereditary osteodystrophy detected by denaturing gradient gel electrophoresis. Proc Natl Acad Sci USA. 1990;87:8287–90.
53. Yu S, Yu D, Hainline BE, Brener JL, Wilson KA, Wilson LC, Oude-Luttikhuis ME, Trembath RC, Weinstein LS. A deletion hot-spot in exon 7 of the $G_s\alpha$ gene (GNAS1) in patients with Albright hereditary osteodystrphy. Hum Mol Genet. 1995;4:2001–2.
54. Wilson LC, Oude-Luttikhuis MEM, Clayton PT, et al. Parental origin of Gsα gene mutations in Albright's hereditary osteodystrophy. J Med Genet. 1994;31:835–9.
55. Schipani E, Weinstein LS, Bergwitz C, et al. Pseudohypoparathyroidism type Ib is not caused by mutations in the coding exons of the human parathyroid hormone (PTH)/PTH-related peptide receptor gene. J Clin Endocrinol Metab. 1995;80:1611–21.
56. Jüppner H, Schipani E, Bastepe M, Cole DE, Lawson ML, Mannstadt M, Hendy GN, Plotkin H, Koshiyama H, Koh T, Crawford JD, Olsen BR, Vikkula M. The gene responsible for pseudohypoparathyroidism type Ib is paternally imprinted and maps in four unrelated kindreds to chromosome 20q13.3. Proc Natl Acad Sci USA. 1998;95:11798–803.
57. Thakker RV. Parathyroid disorders: molecular genetics and physiology. In: Morris PJ, Wood WC, editors. Oxford Textbook of Surgery. Oxford: Oxford University Press; 2000. p. 1121–9.

Primary Hyperparathyroidism in Neonates and Children

15

Eric Mallet and Mireille Castanet

Abstract

This rare disorder in children is presented across the spectrum of ages from birth to the adolescence. The chapter concentrates on the chemical abnormalities of the problem. It tabulates an extensive differential of calcium disorders and gives up-to-date information about chromosomal abnormalities for all of them. The chapter concludes with information about the management of primary hyperparathyroidism in children both from a medical and surgical point of view and focuses on some of the surgical complexities in patient care.

Keywords

Primary hyperparathyroidism • Cellular hyperplasia • Rickets • Vitamin D adolescents • Malabsorption syndromes • Celiac disease • Renal insufficiency • 1,25 Dihydroxyvitamin D • 1,25-(OH)2D3 • Gs alpha mutation • Pseudohypoparathyroidism • Demineralization • Hypotonia • Feeding difficulties • Respiratory problems • Radiological abnormality • Subperiosteal erosions • Fractures • Thoracic deformities • Nephrolithiasis • Hematuria • Polyuropolydipsic syndrome • Nausea • Vomiting • Asthenia • Weight loss • Hypercalcemia • Lamina dura • Intact PTH 1-84 • Hypophosphatemia • Alkaline phosphatase • 25-Hydroxyvitamin-D • Neonatal hyperparathyroidism • Familial hypocalciuric hypercalcemia • G-protein receptor • Receptor gene • Chromosome 3 (3q21.1) • Allelic deletion 11q13 • Somatic mutation • Calcium receptor CaSR • Phenotype • Genotype • Codon 58 • Neuroendocrinopathies • Multiple neuroendocrinopathies type 1 • Adrenal cortex • Pancreas • Gastrointestinal tract • Hyperplasia • MEN type 2A

E. Mallet, MD, PhD (✉)
Department of Pediatrics and CIC INSERM 204,
Rouen University Hospital, 1, Rue de Germont,
Rouen 76031, France
e-mail: eric.mallet@chu-rouen.fr

M. Castanet, MD, PhD
Department of Pediatrics, Rouen University Hospital,
Rouen, France

A.A. Licata and E.V. Lerma (eds.), *Diseases of the Parathyroid Glands*,
DOI 10.1007/978-1-4419-5550-0_15, © Springer Science+Business Media, LLC 2012

(Sipple syndrome) • Medullary cancer of thyroid • Pheochromocytoma • Protooncogene RET • Chromosome 10 (10q11.2) • HPT-JT syndrome • Mandibular/maxillary fibrobone lesions • Suppressor gene HTPR2 • Chromosome 1 (1q25–q31) • Parafibromin • Oncogene cyclin D1 • Menin • Inhibitory kinase • Medical treatment • Bisphosphonates • Pamidronate (AREDIA®) • Cinacalcet • Ultrasound nodules • Doppler imaging • MIBI technetium scintigraphy • Thallium/Tc scintigraphy • Minimal invasive parathyroidectomy • Gland grafts • Hungry bone syndrome

Introduction

Hyperparathyroidism is defined by an excessive production of parathyroid hormone (PTH). Primary parathyroid (HP1) disorder leading to inappropriate or unregulated overproduction of PTH due to adenoma or cellular hyperplasia which characterizes primary hyperparathyroidism, whereas increased production of PTH follow-up to hypocalcemia occurring most frequently in childhood, is that which characterizes secondary hyperparathyroidism. In this group, diverse causes could lead to hypocalcemia such as rickets secondary to low vitamin D still frequently occurring in adolescents, or malabsorption syndromes (celiac disease for example) where intestinal calcium absorption is deficient. Renal insufficiency at early stage of the disease could also lead to an increased PTH secretion secondary to hypocalcemia (and/or hyperphosphoremia). At a later stage, the production of the active metabolite 1, 25-dihydroxyvitamin D (1,25-(OH)2D3) is diminished, leading to severe hypocalcemia, and thus to an increased production of PTH that could become autonomous (i.e., third hyperparathyroidism). In some cases, PTH level could be elevated without true hyperparathyroidism due to PTH resistance mostly due to Gs alpha mutations (i.e., pseudohyporparathyroidism).

In the present chapter, only primary hyperparathyroidism will be discussed. HP1 is a rare disorder in children. A French multicenter retrospective study (nonexhaustive) collected 55 cases over a 20-year period, which allowed to estimate an incidence at 1/200,000–300,000 live births [1].

Clinical and Radiological Manifestations of Primary Hyperparathyroidism

In primary hyperparathyroidism, clinical signs are due to hypercalcemia secondary to excess PTH production.

Neonatal HP1

In neonates, clinical signs are present at diagnosis mostly hypotonia, and more rarely feeding difficulties and respiratory problems. Mild demineralization is a frequent radiological abnormality but more severe forms could appear such as metaphysic irregularities, cortical dualization, subperiosteal erosion, marked skeletal demineralization with multiple fractures or a bell-shaped thoracic deformation (Fig. 15.1).

HP1 in Children and Adolescents

In children, diagnosis of HP1 is usually made between 12 and 16 years. Clinical signs are predominantly those related to nephrolithiasis: kidney stones, hematuria, and/or polyuropolydipsic syndromes. More rarely bone pain, and articular or muscles aches responsible for walking problems such as limping can also be observed. In addition, according to the degree of hypercalcemia, digestive signs (such as nausea–vomiting or abdominal pain), or general signs (i.e., asthenia, weight loss) and/or neuropsychological disorders (from headache to depression) can also be observed. In some cases, hypercalcemia is detected by routine serum calcium measurements and patients are totally asymptomatic.

The delay between the occurrence of early signs and the diagnosis of hyperparathyroidism vary greatly. It is shorter in cases of acute hypercalcemia or kidney stones, and longer when nonspecific digestive disorders or gradually occurring osteomuscular pains are observed, ranging from a few weeks to several years [1].

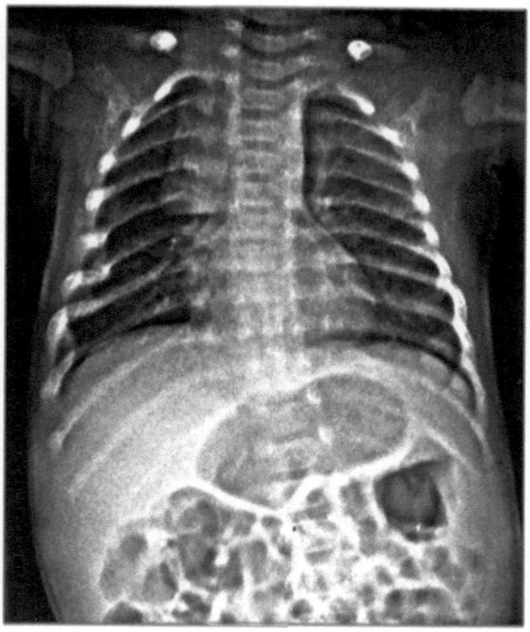

Fig. 15.1 Skeletal demineralization and bell-shaped thoracic deformation in a neonate affected by HP1

With regard to radiological investigations, subperiosteal erosions (microgeodes) can be detected in the phalanx or epiphyses when the diagnosis is late. In severe forms, the tuft of the third phalange is frequently reabsorbed and lamina dura irregularities can be observed. Importantly, in children, kidney ultrasound must be routinely performed to search for nephrolithiasis whatever the clinical signs are (Fig. 15.2).

Biological Data in HP1

The dosage of the PTH, mostly using the detection of the intact PTH 1-84 (iPTH Nichols), is essential for the diagnosis of hyperparathyroidism [2]. However, this data is not sufficient and the PTH level needs to be interpreted depending to the level of calcemia. Indeed, a high PTH level associated to a high level of calcemia usually defines a primary hyperparathyroidism, but a normal or subnormal PTH level in regard to

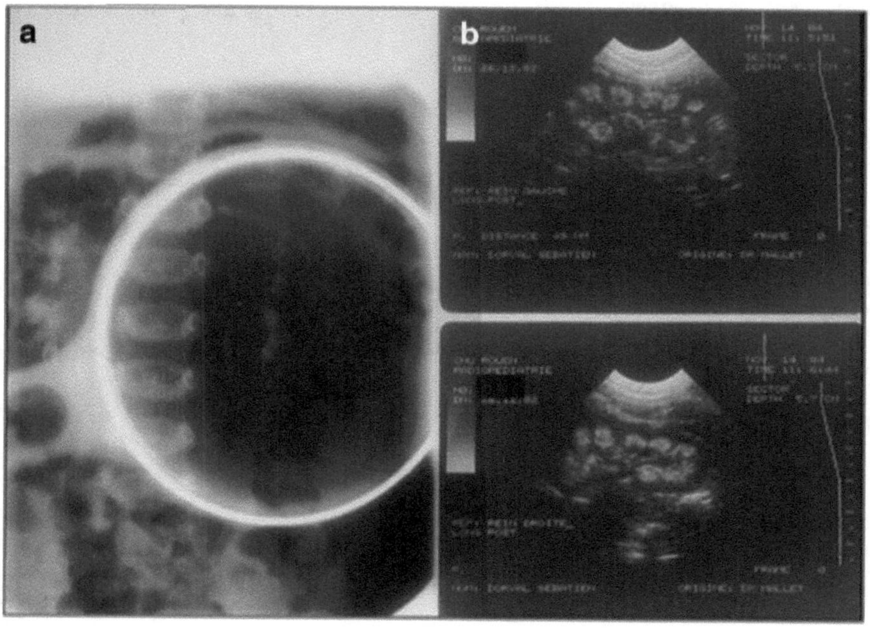

Fig. 15.2 Radiologic (**a**) and echographic (**b**) aspect of nephrolithiasis in neonate affected by HP1

hypercalcemia (>2.6 mmol/L), can also be regarded as primary hyperparathyroidism as under normal conditions, hypercalcemia physiologically suppresses the PTH production. In addition, whereas the level of calcemia is usually elevated in HP1, a normal or false elevated level of calcemia can also occur and does not reject the diagnosis of HP1, particularly in cases of protidic defects or acidosis, that may mask a mild elevated calcium level. In such cases, the ionized calcium level that reflects the reserve in calcium is required. In cases of hyperparathyroidism, ionized calcium level is elevated, while the total calcium is normal or low.

Note that in borderline situations, repeat serum PTH and calcium levels need to be performed for accurate diagnosis.

The other biological abnormalities in HP1 are due to the physiological actions of the parathormone:

- Calciuria is mildly elevated due to the stimulation by PTH on tubular calcium reabsorption and is unadapted to the hypercalcemia.
- Serum phosphatemia is decreased (according to age and blood taking condition), as phosphate and potassium are intracellular components.
- The phosphate renal reabsorption level that is recommended to measure in hypophosphatemic cases is also decreased (<85%).
- The serum activity of alkaline phosphatases, interpreted according to the norm for age, can be elevated in relation to the bone metabolism.
- Low serum 25-hydroxyvitamin D (25-OH-D) can reveal a neonatal deficiency that could aggravate the hyperparathyroidism. Note that in this condition, the dosage of the 1, 25 $(OH)_2$ D_3 is not important, as the values vary greatly .

Etiologies of HP1

Recent research based on molecular biology has allowed for better understanding of the physiological mechanisms responsible for primary hyperparathyroidism in children and addressed the hereditary forms of HP1 (Table 15.1).

Familial Hypocalciuric Hypercalcemia and Severe Neonatal Hyperparathyroidism

The CaSR, a receptor expressed in the parathyroid and renal cells, has recently been involved in HP1. It belongs to the coupled G-protein receptors family and controls the PTH secretion

Table 15.1 Presentation of the HP1 cases in four published pediatric studies

	Johns Hopkins [5]	Mayo Clinic [4]	Mayo Clinic [6]	French Series [1]
Period	1984–2001	1976–1998	1970–2000	1984–2004
Number of cases	24	33	52	44 (+11 neonates)
Age (interval in years)	10.5–20	9–19	4–18.9	6–18
Calcemia (mmol/l)	2.98 [2.65–3.45]	3.02	6.2 [3.2–7.6][a]	3.27 [2.6–4.33]
Frequency of clinical symptoms %	77	94	79	82
Frequency of lithiasis %	83	42	33	41
Frequency of bone and muscular signs	29	27	34	16
Histology				
Adenoma	11	31	35	29
Hyperplasia	4	–	16	11
Search for MEN cases	1 case of MEN 2A	MEN excluded	10 cases of MEN1 and 2 cases of MEN-2A	2 cases of MEN1 and 1 polymorphism in the menin gene

[a]Ionized calcium (mg/dl), *MEN* multiple neuroendocrinopathies

and calcium tubular reabsorption and thus plays a key role in the maintenance of the normal extracellular ionized calcium concentration. The gene encoding for this receptor is located on chromosome 3 (3q21.1). More than 20 loss-of-function CaSR mutations leading to partial resistance of calcium on kidney and/or parathyroid have been reported so far in HP1 cases. *CaSR* mutations are mostly identified at heterozygous stage and are responsible for *benign forms of familial hypocalciuric hypercalcemia* usually diagnosed in childhood [3]. The most frequent mutation (25–40% of adenoma) is an 11q13 allelic deletion (LOH) associated to a somatic mutation within the second allele. Homozygous CaSR mutations are observed in severe neonatal hyperparathyroidism. However, no phenotype–genotype correlation can be established and heterozygous mutations such as those affecting the codon 58 (C58Y) could be also responsible of severe neonatal disorder. Moreover, a great phenotypic variability could be observed in cases affected by a similar mutation even in the same family. Note that based on the dominant autosomal inheritance, the diagnosis in neonates can be made when both heterozygous parents are diagnosed.

Neuroendocrinopathies

In addition to the isolated familial HP1, hyperparathyroidism can be observed in association to other endocrine disorders defining multiple neuroendocrinopathies (MEN). Manifestations of these disorders are observed in neonates as well as later during childhood or adolescence. The mode of revelation and the etiologies in childhood and adolescence are quite similar in the literature [1, 4–6] (Table 15.2).

MEN type 1 is characterized in childhood or adolescence by association of tumors in neuroendocrinogastroenteropancreatic tissues in the adrenal cortex. This disorder usually affects the parathyroid glands (in 90% of cases), parathyroid hyperplasia of the four glands, or multiple adenomas of the endocrine pancreas and/or the pituitary gland. Parathyroid hyperplasia of the four

Table 15.2 Principal causes of primary hyperparathyroidism with hypercalcemia in children

In neonates
• Maternal vitamin D deficiency
• Maternal uncompensated hypoparathyroidism
• Health heterozygous and homozygous mutations of the calcium sensor receptor (CaSR) (hypercalcemia–hypocalciuria syndrome)
In children and adolescents
• Isolated adenoma
• Multiple polyendocrinopathy 1 and 2A (Sipple syndrome)

glands or multiple adenomas are the predominant disorders, but these tumors could also be monoclonal and thus develop isolated adenoma. MEN 1 occurs in about 1/200,000 live births, and the mode of transmission is autosomal dominant with high penetration. The frequency of MEN 1 is approximately 1 % of HP1 in adults, and mutations in the gene encoding for the menin (located in 11q13) are the main cause [7].

MEN type 2A, or Sipple syndrome, is mainly characterized by medullary cancer of the thyroid associated to chromocytomas (50% of cases). Primary hyperparathyroidism, due to cellular C hyperplasia, occurs in only 30% of cases. The protooncongene RET, located within the long arm of chromosome 10 (10q11.2), is involved in this disorder with an autosomal dominant mode of inheritance. Several germinal dominant gain-of-function mutations have been reported with a relatively good genotype–phenotype correlation [8].

HPT-JT Syndrome

Another but rare form of familial hyperparathyroidism syndrome is the *HPT-JT syndrome*, characterized by hyperparathyroidism due to multiple adenomas, mostly revealed at adolescence, and mandibular or maxillary fibro-bone lesions. This disorder is due to a defect in the suppressor tumor gene *HTPR2*, located on chromosome 1 (1q25-q31), a gene encoding for the parafibromin [9] and the mode of transmission is autosomal dominant.

Primary Parathyroid Adenoma

In cases of primary parathyroid adenoma, though the role of the oncogene encoding for the cyclin D1 (*CCND1*), located within the long arm of the chromosome 11 (11q13) is well known, other genes such as the protooncogene RET, the suppressor tumor genes encoding for the menin or parafibromin, the genes encoding for the calcium-sensing receptor (CaSR) and its encoding for the inhibitory kinase CDK11B/p27 have only recently been implicated especially in familial parathyroid hyperplasia [10].

To date, in parathyroid adenomas, mutations have been identified within the oncogenes *CCND1/PRAD1* and the menin gene (*MEN1*) only, and no mutation has been found in the other genes involved in HP1 so far (i.e., CaSR or RET).

In isolated familial hyperparathyroidism, mutations have been found in the CaSR, the menin, and more rarely the *HRPT2* gene. However, many cases remain to be elucidated. Recent genetic studies using the Comparative Genomic Hybridization technique (CGH array) and/or familial studies pointed to new candidate loci, but further studies are required to better understand their involvement in HP1 [11, 12].

In addition to the severe form due to *CaSR* homozygous mutation, there is a moderate form of congenital hyperparathyroidism due to a vitamin D deficit or a noncompensated maternal hypoparathyroidism. These conditions lead to diffuse hyperplasia of fetal parathyroid glands in reaction to the decrease of the calcium flow through the placenta, resulting in excessive PTH production in neonates. This disorder progressively disappears within the first 2 months of life after hydration and vitamin D supplementation [13].

Management of HP1 in Children

Knowledge of clinical forms of variable severity, the molecular elucidation of several forms of HP1 has permitted better understanding of the pathophysiology, and the recent use of bisphosphonates has led to an important change in the management of HP1 in children, especially in neonatal presentation. Routine emergency surgery, usually performed until recently, has decreased in profit to bisphosphonates to control hypercalcemia, and mild symptomatic forms may benefit from monitoring alone, whereas surgery should be reserved for severe forms with poor clinical tolerance.

Medical Treatment

Medical treatment is usually initiated to treat severe and/or symptomatic hypercalcemia by restoring the metabolic balance prior to surgery and moderate or mild forms of HP1 with good clinical tolerance do not now require surgery in the majority of cases.

Bisphosphonates, particularly pamidronate (AREDIA®), are now largely used showing good efficacy in primary intention [14], especially before surgery or in cases of failure of parathyroidectomy before the second surgery [15]. No significant adverse effects have been reported.

CINACALCET® is another therapeutic key usually used in adolescents affected by renal insufficiency with severe secondary hyperparathyroidism [16].

Note that hyperhydration combined with diuretics has frequently been ineffective.

Surgical Treatment

Preoperative Investigations

Preoperative localization of parathyroid adenoma(s) is a major concern. Ultrasound is usually used in first intention but does not discriminate between thyroid or ectopic nodules and does not detect ectopic (retrotracheal or esophagus) parathyroid adenomas. Combining it with Doppler exploration provides better adenoma differentiation [17] (Fig. 15.3).

MIBI scintigraphy, that has recently replaced thallium/Tc scintigraphy, is also an effective tool for the diagnosis of parathyroid adenoma. It is able to detect ectopic glands and discriminate thyroid from parathyroid gland as complex MIBI-technetium is fixed in 15 min in both thyroid and parathyroid glands and is retained longer within

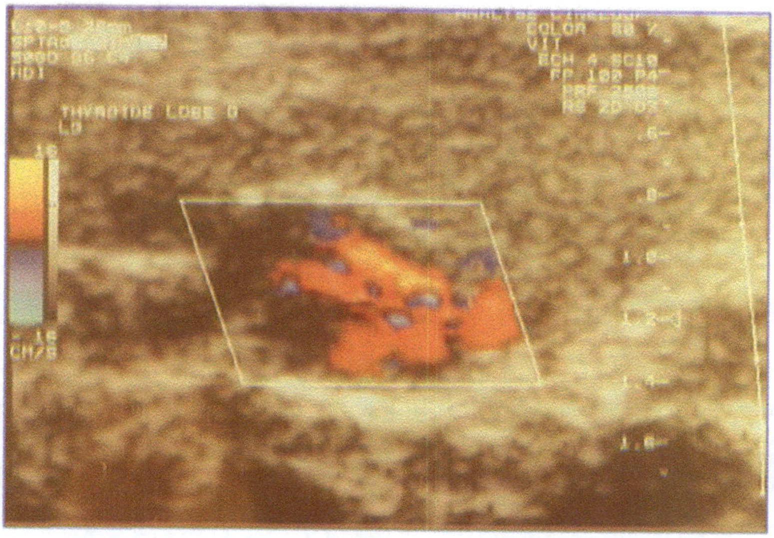

Fig. 15.3 Parathyroid adenoma detected by echography combined with Doppler in a child

the parathyroid glands. Note that the high sensitivity of this technique depends on the size of the lesion [18] (Fig. 15.4).

Combining echography to Doppler and MIBI scintigraphy has greatly improved the preoperative localization of the adenoma [19] allowing thus to propose only unilateral cervical exploration in cases of concordance in the results. This strategy is reserved for cases where preoperative identification of a single adenoma is almost certain and should be combined with preoperative PTH assay. This strategy is now widely used in adults and allows less invasive surgical technique, i.e., microinvasive parathyroidectomy (minimal invasive parathyroidectomy or MIP).

Surgical Treatment

In neonatal hyperparathyroidism, the management depends on the clinical tolerance, degree of hypercalcemia and molecular biology results. In severe forms (i.e., with poor clinical tolerance), subtotal thyroidectomy is performed with insertion of hemiparathyroid gland grafting within the arm.

In children, unilateral cervicotomy following preoperative investigations has recently become the method of choice rather than the classical bilateral surgical treatment. However, such surgical strategy cannot be used in cases of polyglandular disorder (i.e., multiple endocrine neoplasias). Therefore, molecular biology tests should be routinely performed in children as bilateral cervicotomy for subtotal parathyroidectomy (7/8) or total ablation with reimplantation is still debated in such cases because of high risk of HP1 recurrence [20].

In single adenoma, when preoperative investigations have localized the lesions, microinvasive parathyroidectomy (MIP) can be used. This technique uses a small subcutaneous incision, to maintain an esthetic effect, and a camera through the incision in order to determine the level of radioactivity. After the surgical removal, the perioperative PTH assay combining with perioperative scintigraphy should be performed to control the total removal of the lesion [21]. Indeed, despite the high success of surgical treatment, a number of failures can occur which frequently require difficult reintervention. PTH secretion by normal parathyroid glands is almost suppressed because of overproduction of hyperfunctional parathyroid tissue. Preoperative combined with perioperative PTH assay should therefore be used to confirm hyperfunctional tissue resection to assess the effectiveness of surgery. A 50% decreasing PTH at 10 min or more than 60% at 20 min appear to be accurate predictors of surgical efficacy [22] (Fig. 15.5).

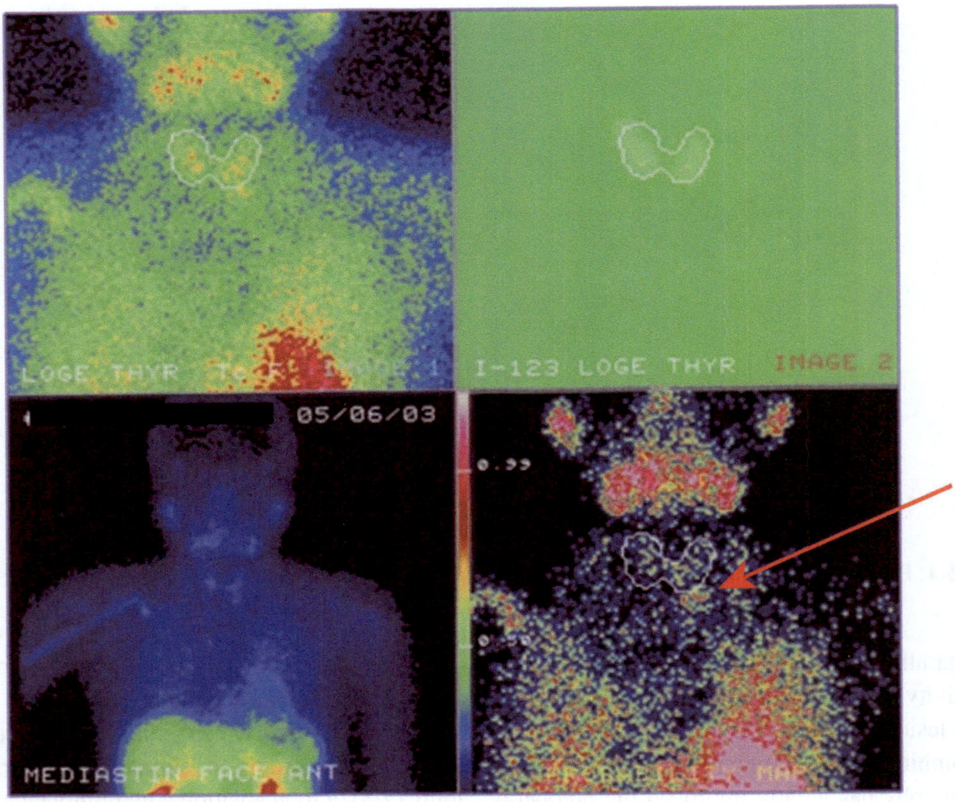

Fig. 15.4 Parathyroid adenoma detected by MIBI scintigraphy in a child (*arrow*)

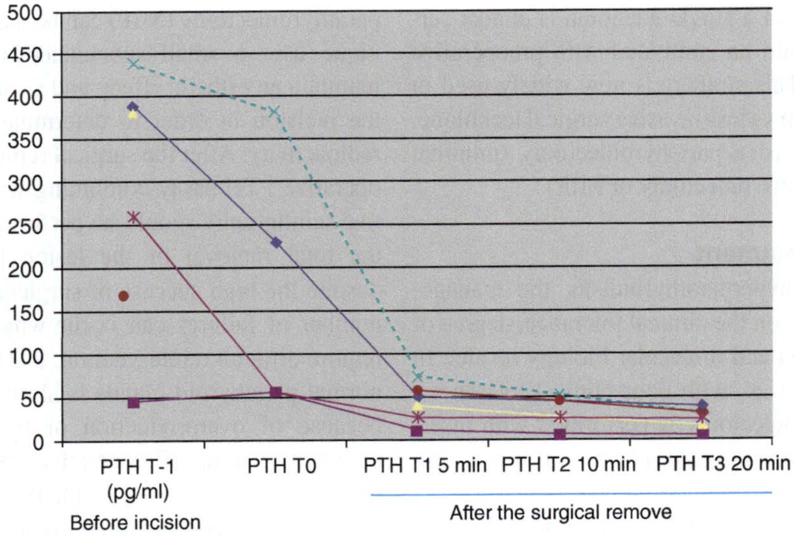

Fig. 15.5 Course of perioperative PTH immunoreactive assays in six patients from the French series [1]

Note that after surgical removal, transitory hypocalcemia can appear, as PTH activity was suppressed because of overproduction of hyperfunctional parathyroid tissue. Therefore, calcium supplementation along with 1-25 OH vitamin D should be added. In cases with major bone lesions, hypocalcemia could be long because of "hungry bone syndrome" [23], especially in cases of vitamin D deficiency that delays the calcium recovery [24].

Conclusion

Primary hyperparathyroidism regroup two distinct entities: (1) neonatal primary hyperparathyroidism linked to hyperplasia of the four parathyroid glands, with early clinical symptoms mainly due to inactive mutations in the calcium-sensing receptor and (2) later occurring primary hyperparathyroidism mainly due to parathyroid adenomas or hyperplasia that could be included in MEN disorder.

In neonatal forms, effective management is now conditioned by clinical tolerance, degree of hypercalcemia and molecular biology results. Molecular investigations should be routinely performed, as identification of mutations within the calcium-sensing receptor has led to an important change in the management of HP1 and avoidance of surgery in many cases. Treatment of hypercalcemia with bisphosphonate drugs is the initial approach.

In forms that occur later, i.e., in adolescence, the use of bisphosphonates as preoperative treatment, as well as improvements in techniques, the sensitivity of preoperative localization procedures, such as Doppler echography and MIBI scintigraphy, and the quick preoperative PTH assay can contribute to more accurate surgery. Currently in children, unilateral surgery replaces the classical bilateral cervicotomy. In pluriglandular pathology (i.e., MEN), bilateral cervicotomy with subtotal parathyroidectomy is the approach. Therefore, molecular biology testing prior to surgery is routinely performed to diagnose MEN [25].

Acknowledgment The authors are most grateful to Richard Medeiros, Rouen University Hospital Medical Editor, for editing the manuscript.

References

1. Mallet E. Primary hyperparathyroidism in neonates and childhood. The French experience (1984-2004). Horm Res. 2008;69(3):180–8.
2. Mallet E, Basuyau JP. Value of the determination of intact parathyroid hormone in calcium metabolism disorders in children. Arch Fr Pediatr. 1988;45(8):599.
3. Pearce SH, et al. Calcium-sensing receptor mutations in familial benign hypercalcemia and neonatal hyperparathyroidism. J Clin Invest. 1995;96(6):2683–92.
4. Harman CR, et al. Sporadic primary hyperparathyroidism in young patients: a separate disease entity? Arch Surg. 1999;134(6):651–5. discussion 655–6.
5. Hsu SC, Levine MA. Primary hyperparathyroidism in children and adolescents: the Johns Hopkins Children's Center experience 1984-2001. J Bone Miner Res. 2002;17 Suppl 2:N44–50.
6. Kollars J, et al. Primary hyperparathyroidism in pediatric patients. Pediatrics. 2005;115(4):974–80.
7. Marx S, et al. Multiple endocrine neoplasia type 1: clinical and genetic topics. Ann Intern Med. 1998;129(6):484–94.
8. Szinnai G, Sarnacki S, Polak M. Hereditary medullary thyroid carcinoma: how molecular genetics made multiple endocrine neoplasia type 2 a paediatric disease. Endocr Dev. 2007;10:173–87.
9. Carpten JD, et al. HRPT2, encoding parafibromin, is mutated in hyperparathyroidism-jaw tumor syndrome. Nat Genet. 2002;32(4):676–80.
10. DeLellis RA, Mazzaglia P, Mangray S. Primary hyperparathyroidism: a current perspective. Arch Pathol Lab Med. 2008;132(8):1251–62.
11. Palanisamy N, et al. Novel chromosomal abnormalities identified by comparative genomic hybridization in parathyroid adenomas. J Clin Endocrinol Metab. 1998;83(5):1766–70.
12. Warner JV, et al. Familial isolated hyperparathyroidism is linked to a 1.7 Mb region on chromosome 2p13.3-14. J Med Genet. 2006;43(3):e12.
13. Vidailhet M, et al. Neonatal hyperparathyroidism secondary to maternal hypoparathyroidism (author's translation). Arch Fr Pediatr. 1980;37(5):305–12.
14. Waller S, et al. Neonatal severe hyperparathyroidism: genotype/phenotype correlation and the use of pamidronate as rescue therapy. Eur J Pediatr. 2004;163(10):589–94.
15. Allgrove J. Use of bisphosphonates in children and adolescents. J Pediatr Endocrinol Metab. 2002;15 Suppl 3:921–8.
16. Silverstein DM, et al. Cinacalcet is efficacious in pediatric dialysis patients. Pediatr Nephrol. 2008;23(10):1817–22.
17. Grall Lerosey M, et al. Current methods for the localization of parathyroid adenoma in children. Arch Pediatr. 1997;4(8):802–3.

18. Sekiyama K, et al. Usefulness of diagnostic imaging in primary hyperparathyroidism. Int J Urol. 2003; 10(1):7–11. discussion 12.
19. De Feo ML, et al. Parathyroid glands: combination of (99m)Tc MIBI scintigraphy and US for demonstration of parathyroid glands and nodules. Radiology. 2000;214(2):393–402.
20. Zhou GW, et al. Diagnosis and surgical treatment of multiple endocrine neoplasia. Chin Med J (Engl). 2009;122(13):1495–500.
21. Sackett WR, et al. Minimal access thyroid surgery: is it feasible, is it appropriate? ANZ J Surg. 2002; 72(11):777–80.
22. Nussbaum SR, et al. Intraoperative measurement of parathyroid hormone in the surgical management of hyperparathyroidism. Surgery. 1988;104(6): 1121–7.
23. Kale N, et al. Hungry bone syndrome in a child following parathyroid surgery. J Pediatr Surg. 1992;27(12):1502–3.
24. Kone-Paut I, et al. Parathyroid adenoma in a child. Pediatrie. 1993;48(6):469–72.
25. Falchetti A, et al. DNA-based test: when and why to apply it to primary hyperparathyroidism clinical phenotypes. J Intern Med. 2009;266(1): 69–83.

Hypoparathyroidism in Children

16

Anne Lienhardt-Roussie and Agnès Linglart

Abstract

This chapter focuses on the rare disorder of hypoparathyroidism in children. It details the clinical features, pathophysiology, and biochemical abnormalities of the many forms seen clinically. Up-to-date information about the genetics of these disorders is provided along with the abnormalities in gene function. The chapter concludes with a summary of current treatment options for children with these disorders.

Keywords

Hypoparathyroidism • Ionized calcium • Hypocalcemia • Parathyroid hormone • Distal renal tubular reabsorption • Urinary calcium • Renal 1 alpha hydroxylase • 1,25 Dihydroxy vitamin D • Seizures • Laryngospasm • Cardioversion disturbances • Neuromuscular irritability • Currently • Paresthesias • Chvostek sign • Trousseau sign • Mental retardation • Dental hypoplasia • Psychological manifestations • Radiological signs • Metaphysis • Basal ganglia • Calcifications of basal ganglia • FARR syndrome • Phosphatemia • Hypomagnesemia • Embryological development • Transcription factors • Calcium sensing receptors • DiGeorge syndrome • Fluorescent in situ hybridization • TBX.1 gene • Microcephaly • Hypertelorism • Cleft palate • Micrognathia • Philtrum • Thymic aplasia • Immunological disorders • Urogenital, skeletal, ocular malformations • Behavioral problems • Glial cell missing B transcription factor • Hypoparathyroidism • Deafness • Renal dysplasia syndrome • Hypoparathyroidism • Retardation • Dysmorphism • Kenny-Caffey syndrome

A. Lienhardt-Roussie, MD, PhD (✉)
Department of Pediatric, National Reference Center for Calcium/Phosphorus metabolic diseases, Limoges, France
e-mail: Anne.lienhardt@chu-limoges.fr

A. Linglart, MD, PhD
Department of Pediatric Endocrinology, Bicêtre-Paris-Sud hospital, French Center of Reference for rare disorders of calcium and phosphate metabolism and INSERM unit U986, 94000 le Kremlin-Bicêtre, France

A.A. Licata and E.V. Lerma (eds.), *Diseases of the Parathyroid Glands*,
DOI 10.1007/978-1-4419-5550-0_16, © Springer Science+Business Media, LLC 2012

• Sanjad–Sakati syndrome • Familial hypoparathyroidism X linked length recessive transmission • SOX3 • Deficiency of PTH production • Heart is normal dominant hypocalcemia • G protein coupled receptors • Activating and inhibiting mutations • Pseudo-Bartter syndrome • Mutation in PTH gene • Mitochondrial disease • Kearns–Sayre syndrome • Acquired hypoparathyroidism • Calcium receptor antibodies • APECED syndrome • NA LP 5 protein • Surgery • Maternal hyperparathyroidism and neonatal hypoparathyroidism • Iatrogenic causes of hypocalcemia • Antiepileptic drugs • Ketoconazole • Aluminum hydroxide • Laxatives • Acute pancreatitis • Rhabdomyolysis • Treatment • Increased urinary calcium excretion • Nephrocalcinosis • Calcium chelators • Septic shock • Infectious syndromes • Chemotherapy • Invasive tumors • Alfacalcidol • Lithiasis • Exogenous PTH • Teriparatide • Osteosarcoma • Autosomal dominant hypoparathyroidism • Cytochrome P450

Introduction

Hypoparathyroidism is a rare disorder due to a deficient secretion of parathyroid hormone (PTH) by the parathyroid glands, and hence the incapacity to maintain normal extracellular ionized calcium levels. It may cause clinical symptoms which upon further investigation will show hypocalcemia, hyperphosphatemia, and an inappropriately low PTH level. In contrast to hypoparathyroidism in adulthood, usually secondary to thyroid surgery, hypoparathyroidism in childhood is mostly due to a congenital disorder, even if symptoms are not present during the neonatal period. In most cases, the diagnosis is made or suspected during infancy or puberty. Those periods are marked by an increase in growth velocity and therefore an increase in calcium requirements. As a consequence, mild or persistent hypocalcemia may become symptomatic.

Clinical Features

Symptoms

Whatever the cause, the symptoms of hypoparathyroidism are due to hypocalcemia. Deficient PTH secretion prevents resorption of calcium from the skeleton and diminished absorption of intestinal calcium due to decreased production of 1,25 dihydroxyvitamin D (from lower activity of renal 1α-hydroxylase), and decreased renal tubular reabsorption.

Symptoms of hypocalcemia vary with age and acuteness of the disease. Hypocalcemia can manifest acutely through generalized seizures, laryngospasm, and cardiac rhythm disturbances. However, symptoms may be milder and nonspecific: neuromuscular irritability (tetany, muscles cramps, paresthesia, increased muscular contractility assessed by Chvostek's sign and Trousseau's maneuver), cardiac rhythm disturbances, attention deficit disorders, poor academic performance, mental retardation, poor dental condition such as enamel hypoplasia. In rare cases, hypocalcemia may be found on routine blood screening for unrelated issues. In older children, hypocalcemia may present as psychological manifestations (depression and sleeping disturbances).

Biochemistry

In patients affected with hypoparathyroidism, serum calcium is low (<2.2 mM), by definition less than the lower limit of the reference laboratory being used. Whatever the age, ionized calcium is also reduced to less than 1 mM. PTH levels are low, often undetectable, or inappropriately normal in presence of hypocalcemia (the absence of PTH rise in response to hypocalcemia asserts the hypoparathyroidism). Because calcium

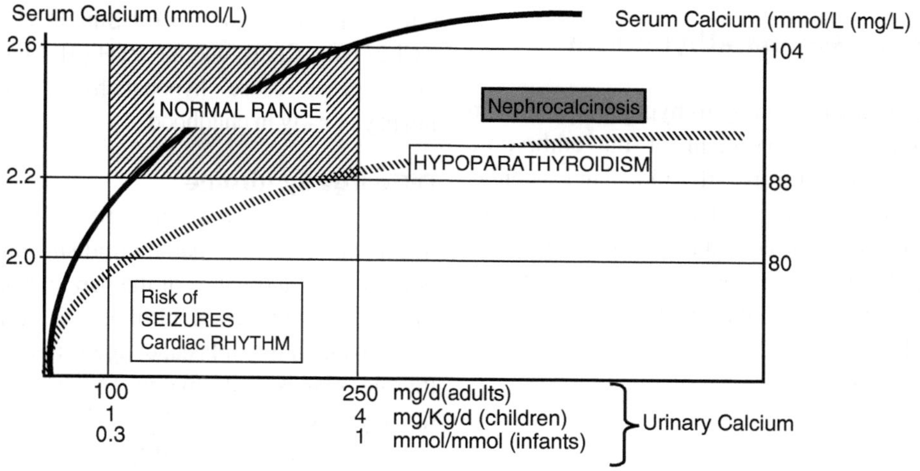

Fig. 16.1 Clinical consequences of hypocalcemia in presence of hypoparathyroidism. Because of PTH lack, relationship between serum and urinary calcium is lowered and shifted toward the right (normal condition: *black line*; hypoparathyroidism: *dotted line*). Therefore, nephrocalcinosis would rapidly appear for lower serum calcium values than in healthy patient

levels are low, the urinary calcium excretion is usually low or undetectable at the time of diagnosis. However, elevated urinary calcium excretion can be found in some rare cases of hypoparathyroidism due to an activation of the calcium sensing receptor (CaSR) or in patients with low–normal calcium levels (Fig. 16.1).

Serum phosphorus is elevated due to the deficient excretion of phosphates in absence of PTH. This observation is often confounded by the natural occurrence of higher levels of phosphorus in infants and young children, but attention to the ambient calcium helps determine the significance. Magnesium levels are normal or low–normal in patients with hypoparathyroidism. However, severe hypomagnesemia, found in patients affected with a genetic defect in magnesium transport, impairs the PTH secretion and mimics the genetic causes of hypoparathyroidism. Although vitamin D levels (25-OH vitamin D) are often low at the time of diagnosis, this alone is not sufficient to cause the symptoms since the normal physiological response to vitamin D deficiency is an increased secretion of PTH and production of hydroxylated vitamin D. Obviously, this counterresponse to low vitamin D and serum calcium is impaired in patients with hypoparathyroidism leading to hypocalcemia.

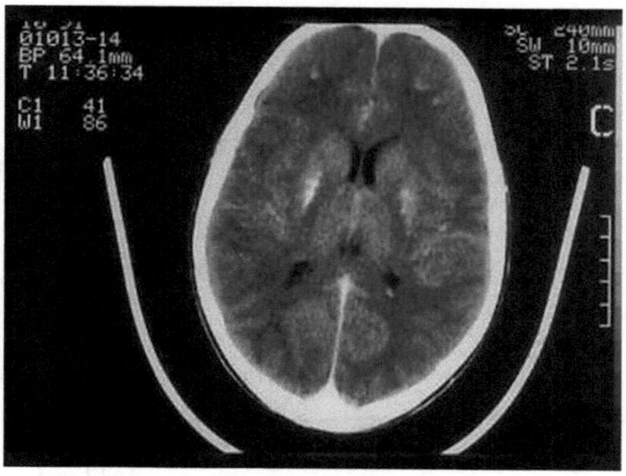

Fig. 16.2 Farr syndrome

Radiological Findings

Because PTH is involved in bone turnover, PTH deficiency, as seen in hypoparathyroidism, is associated with an increase in bone density, dense metaphyseal striae, and cortical thickening [1] (Fig. 16.2). Calcifications of the basal ganglia or widespread calcifications in other intracranial structures assessed through computed tomography imaging of the head may be associated with chronic hypocalcemia (Fahr syndrome) [2].

Causes of Hypoparathyroidism

The mechanisms leading to hypoparathyroidism are numerous: impairment of the embryonic development of the parathyroid glands, abnormal regulation of the PTH synthesis and/or secretion, or acquired injury of the parathyroid glands. Some of the genetic determinants of parathyroid glands embryogenesis, PTH synthesis and secretion, or autoimmunity are now known (Table 16.1).

Impaired Embryonic Development of the Parathyroid Glands

Animal studies have shown that embryogenesis of the parathyroid glands is controlled through a genetic cascade comprising different transcription factors (Hoxa3-Pax1/9-Eya1-Six1/4-Shh-Tbx1-Gcmb2-CCL21), the CaSR, and the PTH [3]. Mutations in those genes cause hypoparathyroidism during infancy or early in childhood.

DiGeorge Syndrome

To date, the DiGeorge syndrome is the most frequent cause of hypoparathyroidism among the embryologic anomalies of the parathyroid glands (around 1/4,000 living births). It is responsible for congenital hypoplasia, or agenesis of the parathyroid glands and thymus. A recurrent large hemizygotic deletion of the 22q11.21-q11.23 region, removing about forty genes, is identified by fluorescent in situ hybridization (FISH) in more than 95% of the patients affected with DiGeorge syndrome. In addition to this autosomal dominant transmission, the deletion may occur de novo [4].Patients affected with the DiGeorge syndrome without the 22q11.21-q11.23 deletion

Table 16.1 Etiologies of hypoparathyroidism

Syndrome	Transmission	Gene(s); chromosome	Alteration	Clinical symptoms
APECED	RA	AIRE; 21q22.3	Immunologic tolerance	Neonatal candidosis, hypoparathyroidism (6–7 years), Addison disease (12–15 years)
DiGeorge (CATCH-22)	Sporadic/DA	rnex40/nex2,2, TBX1 UDFL1; 22q11	Branchial pouches	Dysmorphy, thymus agenesis, heart malformations, immunological abnormalities, mental retardation
Kearns–Sayre	Maternal/ sporadic	Mitochondrial DNA	Energy production	Isolated hypoparathyroidism, mitochondrial disease
Kenny-Caffey	RA	TBCE; 1q42-q43	Tubulin chaperone	Osteosclerosis, short stature, eyes abnormalities
Sanjad–Sakati	RA	TBCE; 1q42-q43	Tubulin chaperone	Short stature, mental retardation
Hypoparathyroidism deafness, renal defect (HDR)	DA	GATA3; 10p14-10p15.1	TF embryologic development	PT agenesis or hypoplasia, neurosensorial deafness, renal dysplasia
Hypoparathyroidism, retardation, dysmorphia (HRD)	RA	TBCE; 1q42-q43	Tubulin chaperone	Mental retardation, microcephaly, IUGR, micropenis, dysmorphy
Autosomal dominant hypocalcemia	DA	CaSR; 3q13.3-q21	PTH synthesis	Unadapted urinary calcium excretion
Isolated hypoparathyroidism	DA/RA	PTH; 11q15.3-p15.1	PTH synthesis	
Isolated hypoparathyroidism	RA/DA	GCMB; 6p24.2	TF PT embryology	PT agenesis

APECED autoimmune endocrinopathy–candidiasis–ectodermal dystrophy, *CaSR* calcium-sensing receptor, *DA* dominant autosomal, *IUGR* intrauterine growth restriction, *RA* recessive autosomal, *TF* transmission factor, *TBCE* tubulin cofactor E, *PT* parathyroid gland

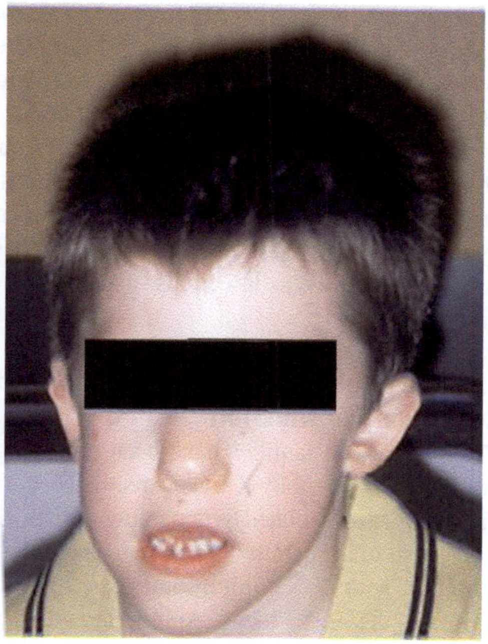

Fig. 16.3 Facial dysmorphia in DiGeorge syndrome

have been described. These patients carry mutations in the *TBX1* gene, located within the 22q11 region, suggesting that *TBX1* is responsible for the main features of the syndrome [5, 6]. Furthermore, a deletion in the 10p13-p14 region, close to the HDR (hypoparathyroidism, deafness, and renal dysplasia) syndrome locus, has been described in patients with a DiGeorge-like phenotype [7].

The phenotypical spectrum of the DiGeorge syndrome is wide and results from a developmental defect of the third and fourth pharyngeal pouches and the facial neural crest. According to the age at diagnosis, symptoms will be more or less prominent [8, 9].

- *Facial dysmorphia* includes microcephaly, narrow palpebral fissures, hypertelorism, small mouth, cleft palate, micrognathia, and smooth philtrum (Fig. 16.3).
- *Various congenital cardiac malformations* are frequent (80–85%). They are most often diagnosed during the fetal or neonatal period: aortic arch anomalies, tetralogy of Fallot, conotruncal anomalies such as truncus arteriosus, interrupted aorta, hypoplasia of the pulmonary artery. In both animal and humans, these defects are attributed to a deficiency inTBX1 [6, 10].
- *Hypoparathyroidism* due to the hypo- or aplasia of the parathyroid glands may be the sole clinical feature.
- *Infectious diseases* during early childhood are frequent because of thymic hypo- or aplasia.
- *Dysimmunity* (celiac disease, Graves' disease, and arthritis) may appear later in adulthood.
- *Malformations* can be present: urogenital (agenesis or renal dysplasia, multicystic kidney, obstructive uropathy, and cryptorchidism), skeletal (scoliosis), and ocular anomalies (coloboma, cataract, and microphthalmia).
- *Behavioral problems* (personality disturbances) have been attributed to the haploinsufficiency of the catechol-*O*-methyl transferase gene [11].

Follow-up of patients affected with the DiGeorge syndrome has to be adjusted to the patient's age: neonatal period—hypocalcemia, heart disease, eating problems; early childhood—hypocalcemia, heart disease, psychomotor retardation, infection; school age—infection, psychomotor retardation, personality disturbances; adult age—autoimmune diseases.

Hypoparathyroidism Associated with a Defect in the Glial Cell Missing B Gene

Glial cell missing B (GCMB) is a transcription factor initially identified in the Drosophila where it is necessary to glial cell differentiation. In mice, *Gcm1* is expressed in the placenta and *Gcm2* in the parathyroid glands and ovaries [3]. The identification of biallelic mutations or monoallelic dominant negative mutations in the *GCMB* gene in families with autosomal recessive and autosomal dominant neonatal hypoparathyroidism, respectively, has demonstrated the importance of GCMB for the embryogenesis and maintenance of parathyroid cells in humans [12–14]. *Gcm* probably contributes to the PTH synthesis by controlling the expression of the calcium sensing receptor [15, 16]

To summarize, mutations in the *GCMB* gene are found in patients affected with isolated hypoparathyroidism, especially when the disease is hereditary.

HDR Syndrome

HDR syndrome, also known as Barakat syndrome, is inherited as an autosomal dominant trait. Haploinsufficiency of GATA3, a member of the GATA family of transcription factors, either through a large deletion in the 10p14-10p15 region or through point mutations of the *GATA3* gene, is responsible for the disease [17–19]. Noteworthy, gene duplications have been also described [20]. GATA3 is a transcription factor belonging to the large GATA family. It is involved in the embryogenesis of the parathyroid glands, kidney, and internal ear, as well as in the differentiation of lymphocytes T_H1 and T_H2 [17].

Hypoparathyroidism secondary to a GATA3 mutation is often severe. Associated features allow the diagnosis of the syndrome [20] sometimes described as a pseudo DiGeorge syndrome: slanted palpebral fissures, hypertelorism, blepharophimosis, narrow nose root, anteverted nostrils, micrognathia, and arched palate. Other cardinal signs are required for the diagnosis: enlargement of the nipple distance, clinodactyly, syndactyly, hypotony, bilateral neurosensitive deafness and renal malformations: multicystic kidneys, nephrotic syndrome, renal dysplasia (hypoplasia), vesicoureteral reflux, chronic renal insufficiency, hematuria, proteinuria, and characteristic bone impairment.

Hypoparathyroidism Retardation Dysmorphism Syndrome

HRD syndrome (hypoparathyroidism retardation dysmorphism) unifies two previously described syndromes: the Kenny-Caffey syndrome, in its autosomal recessive form, and the Sanjad–Sakati syndrome, both due to a defect in the *TBCE* (Tubulin specific Chaperone E) gene, localized in 1q42-q43, and coding for a protein involved in the polymerization of the α and β tubulin subunits. This protein is allows the formation of intracellular microtubules; as a result of genetic abnormalities in the gene coding TBCE, a large amount of intracellular functions are impaired in affected patients [21]. In 4q35, a different gene is likely involved in a phenocopy of the HRD syndrome [22].This syndrome of autosomal recessive inheritance was initially described in the Bedouin families originating from Saudi Arabia affected with hypoparathyroidism and associated symptoms such as intrauterine growth restriction (80% of the cases), extreme growth retardation, mental retardation, microcephaly, facial dysmorphy including hollow eyes, pronounced nasal bridge, small turned-up nose, thin upper lip and micrognathy, short feet and hands, hypogonadism, susceptibility to infections, and dysimmunity [21, 23].

Familial Hypoparathyroidism of X-linked Recessive Transmission

Three American families have been reported as presenting a possible X-linked recessive transmission form of isolated hypoparathyroidism due to agenesis of the parathyroid glands. The patients presented with an X chromosome rearrangement involving the *SOX3* locus. Animal models have demonstrated the role of *SOX3* in the embryogenesis of parathyroid glands [24].

Deficiency in PTH Production and Secretion

Autosomal Dominant Hypocalcemia

Autosomal dominant hypocalcemia (ADH) was described in the 1990s following the cloning of the CaSR. CaSR is a transmembrane receptor belonging to the super family of G-protein coupled receptors (GPCR). The CaSR is expressed, among other tissues, on the cell surface membrane of the parathyroid cells and the renal tubular cells. Extracellular calcium ions are the main ligands of the CaSR. The CaSR controls the PTH synthesis as well as renal tubular calcium reabsorption. Hypocalcemia activates to the receptor and increases PTH synthesis and urinary calcium reabsorption and ultimately in an increase in serum calcium. As for numerous GPCRs, mutations of the CaSR gene have been shown to cause mirror pathologies: activating and inhibiting mutations producing activation and loss of function of the receptor, respectively [25].

Autosomal dominant hypocalcemia results from a heterozygous activating mutation of the CaSR. It is to date the main genetic cause of

Table 16.2 Frequency of hypoparathyroidism etiologies

	Lund [46] 1980	Markowitz [47] 1982	Kruse [48] 1989	Halabe [49] 1994	Winer [42] 2003	Winer [43] 2008	Lienhardt[a] 2009
n	14	10 (Children)	29	17	27 (Adults)	14 (Children)	50 (Children)
CaSR					6 (22%)	1	19 (38%)
22q11				17			13 (26%)
APECED			1 (3%)		2 (7%)	5	7 (14%)
Postsurgery	9	1	2 (7%)	15	11 (41%)	1	1 (2%)
Idiopathic	4	7	26 (90%)	2	8 (30%)	7	7 (14%)
Other causes		2					2 (4%)

APECED autoimmune endocrinopathy–candidiasis–ectodermal dystrophy, *CaSR* calcium-sensing receptor
[a]Personal data

hypoparathyroidism (Table 16.2). Germ-line activating mutations of the CaSR increase the receptor sensitivity to circulating concentrations of ionized calcium in all target tissues and repress both the PTH synthesis and the urinary calcium reabsorption. The resultant hypocalcemia is most often fortuitously discovered in children or in adults. The biochemical phenotype is quite characteristic: hypocalcemia below 2 mM, normal or hyperphosphatemia; normal or high urinary calcium; normal or low PTH. The level of urinary calcium can drop in cases of severe and/or prolonged hypocalcemia: the existence of a low urinary calcium excretion does not therefore necessarily infer the hypothesis of an activating CaSR mutation. When a mutation is found in an index case, the measurement of the calcium level is sufficient for the genetic counseling. Autosomal dominant hypocalcemia can be diagnosed at any age of life and may present with various clinical symptoms, even within the same family. This absence of genotype–phenotype correlation suggests the importance of environmental factors already mentioned above [26]. One patient was described as having an activating homozygote mutation without presenting severe hypoparathyroidism [27]. It should be noted that some patients present with a pseudo-Bartter syndrome. In these patients, the CaSR activation induces not only an increase of the urinary calcium excretion but also a defect in sodium, potassium, and chlorine reabsorption, and a decrease of the transepithelial gradient [28, 29].

Hypoparathyroidism Due to Mutation Within the PTH Gene

Mutations in the PTH gene are extremely rare. Only three mutations have been described so far: two are autosomal recessive inheritance, and one is dominant. All are localized within the PTH coding region for the peptide precursor, the pre-proPTH, and disturb the maturing processing of PTH [30, 31].

Mitochondrial Diseases

The Kearns–Sayre syndrome is the most frequent manifestation of mitochondrial diseases associated with hypoparathyroidism. In 90% of cases, it is secondary to a large deletion of the mitochondrial DNA, but duplications have also been reported. Its transmission is maternal. The Kearns–Sayre syndrome is usually diagnosed during childhood but may also occur later on in adolescence or in early adulthood. The clinical manifestations are variable: impairments of the central (ataxia, mental retardation) or peripheral nervous system, ocular signs (ptosis, retinitis, ophthalmoplegia, and optic atrophy), myopathy, cardiac impairment (conduction disturbances, cardiomyopathy), neurosensorial deafness, endocrine disturbances (hypoparathyroidism, insufficient insulin secretion eventually leading to diabetes, hypogonadism, and hypomagnesemia), and renal tubulopathy. Endocrine impairments, notably hypoparathyroidism, are usually preceded by the neurological impairment. The deficiency in the PTH synthesis appears to be secondary to the low mitochondrial energy production in the parathyroid cell, as this synthesis is very energy-costly [32]. MELAS syndrome and mitochondrial trifunctional protein (MTP) deficit can also be associated with hypoparathyroidism [33, 34].

Acquired Hypoparathyroidism

Hypoparathyroidism with Anti-CaSR Antibodies

Soon after the cloning of the CaSR gene, several teams suggested the possible existence of antibodies directed against the CaSR receptors. They subsequently identified a patient with acquired hypoparathyroidism [35]. Mayer et al. reported anti-CaSR antibodies in five out of 17 patients with isolated hypoparathyroidism, and in two out of 14 patients with hypoparathyroidism and polyendocrinopathy [36].

APECED Syndrome

APECED syndrome (autoimmune polyendocrinopathy candidiasis ectodermal dystrophy) is from a rare autosomal recessive pathology (1/80,000), manifesting early in childhood. Mutations have been found on both alleles of the *AIRE1* (autoimmune regulator) gene, which regulates the transcription of autoantibodies at the thymic level, in affected patients and families [37].

The patients progressively develop autoimmunity toward diverse organs, which include numerous endocrine glands [38]. This pathology evolves throughout life. Hypoparathyroidism is the most frequent symptom (80–95% of cases), often the first, and is due in 49% of cases to autoantibodies directed toward the NALP5 (NACHT leucine-rich-repeat protein 5) protein [39]. The identification of the anti-NALP5 antibody in patient sera could become the first-line diagnostic tool in suspected APECED, before any gene sequencing. To confirm the diagnosis, two out of three of the following clinical impairments are sufficient: chronic mucous–cutaneous candidosis, as soon as early childhood—hypoparathyroidism, with a peak of occurrence around 10 years of age—adrenal insufficiency, appearing around 15 years of age. The other clinical features appear throughout the patient's lifetime, including Graves' disease, autoimmune thyroiditis, active chronic hepatitis, alopecia, autoimmune anemia, malabsorption, vitiligo, insulin dependent diabetes, hypergonadotropic hypogonadism, bronchiolitis [40]—all of these symptoms being related to an organ-targeted autoimmunity. These patients require lifelong monitoring of these autoimmune pathologies.

Surgery

Any cervical, parathyroid, or thyroid surgery can cause hypoparathyroidism. This iatrogenic consequence (3–4% of interventions) essentially depends on the experience of the surgical team and the extension of the intervention. In fact, hypoparathyroidism has been found more frequently after thyroid surgery for invasive thyroid cancer, large multinodular goiters or Graves' disease. It is less frequent, and usually temporary, after surgery on a solitary parathyroid adenoma, or a subtotal parathyroidectomy. The stimulation of the remaining glandular tissue or of the reimplanted tissue prevents hypocalcemia. This cause of hypoparathyroidism is not very common in children [41].

Neonatal Hypoparathyroidism Secondary to Maternal Hyperparathyroidism

Hyperparathyroidism in pregnant women slows down the development of the fetal PTH synthesis as the fetus becomes hypercalcemic. At birth, there is a risk of acute neonatal hypocalcemia due to suppressed parathyroid gland function. This hypocalcemia resolves within a few weeks.

Frequency of Different Etiologies

There is no reliable study regarding the frequency of pediatric hypoparathyroidism etiologies—numerous cases being undiagnosed due to mild clinical expression (ADH) or to the recent discovery of the other genes involved in the appearance of hypoparathyroidism, such as GCMB. We have undertaken in France, with physicians from the National Reference Centre for Rare Diseases of the Calcium and Phosphorus Metabolism, a retrospective study of patients affected with hypoparathyroidism, which outlines some epidemiological tendencies (Table 16.2). Based on this data, the molecular studies that we offer to patients affected with hypoparathyroidism are 22q, CaSR, PTH, and GCMB.

Differential Diagnosis

There are many causes of hypocalcemia besides what has been mentioned above:

- PTH resistance (genetic defect downstream to the PTH receptor) or chronic renal insufficiency—in these cases, PTH levels are elevated.
- Drugs: *Antiepileptic drugs* increase the vitamin D catabolism, *ketoconazole* inhibits the renal 1α-hydroxylase, prolonged use of *aluminum hydroxides* or of *calcium chelators*, such as citrate, and *laxatives*.
- Drugs used for the treatment of hypercalcemia, such as bisphosphonates, calcitonin, or chemotherapies.
- Miscellaneous:
  Acute pancreatitis—hypocalcemia results from the accumulation of calcium deposits in necrotic tissue.
  Hypomagnesemia, hypoalbuminemia.
  Septic shock and infectious syndrome.
- Causes of hyperphosphatemia.

Treatment

The conventional treatment will aim at correcting the hypocalcemia using 1-alpha hydroxylated vitamin D, through the forced intestinal absorption of calcium. The goals of the treatment may differ according to the clinical severity and etiology of the hypoparathyroidism [42].

Treatment and Monitoring

Diminished renal production of 1.25-$(OH)_2D$ is the main cause of hypocalcemia in patients with hypoparathyroidism. Therefore, treatment with a 1α-hydroxylated vitamin D derivative (calcitriol or alfacalcidol) is the reference treatment. The dosage depends on the serum calcium and, above all, on urinary calcium excretion, which must be maintained within normal ranges to avoid urinary calcium intoxication and the development of lithiasis and/or nephrocalcinosis. We have established the following threshold in patients affected with hypoparathyroidism: 24 h-urinary calcium excretion below 5 mg/kg/d or urinary calcium/urinary creatinine <1 mmol/mmol (0.35 mg/mg) under the age of 5 years or <0.5 mmol/mmol (0.17 mg/mg) over the age of 5 years. Yearly renal ultrasonography is also recommended. The initial dose of 1α-hydroxylated vitamin D is 2–8 μg/day once or twice a day (1–4 μg/day of 1α/25-hydroxylated vitamin D twice per day) depending on the severity of the hypocalcemia. When the serum calcium reaches 2.2 mM or higher, the dosage is then reduced by 30–50%, to minimize the excreted urinary calcium levels and yet provide symptomatic relief. The lowest possible effective dose is often between 1 and 2 μg/day, but this has to be individually determined. This is a compromise between clinical symptomatology (prevention of seizures, absence of paresthesia, etc.) and prevention of nephrocalcinosis [43, 44].

We maintain in those children the 25 OH vitamin D in the normal range (above 40–50 nM or 16–20 ng/ml). This threshold should be upgraded in patients receiving antiepileptic drugs, which increase the risk of vitamin D deficiency, as well as in patients receiving recombinant PTH. In fact, in patients affected with hypoparathyroidism, the use of PTH will restore the renal 1 alpha hydroxylase activity and induce the hydroxylation of 25-(OH)D to 1.25-$(OH)_2D$.

Calcium supplementation is carried out intravenously during the acute phase of hypocalcemia and/or in case of high risk of seizures, until the serum calcium reaches approximately 2.2 mM. We recommend the dose of 1,000 mg/m^2 of body surface. The removal of the IV infusion always induces a drop of 0.2 mM of the calcium level. An oral calcium supplementation should be considered as an adjuvant only. It is used at the start of the treatment until total restoration of the calcium pool (4–6 months), after which alimentary contribution (depending on the age) is sufficient. In France, daily dietary calcium needs are 500 mg/day up to 3 years, 700 mg/day up to 6 years, 900 mg/day up to 9 years, and 1,200 mg/day up to 19 years.

The off-label use of synthetic exogenous PTH (teriparatide) has shown its efficiency and is an interesting alternative in cases of hypoparathyroidism resistant to the conventional treatment. The dose for adults is about 30–40 μg/day via two subcutaneous injections [45]. We have recently reported doses of 5–15 μg/day given continuously with the aid of a pump in children, but this remains to be validated [46]. Osteosarcoma has been observed in rodent models at pharmacological doses greater than those used for humans [47]. Two reported cases of osteosarcoma in patients have been reported, but significance is not clear.

Monitoring of Specific Etiologies

In the case of *Autosomal Dominant Hypoparathyroidism*, iatrogenic complications such as increased urinary calcium excretion or nephrocalcinosis are frequent. Treatment must therefore be considered with caution and must only be used when calcium levels are lower than 1.80 mM, or when the symptoms are devastating. To avoid nephrocalcinosis, serum calcium is kept in the lower normal range while maintaining normal urinary calcium excretion. In rare cases, where this balance cannot be established, treatment by recombinant PTH has been proven effective [46, 48].

Patients affected with *APECED* may require higher doses of 1-hydroxylated vitamin D, as well as oral calcium supplementation, because of their digestive malabsorption. Alternatively, in these patients, worsening of the hypocalcaemia and/or elevated urinary calcium excretion may be due to an adrenal insufficiency. Moreover, antiepileptic drugs or liver diseases may inhibit the activity of the liver 25-hydroxylase. In this case, 1-hydroxylated vitamin D has to be replaced by 1.25-(OH)-2D if it is available. Finally, if the patients require an anticandidiasis treatment, it is necessary to closely monitor the serum calcium. Indeed, ketoconazole reduces the activity of several steroid P450-dependant cytochrome hydroxylases and may therefore induce a reduction in the concentration of 1.25-$(OH)_2$D.

For patients with hypoparathyroidism (DiGeorge syndrome in particular), *infectious episodes* may trigger acute hypocalcemia and seizures. Implementing a calcium perfusion during such episodes or temporarily increasing the dose of the 1-hydroxylated vitamin D derivatives may prevent incidents.

The genetic factors causing hypoparathyroidism have been discovered during the past few years. The main treatment is the 1α-hydroxylated vitamin D derivatives and oral calcium supplementation. In very rare cases, especially in cases of refractory hypoparathyroidism, the use of teriparatide, the recombinant PTH, is an interesting alternative.

Acknowledgment The authors thank Richard Medeiros, Rouen University Hospital Medical Editor, for editing the manuscript.

References

1. Abugassa S, Nordenström J, Eriksson S, Sjödén G. Bone mineral density in patients with chronic hypoparathyroidism. J Clin Endocrinol Metab. 1993;76:1617–21.
2. Fukunaga M, Otsuka N, Ono S, Kajihara Y, Nishishita S, Nakano Y, Yamamoto I, Torizuka K, Morita R. Computed tomography of basal ganglia calcifications in pseudo- and idiopathic hypoparathyroidism. Radiat Med. 1987;5:187–90.
3. Gordon J, Bennett AR, Blackburn CC, Manley NR. Gcm2 and Foxn1 mark early parathyroid- and thymus-specific domains in the developing third pharyngeal pouch. Mech Dev. 2001;103:141–3.
4. Iascone MR, Vittorini S, Sacchelli M, Spadoni I, Simi P, Giusti S. Molecular characterization of 22q11 deletion in a three-generation family with maternal transmission. Am J Med Genet. 2002;108:319–21.
5. Merscher S, Funke B, Epstein JA, Heyer J, Puech A, Lu MM, Xavier RJ, Demay MB, Russell RG, Factor S, Tokooya K, Jore BS, Lopez M, Pandita RK, Lia M, Carrion D, Xu H, Schorle H, Kobler JB, Scambler P,

Wynshaw-Boris A, Skoultchi AI, Morrow BE, Kucherlapati R. TBX1 is responsible for cardiovascular defects in velo-cardio-facial/DiGeorge syndrome. Cell. 2001;104:619–29.
6. Yagi H, Furutani Y, Hamada H, Sasaki T, Asakawa S, Minoshima S, Ichida F, Joo K, Kimura M, Imamura S, Kamatani N, Momma K, Takao A, Nakazawa M, Shimizu N, Matsuoka R. Role of TBX1 in human del22q11.2 syndrome. Lancet Engl. 2003;362(9393): 1366–73.
7. Van Esch H, Groenen P, Nesbit M, Schuffenhauer S, Lichtner P, Vanderlinden G, Harding B, Beetz R, Bilous R, Holdaway I, Shaw N, Fryns J, Van de Ven W, Thakker R, Devriendt K. GATA3 haplo-insufficiency causes human HDR syndrome. Nature. 2000;406:419–22.
8. Kobrynski LJ, Sullivan KE. Velocardiofacial syndrome, DiGeorge syndrome: the chromosome 22q11.2 deletion syndromes. Lancet. 2007;370:1443–52.
9. Paylor R, Glaser B, Mupo A, Ataliotis P, Spencer C, Sobotka A, Sparks C, Choi CH, Oghalai J, Curran S, Murphy KC, Monks S, Williams N, O'Donovan MC, Owen MJ, Scambler PJ, Lindsay E. Tbx1 haploinsufficiency is linked to behavioral disorders in mice and humans: implications for 22q11 deletion syndrome. Proc Natl Acad Sci USA. 2006;103:7729–34.
10. Momma K. Cardiovascular anomalies associated with chromosome 22q11.2 deletion syndrome. Am J Cardiol. 2010;105:1617–24.
11. Prasad SE, Howley S, Murphy KC. Candidate genes and the behavioral phenotype in 22q11.2 deletion syndrome. Dev Disabil Res Rev. 2008;14:26–34.
12. Ding C, Buckingham B, Levine MA. Familial isolated hypoparathyroidism caused by a mutation in the gene for the transcription factor GCMB. J Clin Invest. 2001;108:1215–20.
13. Mannstadt M, Bertrand G, Muresan M, Weryha G, Leheup B, Pulusani SR, Grandchamp B, Jüppner H, Silve C. Dominant-negative GCMB mutations cause an autosomal dominant form of hypoparathyroidism. J Clin Endocrinol Metab. 2008;93:3568–76.
14. Thomée C, Schubert SW, Parma J, Lê PQ, Hashemolhosseini S, Wegner M, Abramowicz MJ. GCMB mutation in familial isolated hypoparathyroidism with residual secretion of parathyroid hormone. J Clin Endocrinol Metab. 2005;90:2487–92.
15. Liu Z, Yu S, Manley NR. Gcm2 is required for the differentiation and survival of parathyroid precursor cells in the parathyroid/thymus primordia. Dev Biol. 2007;305:333–46.
16. Kebebew E, Peng M, Wong MG, Ginzinger D, Duh QY, Clark OH. GCMB gene, a master regulator of parathyroid gland development, expression, and regulation in hyperparathyroidism. Surgery. 2004; 136:1261–6.
17. Ali A, Christie PT, Grigorieva IV, Harding B, Van Esch H, Ahmed SF, Bitner-Glindzicz M, Blind E, Bloch C, Christin P, Clayton P, Gecz J, Gilbert-Dussardier B, Guillen-Navarro E, Hackett A, Halac I, Hendy GN, Lalloo F, Mache CJ, Mughal Z, Ong AC, Rinat C, Shaw N, Smithson SF, Tolmie J, Weill J, Nesbit MA, Thakker RV. Functional characterization of GATA3 mutations causing the hypoparathyroidism-deafness-renal (HDR) dysplasia syndrome: insight into mechanisms of DNA binding by the GATA3 transcription factor. Hum Mol Genet. 2007;16:265–75.
18. Benetti E, Murer L, Bordugo A, Andreetta B, Artifoni L. 10p12.1 Deletion: HDR phenotype without DGS2 features. Exp Mol Pathol. 2009;86:74–6.
19. Nesbit MA, Bowl MR, Harding B, Ali A, Ayala A, Crowe C, Dobbie A, Hampson G, Holdaway I, Levine MA, McWilliams R, Rigden S, Sampson J, Williams AJ, Thakker RV. Characterization of GATA3 mutations in the hypoparathyroidism, deafness, and renal dysplasia (HDR) syndrome. J Biol Chem. 2004;279:22624–34.
20. Bernardini L, Sinibaldi L, Capalbo A, Bottillo I, Mancuso B, Torres B, Novelli A, Digilio MC, Dallapiccola B. HDR (hypoparathyroidism, deafness, renal dysplasia) syndrome associated to GATA3 gene duplication. Clin Genet. 2009;76:117–9.
21. Parvari R, Diaz GA, Hershkovitz E. Parathyroid development and the role of tubulin chaperone E. Horm Res. 2007;67:12–21.
22. Courtens W, Wuyts W, Poot M, Szuhai K, Wauters J, Reyniers E, Eleveld M, Diaz G, Nöthen MM, Parvari R. Hypoparathyroidism-retardation-dysmorphism syndrome in a girl: a new variant not caused by a TBCE mutation – clinical report and review. Am J Med Genet A. 2006;140:611–7.
23. Hershkovitz E, Parvari R, Diaz GA, Gorodischer R. Hypoparathyroidism-retardation-dysmorphism (HRD) syndrome – a review. J Pediatr Endocrinol Metab. 2004;17:1583–90.
24. Bowl MR, Nesbit MA, Harding B, Levy E, Jefferson A, Volpi E, Rizzoti K, Lovell-Badge R, Schlessinger D, Whyte MP, Thakker RV. An interstitial deletion–insertion involving chromosomes 2p25.3 and Xq27.1, near SOX3, causes X-linked recessive hypoparathyroidism. J Clin Invest. 2005;115:2822–31.
25. Thakker RV. Diseases associated with the extracellular calcium-sensing receptor. Cell Calcium. 2004;35:275–82.
26. Lienhardt A, Bai M, Lagarde JP, Rigaud M, Zhang Z, Jiang Y, Kottler ML, Brown EM, Garabédian M. Activating mutations of the calcium-sensing receptor: management of hypocalcemia. J Clin Endocrinol Metab. 2001;86:5313–23.
27. Lienhardt A, Garabédian M, Bai M, Sinding C, Zhang Z, Lagarde JP, Boulesteix J, Rigaud M, Brown EM, Kottler ML. A large homozygous or heterozygous in-frame deletion within the calcium-sensing receptor's carboxylterminal cytoplasmic tail that causes autosomal dominant hypocalcemia. J Clin Endocrinol Metab. 2000;85:1695–702.
28. Gamba G, Friedman PA. Thick ascending limb: the Na(+):K (+):2Cl (–) co-transporter, NKCC2, and the calcium-sensing receptor, CaSR. Pflugers Arch. 2009;458:61–76.

29. Watanabe S, Fukumoto S, Chang H, Takeuchi Y, Hasegawa Y, Okazaki R, Chikatsu N, Fujita T. Association between activating mutations of calcium-sensing receptor and Bartter's syndrome. Lancet. 2002;360:692–4.
30. Ahn TG, Antonarakis SE, Kronenberg HM, Igarashi T, Levine MA. Familial isolated hypoparathyroidism: a molecular genetic analysis of 8 families with 23 affected persons. Medicine (Baltimore). 1986;65:73–81.
31. Arnold A, Horst SA, Gardella TJ, Baba H, Levine MA, Kronenberg HM. Mutation of the signal peptide-encoding region of the preproparathyroid hormone gene in familial isolated hypoparathyroidism. J Clin Invest. 1990;86:1084–7.
32. D'Amour P, Palardy J, Bahsali G, Mallette LE, DeLean A, Lepage R. The modulation of circulating parathyroid hormone immunoheterogeneity in man by ionized calcium concentration. J Clin Endocrinol Metab. 1992;74:525–32.
33. Katsanos KH, Elisaf M, Bairaktari E, Tsianos EV. Severe hypomagnesemia and hypoparathyroidism in Kearns-Sayre syndrome. Am J Nephrol. 2001;21:150–3.
34. Wilichowski E, Grüters A, Kruse K, Rating D, Beetz R, Korenke GC, Ernst BP, Christen HJ, Hanefeld F. Hypoparathyroidism and deafness associated with pleioplasmic large scale rearrangements of the mitochondrial DNA: a clinical and molecular genetic study of four children with Kearns-Sayre syndrome. Pediatr Res. 1997;41:193–200.
35. Brown EM. Anti-parathyroid and anti-calcium sensing receptor antibodies in autoimmune hypoparathyroidism. Endocrinol Metab Clin N Am. 2009;38:437–45. x.
36. Mayer A, Ploix C, Orgiazzi J, Desbos A, Moreira A, Vidal H, Monier JC, Bienvenu J, Fabien N. Calcium-sensing receptor autoantibodies are relevant markers of acquired hypoparathyroidism. J Clin Endocrinol Metab. 2004;89:4484–8.
37. Gardner JM, Fletcher AL, Anderson MS, Turley SJ. AIRE in the thymus and beyond. Curr Opin Immunol. 2009;21:582–9.
38. Wolff AS, Erichsen MM, Meager A, Magitta NF, Myhre AG, Bollerslev J, Fougner KJ, Lima K, Knappskog PM, Husebye ES. Autoimmune polyendocrine syndrome type 1 in Norway: phenotypic variation, autoantibodies, and novel mutations in the autoimmune regulator gene. J Clin Endocrinol Metab. 2007;92:595–603.
39. Alimohammadi M, Björklund P, Hallgren A, Pöntynen N, Szinnai G, Shikama N, Keller MP, Ekwall O, Kinkel SA, Husebye ES, Gustafsson J, Rorsman F, Peltonen L, Betterle C, Perheentupa J, Akerström G, Westin G, Scott HS, Holländer GA, Kämpe O. Autoimmune polyendocrine syndrome type 1 and NALP5, a parathyroid autoantigen. N Engl J Med. 2008;358:1018–28.
40. Alimohammadi M, Dubois N, Sköldberg F, Hallgren A, Tardivel I, Hedstrand H, Haavik J, Husebye ES, Gustafsson J, Rorsman F, Meloni A, Janson C, Vialettes B, Kajosaari M, Egner W, Sargur R, Pontén F, Amoura Z, Grimfeld A, De Luca F, Betterle C, Perheentupa J, Kämpe O, Carel JC. Pulmonary autoimmunity as a feature of autoimmune polyendocrine syndrome type 1 and identification of KCNRG as a bronchial autoantigen. Proc Natl Acad Sci USA. 2009;106:4396–401.
41. Page C, Strunski V. Parathyroid risk in total thyroidectomy for bilateral, benign, multinodular goitre: report of 351 surgical cases. J Laryngol Otol. 2007;121:237–41.
42. Lienhardt-Roussie A, Linglart A, Garabedian M. Treatment of chronic hypocalcaemia during childhood. Arch Pediatr. 2008;15:650–2.
43. Misselwitz J, Hesse V, Markestad T. Nephrocalcinosis, hypercalciuria and elevated serum levels of 1,25-dihydroxyvitamin D in children. Possible link to vitamin D toxicity. Acta Paediatr Scand. 1990;79:637–43.
44. Weber G, Cazzuffi MA, Frisone F, de Angelis M, Pasolini D, Tomaselli V, Chiumello G. Nephrocalcinosis in children and adolescents: sonographic evaluation during long-term treatment with 1,25-dihydroxycholecalciferol. Child Nephrol Urol. 1988;9:273–6.
45. Winer KK, Sinaii N, Peterson D, Sainz B, Cutler GB. Effects of once versus twice-daily parathyroid hormone 1–34 therapy in children with hypoparathyroidism. J Clin Endocrinol Metab. 2008;93:3389–95.
46. Linglart A, Rothenbuhler A, Gueorgieva I, Lucchini P, Silve C, Bougnères P. Long-term results of continuous subcutaneous recombinant PTH (1–34) infusion in children with refractory hypoparathyroidism. J Clin Endocrinol Metab. 2011;96(11):3308–12.
47. Subbiah V, Madsen VS, Raymond AK, Benjamin RS, Ludwig JA. Of mice and men: divergent risks of teriparatide-induced osteosarcoma. Osteoporos Int. 2010;21:1041–5.
48. Theman TA, Collins MT, Dempster DW, Zhou H, Reynolds JC, Brahim JS, Roschger P, Klaushofer K, Winer KK. PTH(1–34) replacement therapy in a child with hypoparathyroidism caused by a sporadic calcium receptor mutation. J Bone Miner Res. 2009; 24:964–73.

Parathormone Resistance in Children

17

Agnès Linglart and Eric Mallet

Abstract

This chapter describes the spectrum of problems in children in which there is resistance to parathyroid hormone. This is described by the term pseudohypoparathyroidism. The authors describe the clinical presentation of all of the various parathyroid hormone resistant syndromes and their associated general endocrine abnormalities and skeletal changes. The known genetic abnormalities are highlighted in each of these disorders. The chapter concludes with a detailed presentation of the clinical management of all these problems.

Keywords

Renal phosphate transporters—NaPi2c, NaPi2a • PTH or parathormone • Hypocalcemia • Hyperphosphatemia • Receptor PTHR1, PTH/PTHrp • G receptor coupled • Chondrocytes • Pseudohypoparathyroidism • Blomstrand chondrodysplasia • Alpha stimulatory subunit of G protein—Gsa • Heterotrimers • Nephrogenic cyclic AMP—cAMP • PHP1a, PHP1b, PHP1c • Parental imprinting • DMR • Bone dysplasia • Brachymetacarpia • Brachymetatarsia • Chondrogenesis • GHRH resistance • IGF1 • Heterotopic ossification • Fuller Albright osteodystrophy • 1 Alpha hydroxylase • Calcitriol • 1,25 Dihydroxyvitamin D • TSH resistance • LH • ACTH • Loss of function mutation • Pseudopseudohypoparathyroidism • Progressive osseous heteroplasia • Phenotypes • GNAS • Alfacalcidiol • Hypercalciuria

A. Linglart, MD, PhD (✉)
Department of Pediatric Endocrinology, Bicêtre-Paris-Sud hospital, French Center of Reference for rare disorders of calcium and phosphate metabolism and INSERM unit U986, 94000 le Kremlin-Bicêtre, France
e-mail: agnes.linglart@inserm.fr

E. Mallet, MD, PhD
Department of Pediatrics and CIC INSERM 204, Rouen University Hospital, 1, Rue de Germont, Rouen 76031, France
e-mail: eric.mallet@chu-rouen.fr

A.A. Licata and E.V. Lerma (eds.), *Diseases of the Parathyroid Glands*,
DOI 10.1007/978-1-4419-5550-0_17, © Springer Science+Business Media, LLC 2012

Abbreviations

GNAS	Guanine nucleotide binding protein (G protein), alpha stimulating activity polypeptide
NaPi2c	Sodium phosphate cotransporter type 2a
NaPi2a	Sodium phosphate cotransporter type 2c
PTHR1	PTH receptor type 1
PTHLH	Parathyroid hormone-like hormone
NESP	Neurosecretory protein
AS	Antinsense
GHRH	Growth hormone releasing hormone
IGF1	Insulin-like growth factor 1
FSH	Follicle stimulating hormone
LH	Luteinizing hormone
ACTH	Adrenocorticotropic hormone
STX16	Syntaxin 16

Introduction

Parathormone or PTH is a 84-amino-acid peptide maintaining the blood calcium level between 2.25 and 2.65 mM. Besides its crucial role in calcium homeostasis, PTH controls the urinary excretion of phosphate through the repression of the expression of the renal phosphate transporters (NaPi2c and NaPi2a) at the apical border of the tubular cell. As a consequence, PTH secretion or action deficiency results in hypocalcemia, hyperphosphatemia, and increased tubular reabsorption of phosphates. However, defects of PTH secretion are revealed by low levels of PTH, whereas PTH resistance due to a deficient action of the PTH is associated with high levels of PTH. PTH action on target tissues (bone and kidney) requires the binding to its receptor (PTHR1 or PTH/PTHrp receptor), a G-protein-coupled receptor (GPCR). PTHrp- or PTH-related peptide is an alternative ligand for PTHR1 that is necessary for chondrocyte differentiation.

Failure in PTH action through its receptor is termed pseudohypoparathyroidism (PHP) because of the association of hypocalcemia and hyperphosphatemia reminiscent of hypoparathyroidism, but in this case the PTH levels are elevated.

Several causes of PHP have been now identified, all of them being consequences of a deficient signaling of the PTHR1:

- Loss of function of the PTHR1. Blomstrand chondrodysplasia is a recessive autosomal rare disease due to a mutation on both alleles of the PTHR1 [1].
- Deficient expression or function of the alpha stimulatory subunit of the G protein (or Gsa) that is necessary for the signaling of PTHR1. G proteins are heterotrimers (alpha, beta, and gamma), which, after ligand-binding, induce the production of intracellular cAMP through the activation of adenylate cyclase (AC). In vivo, absent or deficient Gsa prevents the response to the injection of exogenous PTH, which, in physiological conditions, increases nephrogenic cAMP and decreases phosphate tubular reabsorption. Such PHP are classified as PHP type I.
- A defect downstream of the cascade PTHR1/Gsa/AC. Those PHP are classified as type II as the injection of exogenous PTH induces an increase in nephrogenic cAMP, although with no phosphaturic response.

This chapter focuses on the description of PHP type I, the most common and recently deciphered form of PHP. Most of them are due to genetic or epigenetic defects at the *GNAS* locus encoding Gsa.

Parental Imprinting at the *GNAS* Locus

Parental imprinting refers to mechanisms that lead to the repression of gene expression from one parental allele. Genes subjected to parental imprinting are usually clustered in regions rich in CpG dinucleotides and contain imprinting control elements in differentially methylated regions (DMRs). In most loci, the parent-specific expressed transcripts are associated with a pattern of non- or low-methylated DNA, whereas the nonexpressed transcripts are associated with a pattern of methylated DNA [1].

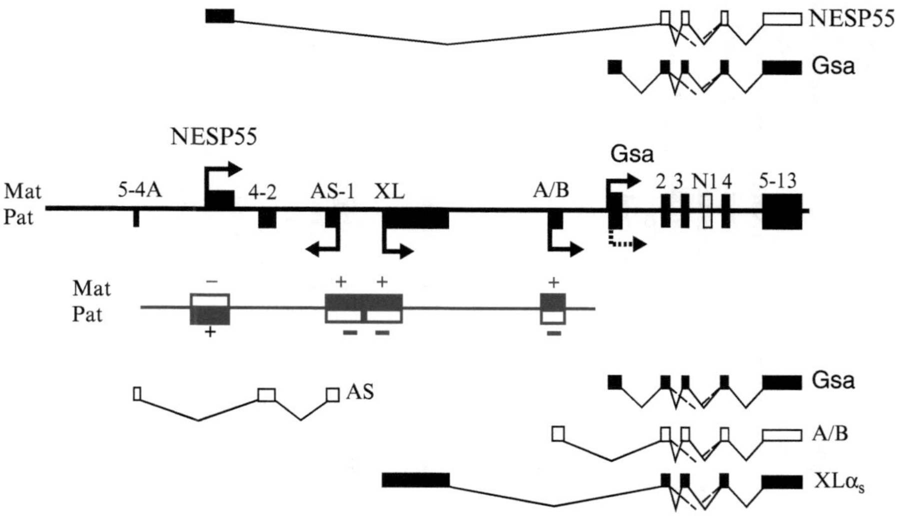

Fig. 17.1 Schematic drawing of the *GNAS* locus. The *GNAS* locus is not scaled. The four DMRs mentioned in this chapter are represented below the genomic line by *gray boxes* (+ or methylated) or *white boxes* (– or unmethylated) on the paternal (Pat) or maternal (Mat) allele. Exons are indicated as *black rectangles* and allelic origin of transcription as *broken arrows* on the paternal (Pat) or maternal (Mat) allele. Transcripts arising from the locus are depicted above (maternal) or below (paternal) the genomic line

GNAS is an imprinted locus that produces several transcripts comprising Gsa, the alpha stimulatory subunit of the G protein, XL, A/B (also referred as 1A), NESP, and the antisense transcript AS. Due to differential methylation of their promoters, most transcripts of this locus originate from one parental allele only. XL, A/B, and AS are transcribed from the paternal allele; NESP is transcribed from the maternal allele only [2, 3]. The promoter of Gsa is not differentially methylated and therefore, Gsa expression arises from both alleles in most tissues (Fig. 17.1). However, due to a yet incompletely understood imprinting mechanism, Gsa is expressed from the maternal allele only in several tissues including the renal proximal tubule, the thyroid, the pituitary, and the gonads [4–6]. For a detailed review on genomic imprinting at the *GNAS* locus, see [2].

PHP Type I

As mentioned above, the biochemical properties of an acute injection of PTH in vivo have delineated the main PHP subtypes (I and II) and pinpointed Gsa as the main candidate-gene for the PHP type I. Based on clinical and in vitro assays (G protein activity measured in red blood cells or in Cyc cells), PHP type I has been subdivided into type Ia (Albright osteodystrophy and diminished G protein activity), type Ib (absence of Albright osteodystrophy and normal G protein activity), and type Ic (Albright osteodystrophy and normal G protein activity) [3–6]. Molecular genetics has shown that those three subtypes overlap and suggested that a new classification based on the molecular mechanism of the disease may be more appropriate (Table 17.1).

PHP-Ia

PHP type Ia is a rare autosomal dominant disease due to a defect in the expression or function of Gsa. The maternal inheritance of the disease is due to the allele-specific expression of Gsa in certain tissues. Clinical features depend on the mono- or biallelic transcription of Gsa in tissues (maternal-specific expression in renal proximal tubules, thyroid or gonads; biallelic expression in lymphocytes, fibroblasts, adipocytes, and bone).

Table 17.1 Classifications of pseudohypoparathyroidism type I

	Clinical classification				Molecular classification				
	PHP-Ia	PHP-Ib	PHP-Ic	pPHP	PHP-Ia	PHP-Ib	pPHP	POH	Syndrome of severe pre- and postnatal growth retardation
Clinical features	Albright osteodystrophy	–	Albright osteodystrophy	Albright osteodystrophy[a]	Albright osteodystrophy	Some features of the Albright osteodystrophy may be present	Albright osteodystrophy[a]	Albright osteodystrophy[a] and heterotopic progressive ossifications, small for gestational age	Severe intrauterine growth retardation, feeding difficulties, and severe postnatal growth retardation
Hormonal resistances	PTH, TSH, calcitonin, epinephrin, gonadotropins, GHRH resistances	PTH resistance	PTH, TSH, calcitonin, epinephrin, gonadotropins, GHRH resistances	–	PTH, TSH, calcitonin, epinephrin, gonadotropins, GHRH resistances	PTH resistance, mild TSH, and calcitonin resistances[b]	–	–	–
Biological activity of the G protein, in vitro	Low	Normal	Normal	Low	Low or normal	Normal	Low or normal	Low or normal	Normal
Molecular analysis	Heterozygous loss of function maternal mutation in the coding sequence of the GNAS gene (exons 1–13) in about 70–80% of the patients Loss of methylation at the A/B promoter of GNAS in about 10–15% of the patients[b]	Loss of methylation at the A/B promoter of GNAS Deletion Ile382 in the Gsa coding sequence	Heterozygous loss of function maternal mutation in the exon 13 of the GNAS gene	Heterozygous loss of function paternal mutation in the coding sequence of the GNAS gene (exons 1–13)	Heterozygous loss of function maternal mutation in the coding sequence of the GNAS gene (exons 1–13)	Loss of methylation at the A/B promoter of GNAS	Heterozygous loss of function paternal mutation in the coding sequence of the GNAS gene (exons 1–13)	Heterozygous loss of function paternal mutation in the coding sequence of the GNAS gene (exons 1–13)	Paternal deletion of the GNAS locus removing the XL exon

[a] Mild features of Albright osteodystrophy, see text
[b] In our experience

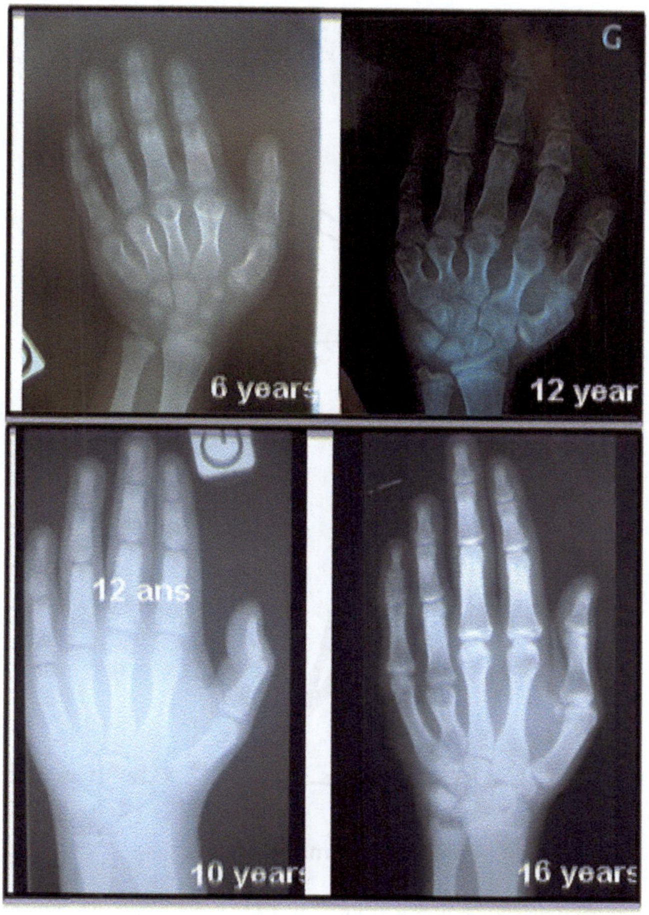

Fig. 17.2 Progressive development of the brachymetacarpy and brachydactyly in a girl (*upper panels*) and a boy (*lower panels*) affected with PHP-Ia

In addition to the resistance to hormones that signal through GPCRs, patients affected with PHP-Ia present with a collection of features, first described by Fuller Albright in 1942, the Albright hereditary osteodystrophy.

- Bone dysplasia comprises a brachymetacarpia (mainly fourth and fifth metacarpals), brachydactyly (Fig. 17.2) and/or brachymetatarsia (present in all patients albeit at variable degrees), narrowed lumbar shaft, and underdeveloped femoral necks. Absent at birth, the bone dysplasia develops overtime, especially at puberty and likely results from the deficient action of the PTHrp during chondrogenesis. In fact, loss of function mutations of the *PTHLH* (the gene coding PTHrp) are associated with similar bone shape abnormalities. The bone density of the patients is roughly normal, yet they are prone to rheumatologic complications such as femoral slipped epiphysis or osteoarthritis [7, 8].
- Adult patients affected with PHP-Ia have short final heights as shown by height *z*-score (−2.5 ± 0.3 and −3.0 ± 0.9 in Long's and our series of patients, respectively). Most children with PHP-Ia have normal stature until they undergo premature closure of the epiphyses which occurs mainly between 10 and 15 years of age. Short stature results from both the deficient chondrogenesis and the GHRH resistance assessed by the insufficient secretion of growth hormone in response to stimulation

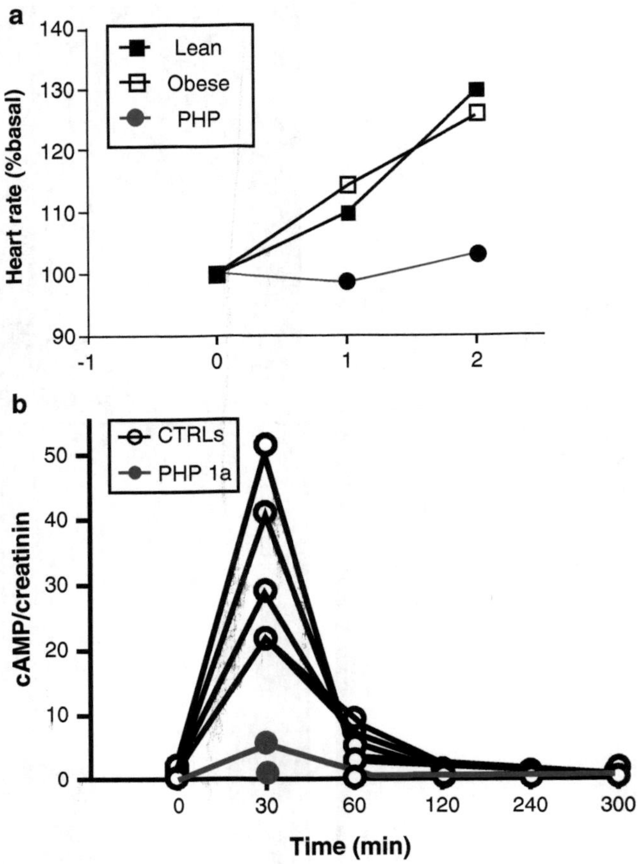

Fig. 17.3 (**a**) The epinephrine resistance is shown by the absence of increase in the heart rate during the IV infusion of epinephrine in six patients affected with PHP-Ia compared to lean and obese controls. (**b**) The resistance to PTH is shown by the absence of increase in urinary cAMP after IV infusion of recombinant PTH in two patients affected with PHP-Ia (*gray*) compared to controls (CTRLs)

and the low normal IGF1 levels in about 70% of the patients [9]. Finally, the gonadotropin resistance, by limiting the sex steroid production during adolescence, may also participate in the height deficit.

- Obesity is one of the main features of the disease. In our series, 42% of the patients (children and adults) had a body mass index (BMI) over 2 SD compared to the age-reference. The mean *z*-score BMI of 40 patients reported by Long and colleagues was 2.3±0.2 SD, including two adults with a BMI over 40 kg/m^2 thereby affected by severe obesity [10]. Two contributing factors have been identified as favoring obesity in PHP-Ia. One is the resistance to epinephrine, a lipolysis stimulating hormone that acts through GPCRs (Fig. 17.3) [11], and the second is the potent antiadipogeneic effect of Gsa in vitro [12].
- Heterotopic ossifications (*osteoma cutis*) in children, inadequately called heterotopic calcifications, compose a specific feature of Gsa loss of function. They are usually superficial (dermal or subcutaneous fat), made of endochondral bone, and may progress unforeseeably superficially or within deeper tissues [13]. In contrast with progressive osseous heteroplasia (see below), heterotopic ossification in patients affected with PHP-Ia may appear after a trauma or at friction zones. Consequences of these ossifications depend on their localization, pain, limited movements [13], etc.
- Developmental delay and cognitive dysfunction have been reported repeatedly in textbooks

since the first description by Fuller Albright in 1942. In 2008, Mouallem and colleagues have shown that approximately 70% of the patients affected with PHP-Ia exhibit a moderate-to-severe cognitive impairment (i.e., that 30% do not have any impairment). Prolonged hypocalcemia or hypothyroidism due to PTH and TSH resistances, respectively, may be partly involved [14].

In our experience, PHP-Ia is diagnosed early (6 years and a half on average) during the investigation of symptomatic hypocalcemia (48%), heterotopic ossifications (9.5%), growth retardation (9.5%), familial screening (14%), hypothyroidism (9.5%), or developmental delay (9.5%).

The resistance to PTH is defined by the association of low calcium level (2.05 ± 0.27 mM), elevated phosphate level (1.93 ± 0.45 mM), elevated circulating intact PTH (333 ± 178 pg/ml), and undetectable urinary calcium excretion. Absent at birth, the PTH resistance gradually develops during the first months or years of life [15, 16]. Phosphate and PTH levels increase first, followed by a decrease in calcemia due to the defect in the PTH-dependant 1 alpha hydroxylation of vitamin D. In the renal proximal tubule, the defect in PTH signaling induces (1) the lack of 1 alpha hydroxylase transcription and 1,25 $(OH)_2$ vitamin D production, and (2) an increased expression of the phosphate transporters, therefore an increase in tubular phosphate reabsorption. In the distal tubule, the calcium reabsorption depends also on the PTH-driven intracellular cAMP production. However, likely due to the biallelic expression of Gsa in the distal tubule, urinary calcium reabsorption seems close to normal in patients with PHP-Ia (personal data) and may be involved in the long-term tolerance of the PTH resistance in patients before they develop hypocalcemia. Events requiring increasing amounts of calcium like vitamin D deficiency or pubertal growth spurt may worsen the hypocalcemia and reveal the disease. In fact, low vitamin D is often present at the time of diagnosis. Hyperphosphatemia, Albright osteodystrophy, and TSH resistance allow the differential diagnosis with secondary hyperparathyroidism due to vitamin D deficiency. In rare cases, the examination of the renal response to the infusion of PTH (or Ellsworth-Howard test) is required and shows the absence of nephrogenic cAMP production and of increase in phosphaturia (Fig. 17.3).

The resistance to TSH is found in most, if not all, patients affected and is, in our experience, a contributive element for the diagnosis of PHP-Ia [17]. TSH resistance is characterized by elevated TSH (15.1 mUI/L on average in our series, 4.9 mUI/L in Balavoine's), low normal free T4 (11.1 ± 2.5 pmol/L), and small or normal thyroid volume. Usually present at birth, the TSH resistance is sometimes revealed through the neonatal screening program. Jean-Louis Wemeau's group has shown in 2008 and 2001 that the patients affected with PHP-Ia also display resistances to TRH and calcitonin [18, 19] with no clinical symptoms.

Gonadotropins signal through GPCRs and their actions are likely modified in patients with Gsa loss of function. In fact, cryptorchidism, even bilateral, is frequent in boys; menarche may be delayed and elevated FSH levels (150–200% of the upper normal range in our experience), yet normal LH levels, have been measured in affected girls [20, 21].

ACTH resistance has not been found in patients, may be because Gsa does not seem to be imprinted in human adrenals [22]. GHRH and catecholamine resistances have previously been mentioned.

The diagnosis of PHP-Ia relies on the identification of a loss of function mutation on the maternal allele of the coding sequence of *GNAS* (exons 1–13). All types of mutations can be found such as deletion, insertion, amino-acid substitution or stop codon; three hot-spots, not exclusive, are located in exons 6, 7, and 13, respectively. Note that the alternatively spliced exon 3 may also be mutated [23]. We will mention here only mutations associated with specific phenotypes:

- The A366S mutation was identified in a patient affected with PHP-Ia and testotoxicosis [24].
- Although mutations in the first exon of Gsa do not modify the sequence nor the function of XLas, the alternative transcript of Gsa able to stimulate the cAMP production, the

phenotype of mutated patients do not appear different from those harboring mutations in exons 2–13 [25].

- Mutations located at the 3' end of the exon 13 modify the domain of interaction between Gsa and the GPCRs. However, those mutations do not affect the GTPase activity nor the interaction with the AC, two characteristics assayed when measuring the G protein biological activity in vitro. Therefore, those mutations are characterized by an in vitro biological activity of the G protein close to controls [26, 27].
- A deletion of isoleucine at position 382 of Gsa was found in two brothers exhibiting isolated PTH resistance and improperly diagnosed with PHP-Ib. Later on, the functional characterization of the mutation was performed in vitro and showed the deficient coupling of the mutated Gsa to the PTHR1 [26].
- Finally, large deletions of the *GNAS* locus may be inaccessible to current molecular biology techniques and misinterpreted as methylation changes, i.e., PHP-1b [28].

In our center, the measure of the biological activity of the G protein is not required for the diagnosis of PHP-Ia; however, it may be necessary for a better understanding of the genotype–phenotype relationship. Note that this in vitro assay has to be performed after correction of vitamin D deficiency which artificially decreases the Gsa biological activity.

Pseudopseudohypoparathyroidism or pPHP or Isolated Albright Osteodystrophy

Patients affected with pPHP have been first identified within relatives of PHP-Ia patients. They present with Albright osteodystrophy and no hormonal resistances, and harbor the exact same loss of function mutation of Gsa than their relatives albeit on the paternal allele. Very few studies have attempted to delineate their phenotypes. However, recent observations have shown that patients affected with pPHP are not obese (average BMI of 0.1 ± 0.5, significantly inferior to that in PHP-Ia ($p=0.02$) [10]) and do not have cognitive impairment [14]. Nonetheless, they exhibit short final height and heterotopic ossifications sometimes more severe than their PHP-Ia counterparts [29]. The search for a mutation in the Gsa coding sequence in sporadic patients with short stature, brachydactyly, and obesity has proven to be frequently unsuccessful.

Progressive Osseous Heteroplasia or POH

POH is a rare disorder of osteogenesis characterized by a single characteristic manifestation (progressive heterotopic ossification) that can vary in its degree of severity. POH appears during infancy with heterotopic bone in the derma and subcutaneous fat. Bone plaques eventually fuse and progress deeper into fascia, skeletal muscle, tendons, and ligaments, leading to ankylosis and preventing the natural limb growth. In some patients, Kaplan and colleagues noted features of Albright osteodystrophy and subsequently identified *GNAS* as the causing-disease gene [29, 30]. Mutations in the coding sequence of Gsa found in patients affected with POH are also found in patients with PHP-Ia or pPHP, although they are exclusively located on the paternal allele and are mostly severely affecting the protein function [31]. We believe that pPHP and POH are both extremes of a common disease.

PHP-Ib

PHP-Ib is a rare disease due to the defective signaling through Gsa in selected tissues like the renal proximal tubule or the thyroid. Because of an abnormal methylation at the maternal A/B promoter of *GNAS*, the Gsa expression is limited in those tissues resulting in hormonal resistances.

The mean age at diagnosis is about 13 years of age, mostly because of hypocalcemic symptoms. In our experience, patients diagnosed after the age of 20 represent at least 20% of our cohort.

The PTH resistance is the main symptom of the disease (for a long time considered as the single one). This is likely because of the absence of physical features allowing an earlier diagnosis in PHP-Ia. Patients affected with PHP-Ib usually show a very low calcium level at the time of diagnosis (1.6±0.3 mM), high phosphate level (2.2±0.2 mM) due to an increased tubular reabsorption of phosphates, elevated intact PTH levels (530±304 pg/ml), undetectable urinary calcium excretion, and, in most patients, vitamin D deficiency that triggered the symptoms [4, 32]. Like in PHP-Ia, the PTH resistance develops overtime [16]. In contrast to PHP-Ia, in which haploinsufficiency ensures end-organ resistance in all tissues, patients affected with PHP-Ib maintain a biallelic expression of Gsa in most tissues (lymphocytes and bone). Consequently, their bone responds adequately to the elevated PTH levels through an increased bone resorption and demineralization resembling severe primary hyperparathyroidism [33, 34].

It is now widely accepted that PTH resistance is not the sole manifestation of PHP-Ib. In fact, resistances to several hormones signaling through GPCRs have been found in patients affected with PHP-Ib. The TSH resistance is not always present in patients affected with PHP-Ib, and usually mild (in our 35 patients, the mean TSH was 4.6±1.0 mUI/L, minimum 2.5, and maximum 10.0 mUI/L; in Liu's report TSH ranged between 2.4 and 9.5 mUI/L; in Levine's report TSH level was 4.5 mUI/L) [35, 36]. Despite high TSH, we could not detect any symptoms of hypothyroidism and free T4 levels were within the normal range. As in PHP-Ia, we found elevated calcitonin levels in eight out of ten patients investigated. Mantovani et al.'s group failed to identify neither gonadotropin nor GHRH resistance in those patients [37].

It is noteworthy that several features of Albright osteodystrophy might be present, rarely all of them in a single patient. Some patients present with a typical brachymetacarpy [38] or slender heterotopic ossifications [39]. In our series of patients, the BMI, especially in girls, was significantly higher than that of the general population (1.0±0.4 SD, $p=0.019$), yet the final height was normal. In fact, Mantovani et al.'s group had shown that patients affected with PHP-Ib are frequent among the samples send for PTH resistance and AHO yet having no mutation in the *GNAS* coding sequence [40].

In patients affected with an isolated PTH resistance or with PTH resistance and few associated features (TSH resistance or mild AHO), we would first look for methylation changes at the *GNAS* promoters. Patients affected with PHP-Ib typically show a loss of cytosine methylation of the maternal A/B promoter (often referred in molecular biology articles as the A/B differentially methylated region or DMR) [41]. The A/B DMR is located just upstream of the Gsa promoter and first exon and controls the tissue-specific expression of Gsa. Consequently, a loss of methylation at A/B leads to a suppression of Gsa expression in the renal proximal tubule and the thyroid, hence, PTH and TSH resistance, respectively.

Several subtypes of PHP-Ib have now been recognized:

- The autosomal dominant form of PHP-Ib or AD-PHP-Ib. It represents most of the familial form of PHP-Ib, and about 15% of the patients affected with PHP-Ib. These patients show a loss of methylation restricted to the maternal A/B DMR (the methylation at the rest of the *GNAS* locus is preserved). Most of the patients, except one family worldwide, carry an identical maternal deletion of 3,6-kb at the neighboring *STX16* gene, 220-kb upstream of *GNAS* [16, 42]. This deletion likely removes a genomic element that is necessary for the proper methylation at the A/B DMR of *GNAS*. The phenotype of AD-PHP-Ib is associated with the maternal transmission of the deletion, whereas no phenotype, including no methylation abnormality, is associated with the paternal transmission of the disease (healthy carriers).
- In three families affected with AD-PHP-Ib, Murat Bastepe and HaraldJueppner's group has identified deletions removing the exons 3 and 4 of the antisense transcript of *GNAS*. The patients differed from the most frequent AD-PHP-Ib patients because they harbored methylation changes spanning the entire maternal *GNAS* locus (loss of methylation at A/B, AS, and XL DMRs, gain of methylation at the NESP DMR). As mentioned previously, we

believe that those deletions removed a genomic sequence that is required for the methylation over the whole *GNAS* locus [43, 44].

- The sporadic form of PHP-Ib is the by far the most frequent. The patients do not have any affected siblings. In those patients, the methylation defect is not restricted to A/B (it always includes a loss of methylation at A/B) but spreads to the other DMRs of *GNAS* comprising AS, XL, and NESP. The cause of these methylation changes is still unknown. Researchers failed to identify deletions in STX16 or in AS in those patients [40, 41, 45].

There is no major difference in the phenotypes of patients affected with the familial or the sporadic form of PHP-Ib[32]. Therefore, the diagnosis of PHP-Ib relies on (1) the identification through molecular biology of the loss of methylation at the A/B DMR of *GNAS* and (2) its characterization through the search for the common deletion at *STX16* and the analysis of the methylation at the entire *GNAS* locus.

Treatment

The objectives of the treatment of the PTH resistance could be defined as (1) maintain calcemia within the low normal range (2.0–2.5 mM), (2) prevent hypercalciuria, (3) prevent the bone resorption due to elevated PTH levels (lower PTH below 150 pg/ml). In children, the key treatment is the 1 alpha hydroxylated vitamin D (calcitriol twice a day or alfacalcidol once a day). The dose does not depend on the weight; most patients have 1–2 μg/day of alfacalcidol or 0.5–1 μg of calcitriol. Highest doses may be needed during periods of high growth velocity (infancy and puberty). The treatment with calcitriol or alfacalcidol permits to recover a normal calcium level and lowers the PTH levels to the normal or upper normal range. Usually, phosphate levels remain slightly elevated as they do not depend on 1,25 $(OH)_2$ vitamin D, but on PTH signaling alone. As mentioned before, the ability of the distal tubule to maintain, at least in part, the urinary calcium reabsorption prevents excessive excretion of calcium in the urine; in contrast to patients affected with hypoparathyroidism, the treatment with alfacalcidol or calcitriol in patients with PTH resistance rarely leads to hypercalciuria.

Calcium supplements, 500–1,000 mg daily according to age, are recommended during the first year following the diagnosis of PTH resistance.

The TSH resistance is usually treated in patients affected with PHP-Ia by oral thyroxin according to the weight. Except during pregnancy, patients affected with PHP-Ib do not require a treatment for their TSH resistance.

Off-label use of growth hormone has been done in patients affected with PHP-Ia and short stature with variable results. Unfortunately, clinical trials are lacking to prove the efficacy of the drug [46].

The treatment of the heterotopic ossifications is one of the most important challenges of this disease. Small and non-problematic ossifications should remain untouched as they easily recur after surgery. Orthopedic measures or surgery may be necessary to maintain the mobility of the joints. Several treatments like nonsteroidal anti-inflammatory drugs or bisphosphonates have been reported in case reports yet are not considered as fully effective[47].

At birth, the molecular diagnosis for the newborn may be done on cord blood [16]. Because of the absent PTH resistance during the first months of life, affected newborn babies do not risk hypocalcemia. However, TSH resistance may be present at birth, especially in PHP-Ia. Therefore, a blood test is recommended for those babies at day 3 of life, and a treatment with thyroxin should be started in newborns with elevated TSH even before the result of the molecular biology analysis.

Conclusion

PHP type I is a rare disease that has been characterized at the clinical, genetic, and epigenetic level in the last 20 years. We propose that the classification of the PHP subtypes should now include the molecular biology analysis as it has been shown that the different phenotypes overlap significantly. The treatment of the hormonal resistance in PHP, whatever the subtype, is fairly easy; we feel, however, that a specific therapy is needed for at least three specific features of the disease: heterotopic ossifications, obesity, and short stature.

Acknowledgment The authors are most grateful to Richard Medeiros, Rouen University Hospital Medical Editor, for editing the manuscript.

References

1. Blomstrand S, Claësson I, Säve-Söderbergh J. A case of lethal congenital dwarfism with accelerated skeletal maturation. Pediatr Radiol. 1985;15:141–3.
2. Kelsey G. Imprinting on chromosome 20: tissue-specific imprinting and imprinting mutations in the GNAS locus. Am J Med Genet C Semin Med Genet. 2010;154C:377–86.
3. Levine MA, Downs Jr RW, Singer M, Marx SJ, Aurbach GD, Spiegel AM. Deficient activity of guanine nucleotide regulatory protein in erythrocytes from patients with pseudohypoparathyroidism. Biochem Biophys Res Commun. 1980;94:1319–24.
4. Marguet C, Mallet E, Basuyau JP, Martin D, Leroy M, Brunelle P. Clinical and biological heterogeneity in pseudohypoparathyroidism syndrome. Results of a multicenter study. Horm Res. 1997;48:120–30.
5. Albright F, Burnett CH, Smith PH, Parson W. Pseudohypoparathyroidism—an example of "seabright-bantam syndrome". Endocrinology. 1942;30:922–32.
6. Weinstein LS, Yu S, Warner DR, Liu J. Endocrine manifestations of stimulatory G protein a-subunit mutations and the role of genomic imprinting. Endocr Rev. 2001;22:675–705.
7. Long DN, Levine MA, Germain-Lee EL. Bone mineral density in pseudohypoparathyroidism type 1a. J Clin Endocrinol Metab. 2010;95(9):4465–75.
8. Linglart A. Consequences of PTH resistance on adult bone. Arch Pediatr. 2007;14:546–8.
9. Mantovani G, Maghnie M, Weber G, De Menis E, Brunelli V, Cappa M, et al. Growth hormone-releasing hormone resistance in pseudohypoparathyroidism type ia: new evidence for imprinting of the Gs alpha gene. J Clin Endocrinol Metab. 2003;88:4070–4.
10. Long DN, McGuire S, Levine MA, Weinstein LS, Germain-Lee EL. Body mass index differences in pseudohypoparathyroidism type 1a versus pseudopseudohypoparathyroidism may implicate paternal imprinting of Galpha(s) in the development of human obesity. J Clin Endocrinol Metab. 2007;92:1073–9.
11. Carel JC, Le Stunff C, Condamine L, Mallet E, Chaussain JL, Adnot P, et al. Resistance to the lipolytic action of epinephrine: a new feature of protein Gs deficiency. J Clin Endocrinol Metab. 1999;84:4127–31.
12. Wang HY, Watkins DC, Malbon CC. Antisense oligodeoxynucleotides to GS protein alpha-subunit sequence accelerate differentiation of fibroblasts to adipocytes. Nature. 1992;358:334–7.
13. Kaplan FS, Shore EM. Progressive osseous heteroplasia. J Bone Miner Res. 2000;15:2084–94.
14. Mouallem M, Shaharabany M, Weintrob N, Shalitin S, Nagelberg N, Shapira H, et al. Cognitive impairment is prevalent in pseudohypoparathyroidism type Ia, but not in pseudopseudohypoparathyroidism: possible cerebral imprinting of Gsalpha. Clin Endocrinol (Oxf). 2008;68:233–9.
15. Linglart A. Progressive PTH resistance in pseudohypoparathyroidism (PHP) type Ia and Ib stéphanie méhouas jean-claude carel, marie laure kottler and Agnès Linglart ESPE meeting, sept 2008, ISTANBUL.
16. Linglart A, Gensure RC, Olney RC, Juppner H, Bastepe M. A novel STX16 deletion in autosomal dominant pseudohypoparathyroidism type Ib redefines the boundaries of a cis-acting imprinting control element of GNAS. Am J Hum Genet. 2005;76: 804–14.
17. Germain-Lee EL, Groman J, Crane JL, Jan de Beur SM, Levine MA. Growth hormone deficiency in pseudohypoparathyroidism type 1a: another manifestation of multihormone resistance. J Clin Endocrinol Metab. 2003;88:4059–69.
18. Balavoine AS, Ladsous M, Velayoudom FL, Vlaeminck V, Cardot-Bauters C, d'Herbomez M, et al. Hypothyroidism in patients with pseudohypoparathyroidism type Ia: clinical evidence of resistance to TSH and TRH. Eur J Endocrinol. 2008;159:431–7.
19. Vlaeminck-Guillem V, D'Herbomez M, Pigny P, Fayard A, Bauters C, Decoulx M, et al. Pseudohypoparathyroidism Ia and hypercalcitoninemia. J Clin Endocrinol Metab. 2001;86:3091–6.
20. Herman-Giddens ME, Slora EJ, Wasserman RC, Bourdony CJ, Bhapkar MV, Koch GG, et al. Secondary sexual characteristics and menses in young girls seen in office practice: a study from the pediatric research in office settings network. Pediatrics. 1997;99:505–12.
21. Namnoum AB, Merriam GR, Moses AM, Levine MA. Reproductive dysfunction in women with Albright's hereditary osteodystrophy. J Clin Endocrinol Metab. 1998;83:824–9.
22. Mantovani G, Ballare E, Giammona E, Beck-Peccoz P, Spada A. The Gsa gene: predominant maternal origin of transcription in human thyroid gland and gonads. J Clin Endocrinol Metab. 2002;87:4736–40.
23. Thiele S, Werner R, Ahrens W, Hoppe U, Marschke C, Staedt P, et al. A disruptive mutation in exon 3 of the GNAS gene with Albright hereditary osteodystrophy, normocalcemic pseudohypoparathyroidism, and selective long transcript variant Gsalpha-L deficiency. J Clin Endocrinol Metab. 2007;92:1764–8.
24. Nakamoto JM, Zimmerman D, Jones EA, Loke KY, Siddiq K, Donlan MA, et al. Concurrent hormone resistance (pseudohypoparathyroidism type Ia) and hormone independence (testotoxicosis) caused by a unique mutation in the G alpha s gene. Biochem Mol Med. 1996;58:18–24.
25. Thiele S, Werner R, Ahrens W, Hubner A, Hinkel KG, Hoppner W, et al. Selective deficiency of Gsalpha and the possible role of alternative gene products of

GNAS in Albright hereditary osteodystrophy and pseudohypoparathyroidism type Ia. Exp Clin Endocrinol Diabetes. 2010;118:127–32.
26. Linglart A, Mahon MJ, Kerachian MA, Berlach DM, Hendy GN, Juppner H, et al. Coding GNAS mutations leading to hormone resistance impair in vitro agonist- and cholera toxin-induced adenosine cyclic 3′,5′-monophosphate formation mediated by human XLalphas. Endocrinology. 2006;147:2253–62.
27. Al-Salameh A, Despert F, Kottler ML, Linglart A, Carel JC, Lecomte P. Resistance to epinephrine and hypersensitivity (hyperresponsiveness) to CB1 antagonists in a patient with pseudohypoparathyroidism type Ic. Eur J Endocrinol. 2010;162:819–24.
28. Fernandez-Rebollo E, Garcia-Cuartero B, Garin I, Largo C, Martinez F, Garcia-Lacalle C, et al. Intragenic GNAS deletion involving exon A/B in pseudohypoparathyroidism type 1A resulting in an apparent loss of exon A/B methylation: potential for misdiagnosis of pseudohypoparathyroidism type 1B. J Clin Endocrinol Metab. 2010;95:765–71.
29. Schimmel RJ, Pasmans SG, Xu M, Stadhouders-Keet SA, Shore EM, Kaplan FS, et al. GNAS-associated disorders of cutaneous ossification: two different clinical presentations. Bone. 2010;46:868–72.
30. Shore EM, Ahn J, Jan de Beur S, Li M, Xu M, Gardner RJ, et al. Paternally inherited inactivating mutations of the GNAS1 gene in progressive osseous heteroplasia. N Engl J Med. 2002;346:99–106.
31. Lebrun M, Richard N, Abeguile G, David A, Coeslier Dieux A, Journel H, et al. Progressive osseous heteroplasia: a model for the imprinting effects of GNAS inactivating mutations in humans. J Clin Endocrinol Metab. 2010;95:3028–38.
32. Linglart A, Bastepe M, Juppner H. Similar clinical and laboratory findings in patients with symptomatic autosomal dominant and sporadic pseudohypoparathyroidism type Ib despite different epigenetic changes at the GNAS locus. Clin Endocrinol (Oxf). 2007; 67:822–31.
33. Burnstein MI, Kottamasu SR, Pettifor JM, Sochett E, Ellis BI, Frame B. Metabolic bone disease in pseudohypoparathyroidism: radiologic features. Radiology. 1985;155:351–6.
34. Mahmud FH, Linglart A, Bastepe M, Jüppner H, Lteif AN. Molecular diagnosis of pseudohypoparathyroidism type Ib in a family with presumed paroxysmal dyskinesia. Pediatrics. 2005;115:e242–4.
35. Liu J, Erlichman B, Weinstein LS. The stimulatory G protein a-subunit Gsa is imprinted in human thyroid glands: implications for thyroid function in pseudohypoparathyroidism types 1a and 1b. J Clin Endocrinol Metabol. 2003;88:4336–41.
36. Germain-Lee EL, Ding CL, Deng Z, Crane JL, Saji M, Ringel MD, et al. Paternal imprinting of Galpha(s) in the human thyroid as the basis of TSH resistance in pseudohypoparathyroidism type 1a. Biochem Biophys Res Commun. 2002;296:67–72.
37. Mantovani G, Bondioni S, Linglart A, Maghnie M, Cisternino M, Corbetta S, et al. Genetic analysis and evaluation of resistance to thyrotropin and growth hormone-releasing hormone in pseudohypoparathyroidism type Ib. J Clin Endocrinol Metab. 2007;92: 3738–42.
38. Mariot V, Maupetit-Mehouas S, Sinding C, Kottler ML, Linglart A. A maternal epimutation of GNAS leads to Albright osteodystrophy and parathyroid hormone resistance. J Clin Endocrinol Metab. 2008;93: 661–5.
39. de Nanclares GP, Fernandez-Rebollo E, Santin I, Garcia-Cuartero B, Gaztambide S, Menendez E, et al. Epigenetic defects of GNAS in patients with pseudohypoparathyroidism and mild features of Albright's hereditary osteodystrophy. J Clin Endocrinol Metab. 2007;92:2370–3.
40. Mantovani G, de Sanctis L, Barbieri AM, Elli FM, Bollati V, Vaira V, et al. Pseudohypoparathyroidism and GNAS epigenetic defects: clinical evaluation of Albright hereditary osteodystrophy and molecular analysis in 40 patients. J Clin Endocrinol Metab. 2010;95:651–8.
41. Liu J, Litman D, Rosenberg M, Yu S, Biesecker L, Weinstein L. A GNAS1 imprinting defect in pseudohypoparathyroidism type Ib. J Clin Invest. 2000; 106:1167–74.
42. Bastepe M, Fröhlich LF, Hendy GN, Indridason OS, Josse RG, Koshiyama H, et al. Autosomal dominant pseudohypoparathyroidism type Ib is associated with a heterozygous microdeletion that likely disrupts a putative imprinting control element of GNAS. J Clin Invest. 2003;112:1255–63.
43. Bastepe M, Fröhlich LF, Linglart A, Abu-Zahra HS, Tojo K, Ward LM, et al. Deletion of the NESP55 differentially methylated region causes loss of maternal GNAS imprints and pseudohypoparathyroidism type Ib. Nat Genet. 2005;37:25–7.
44. Chillambhi S, Turan S, Hwang DY, Chen HC, Juppner H, Bastepe M. Deletion of the noncoding GNAS antisense transcript causes pseudohypoparathyroidism type Ib and biparental defects of GNAS methylation in cis. J Clin Endocrinol Metab. 2010;95(8):3993–4002.
45. Maupetit-Mehouas S, Mariot V, Reynes C, Bertrand G, Feillet F, Carel JC, et al. Quantification of the methylation at the GNAS locus identifies subtypes of sporadic pseudohypoparathyroidism type Ib. J Med Genet. 2011;48(1):55–63.
46. Mantovani G, Ferrante E, Giavoli C, Linglart A, Cappa M, Cisternino M, et al. Recombinant human GH replacement therapy in children with pseudohypoparathyroidism type Ia: first study on the effect on growth. J Clin Endocrinol Metab. 2010;95:5011–7.
47. Kovalovsky D, Refojo D, Liberman AC, Hochbaum D, Pereda MP, Coso OA, et al. Activation and induction of NUR77/NURR1 in corticotrophs by CRH/cAMP: involvement of calcium, protein kinase A, and MAPK pathways. Mol Endocrinol. 2002;16:1638–51.

The Use of Ultrasonography in the Management of Parathyroid Diseases

18

Zvonimir L. Milas and Mira Milas

Abstract

Ultrasound affords certain key advantages in general and specifically for parathyroid disease management. It can be readily performed in the office and even portably in the operating room, allows real-time examination that is noninvasive and comfortable for the patient, identifies co-existing thyroid pathology that may require treatment, and can be performed by a clinician who is evaluating the patient with access to all relevant clinical information. Recognizable sonographic features allow identification of abnormal parathyroid glands, can be readily learned, and make ultrasound a powerful tool especially when performed by clinicians with access to comprehensive information about the patient's parathyroid disease. Ultrasound can guide appropriate interventions to clarify challenging diagnostic scenarios, although ultimately it should not be viewed as a diagnostic test for hyperparathyroidism. It has a demonstrated history of valuable clinical use.

The following review highlights these advantages, describes the technical and anatomical findings expected with parathyroid ultrasound, relates the specific indications for its use, and presents an overview of reported performance as a localizing study in the management of hyperparathyroidism.

Keywords

Ultrasonography • Mibi scan • Parathyroid • Hyperparathyroidism • Ultrasound

Z.L. Milas, MD (✉)
Head and Neck Surgical Oncology, MD Anderson Cancer Center, 1400 S. Orange Ave., MP 760, Orlando, FL 82806, USA
e-mail: zvonimir.milas@orlandohealth.com

M. Milas, MD
The Thyroid Center, Department of Endocrine Surgery, Cleveland Clinic, 9500 Euclid Ave F20, Cleveland, OH 44195, USA

A.A. Licata and E.V. Lerma (eds.), *Diseases of the Parathyroid Glands*,
DOI 10.1007/978-1-4419-5550-0_18, © Springer Science+Business Media, LLC 2012

The Modern Context of Parathyroid Ultrasound

Neck ultrasound evolved into its current role as the primary imaging modality for the evaluation of thyroid diseases and thyroid cancer over the last decade [1]. During this time period, ultrasound has also become an increasingly used tool in the management of parathyroid diseases. A query of publications indexed with the US National Library of Medicine shows fewer than 80 devoted to ultrasound and parathyroid disease in the period 1990–2000, compared to nearly 900 in the decade since[2]. Viewed from the vantage point of modern-day parathyroid surgery, this application of ultrasound is not surprising and has come as part of a paradigm shift in the treatment of primary hyperparathyroidism. Although ultrasound as a technology was available in the 1980s, the philosophy of treating parathyroid disease was quite different. Symptomatic patients with obvious primary hyperparathyroidism constituted the vast majority of those with parathyroid diseases. Operative rather than medical treatment was logical and rarely questioned, and the strategy at surgery was a mandatory four-gland parathyroid exploration with removal of the gland or glands which appeared abnormal. Parathyroid localization procedures were rarely used, since surgery was successful in >95% of patients without them [3, 4].

A sequence of technological innovations occurred by the mid-1990s to change the paradigm from bilateral parathyroid examination to focused surgery targeted to a single area of suspected parathyroid disease [5]. These innovations included the use of other radiologic modalities, most notably 99-technetium Sestamibi (Mibi) scans, and the intraoperative measurement of parathyroid hormone (PTH) as a metric of disease cure [6, 7]. Additionally, the landscape of parathyroid disease broadened to include significantly more patients with incidentally discovered, asymptomatic hyperparathyroidism for whom the benefits of surgery came be viewed as controversial, prompting the development of treatment guidelines [8–11]. It is in this context and from the need for reliable, noninvasive localization methods that ultrasound was incorporated into the management of parathyroid disease.

It is also not surprising, then, that surgeons have in large part driven the use of ultrasound in parathyroid disease [12–20]. Most patients with endocrine diseases, such as primary hyperparathyroidism, have received extensive biochemical diagnostic evaluation before referral to a surgeon. Indeed, ultrasound is not a diagnostic tool for primary hyperparathyroidism, but a tool to refine intended surgical treatment. Surgeons bring unique dimensions to a parathyroid ultrasound examination: images are interpreted by those who encounter the relevant anatomy daily and directly in the operating room and can recognize subtle findings; available to them are the full history, physical exam, and laboratory findings to complete an assessment of hyperparathyroidism; and the ultrasound images can give a mental picture of expected findings in the operating room for that particular patient. Not all surgeons perform parathyroid ultrasound. That expertise may reside with other specialists as well, whose contributions are essential and enormous in providing valuable information to guide patient care, particularly in collaboration with other treating physicians [21–24].

Ultrasound affords certain key advantages in general and specifically for parathyroid disease management. It can be readily performed in the office and even portably in the operating room, allows real-time examination that is noninvasive and comfortable for the patient, identifies co-existing thyroid pathology that may require treatment, and can be performed by a clinician who is evaluating the patient with access to all relevant clinical information. The following review highlights these advantages, describes the technical and anatomical findings expected with parathyroid ultrasound, relates the specific indications for its use, and presents an overview of reported performance as a localizing study in the management of hyperparathyroidism.

Equipment and Technique of Parathyroid Ultrasound

Parathyroid ultrasound should be performed with a high-resolution, real-time ultrasound with both gray scale and color Doppler resolution. Because of the relatively superficial location of the thyroid and parathyroid glands, the anatomic imaging can be remarkably detailed. Although a variety of ultrasounds are commercially available, a key feature is the use of high-frequency transducers at 7.5–15 MHz. These can be linear or small curvilinear ("fingerprint") transducers. Other helpful features of the ultrasound equipment include the ability to adjust focal zones, the ability to evaluate the vascular pattern of the abnormal findings with the color Doppler function, and the ability to store images for documentation.

For ultrasound examination, the patient is positioned supine with a small pillow below the shoulders to achieve gentle extension of the neck, mimicking the position during surgery (Fig. 18.1a, b). This allows abnormally enlarged parathyroids that reside in deeper neck planes to be brought into more prominent view on ultrasound. Parathyroid abnormalities can be appreciated upon even further degrees of neck hyperextension achieved during surgery in an anesthetized patient, which might be impractical or uncomfortable during an office-based exam. This supports the virtue of repeating a parathyroid ultrasound in the operating room, especially if office-based ultrasound was negative, and demonstrates its versatility as a stethoscope-like tool. The sonographer usually stands on the patient's right side (as illustrated in Fig. 18.1b) and faces the ultrasound machine.

The region of the thyroid and the central neck should be examined in transverse and longitudinal planes (Fig. 18.2a, b). The lateral cervical regions, particularly along the carotid and jugular vasculature and the region adjacent to the submandibular gland, should likewise be examined, for the purpose of identifying ectopic parathyroids (Fig. 18.2c). For the same purpose, tilting the transducer toward the upper mediastinum can identify abnormal parathyroids in the upper mediastinum or cervical thymus. As with thyroid ultrasound, the sequence of examination should ideally be performed in a step-wise and systematic fashion that visualizes all anatomic regions of the thyroid and immediately adjacent soft tissue. Additionally, regions along the posterior border of the thyroid, and the paratracheal, retroesophageal, and pretracheal spaces, require careful evaluation. In these regions, graded pressure or a balloting motion applied by the

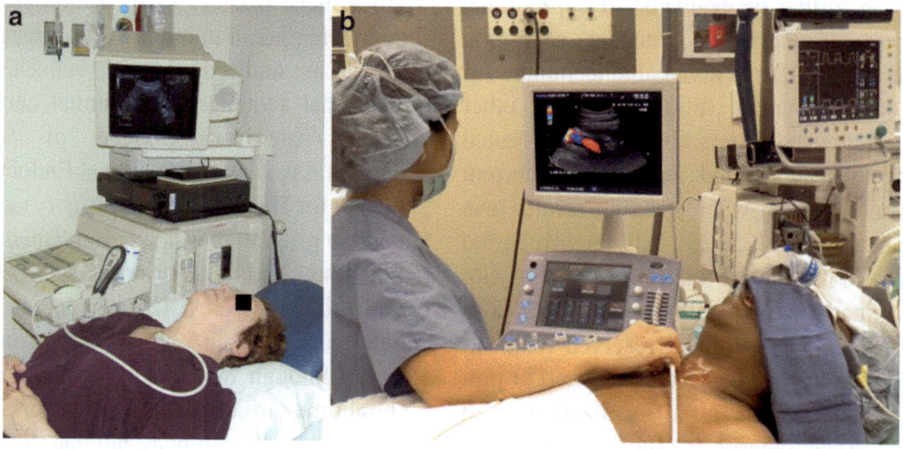

Fig. 18.1 Patient positioning for parathyroid ultrasound examination in an office-based setting (**a**) and in the operating room (**b**)

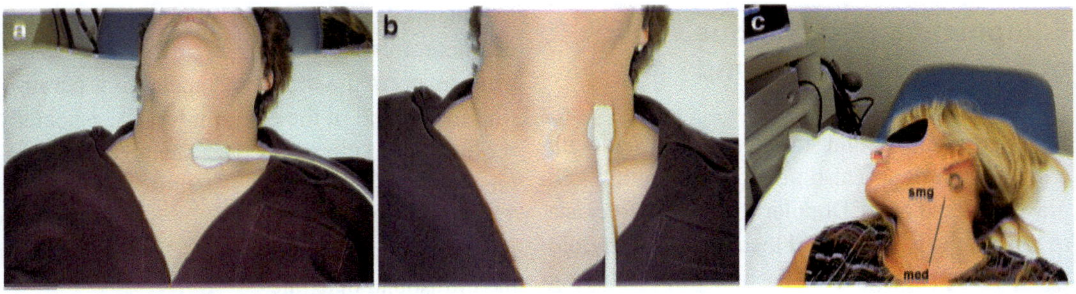

Fig. 18.2 Ultrasound examination is oriented in transverse (**a**) and longitudinal (**b**) planes in the area immediately adjacent to the thyroid. To detect abnormal parathyroid glands in ectopic cervical regions, the lateral aspects of the neck (**c**) along the carotid and jugular vasculature (*line*) and submandibular glands (*smg*) should also sonographically imaged, and the probe directed toward the upper mediastinum (*med*) as well

transducer can sometimes cause an abnormal parathyroid to "pop out" or shift with respect to surrounding structures. Swallowing by the patient may also aid in abnormal parathyroid identification. A patient with hyperparathyroidism may bring medical records of a thyroid ultrasound that fails to describe an obvious parathyroid abnormality. This may be understandable in the context that a thyroid ultrasound focuses solely on the thyroid parenchyma and potential thyroid nodular disease. Communicating a specific request to the sonographer, however, to perform dedicated ultrasound examination for parathyroid abnormalities is crucial.

An abnormality detected by ultrasound to be suspicious but not convincing for parathyroid disease can further be evaluated, if appropriate, by ultrasound-guided fine needle aspiration biopsy (FNAB). This is a valuable technique for evaluation of potential intrathyroidal or other ectopic parathyroid glands, abnormalities located in a previously operated neck, and recurrent hyperparathyroidism when imaging results give discordant findings [25, 26]. Although reported by some as a routine procedure for patients with initial primary hyperparathyroidism [27, 28], parathyroid FNAB is usually reserved for challenging scenarios and is not the preferred or prevailing approach with initial localization, as it can affect tissue integrity for subsequent surgery [29]. The FNAB aspirate is examined both cytologically and for PTH measurement [25]. It is important to alert the pathologist that the source of the FNAB was a potentially abnormal parathyroid, as the cytologic appearance can mimic a thyroid follicular neoplasm [30]. It is also important to alert the laboratory that the PTH sample is a nonserum sample. A number of methods for PTH measurement have been described [25, 31]; simply drawing up 5 ml of sterile saline into the syringe used for the biopsy, then submitting this aliquot for testing usually yields enormously elevated PTH values that leave no diagnostic uncertainty; one study suggested that a PTH aspirate value of 42 or higher gave no false-negative findings [25]. The typical finding of a parathyroid cyst is the aspiration of a perfectly clear, colorless fluid, described by some to appear as water or ethyl alcohol [32, 33].

To achieve mastery of the parathyroid ultrasound technique, a number of resources exist as publications and educational venues. Several professional societies offer annual certification courses (American College of Surgeons, American Association of Clinical Endocrinology, Societies for Head and Neck Surgery) and a collaborative program has been established between radiologists and endocrinologists (Endocrine Certification in Neck Ultrasound, ECNU) to enhance expertise in clinician-performed ultrasound. Although many publications deservedly highlight the virtues of surgeon-performed ultrasound, it should be emphasized that the ability to perform highly accurate parathyroid ultrasound rests with any clinician who invests dedicated focus and practice to this application.

Survey of Normal and Abnormal Parathyroid Anatomy with Ultrasound

Parathyroid Anatomy

Ultrasonographic examination relies on knowledge of the anatomy and embryology of parathyroid glands to detect expected locations of abnormal glands. Most individuals have four parathyroid glands situated on the capsule of the thyroid, but 10% can have supranumerary glands and 5% can be ectopic (Fig. 18.3) [34]. Normal parathyroid glands are typically not seen by ultrasound. They are too tiny (6×3×2 mm oval shape or smaller). They also have a somewhat fatty consistency, may be encased in a purely fatty halo of tissue and kept flattened close to the thyroid surface under a thin adventitial veil. Thus, as ultrasound waves penetrate this region, normal parathyroid glands may not reflect waves sufficiently differently from either adjacent fat or thyroid tissue to appear as discreet entities.

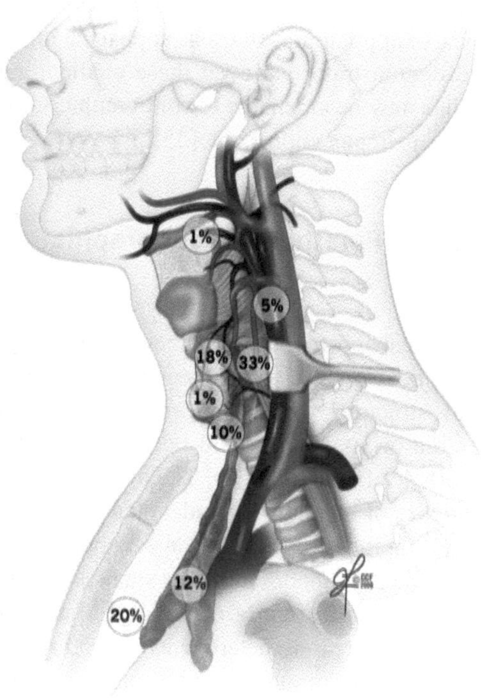

Fig. 18.3 Ectopic distribution of abnormal parathyroid glands in patients with primary hyperparathyroidism. Reprinted with permission, Cleveland Clinic Center for Medical Art & Photography © 2008–2011. All Rights Reserved

Superior parathyroids are located on the posterior thyroid surface, generally on the medial aspect close to the tracheoesophageal groove (Fig. 18.4a). Most are within a 2 cm diameter region centered around the intersection between the recurrent laryngeal nerve (usually not seen on ultrasound) and the inferior thyroid artery and its most distal branches (typically seen clearly on ultrasound in both transverse and longitudinal views). The inferior thyroid artery usually enters the midportion of the thyroid and gives an arterial branch to the superior and inferior parathyroids. When imaged longitudinally, an enlarged parathyroid centered on the posterior midportion of the thyroid gland, or higher toward the upper pole of the thyroid, is typically an abnormal superior parathyroid. Because the normal superior parathyroid glands favor a posteromedial position, when they become enlarged, they track downward along the tracheoesophageal groove, to become situated even more posteriorly or inferiorly. In these deep positions, which can extend even to the upper mediastinum, enlarged superior parathyroids may not be discernible on ultrasound. It is here that the technical maneuvers described above (neck extension, transducer pressure, or balloting) may become helpful. Superior parathyroid glands also have ectopic locations and knowledge of these is useful for sonographic examination. Most enlarged superior parathyroid in these ectopic regions are detectable by ultrasound, particularly those where the gland is situated higher than the superior pole of the thyroid gland, among the superior thyroid vessels, or higher in the carotid sheath.

Inferior parathyroid glands are located typically on the lateral tip of the lower thyroid pole and are much more anterior in location, with respect to virtually all reference points, such as the superior parathyroid glands, the course of the recurrent laryngeal nerve and inferior thyroid artery (Fig. 18.4b). They can also be distributed

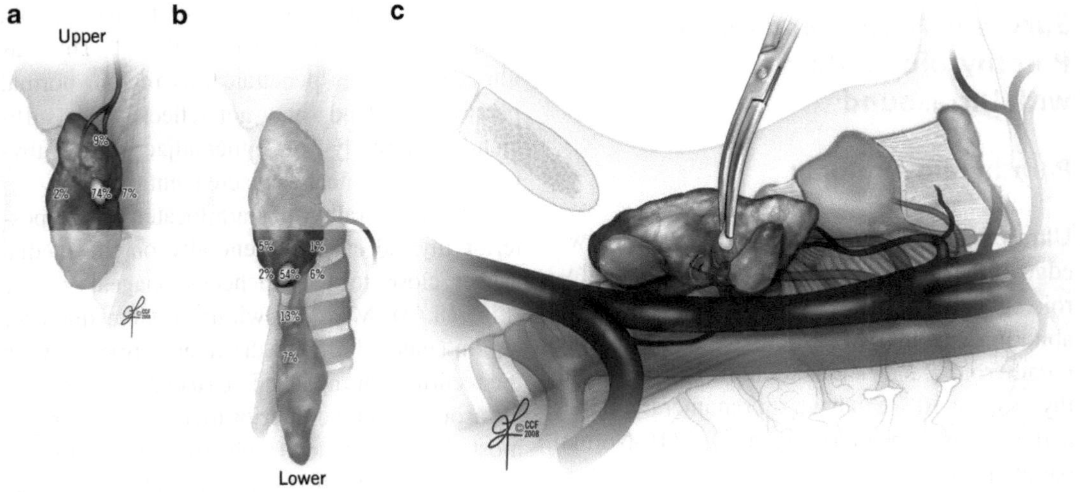

Fig. 18.4 Normal distribution of superior (**a**) and inferior (**b**) parathyroid glands. The drawing in (**b**) demonstrates the entry of the inferior thyroid artery on the posterior midportion of the thyroid gland. Enlarged inferior and superior parathyroids are illustrated in (**c**). Reprinted with permission, Cleveland Clinic Center for Medical Art & Photography © 2008–2011. All Rights Reserved

more widely than superior parathyroid glands and have broader extent of ectopic locations (mediastinum, carotid sheath, and intrathyroidal). They are often within the thyrothymic tract just inferior to the tip of the thyroid gland or within the cervical portion of the thymus. When imaged longitudinally, an enlarged parathyroid just below the strap muscles is typically an inferior parathyroid.

Ectopic parathyroids that can be evaluated with ultrasound include those that are intrathyroidal (3%, typically considered to be inferior parathyroids), intrathymic, located along the carotid sheath or adjacent to the submandibular gland. They tend to have similar features to abnormal parathyroid glands located in typical distributions, and lack the distinctive sonographic architecture of the central vascular hilum of lymph nodes, which may also be found in these regions. Ectopic parathyroids that are difficult to detect with ultrasound include those that are retrotracheal and/or anterior to the cervical spine, and those deep in the mediastinum. Ultrasound is technically limited to identify substernal ectopic parathyroid disease because the acoustic shadows cast by both air-filled (trachea and esophagus) and bony structures obscure surrounding soft-tissue anatomy. However, innovative applications of transesophageal ultrasound demonstrate that even these challenging locations may be amenable to sonographic visualization using an endoscope [35].

Abnormal Parathyroid Sonographic Features

The classical appearance of an abnormal parathyroid can be described as a hypoechoic, teardrop-shaped structure with a hyperechoic line of adventitia on its anterior and posterior surfaces (Figs. 18.4c, 18.5, and 18.6). The average longitudinal size of a parathyroid adenoma is 15 mm, although the teardrop shape can be appreciated with parathyroid abnormalities as small as 8 mm. The hypoechoic texture of the enlarged parathyroid is uniform, rarely heterogeneous, and rarely with hyperechoic or more knobby configurations. Although these variations can be seen (Fig. 18.7), they occur more often with the sclerotic changes and calcifications within parathyroid tissue of patients with secondary and tertiary hyperparathyroidism. The vascular pedicle, a branch of the inferior thyroid artery, can usually be identified

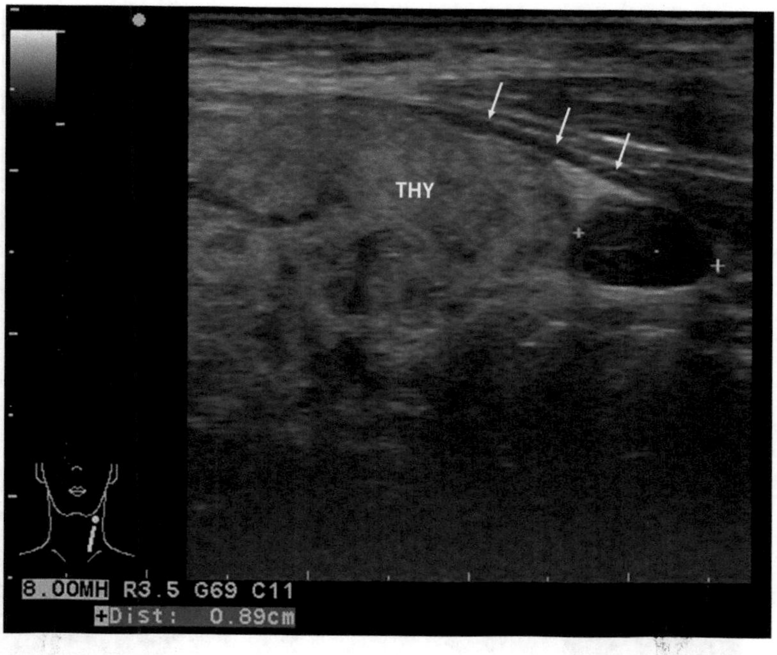

Fig. 18.5 Typical appearance of an abnormally large parathyroid gland. This example demonstrates an enlarged left inferior parathyroid gland adjacent to the lower pole of the thyroid gland (THY) and below the border of the sternothyroid muscle that appears as a hypoechoic dark stripe (below *white arrows*)

to enter the parathyroid at the narrow beginning of the teardrop shape of the abnormal parathyroid. This vascular pedicle may have a tortuous configuration outside of the parathyroid, may in some patients have multiple branching patterns within the parathyroid or just prominent Doppler signal on the parathyroid capsule. A parathyroid vascular pedicle may be difficult to image in some patients, but it rarely, if ever, has the single, clean central hilar vascular stripe that is characteristic of cervical lymph nodes (Fig. 18.8).

In addition to the clues based on anatomic distribution, there are two visual patterns that are distinctive for parathyroid sonography. The "triple circle sign," a term designated by the authors, refers to the presence of three hypoechoic circular entities lateral to the thyroid on transverse imaging: the most lateral circle is the cross section of the jugular vein, the middle circle is the cross section of the common carotid artery, and the medial circle is that of an abnormally large parathyroid (Fig. 18.9). Doppler flow examination demonstrates the distinction between the vascular and parathyroid structures clearly (Fig. 18.10). This pattern on transverse sonographic view is unique for parathyroid disease, and images with this spatial relationship are uncommon with thyroid nodules, abnormal lymph nodes, or other tissues representing the medial circle.

The other visual pattern of identification is the triangularization of the central neck, where the strap muscles (specifically sternothyroid) can be seen as the roof of the central neck space and represents one side of the triangle on a longitudinal section obtained with ultrasound transducer resting just to the side of the trachea (Fig. 18.11). Parathyroids located within this triangle are inferior parathyroid glands. Delineating this triangle helps in the methodical search for parathyroid abnormalities. The differential diagnosis of other sonographic entities in this triangular space is very limited—the only tissues that reside here are normal fibrofatty lobules, normal or abnormal lymph nodes, thymus, and occasionally accessory nodules of thyroid tissue.

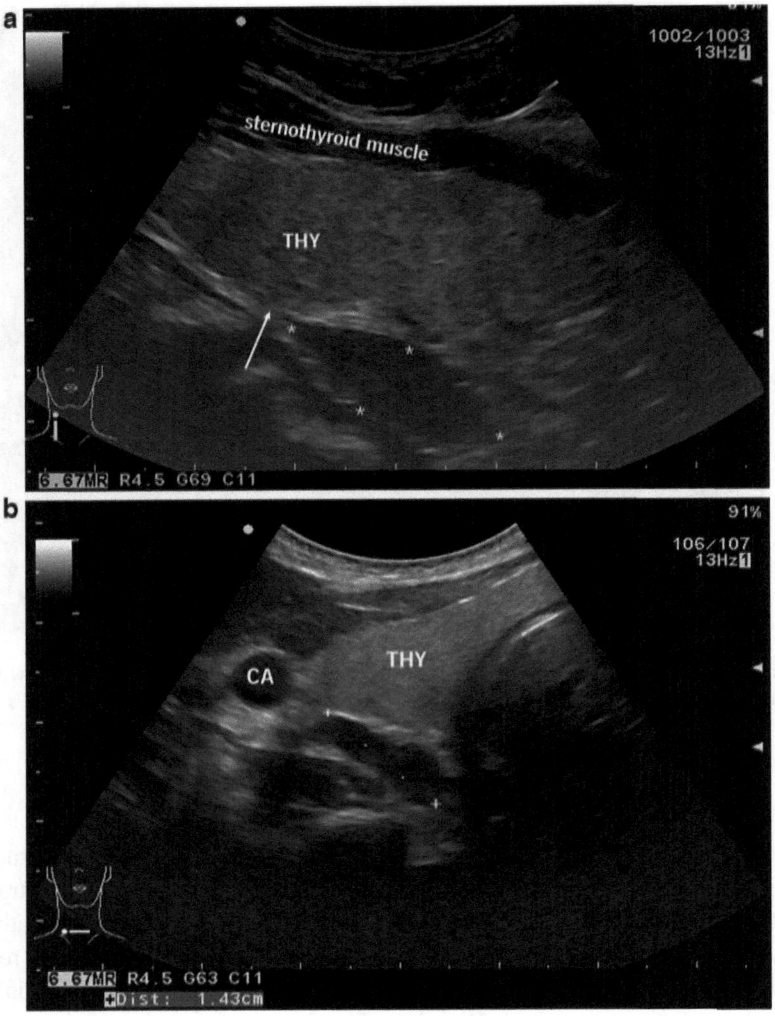

Fig. 18.6 Another illustration of a typical appearance of an abnormally large parathyroid gland, this time a right superior parathyroid in longitudinal view (**a**). The tip of its "teardrop" shape begins at the posterior midportion of the thyroid gland (*arrow*). The extent of the parathyroid is marked at four points (*asterisks*). The transverse image (**b**) measures the abnormal parathyroid as 1.4 cm, compatible with average lengths of a single adenoma. The carotid artery (CA) and right thyroid lobe (THY) are marked

Sonographic Illustrations of Abnormal Parathyroid Disease Entities

The spectrum of parathyroid abnormalities that can be identified with ultrasound is demonstrated in Figs. 18.5–18.15. Represented in this sequence are variations within the major disease manifestations of primary hyperparathyroidism. Thus, for example, a classical parathyroid adenoma is illustrated in Figs. 18.5 and 18.6, with less typical versions seen in Fig. 18.7. The multigland hyperplasia example (Fig. 18.12) is from a patient with primary hyperparathyroidism; although at surgery this patient had four-gland hyperplasia, a double adenoma might have imaged similarly on ultrasound. More subtle abnormalities suggesting parathyroid cancer are seen in Fig. 18.13. Illustrated also are more interesting examples of abnormal parathyroids in ectopic locations, such as in the carotid sheath and as implants in the sternocleidomastoid muscle (Fig. 18.14). Finally, an example of co-existing thyroid and parathyroid pathology is provided to emphasize the utility of parathyroid

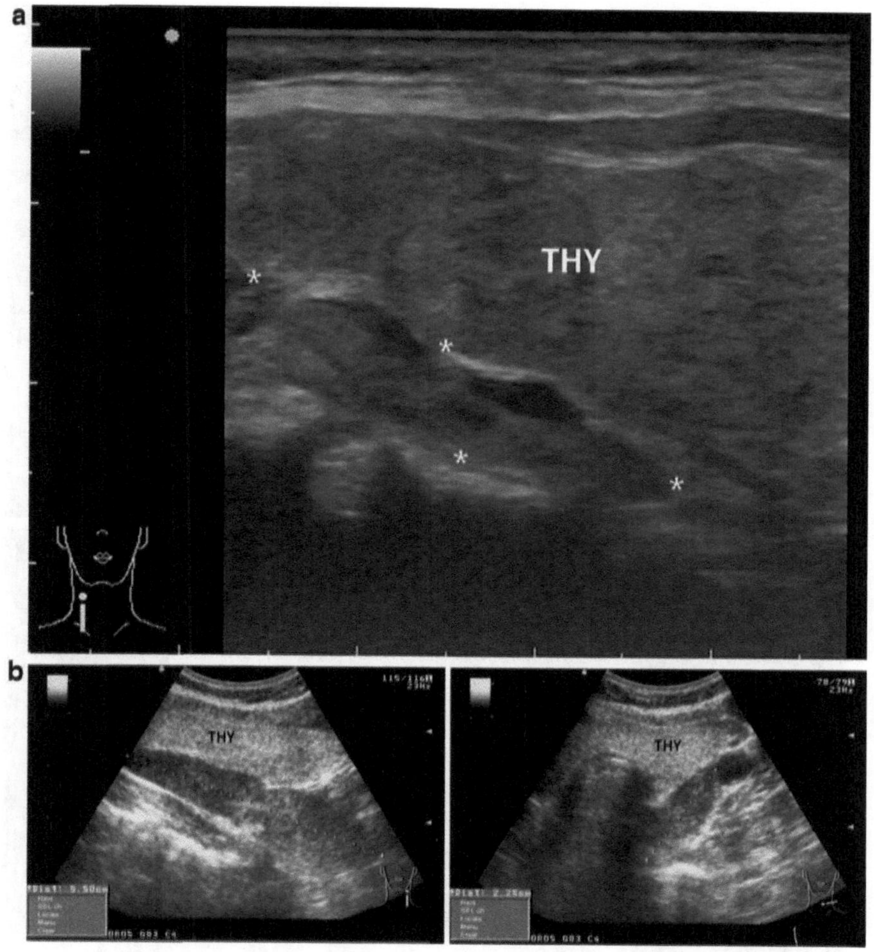

Fig. 18.7 Variations of the sonographic appearance of abnormal parathyroid glands. (**a**) Enlarged parathyroid (*asterisks*) with knobby shape, texture isoechoic with the adjacent thyroid and cystic degeneration within the parathyroid tissue (*black areas*). This was imaged with a linear transducer probe. (**b**) Left upper parathyroid imaged longitudinally to measure nearly 6 cm and be larger than the thyroid (*left panel*) and imaged transversely (*right panel*) using a "fingertip" curvilinear probe. (**c**) Right superior parathyroid (*asterisks*) is shown, imaged longitudinally and located deep to the superior pole of the thyroid gland (*lines*) and adjacent to the spine. Subtle hypoechoic densities such as this one are nevertheless indicative of abnormal parathyroid glands. (**d**) The right superior parathyroid (*asterisks*) located deep in the neck anterior to the spine does not have the typical hypoechoic sonographic texture. The protrusion of the tubercle of Zuckerkandl (tz) provides a valuable preview of an anatomic detail to expect during surgery

ultrasound in detecting adjacent pathology that might require treatment (Fig. 18.15).

The Use of Ultrasound in the Clinical Management of Hyperparathyroidism

Parathyroid ultrasound is intended principally as a localizing rather than diagnostic tool. Thus, the main indications for its use are (1) to identify the site or sites of abnormal parathyroid glands in patients with initial diagnosis of hyperparathyroidism following biochemical confirmation of primary, secondary, or tertiary forms of this disease and (2) to aid localization of persistent or recurrent parathyroid disease. For the first indication, ultrasound can be used as the sole localizing modality or in combination with other radiologic methods, such as Mibi scans and/or computed tomography scans (CT) [16, 36–43]. For the second indication, ultrasound is typically always

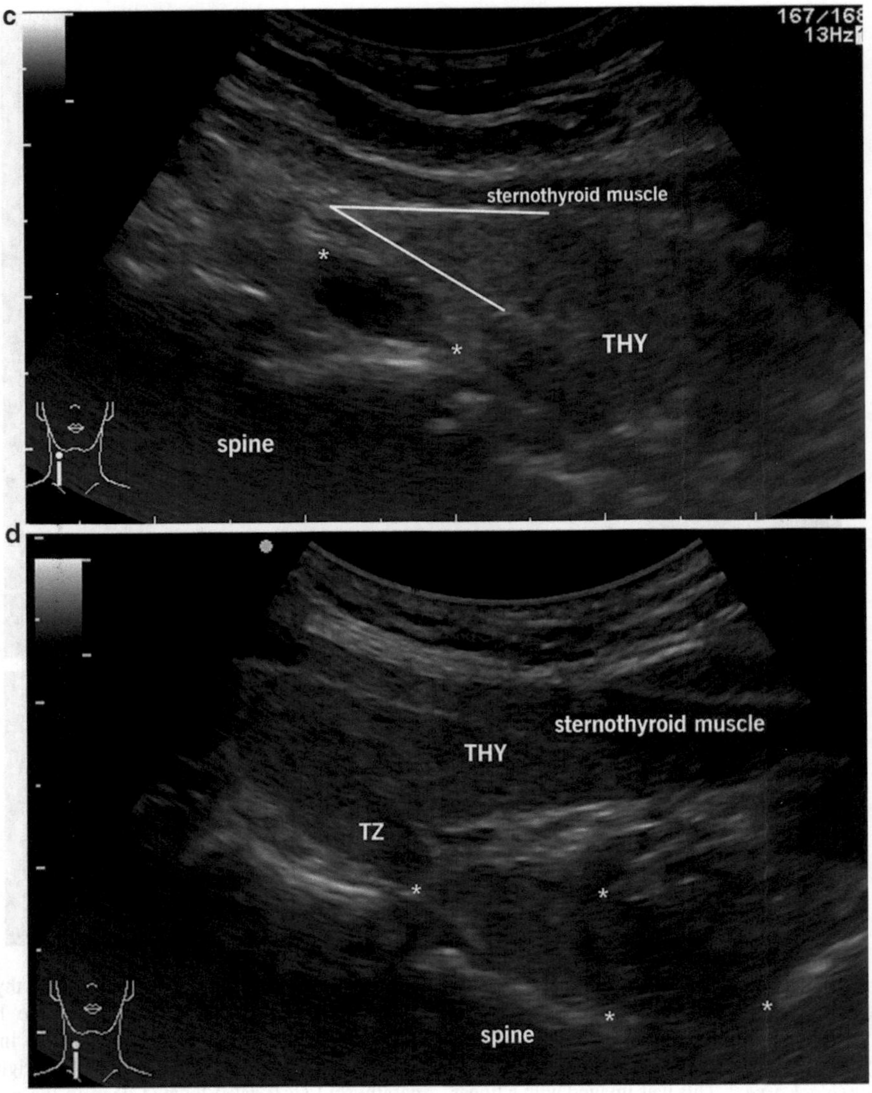

Fig. 18.7 (continued)

part of a sequence of several localizing modalities, usually within an algorithm meant to enhance the accuracy of potential re-operative surgery [44–47]. A negative ultrasound—one that does not reveal any potential sites of parathyroid disease—should not be viewed as excluding the diagnosis of hyperparathyroidism, especially if a complete biochemical work-up has not been performed. A negative ultrasound with confirmed diagnosis of hyperparathyroidism usually raises the likelihood of the presence of multigland hyperplasia (rather than a single adenoma) or the presence of ectopic disease [37, 38, 40, 48].

While principally used for these indications, ultrasound naturally confers some broader functionality and benefits. It can facilitate focal parathyroid exploration or “minimally invasive parathyroid surgery,” particularly when a Mibi scan is unrevealing [29, 42]. Ultrasound identifies co-existing thyroid disease and thyroid cancer, thus refining the surgical management plan so that the patient and surgeon have clearer

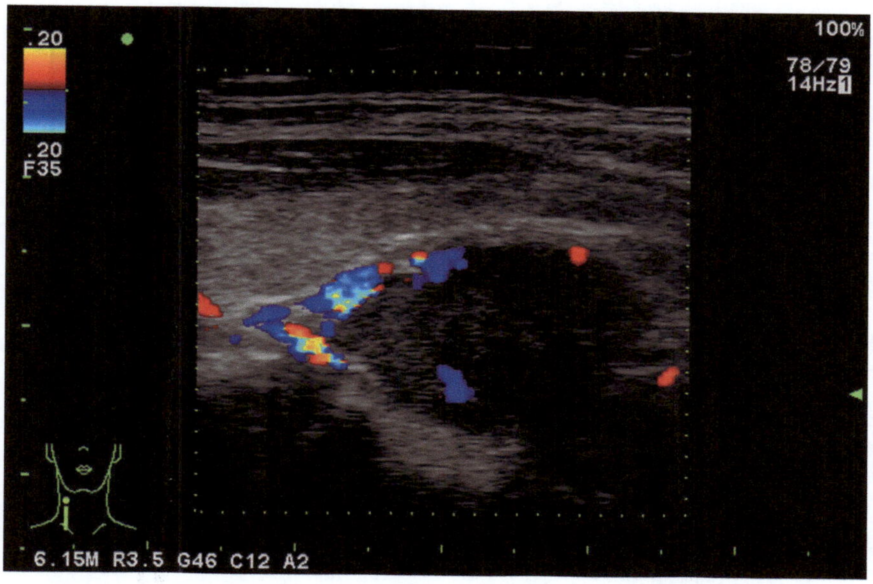

Fig. 18.8 The vascular pedicle of an abnormal parathyroid caps the superior tip of the parathyroid. Unlike the vascular hilar stripe of a lymph node which appears centrally within the lymph node, there is no central, linear vascular signal in this parathyroid, which remains uniformly hypoechoic

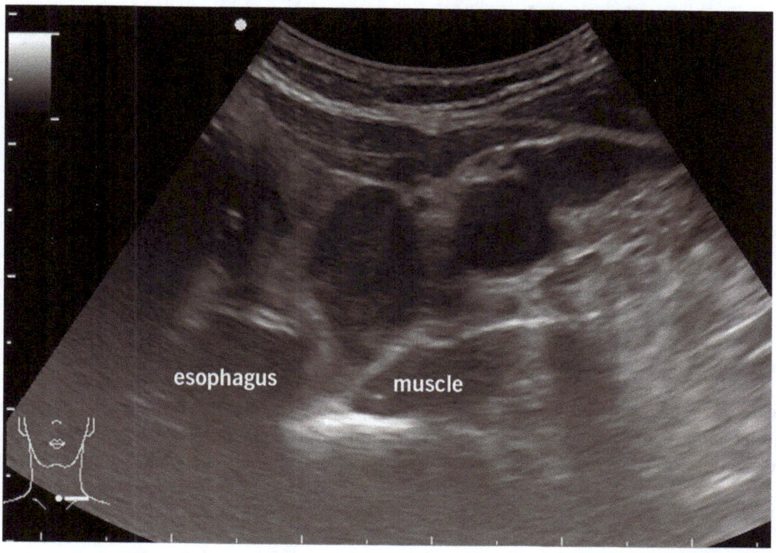

Fig. 18.9 The "triple circle sign" refers to the three dark circles imaged on transverse view during parathyroid ultrasound. These are purposefully unlabeled to be seen in contrast to the esophagus and underlying muscle. The dark circle belonging to the left superior parathyroid adenoma is in the center, the carotid artery cross section is next, and the jugular vein cross section is at far right

expectations of the necessary extent of treatment before surgery [49–51]. One study suggested that the rate of concomitant thyroid surgery during parathyroidectomy was reduced from 30 to 6% by being able to diagnose benign thyroid disease preoperatively [51]. The rate of thyroid cancer diagnosed concurrently with hyperparathyroidism when evaluations involved ultrasound has

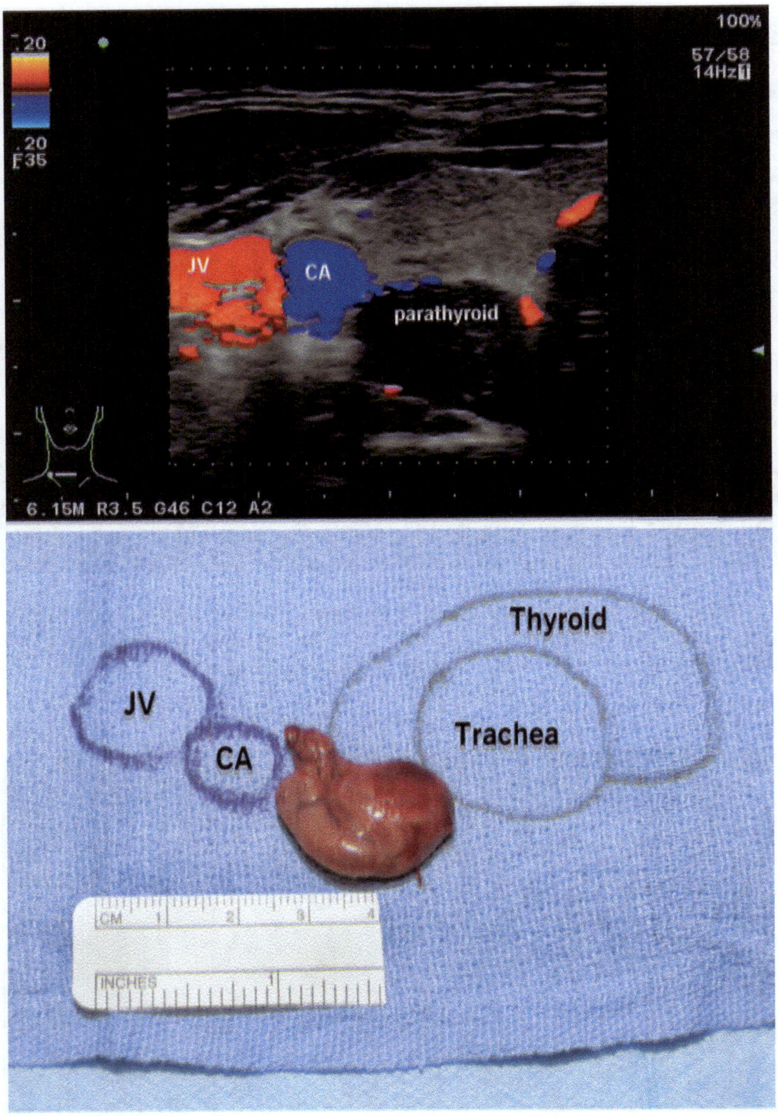

Fig. 18.10 Illustrated is the "triple circle sign" of a right-sided parathyroid adenoma, with marked cross sections of the jugular vein (JV), carotid artery (CA), and enlarged parathyroid gland in the sonographic image (*top*). The specimen photo (*bottom*) orients the large 3-cm right parathyroid adenoma in the anatomical context of these structures

been reported as 5–15% [49–51]. Among other benefits, the awareness of additional concerns improves the informed consent process between patient and surgeon, and reduces the anxiety to the patient and their family of unanticipated findings and duration of surgery. Ultrasound poses no radiation risks and is therefore the main imaging modality in the rare event hyperparathyroidism is diagnosed in pregnant women or in patients with other contraindications for usage of radioisotopes or radiologic dyes. For recurrent hyperparathyroidism, and for unusual and ectopic lesions even with initially diagnosed hyperparathyroidism, ultrasound can help confirm the parathyroid origin of a suspected abnormality by guiding FNAB for cytologic and PTH evaluation. Some authors have even used it to guide aspiration of bilateral jugular vein blood samples for PTH measurement during an office-based visit, helping lateralize the abnormality to the right or left side of the

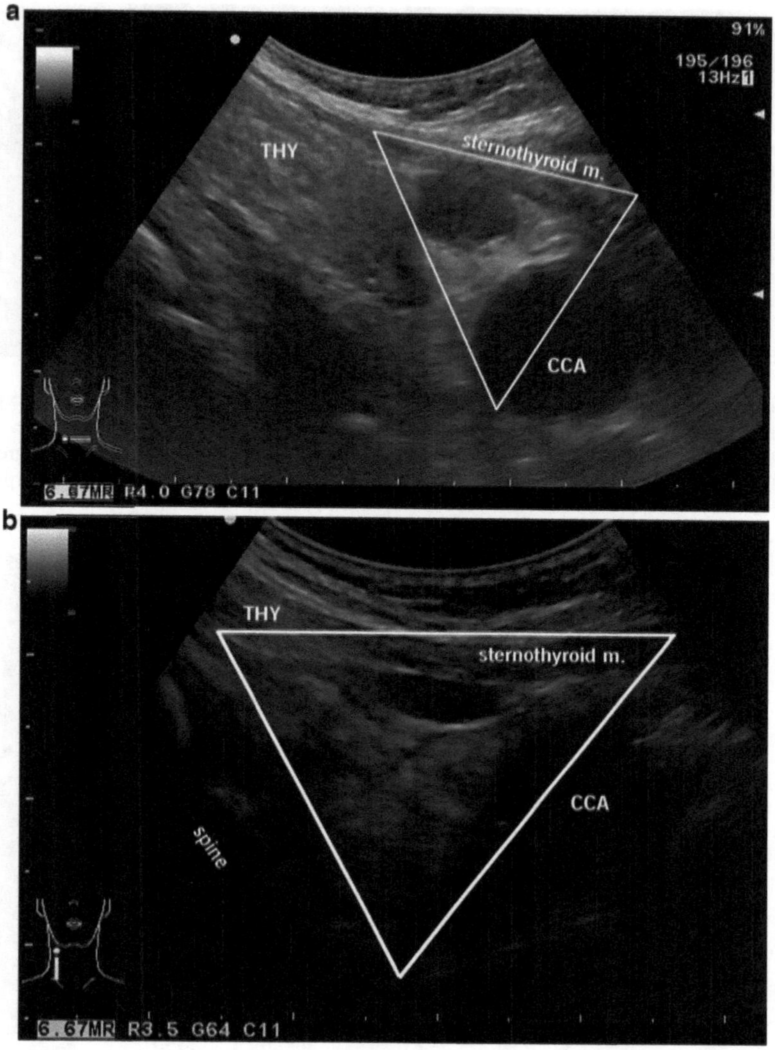

Fig. 18.11 The "triangularization" of the central neck is a view in the longitudinal ultrasound plane that helps define a space where abnormal inferior parathyroids reside. The outlines of the triangle are the sternothyroid muscle, a line paralleling the spine to reach the lower pole of the thyroid gland, and a line across the sternal notch, or in example A, the cross section of the common carotid artery (CCA). The hypoechoic density contained within this triangle is an inferior parathyroid adenoma. Note also that the orientation icon, which requires manual change by the operator, has remained incorrectly designated in a transverse orientation—a reminder that these icons are often not as reliable as what the ultrasound image itself conveys. The anatomy of the sternothyroid muscle clearly establishes a longitudinal view. In example B, the lower parathyroid has classical sonographic features and the icon also indicates a longitudinal view

neck [52]. In rare cases, ultrasound can also guide nontraditional therapy for hyperparathyroidism, such as ethanol injection of parathyroid glands, a procedure that may have limited role in patients with recurrent, inoperable, or challenging parathyroid disease scenarios [53–56]. For an experienced sonographer, ultrasound can function also to preview the anatomy expected at surgery, with nuances that alert to more complex or simple technical details about how to surgically approach the parathyroid. As mentioned previously as well, ultrasound can be performed within the operating room as a procedure prior to start of surgery; if needed, the transducer can also be placed in a

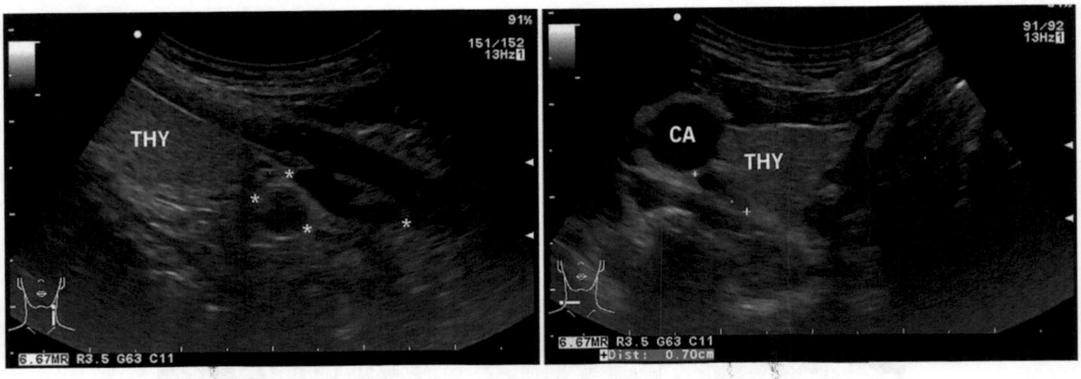

Fig. 18.12 Multigland parathyroid hyperplasia in hyperparathyroidism is more likely to be the underlying etiology when small (0.7–1.0 cm) hypoechoic densities are imaged bilaterally (*asterisks*). In the *left panel*, the left inferior parathyroid was found at surgery to be lobulated, as suggested in the ultrasound image. Similar bilateral distribution but usually with much greater parathyroid enlargement occurs in secondary hyperparathyroidism

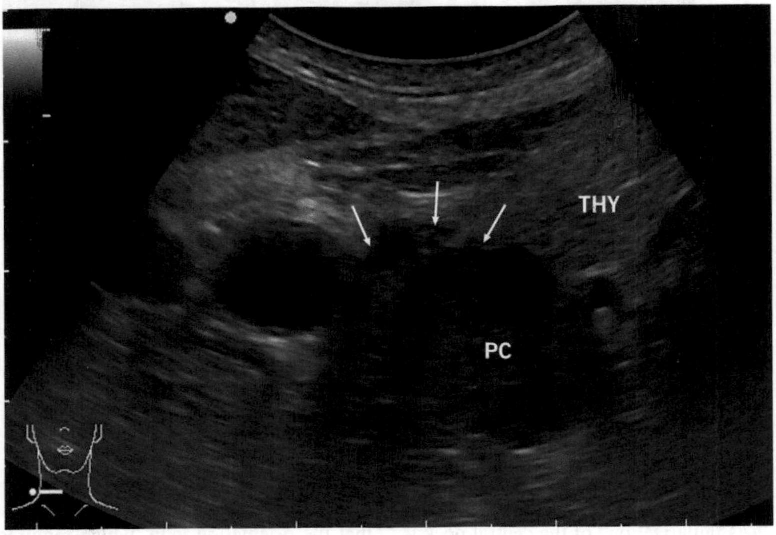

Fig. 18.13 Parathyroid cancer (PC) suspected from a large 3-cm parathyroid with irregular border (*arrows*) adjacent to the thyroid gland, in a patient with primary hyperparathyroidism and preoperative calcium values of 14 mg/dL and PTH 1,200 pg/ml

sterile sheath and used to search for parathyroid densities within the surgically exposed neck space after the incision has been made. These benefits are highlighted in Table 18.1.

An evidence-based review of the literature shows that accuracy of ultrasound varies with the manner used for localization of abnormal parathyroid glands [16, 19–24, 36–38, 42]. It appears from these studies that, on average, 75–80% of abnormal parathyroid glands are correctly detected by ultrasound. However, this performance varies depending on clinical circumstances, type of underlying parathyroid disease, the definition used for successful localization and accuracy, and the specialist conducting the ultrasound exam. When performed by experienced surgeon—sonographers, parathyroid ultrasound was found to be superior to Mibi in all clinical subgroups: single adenomas, double adenomas, hyperplasia, familial hyperparathyroidism, and secondary/tertiary forms of hyperparathyroidism [57]. Ultrasound sensitivity was greater for single

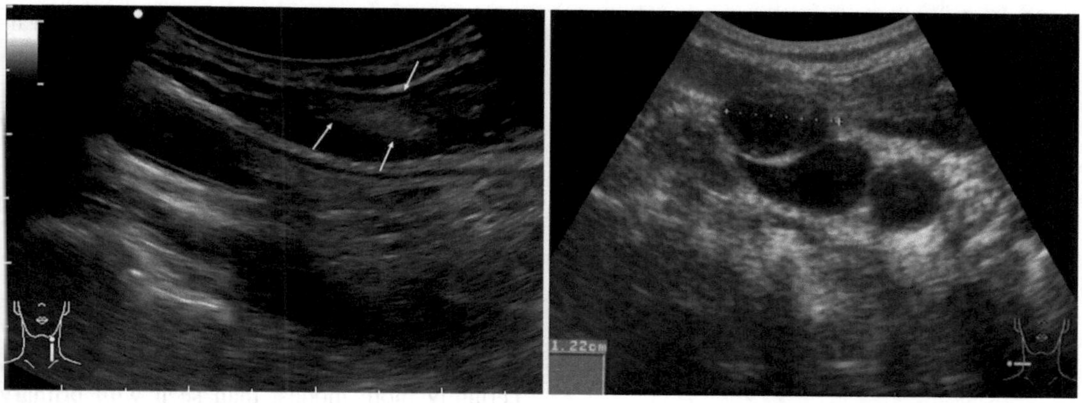

Fig. 18.14 Images of ectopically located abnormal parathyroids in the neck. A hyperechoic and vague density (*arrows*) in the left sternocleidomastoid muscle represents an adenoma that developed at the site of a parathyroid autotransplant performed 20 years previously during thyroid surgery (*left panel*). An ectopic parathyroid adenoma measuring 1.2 cm is situated adjacent to the jugular vein and carotid artery (*right panel*). In both instances, ultrasound-guided FNA was used to confirm parathyroid tissue

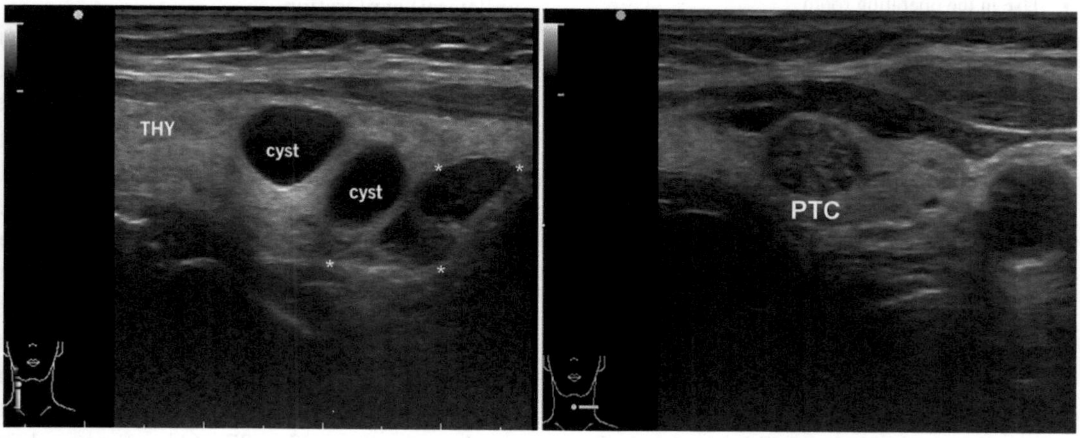

Fig. 18.15 Co-existing thyroid disease with primary hyperparathyroidism. The sonographic image depicts two intrathyroidal cysts and an enlarged right inferior parathyroid gland (*asterisks*). A small papillary thyroid cancer (PTC) was diagnosed in the contralateral thyroid lobe

adenomas than for multigland disease, whereas these rates were more comparable for Mibi scans [57]. When surgeon-performed ultrasound was used as the first localizing test and intended potentially as the only test, it was found to have equal accuracy as Mibi, but was easier to perform, identified concomitant thyroid disease, and was more cost-effective [37]. These authors suggested an algorithm that uses ultrasound as the principal localizing modality for hyperparathyroidism, with application of other interventions only in the setting of equivocal or negative ultrasound [37]. In these circumstances of surgeon-performed ultrasound, especially with stringent and selective criteria applied to operate on patients with clear sonographic findings, a true positive rate as high as 89% was achieved [14, 16, 37]. Taking into considerations that study design and definitions were not necessarily comparable, others have reported higher positive predictive values, such as 99% in a study where ultrasound was performed by interventional radiologists [23].

Table 18.1 The spectrum of advantages seen with the use of parathyroid ultrasound for evaluation of patients with hyperparathyroidism

• Localization of parathyroid disease prior to initial surgery for hyperparathyroidism
• Localization of persistent and recurrent parathyroid disease
• Ability to direct focal or limited parathyroid surgery
• Guidance of diagnostic parathyroid interventions (FNAB, jugular vein PTH sampling)
• Guidance of therapeutic parathyroid interventions (alcohol ablation)
• Identification of concomitant thyroid disease and thyroid cancer
• Reduction in concomitant thyroid surgery during operation for hyperparathyroidism
• Facilitation of surgical planning for patient and surgeon
• Preview of precise anatomical details valuable for surgery
• Convenience of use in office-based practice
• Use in the operating room
• Lack of radiation exposure
• Cost-effectiveness

Ultrasound appears to be particularly helpful following negative Mibi scans, as ultrasound was able to localize an abnormal parathyroid suggestively or conclusively in 56% of patients and surgery confirmed this prediction was correct in 84% of patients [58]. Another study found that ultrasound detected abnormal parathyroid glands in 83% of patients with negative Mibi scans [36]. In this same study, when Mibi scans were found to perform slightly better than ultrasound, this was attributed to Mibi's advantage in detecting mediastinal and multigland disease [36].

The performance of US in re-operative parathyroid surgery has been examined by a number of investigators [25, 26, 36, 44–47]. In this setting, US and Mibi should be viewed as complementary studies and both ideally need to be performed. As alluded to already, ultrasound provides the ability to have tissue or hormonal confirmation of parathyroid disease by guiding FNA of suspected lesions. In the re-operative setting, the sensitivity of ultrasound was 56% and a combined multimodality algorithm allowed a successful focal approach in 60% [44].

The use of parathyroid ultrasound in the evaluation of patients with secondary and tertiary hyperparathyroidism has likewise been described [59, 60]. As with hyperplasia in general, neither ultrasound nor Mibi scans reliably detect parathyroid hyperplasia or visualize all of the involved glands in hyperplasia, an observation consistently reported by several investigators both in the 1990s [12, 48] and more recently [36, 38, 40]. The rate of accurate diagnosis with secondary hyperparathyroidism has been reported as 64%, certainly more modest than seen with primary hyperparathyroidism [59]. In the secondary/tertiary hyperparathyroidism scenario, given that the underlying biology affects all parathyroid glands, bilateral neck exploration is essential; hence, high ultrasound accuracy does not have the same purpose of allowing focal (limited or unilateral) exploration.

A number of factors have been identified to impact detection of abnormal parathyroid glands by ultrasound. These include younger patients [37], body mass index (BMI) [57], parathyroid gland size and gland volume [57], and the skill and experience of the examiner [21, 22, 36]. What determines whether ultrasound should be chosen for initial or exclusive preoperative localization depends on the availability of skilled and experienced examiners perhaps more so than any set of benefits posed by each imaging modality. As summarized by Inabnet et al. and others [36, 37, 61], ultrasound is favored by low cost, convenience, lack of radiation exposure, precise anatomical detail, and detection of concomitant thyroid nodules and thyroid cancer. By contrast, Mibi scans seem to be favored for imaging of ectopic, especially mediastinal disease, and thus may be preferred as the initial test for patients with failed prior parathyroid surgery and suspected ectopic disease. Other imaging modalities, such as computed tomography, pose significantly higher radiation exposures to weigh against unique benefits. The data from the studies presented above seems to point out clearly that, if at all possible, ultrasound should be part of the clinical management of hyperparathyroidism.

Conclusion

Ultrasound is a readily applicable, noninvasive and versatile tool for the evaluation of patients with parathyroid diseases. It aids in the localization of parathyroid abnormalities to direct appropriate parathyroid surgery. It also offers the opportunity to identify and address co-existing thyroid disease, including thyroid cancer. Whether used as the only technique by experienced sonographers for initial localization in first-time hyperparathyroid patients, or as part of a multi-imaging algorithm, ultrasound provides valuable clinical information. Recognizable sonographic features allow identification of abnormal parathyroid glands, can be readily learned, and make ultrasound a powerful tool especially when performed by clinicians with access to comprehensive information about the patient's parathyroid disease. Ultrasound can guide appropriate interventions to clarify challenging diagnostic scenarios, although ultimately it should not be viewed as a diagnostic test for hyperparathyroidism. It has a demonstrated history of valuable clinical use [3, 13, 15, 62]. As it has in the past, ultrasound will continue to have an important role in the management of patients with parathyroid disease.

References

1. Baskin HJ. Thyroid ultrasound-just do it. Thyroid. 2004;14(2):91–2.
2. http://www.ncbi.nlm.nih.gov/sites/entrez?dr=Abstract&holding=ohiolinklib%2Cohccalib_fft_ndi&otool=ohccalib. Accessed December 2009. Entry of keywords "parathyroid ultrasound" for the years 1990–2000 and 2000–present.
3. Harness J, Wisher D. Ultrasound in surgical practice. New York: Wiley; 2001.
4. Phitayakorn R, McHenry CR. Parathyroidectomy: overview of the anatomic basis and surgical strategies for parathyroid operations. Clin Rev Bone Miner Metabol. 2007;5(2):89–102.
5. Greene A, Mitchell J, Davis R, Barbosa G, Tsinberg M, Berber E, et al. National trends in parathyroid surgery from 1997–2007: a decade of change. J Am Coll Surg. 2009;209:332–43.
6. Coakley AJ, Kettle AG, Wells CP, O'Doherty MJ, Collins RE. 99Tcm sestamibi—a new agent for parathyroid imaging. Nucl Med Commun. 1989;10(11):791–4.
7. Irvin 3rd GL, Dembrow VD, Prudhomme DL. Operative monitoring of parathyroid gland hyperfunction. Am J Surg. 1991;162(4):299–302.
8. Mazzaglia PJ, Berber E, Kovach A, Milas M, Siperstein A. The changing presentation of hyperparathyroidism over three decades. Arch Surg. 2008;143:260–6.
9. Udelsman R, Pasieka JL, Sturgeon C, Young JE, Clark OH. Surgery for asymptomatic primary hyperparathyroidism: proceedings of the third international workshop. J Clin Endocrinol Metab. 2009;94(2):366–72.
10. AACE/AAES Task Force on Primary Hyperparathyroidism. The American Association of Clinical Endocrinologists and the American Association of Endocrine surgeons position statement on the diagnosis and management of primary hyperparathyroidism. Endocr Pract. 2005;11(1):49–54.
11. Silverberg S, El-Hajj Fuleihan G. Preoperative localization and surgical therapy of primary hyperparathyroidism. 2009. http://www.uptodate.com/online.
12. Light VL, McHenry CR, Jarjoura D, Sodee DB, Miron SD. Prospective comparison of dual-phase technetium-99 m-sestamibi scintigraphy and high resolution ultrasonography in the evaluation of abnormal parathyroid glands. Am Surg. 1996;62:562–7.
13. Milas M, Stephen A, Berber E, Wagner K, Miskulin J, Siperstein A. Ultrasound for the endocrine surgeon: a valuable clinical tool to enhance diagnostic and therapeutic outcomes. Surgery. 2005;138:1193–201.
14. Solorzano CC, Lee TM, Ramirez MC, Carneiro DM, Irvin GL. Surgeon-performed ultrasound improves localization of abnormal parathyroid glands. Am Surg. 2005;71(7):557–62. discussion 562–3.
15. Orloff L, editor. Head and neck ultrasonography. San Diego, CA: Plural Publishing; 2008.
16. Solorzano CC, Carneiro-Pla DM, Irvin 3rd GL. Surgeon-performed ultrasonography as the initial and only localizing study in sporadic primary hyperparathyroidism. J Am Coll Surg. 2006;202(1):18–24.
17. Terris DJ, Stack Jr BC, Gourin CG. Contemporary parathyroidectomy: exploiting technology. Am J Otolaryngol. 2007;28(6):408–14.
18. Ruda JM, Hollenbeak CS, Stack Jr BC. A systematic review of the diagnosis and treatment of primary hyperparathyroidism from 1995 to 2003. Otolaryngol Head Neck Surg. 2005;132(3):359–72.
19. Arora S, Balash PR, Yoo J, Smith GS, Prinz RA. Benefits of surgeon-performed ultrasound for primary hyperparathyroidism. Langenbecks Arch Surg. 2009;394(5):861–7.
20. Gurney TA, Orloff LA. Otolaryngologist—head and neck surgeon—performed ultrasonography for parathyroid adenoma localization. Laryngoscope. 2008;118(2):243–6.
21. Lloyd MN, Lees WR, Milroy EJ. Preoperative localization in primary hyperparathyroidism. Clin Radiol. 1990;41:239–43.
22. De Feo ML, Colagrande S, Biagini C, Tonarelli A, Bisi G, Vaggelli L, et al. Parathyroid glands: combination of (99 m)Tc MIBI scintigraphy and US for demonstration of parathyroid glands and nodules. Radiology. 2000;214:393–402.

23. Tresoldi S, Pompili G, Maiolino R, Flor N, De Pasquale L, Bastagli A, et al. Primary hyperparathyroidism: can ultrasonography be the only preoperative diagnostic procedure? Radiol Med. 2009;114(7):1159–72.
24. Akinci B, Demir T, Yener S, Comlekci A, Binicier O, Ozdogan O, et al. Beneficial effect of endocrinologist-performed ultrasonography on preoperative parathyroid adenoma localization. Endocr Pract. 2009;15(1): 17–23.
25. Stephen A, Milas M, Garner C, Wagner KE, Siperstein A. Use of surgeon-performed office ultrasound and parathyroid fine needle aspiration (FNA) for complex parathyroid localization. Surgery. 2005; 138:1143–51.
26. Sacks BA, Pallotta JA, Cole A, Hurwitz J. Diagnosis of parathyroid adenomas: efficacy of measuring parathormone levels in needle aspirates of cervical masses. AJR Am J Roentgenol. 1994;163(5):1223–6.
27. Erbil Y, Barbaros U, Salmaslioglu A, Tunaci M, Ozbey N, Bozbora A, et al. Value of parathyroid hormone assay for preoperative sonographically guided parathyroid aspirates for minimally invasive parathyroidectomy. J Clin Ultrasound. 2006;34(9):425–9.
28. Abraham D, Sharma PK, Bentz J, Gault PM, Neumayer L, McClain DA. Utility of ultrasound-guided fine-needle aspiration of parathyroid adenomas for localization before minimally invasive parathyroidectomy. Endocr Pract. 2007;13(4):333–7.
29. Norman J, Politz D, Browarsky I. Diagnostic aspiration of parathyroid adenomas causes severe fibrosis complicating surgery and final histologic diagnosis. Thyroid. 2007;17(12):1251–5.
30. Yoder B, Siperstein A, Milas M, Biscotti C. Parathyroid aspiration: a cytologic analysis of hyperfunctional glands. Acta Cytol. 2004;48:744.
31. Marcocci C, Mazzeo S, Bruno-Bossio G, Picone A, Vignali E, Ciampi M, et al. Preoperative localization of suspicious parathyroid adenomas by assay of parathyroid hormone in needle aspirates. Eur J Endocrinol. 1998;139(1):72–7.
32. McCoy KL, Yim JH, Zuckerbraun BS, Ogilvie JB, Peel RL, Carty SE. Cystic parathyroid lesions: functional and nonfunctional parathyroid cysts. Arch Surg. 2009;144(1):52–6. discussion 56.
33. Cappelli C, Rotondi M, Pirola I, De Martino E, Leporati P, Magri F, et al. Prevalence of parathyroid cysts by neck ultrasound scan in unselected patients. J Endocrinol Invest. 2009;32(4):357–9.
34. Ritter H, Milas M. Parathyroidectomy: bilateral neck exploration. In: Terris D, editor. Operative techniques in otolaryngology. St. Louis, MO: Elsevier; 2009. p. 44–53.
35. Graff-Baker A, Roman SA, Boffa D, Aslanian H, Sosa JA. Diagnosis of ectopic middle mediastinal parathyroid adenoma using endoscopic ultrasonography—guided fine-needle aspiration with real-time rapid parathyroid hormone assay. J Am Coll Surg. 2009;209(3):e1–4.
36. Haber RS, Kim CK, Inabnet WB. Ultrasonography for preoperative localization of enlarged parathyroid glands in primary hyperparathyroidism: comparison with 99mtechnetium sestamibi scintigraphy. Clin Endocrinol (Oxf). 2002;57(2):241–9.
37. Jabiev AA, Lew JI, Solorzano CA. Surgeon-performed ultrasound: a single institution experience in parathyroid localization. Surgery. 2009;146(4):569–77.
38. Siperstein A, Berber E, Wagner K, Alghoul M, Stephen A, Milas M. Prospective evaluation of sestamibi, ultrasound, and rapid PTH to predict the success of limited exploration for sporadic primary hyperparathyroidism. Surgery. 2004;136:872–80.
39. Sharma J, Mazzaglia P, Milas M, Berber E, Schuster D, Halkar R, et al. Radionuclide imaging for hyperparathyrodism: which is the best ^{99}tc-sestamibi modality? Surgery. 2006;140:856–65.
40. Siperstein A, Berber E, Barbosa G, Tsinberg M, Greene A, Mitchell J, et al. Predicting success of limited exploration for primary hyperparathyroidism using ultrasound, sestamibi scan, and intraoperative PTH: analysis of 1,055 cases. Ann Surg. 2008;248(3): 420–8.
41. Rodgers SE, Hunter GJ, Hamberg LM, Schellingerhout D, Doherty DB, Ayers GD, et al. Improved preoperative planning for directed parathyroidectomy with 4-dimensional computed tomography. Surgery. 2006;140(6):932–40. discussion 940–1.
42. Tublin ME, Pryma DA, Yim JH, Ogilvie JB, Mountz JM, Bencherif B, et al. Localization of parathyroid adenomas by sonography and technetium tc 99 m sestamibi single-photon emission computed tomography before minimally invasive parathyroidectomy: are both studies really needed? J Ultrasound Med. 2009;28(2):183–90.
43. Lumachi F, Zucchetta P, Marzola MC, Boccagni P, Angelini F, Bui F, et al. Advantages of combined technetium-99 m-sestamibi scintigraphy and high-resolution ultrasonography in parathyroid localization: comparative study in 91 patients with primary hyperparathyroidism. Eur J Endocrinol. 2000;143(6): 755–60.
44. Yen TW, Wang TS, Doffek KM, Krzywda EA, Wilson SD. Reoperative parathyroidectomy: an algorithm for imaging and monitoring of intraoperative parathyroid hormone levels that results in a successful focused approach. Surgery. 2008;144(4):611–9. discussion 619–21.
45. Feingold DL, Alexander HR, Chen CC, Libutti SK, Shawker TH, Simonds WF, et al. Ultrasound and sestamibi scan as the only preoperative imaging tests in reoperation for parathyroid adenomas. Surgery. 2000;128(6):1103–9. discussion 1109–10.
46. Richards ML, Thompson GB, Farley DR, Grant CS. Reoperative parathyroidectomy in 228 patients during the era of minimal-access surgery and intraoperative parathyroid hormone monitoring. Am J Surg. 2008;196(6):937–42. discussion 942–3.

47. Powell AC, Alexander HR, Chang R, Marx SJ, Skarulis M, Pingpank JF, et al. Reoperation for parathyroid adenoma: a contemporary experience. Surgery. 2009;146(6):1144–55.
48. Heller KS, Attie JN, Dubner S. Parathyroid localization: inability to predict multigland involvement. Am J Surg. 1993;166:357–9.
49. Gul K, Ozdemir D, Korukluoglu B, Ersoy PE, Aydin R, Ugras SN, et al. Evaluation of preoperative and postoperative thyroid pathologies in patients operated for primary hyperparathyroidism. Endocr Pract. 2009;24:1–18.
50. Morita SY, Somervell H, Umbricht CB, Dackiw AP, Zeiger MA. Evaluation for concomitant thyroid nodules and primary hyperparathyroidism in patients undergoing parathyroidectomy or thyroidectomy. Surgery. 2008;144(6):862–6. discussion 866–8.
51. Milas M, Alghoul M, Berber E, Stephen A, Mensah A, Siperstein A, et al. Impact of office neck ultrasonography on reducing unnecessary thyroid surgery in patients undergoing parathyroidectomy. Thyroid. 2005;15:1055–9.
52. Carneiro-Pla D. Effectiveness of "office"-based, ultrasound-guided differential jugular venous sampling (DJVS) of parathormone in patients with primary hyperparathyroidism. Surgery. 2009;146(6): 1014–20.
53. Veldman MW, Reading CC, Farrell MA, Mullan BP, Wermers RA, Grant CS, et al. Percutaneous parathyroid ethanol ablation in patients with multiple endocrine neoplasia type 1. AJR Am J Roentgenol. 2008; 191(6):1740–4.
54. Eisenberg H, Pallotta J, Sacks B, Brickman AS. Parathyroid localization, three-dimensional modeling, and percutaneous ablation techniques. Endocrinol Metab Clin North Am. 1989;18(3):659–700.
55. Montenegro FL, Chammas MC, Juliano AG, Cernea CR, Cordeiro AC. Ethanol injection under ultrasound guidance to palliate unresectable parathyroid carcinoma. Arq Bras Endocrinol Metabol. 2008;52(4): 707–11.
56. Cappelli C, Pelizzari G, Pirola I, Gandossi E, De Martino E, Delbarba A, et al. Modified percutaneous ethanol injection of parathyroid adenoma in primary hyperparathyroidism. QJM. 2008;101(8):657–62.
57. Berber E, Parikh R, Ballem N, Garner C, Milas M, Siperstein A. Why parathyroid localization studies fail: analysis of 1,000 patients. Surgery. 2008;144: 74–9.
58. Davis ML, Quayle FJ, Middleton WD, Acosta LM, Hix-Hernandez SJ, Snyder SK, et al. Ultrasound facilitates minimally invasive parathyroidectomy in patients lacking definitive localization from preoperative sestamibi scan. Am J Surg. 2007;194(6):785–90. discussion 790.
59. Kawata R, Kotetsu L, Takamaki A, Yoshimura K, Takenaka H. Ultrasonography for preoperative localization of enlarged parathyroid glands in secondary hyperparathyroidism. Auris Nasus Larynx. 2009; 36(4):461–5.
60. Vulpio C, Bossola M, De Gaetano A, Maresca G, Di Stasio E, Spada PL, et al. Ultrasound patterns of parathyroid glands in chronic hemodialysis patients with secondary hyperparathyroidism. Am J Nephrol. 2008; 28(4):589–97.
61. Hollenbeak CS, Lendel I, Beus KS, Ruda JM, Stack Jr BC. The cost of screening for synchronous thyroid disease in patients presenting with primary hyperparathyroidism. Arch Otolaryngol Head Neck Surg. 2007;133(10):1013–21.
62. Fine IJ. Parathyroid imaging: its current status and future role. Semin Nucl Med. 1987;17(4):350–9.

Imaging in Parathyroid Diseases

19

Donald R. Neumann and Joyce J. Shin

Abstract

Preoperative imaging studies play an important role in providing successful localization of parathyroid lesions and their use has increased and parallels the recent growth of minimally invasive parathyroidectomy. The development of simple, noninvasive imaging studies and the increasingly popular surgical technique known as minimally invasive parathyroidectomy have greatly expanded the role of preoperative localization procedures. A variety of anatomic and functional imaging techniques can be used to localize parathyroid lesions, including ultrasound, MRI (magnetic resonance imaging), CT, and scintigraphy. The diagnostic imaging algorithms vary between institutions based on local availability and clinical expertise. Initial imaging usually includes ultrasonography and parathyroid scintigraphy. In the evaluation of hyperparathyroidism, tomographic SPECT imaging has been shown to have incremental value over planar scintigraphy for parathyroid lesion localization. MRI and contrast-enhanced CT are usually reserved for problem-solving when initial imaging studies are negative, equivocal or contradictory.

Keywords

Parathyroidectomy • Ultrasonography • Computed tomography • Magnetic resonance imaging • Doppler ultrasonography • Hypoechoic • Selenium • Thallium • SPECT (single photon emission computed tomography) • Parathyroid • Hyperparathyroidism • Imaging

D.R. Neumann, MD, PhD (✉)
Department of Nuclear Medicine,
Cleveland Clinic Imaging Institute,
9500 Euclid Avenue, Jb3, Cleveland, OH 44195, USA
e-mail: neumand@ccf.org

J.J. Shin, MD
Department of Endocrine Surgery,
Endocrinology & Metabolism Institute,
9500 Euclid Avenue, F20, Cleveland, OH 44195, USA

Introduction

Hyperparathyroidism is an endocrine disorder resulting from the overproduction of parathyroid hormone. This excess production of parathormone (PTH) results in hypercalcemia. The most common cause of hyperparathyroidism is a solitary parathyroid adenoma in approximately 85% of

A.A. Licata and E.V. Lerma (eds.), *Diseases of the Parathyroid Glands*,
DOI 10.1007/978-1-4419-5550-0_19, © Springer Science+Business Media, LLC 2012

cases. Less commonly, hyperplasia of all parathyroid glands (13–15%) or double parathyroid adenomas (1–4%) are responsible. Parathyroid carcinoma is a rare cause, typically found in less than 1% in many series [1–4].

Primary hyperparathyroidism is a common endocrinopathy, reported to affect approximately 1 in 1,000 older adults in the general population. Since the advent of preoperative image-based techniques for the localization of pathologic parathyroid glands, the management of primary hyperparathyroidism has changed significantly.

Secondary hyperparathyroidism occurs in response to insufficient levels of calcium, vitamin D, or both. It is usually due to multiglandular parathyroid hyperplasia, although parathyroid adenomas may develop in rare instances. Patients have elevated serum PTH levels and low to normal serum calcium concentrations. The most common underlying cause is end-stage renal failure, with vitamin D deficiency and malabsorption syndromes being less common causes. Medical management is the mainstay of treatment, but surgery may be indicated in severe cases. Prolonged hypocalcemia and hyperphosphatemia, which can occur in end-stage renal disease, may result in the autonomous PTH secretion and subsequent development of hypercalcemia, known as tertiary hyperparathyroidism.

Although hyperparathyroidism can be managed conservatively if the patient's condition is stable, parathyroidectomy is the treatment of choice for patients with primary hyperparathyroidism and may be indicated for patients with secondary or tertiary hyperparathyroidism if they do not respond to medical therapy [5]. Preoperative imaging studies play an important role in providing successful localization of parathyroid lesions, and their use has increased and parallels the recent growth of minimally invasive parathyroidectomy. The development of simple, noninvasive imaging studies and the increasingly popular surgical technique known as minimally invasive parathyroidectomy have greatly expanded the role of preoperative localization procedures [6]. A variety of anatomic and functional imaging techniques can be used to localize parathyroid lesions, including ultrasound, MRI (magnetic resonance imaging), CT, and scintigraphy.

Minimally Invasive Parathyroid Surgery (Please Refer to Chapter on Surgical Management of Parathyroid Diseases for Further Discussion)

Until the mid 1990s, the standard surgical procedure for patients undergoing an initial operation for primary hyperparathyroidism was a bilateral neck dissection and four-gland exploration to identify the pathologic parathyroid gland(s) under general anesthesia. Over the past several years, however, parathyroid surgery has changed dramatically. With the evolution of accurate localization imaging studies and the introduction of intraoperative parathyroid monitoring techniques, limited parathyroid explorations are now far more common. Currently, minimally invasive surgical approach is becoming more common than the more traditional bilateral neck exploration. This minimally invasive approach can be done as outpatient surgery, and often with the use of either local anesthesia or cervical block anesthesia. This shift in surgical treatment is in part due to the improvement of preoperative imaging studies and the development of rapid intraoperative parathyroid hormone (ioPTH) level assay [7, 8].

Typically, the minimally invasive approach involves a unilateral neck exploration and identification of both ipsilateral superior and inferior parathyroid glands [9]. The ability to perform minimally invasive parathyroidectomy has, in part, resulted from the development of more sophisticated imaging modalities. An essential component of this focused surgical approach is the accurate and reliable preoperative localization of parathyroid pathology. Successful preoperative localization permits such a focused surgical approach, thereby decreasing morbidity by avoiding injury to the recurrent laryngeal nerve and normal parathyroid glands [10]. Measurement of ioPTH levels helps determine when hyperfunctioning parathyroid glands have been removed, decreasing failure in patients with multiglandular disease.

Minimally invasive surgical procedures have decreased cost, lower associated rates of morbidity and mortality, and reduced operation time, recovery time, and hospital stay compared to routine bilateral neck explorations [11, 12].

Parathyroid Anatomy, Embryology, and Histology

Knowledge of parathyroid anatomy and embryology is essential for accurate interpretation of various parathyroid imaging modalities. The parathyroid glands are small ellipsoid structures that are generally located immediately dorsal to both thyroid lobes. The normal parathyroid gland measures approximately 5–7 mm in length and 3–4 mm in breadth, weighing approximately 40–60 mg [13]. The parathyroid glands are typically four in number, and are derived from the third and fourth pharyngeal pouches [14].

The superior glands, arising from the fourth pharyngeal pouch, descend from the base of the tongue along with the superior pole of the thyroid gland, eventually coming to lie midway along the posterior border of the thyroid lobe [15]. The location of the superior parathyroid glands is relatively constant, but may prolapse inferiorly, descending behind the midpole of the thyroid or even more inferiorly, typically along the tracheoesophageal groove.

The inferior parathyroid glands, arising from the third pharyngeal pouch, migrate caudally along with the thymus. The location of the inferior glands is considerably more variable than that of the superior glands. The inferior parathyroid glands can be found anywhere from above the carotid bifurcation to the inferior mediastinum. In approximately 40% of the population, these glands are located near the lower poles of the thyroid gland. In another 40%, they are located near the thymic tongue. In 20% of the population, they may be located at any of several sites: at the angle of the mandible, in the retroesophageal and pretracheal regions, along the tracheoesophageal groove, and even in the pericardium [16, 17].

Histologically, the normal parathyroid gland is composed of equal amounts of parenchyma, which consists of interconnecting columns of cells and stroma. The stroma, made of adipose tissue having an abundant vascular supply, provides support for the parenchymal cells. Normal parathyroid parenchyma is composed of two cell types: chief cells and oxyphil cells [18]. The chief, or principal, cells make up the majority of the parenchyma and are responsible for most of the parathyroid hormonal secretion. Oxyphil cells are usually not present until 5–7 years of age and gradually increase in number after puberty. Oxyphil cells are eosinophilic and contain abundant mitochondria, but do not typically possess a significant secretory function. The number of oxyphil cells and amount of adipose tissue tend to increase with age.

Ultrasonography (Please Refer to Chapter on Ultrasonography in Parathyroid Diseases for Further Discussion)

Since the late 1970s, ultrasonography has been used to localize abnormal parathyroid glands [19]. However, its full potential as a powerful imaging modality was recognized in the 1990s with advances in technology [20–22]. Ultrasound as a reliable and accurate preoperative localizing test, in part, led to a paradigm shift in the surgical management of primary hyperparathyroidism, where the availability of localizing studies and intraoperative rapid parathyroid hormone assay allowed surgeons to move away from traditional bilateral parathyroid exploration and perform focused parathyroidectomy [10, 23, 24].

Ultrasound is currently one of the most commonly used techniques for preoperative localization of parathyroid adenomas. The advantages of this imaging modality include low cost, convenience, lack of radiation exposure, precise real-time anatomic detail for facilitation of surgical planning, and ability to detect concomitant thyroid pathology. Recent studies have reported sensitivity and positive predictive value ranging as high as 70–96% and 90–98%, respectively, and have advocated the use of ultrasound as the only localizing study in the management of primary hyperparathyroidism [25–28]. However, to achieve

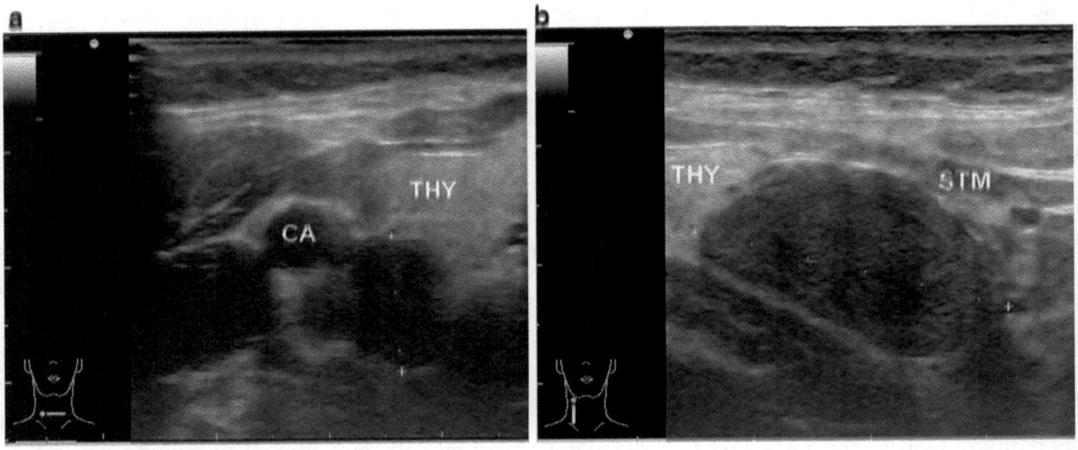

Fig. 19.1 Transverse (**a**) and longitudinal (**b**) ultrasonographic views of an abnormal upper parathyroid gland, located on the posteromedial aspect of the thyroid. When enlarged, it appears as an oval mass with a homogeneous, hypoechoic echotexture. The carotid artery (CA), thyroid gland (THY), and sternothyroid muscle (STM) are marked

these high success rates, it must be performed by skilled and experienced sonographers with extensive knowledge of the cervical anatomy.

Parathyroid ultrasound examination is performed with the patient in a supine position with the neck gently extended. This position aids in the visualization of deeply located parathyroid glands and allows elevation of mediastinal structures. The optimal ultrasound system consists of a high-resolution, real-time ultrasound with both gray scale and color Doppler resolution and a high-frequently transducer (linear or small curvilinear) of 7.5–15 MHz. Color Doppler sonography allows identification of the feeding vessels supplying the parathyroid adenomas, which is useful in differentiating parathyroid glands from other cervical structures [21]. Ultrasound examination should follow a routine and systematic fashion so that all regions of the neck are fully evaluated, first focusing on the region of the thyroid and central neck compartment in transverse and longitudinal planes. Abnormal parathyroids can be found along the posterior border of the thyroid gland (Fig. 19.1) and in the pretracheal, paratracheal, and retroesophageal spaces. The lateral cervical regions (carotid artery and jugular vein), as well as the superior (submandibular gland) and inferior (innominate vessels) aspects of the neck, should also be examined, where ectopic adenomas may be located [29]. Swallowing maneuvers can help separate parathyroid adenomas from the thyroid gland, especially those that are posteriorly located, and also help visualize lesions in the upper mediastinum or cervical thymus [30]. The probe can also be angled inferiorly to identify parathyroids below the sternal notch.

Most individuals have four parathyroid glands, but the percentage of individuals with supernumerary glands varies from 2.5 to 13% [31]. Normal parathyroid glands are typically not seen on ultrasound because they are small (approximately 5×3×1 mm) and have insufficient acoustic difference from surrounding tissues [29]. The superior parathyroids are located on the posteromedial aspect of the thyroid gland near the tracheoesophageal groove, whereas the inferior parathyroids are more widely distributed. They are usually inferior or just posterior to the lower pole of the thyroid and anterior to the superior parathyroid gland and recurrent laryngeal nerve. When enlarged, parathyroids appear typically as an oval or triangular mass with a homogeneous hypoechoic texture and a hyperechoic rim of adventitia (Fig. 19.2). They usually have sharp borders; lesions with irregular borders are suspicious for carcinoma. Microcalcifications may be seen within parathyroid tissue, particularly in patients with secondary and tertiary hyperparathyroidism [29, 30]. Because parathyroid glands have a distinct blood supply (branch of the inferior thyroid artery in 80% of

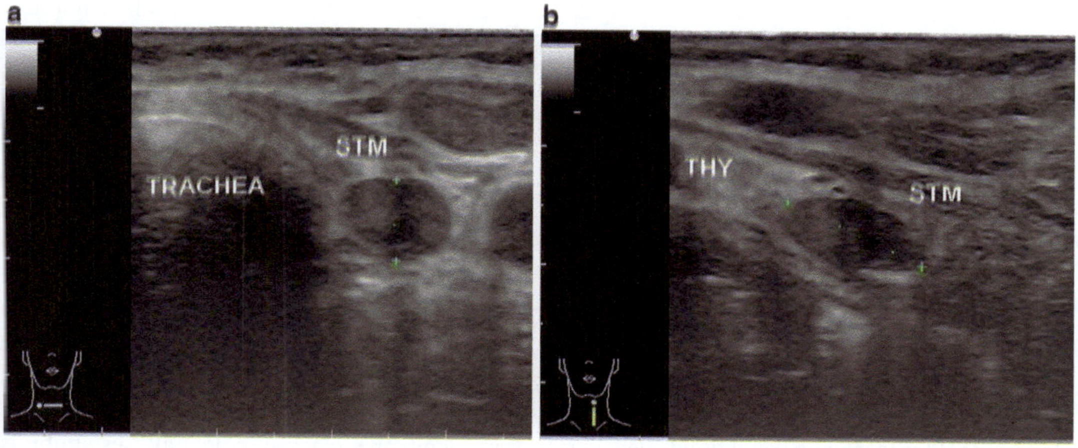

Fig. 19.2 Typical sonographic appearance of an enlarged lower parathyroid gland in transverse (**a**) and longitudinal (**b**) views. It is located inferior to the lower pole of the thyroid gland (THY) and deep to the sternothyroid muscle (STM)

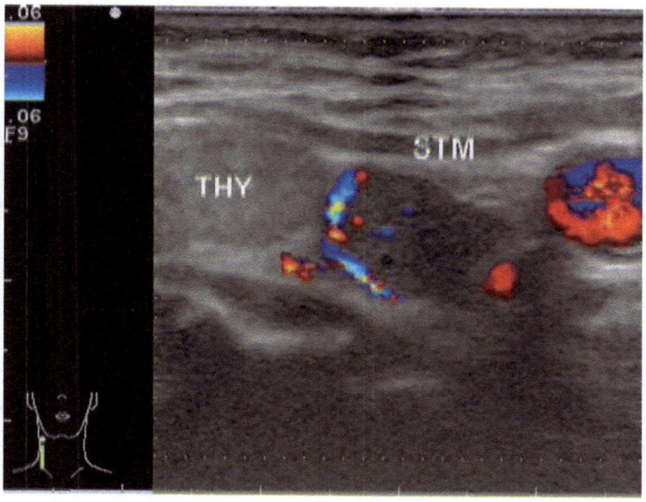

Fig. 19.3 Ultrasonographic demonstration of an arclike vascular pedicle at the superior aspect of an abnormal parathyroid gland. This configuration differs from the central hilar vascular flow pattern of lymph nodes. The thyroid gland (THY) and sternothyroid muscle (STM) are marked

the cases), color Doppler ultrasound can help differentiate parathyroids from lymph nodes. The parathyroid vascular pedicle, which can have a tortuous or arclike configuration, can be seen entering the parathyroid gland, in contrast to the central hilar branching vascular flow pattern of lymph nodes (Fig. 19.3) [21, 27, 30].

When the normal anatomic locations for parathyroid glands are imaged and do not reveal an abnormal parathyroid adenoma, the variable and potential ectopic sites should be examined. The common ectopic locations are in the thyrothymic ligament, on the prevertebral fascia, in a retroesophageal, paraesophageal, or paratracheal position, in the carotid sheath, within the thyroid gland, and in the anterior, or less commonly, in the posterior mediastinum. Intrathyroidal parathyroid glands may be difficult to distinguish from thyroid nodules. However, ultrasound-guided fine-needle aspiration biopsy for cytology and parathyroid hormone assay can be used for diagnostic purposes.

Although parathyroid ultrasound has many useful qualities as a localizing modality, it also has limitations. The accuracy of this technique is highly dependent on the skill and experience of the sonographer. Additionally, ultrasound is limited in its ability to detect multigland parathyroid disease and ectopic parathyroid adenomas, particularly those located in the mediastinum [10, 24]. Other factors have been shown to affect the accuracy of parathyroid ultrasound, which include concomitant thyroid disease, neck thickness, body mass index, gland size, and scarring from prior neck surgeries [10, 24, 27, 32]. Even with these shortcomings, ultrasonography in experienced hands can serve as an accurate, cost-effective tool for localizing parathyroid adenomas.

Parathyroid Scintigraphy

Parathyroid glands are able to concentrate a variety of chemical substances, including vital dyes and several radiopharmaceuticals, and this property has been exploited for localization purposes. Selenium-75-methionine, an amino acid analog of methionine, and thallium-201 are of historical interest. Their use was abandoned because of relatively poor image quality and technical limitations that led to suboptimal diagnostic accuracy.

The first radiotracer to gain widespread acceptance for parathyroid imaging was Tl-201 thallous chloride, which was introduced in the early 1980s. Originally employed for myocardial perfusion imaging, Tl-201 is an inorganic cationic analog of potassium. With the aid of the sodium–potassium ATPase pump, Tl-201 is actively transported into cells where it is rapidly integrated into the intracellular potassium pool. Thallium accumulates in parathyroid tissue and thyroid tissue as well, and consequently distinction from thyroid activity is required to identify parathyroid Tl-201 activity. This is usually accomplished by the administration of either Tc-99m pertechnetate or I-123 sodium iodide, which accumulate in thyroid tissue but not in the parathyroid glands. The Tl-201 and thyroid radiotracer images can be acquired either sequentially or simultaneously, followed by subtraction of the thyroid marker from the Tl-201 image. Postsubtraction residual activity represents activity in abnormal parathyroid tissue.

Currently, Tc-99m-sestamibi is the radiotracer of choice for parathyroid scintigraphy.

In 1989, Coakley and coworkers reported on the use of Tc-99m sestamibi (methoxyisobutylisonitrile) for parathyroid imaging [33]. Because of its superior image quality, more favorable radiation dosimetry, and improved accuracy, Tc-99m sestamibi rapidly replaced Tl-201 as the radiopharmaceutical of choice for parathyroid scintigraphy.

Sestamibi is a lipophilic, monovalent cationic isonitrile compound that diffuses passively across the cell membrane. Because of the large negative transmembrane electric potential, sestamibi is primarily sequestered in the mitochondria and trapped intracellularly [34–36].

Over the years, many different methods of performing parathyroid imaging with sestamibi have been suggested. One of the first proposed methods was introduced by Taillefer and coworkers, referred to as the "single-isotope, double-phase technique" [37]. This technique is based on the observation that sestamibi tends to clear more rapidly from the thyroid than from abnormal parathyroid tissue. The retention of sestamibi in parathyroid lesions is presumably related to the presence of oxyphil cells in these lesions [38]. Oxyphil cells are rich in mitochondria, which are the site of sestamibi sequestration.

This single-isotope double-phase technique is relatively easy to perform, requiring only a single injection of Tc-99m sestamibi followed by imaging approximately 15 min and 1.5–3 h later. A persistent focus of activity on the delayed images, relative to the thyroid activity, is indicative of a parathyroid lesion (Fig. 19.4). The sensitivity of double-phase sestamibi imaging typically ranges from 62 to 90% for solitary parathyroid adenomas and 15 to 50% for multigland disease [39].

There are several limitations to sestamibi scintigraphy, however. For example, images that are limited to the lower neck may overlook ectopic parathyroid lesions. Therefore, scintigraphic images typically extend from the base of the jaw to the apex of the heart.

There are additional limitations of sestamibi imaging. Some parathyroid lesions do not retain sestamibi (Fig. 19.5), whereas some thyroid

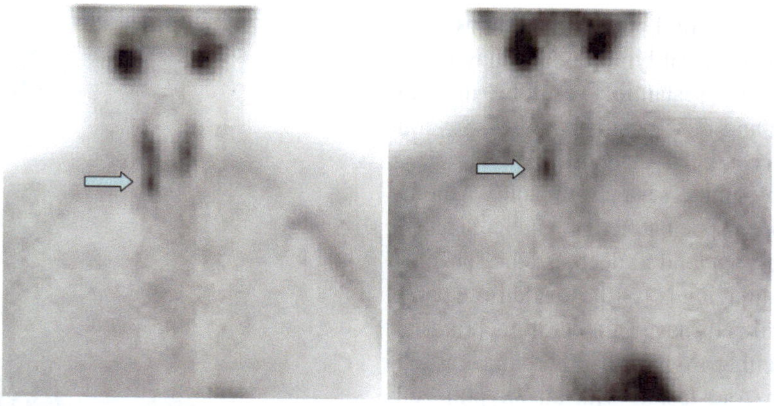

Fig. 19.4 True-positive double-phase sestamibi scan. Focal radiotracer activity in the right superior mediastinum on the early phase (*arrow*, *left image*) shows preferential retention on delayed imaging compared to washout of activity from the thyroid (*arrow*, *right image*). At surgery, a parathyroid adenoma was resected from the right anterior mediastinum

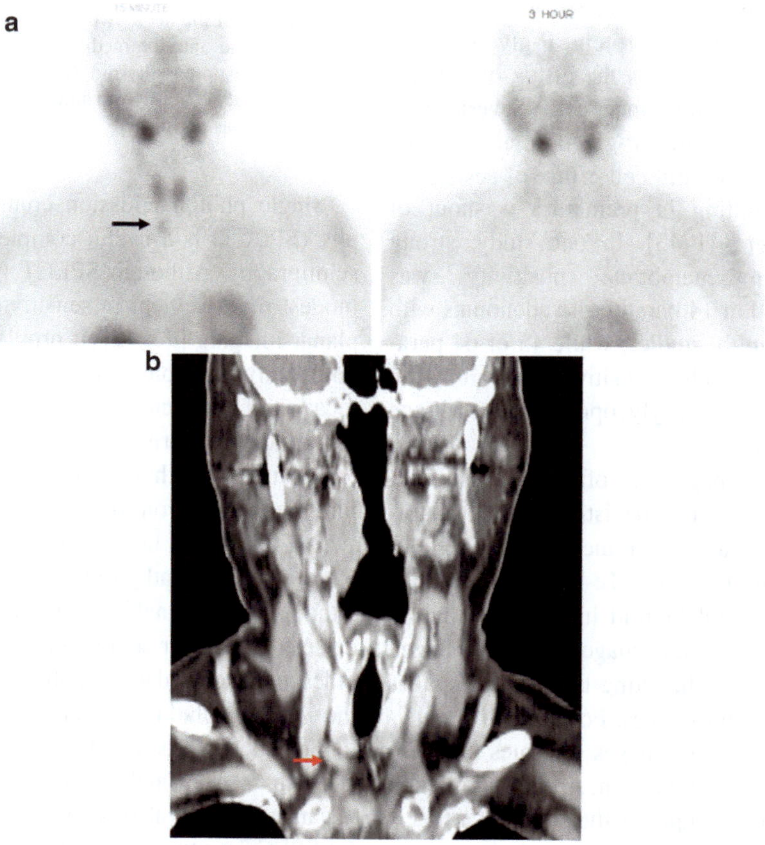

Fig. 19.5 False-negative dual-phase sestamibi scan. (**a**) Focal activity in the right superior mediastinum (*arrow*) is demonstrated on the early postinjection image (*left image*). Delayed imaging at 2 h after radiotracer injection (*right image*) demonstrates clearance of this activity, at a rate similar to that of the nearby thyroid. (**b**) Coronal contrast-enhanced CT tomogram demonstrates an enhancing nodule (*red arrow*) immediately inferior to the lower pole of the right thyroid lobe. Later, at surgery, a parathyroid adenoma was successfully resected from the right superior mediastinum

lesions, such as solid thyroid nodules and thyroiditis, and cervical lymph nodes may accumulate and retain sestamibi, resulting in both false-negative and false-positive studies. Several suggestions have been made to explain false-negative double-phase sestamibi results. Among these, it has been speculated that smaller sizes of parathyroid lesions tend to decrease the sensitivity of nuclear imaging [11, 40]. In addition, parathyroid oxyphil cells have a higher mitochondrial content than either thyroid or other adjacent tissue. A parathyroid lesion with an oxyphil cell predominance is expected to exhibit a higher degree of sestamibi uptake, while a lesion with a chief cell predominance may exhibit less sestamibi accumulation.

It is also speculated that false-negative sestamibi studies might be associated with the presence of an intracellular protein, P-glycoprotein. This lipoprotein increases the efflux of chemotherapeutic drugs from cancer cells. Several studies have suggested that P-glycoprotein may be involved in parathyroid cell efflux of sestamibi, ultimately resulting in premature washout of the radiotracer [41–43]. In one study, strong P-glycoprotein membrane positivity was observed in 10 of 14 parathyroid adenomas with negative sestamibi studies, while 45 of 64 parathyroid lesions with a positive sestamibi scan demonstrated no P-glycoprotein membrane expression [44].

Subtraction imaging is often helpful, especially in patients with coexisting thyroid abnormalities. The subtraction method requires the administration of I-123 or Tc-99m pertechnetate to acquire a digital thyroid image. The thyroid images and sestamibi images are normalized prior to digitally subtracting the thyroid images from the sestamibi images. Focal residual activity on the subtraction images indicates the location of the parathyroid lesion. A major limitation of subtraction techniques is the potential artifacts generated due to patient motion during image acquisition [45]. This type of motion artifact may potentially be avoided by simultaneous, dual-isotope imaging of two different radionuclides, such as the combination of technetium-99m and iodine-123 (Fig. 19.6) [46].

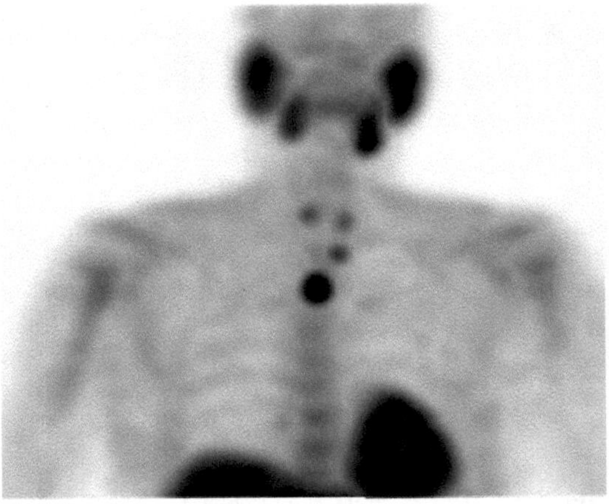

Fig. 19.6 Multiglandular parathyroid hyperplasia. Simultaneous, dual-isotope (I-123/Tc-99m-sestamibi) subtraction imaging. Following the digital subtraction of I-123 activity, the planar image demonstrates the presence of four discrete sites of residual Tc-99m activity: one on the right side of the neck, two in the left side of the neck, and one in the anterior mediastinum. Later, at surgery, four hyperplastic parathyroid glands were resected from these sites, and a parathyroid autotransplant to a left forearm muscle was performed

Single photon emission computed tomography (SPECT) is a useful complement to planar scintigraphy. Although SPECT provides only a modest improvement in sensitivity compared to planar imaging [47–49], it provides information not readily available on planar imaging about the location of a particular abnormality [50, 51]. This tomographic information is useful not only for localizing a parathyroid lesion but also for differentiating a thyroid from a parathyroid lesion.

SPECT is also useful for detecting and localizing ectopic parathyroid lesions. For example, although mediastinal parathyroid lesions may be detected on planar scintigrams, tomography provides more detailed topographic information about the lesion, including its relation to various anatomic structures such as the major salivary glands, sternum, spine, and myocardium. The false-negative rate has also been reported to be lower for SPECT compared to planar imaging [49, 50].

The most frequent cause of false-positive results in sestamibi parathyroid imaging is the solid thyroid nodule, either solitary or in a multinodular thyroid [52]. Other causes of false-positive results include sestamibi accumulation in thyroid carcinoma, thyroiditis, lymphoma, and causes of lymphadenopathy, including metastatic disease, inflammation, and sarcoidosis [46, 53]. Accumulation of sestamibi by brown tumors of hyperparathyroidism has also been observed [54].

Several factors are associated with the failure of sestamibi imaging to identify some parathyroid lesions. Lesion size is certainly important, related to both the spatial resolution of the imaging system and to the total amount of radiotracer uptake by the lesion [55]. Sestamibi tends to be less sensitive for detecting hyperplastic parathyroid glands than for detecting adenomatous lesions.

The presence of mitochondria-rich oxyphil cells presumably accounts for a significant amount of sestamibi uptake in parathyroid lesions. Parathyroid glands with lower concentrations of oxyphil cells, and hence fewer mitochondria, may account for both lower sestamibi uptake and faster washout of sestamibi activity from the parathyroid lesion [36, 38, 56, 57]. Although the mechanism of cellular uptake and retention of sestamibi is not fully elucidated, the lipophilic sestamibi molecule is thought to be concentrated by mitochondria.

In 10–15% of patients, more than one parathyroid lesion is the cause of primary hyperparathyroidism, and data suggests that sestamibi imaging is less sensitive for the detection of multiglandular parathyroid disease [58, 59].

For ectopic parathyroid lesions, sestamibi scanning is much more successful compared to ultrasonography, visualizing those parathyroid lesions in the cervical as well as the mediastinal region with relatively high sensitivity [60]. When ultrasound and sestamibi are positive and both suggest the same site, the accuracy of these combined tests is approximately 90% [61, 62].

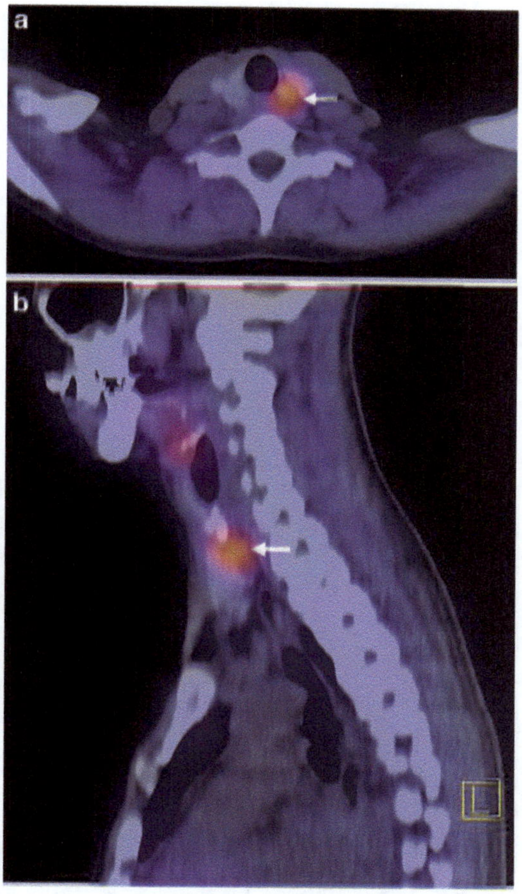

Fig. 19.7 Eutopic parathyroid adenoma. Sestamibi SPECT/CT demonstrates a sestamibi-avid soft tissue nodule (*arrow*) immediately posterior to the superior aspect of the left thyroid lobe. Transverse (**a**) and sagittal (**b**) coregistered SPECT/CT tomograms. Later, a parathyroid adenoma was surgically resected from this site

SPECT/CT

SPECT/CT is a recently developed hybrid imaging modality that combines nuclear medicine and CT technology into a single physically integrated instrument. Both the CT and the SPECT acquisition can be performed in a single imaging session without moving the patient from the imaging bed, providing for near-perfect registration of the SPECT and the CT images (Fig. 19.7). The CT portion provides the structural map to accurately localize the radiotracer uptake demonstrated on the SPECT images. CT provides the added benefit of providing the information needed to correct the effects of tissue attenuation of the single photon emissions. Attenuation correction, in turn, improves the sensitivity for the detection of deeper lesions and also providing the potential to quantitate local radiotracer concentration.

Tc-99m sestamibi scanning with SPECT/CT has been the recent focus of investigation and studies have demonstrated an increase in the

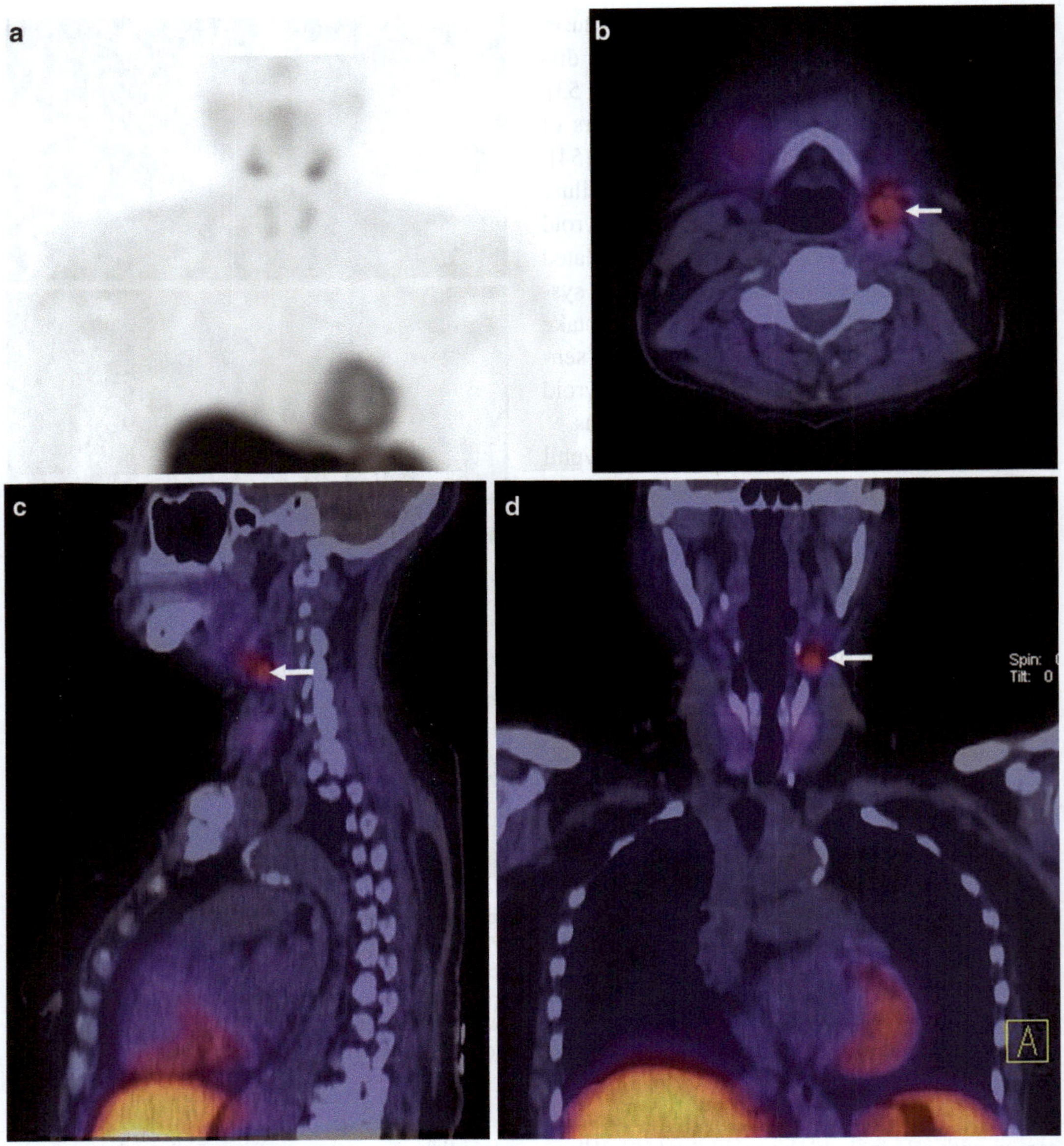

Fig. 19.8 Undescended parathyroid adenoma. (**a**) Planar sestamibi scan appears relatively unremarkable. Sestamibi SPECT/CT demonstrates a sestamibi-avid soft tissue nodule (*arrow*) posterior to the left submandibular gland in the transverse (**b**), sagittal (**c**), and coronal (**d**) planes. A parathyroid adenoma was later surgically resected from this site

detection rate of parathyroid lesions compared to SPECT. SPECT/CT allows visualization of corresponding anatomy, improving the differentiation of abnormal from physiologic sestamibi accumulation (Fig. 19.8). The CT component of SPECT/CT aids in demonstrating the relationship of sestamibi-avid lesions to adjacent anatomic structures (Fig. 19.9). Also important, SPECT/CT improves localization of parathyroid lesions detected in more difficult sites for surgical access, such as retroesophageal adenomas (Fig. 19.10) [63, 64] and mediastinal locations (Figs. 19.11–19.14). In addition, several reports indicate a significant reduction in false-positive findings with SPECT/CT compared to sestamibi SPECT due to the information provided by the CT images [17, 46].

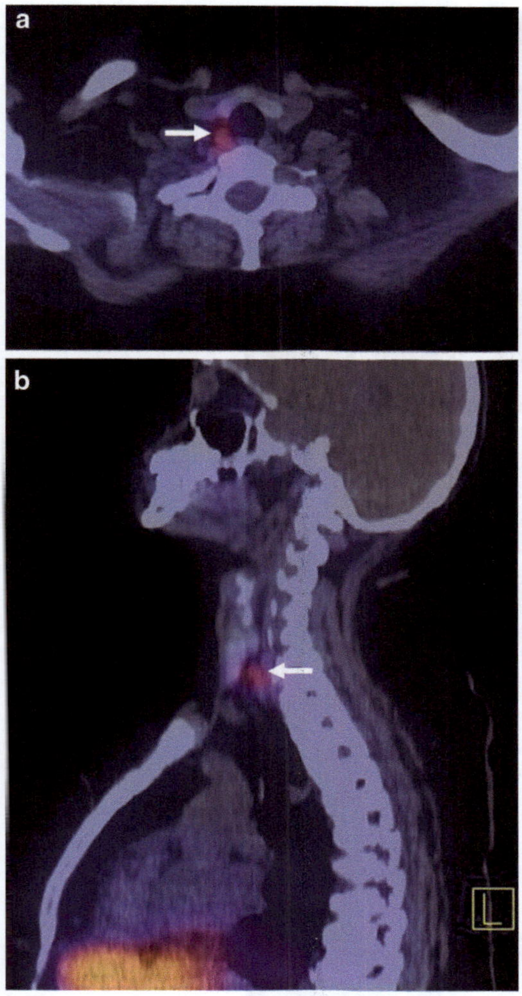

Fig. 19.9 Ectopic parathyroid adenoma (*arrow*) in the right tracheoesophageal groove demonstrated on coregistered sestamibi SPECT/CT tomograms in the transverse (**a**) and sagittal (**b**) planes

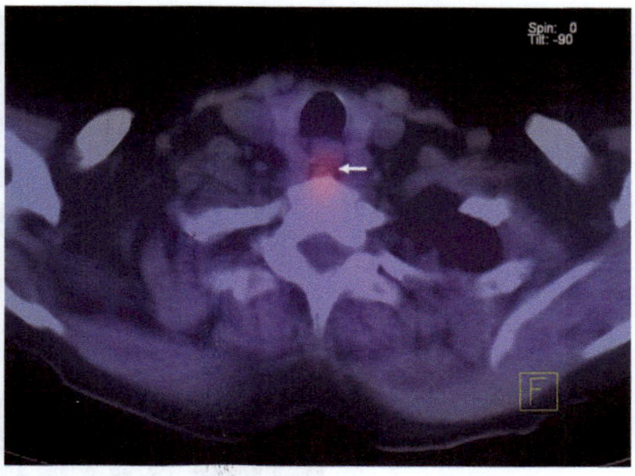

Fig. 19.10 Ectopic retroesophageal parathyroid adenoma (*arrow*) demonstrated on the coregistered transverse sestamibi SPECT/CT tomogram

Computed Tomography

Computed tomography (CT) is not commonly used exclusively for preoperative parathyroid imaging. However, it is occasionally used in conjunction with other imaging modalities to identify enlarged parathyroid glands. In contrast to ultrasonography, CT can examine both the neck and mediastinum. Conventional multirow detector spiral CT imaging for parathyroid localization consists of thin-slice contrast-enhanced imaging from the base of the skull through the superior mediastinum. CT images can be displayed in the transaxial plane, or, by means of multiplanar reconstruction, also be displayed in the sagittal and/or coronal planes, facilitating precise localization of parathyroid lesions and act as a guide for surgical planning (Fig. 19.15).

CT provides contiguous thin-section images, or slices, by obtaining a series of radiographic projections from various angles and reconstructing them in a two-dimensional tomographic fashion. For parathyroid imaging, craniocaudal coverage is obtained from the orbital meatus to 2 cm below the carina.

On conventional single-phase contrast-enhanced CT imaging, density measurements and anatomic location can assist in differentiating parathyroid lesions from lymph nodes and normal thyroid tissue. Parathyroid adenomas are typically seen as well-defined structures having attenuation measurements lower than 80 Hounsfield units (HU), whereas the density of normal thyroid tissue due to its physiologically high iodine content is typically greater than 80 HU [65]. Following the intravenous administration of iodinated radiographic contrast, parathyroid lesions demonstrate intense enhancement greater than 130 HU. This enhancement pattern aids in differentiating parathyroid adenomas from lymph nodes since lymph nodes tend to enhance to a lesser degree, often demonstrating isoenhancement relative to nearby skeletal muscle [66] (Fig. 19.16).

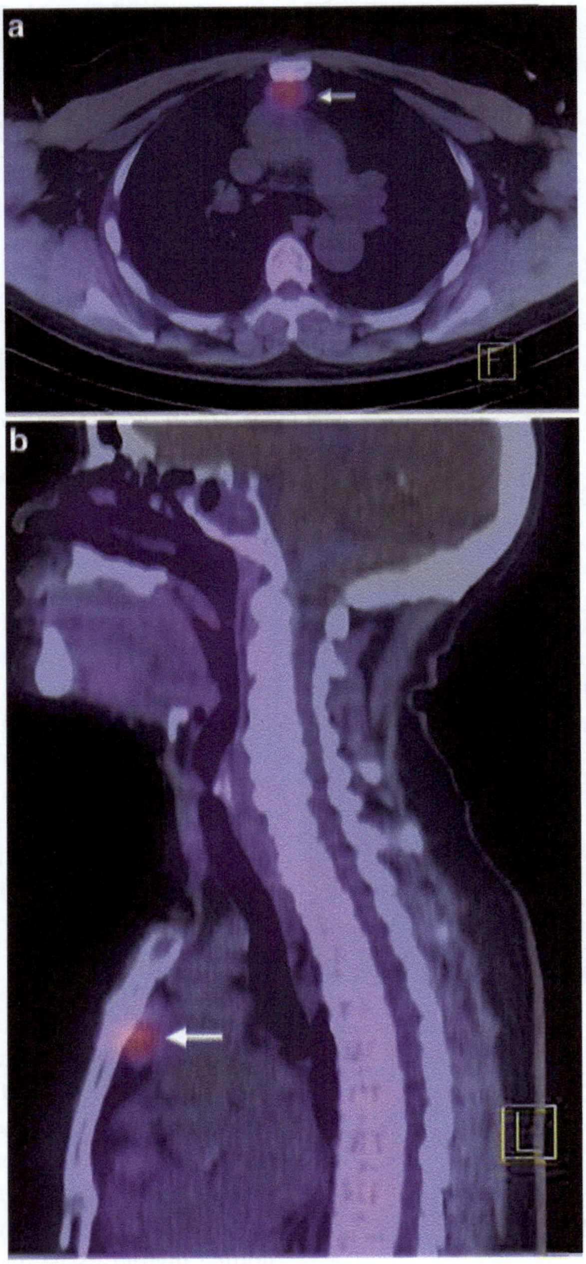

Fig. 19.11 Ectopic parathyroid adenoma (*arrow*) in the anterior superior mediastinum, posterior to the upper sternal body, demonstrated on coregistered sestamibi SPECT/CT tomograms in the transverse (**a**) and sagittal (**b**) planes

In its earlier years, using single-slice instrumentation with relatively thick slice thicknesses, CT had a very low sensitivity for the detection of parathyroid lesions. Recent developments of instrumentation, including multirow detector spiral CT technology with thinner slice collimation and multiplanar reconstruction capability, and improvements in imaging algorithms and scan protocols have increased its sensitivity, reported to range from 46 to 87%. In spite of these improvements, however, the sensitivity of CT still remains lower than both sestamibi and ultrasound [67].

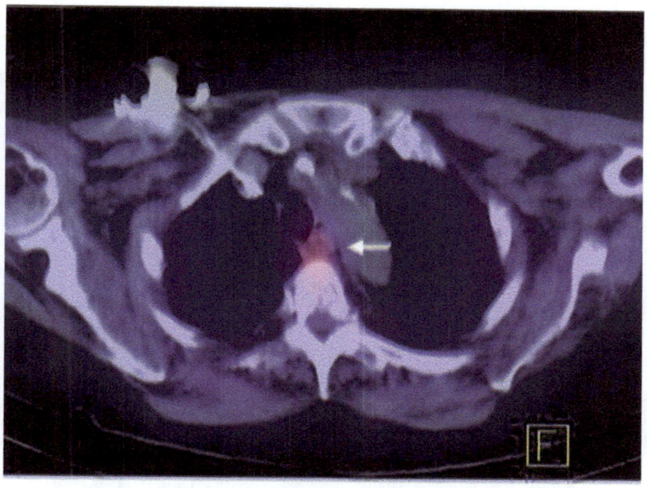

Fig. 19.12 Ectopic parathyroid adenoma (*arrow*) in the posterior mediastinum demonstrated on the transverse sestamibi SPECT/CT. This sestamibi-avid lesion is located anterior to the vertebral body and posterior to the esophagus which shows a small pocket of intraluminal air

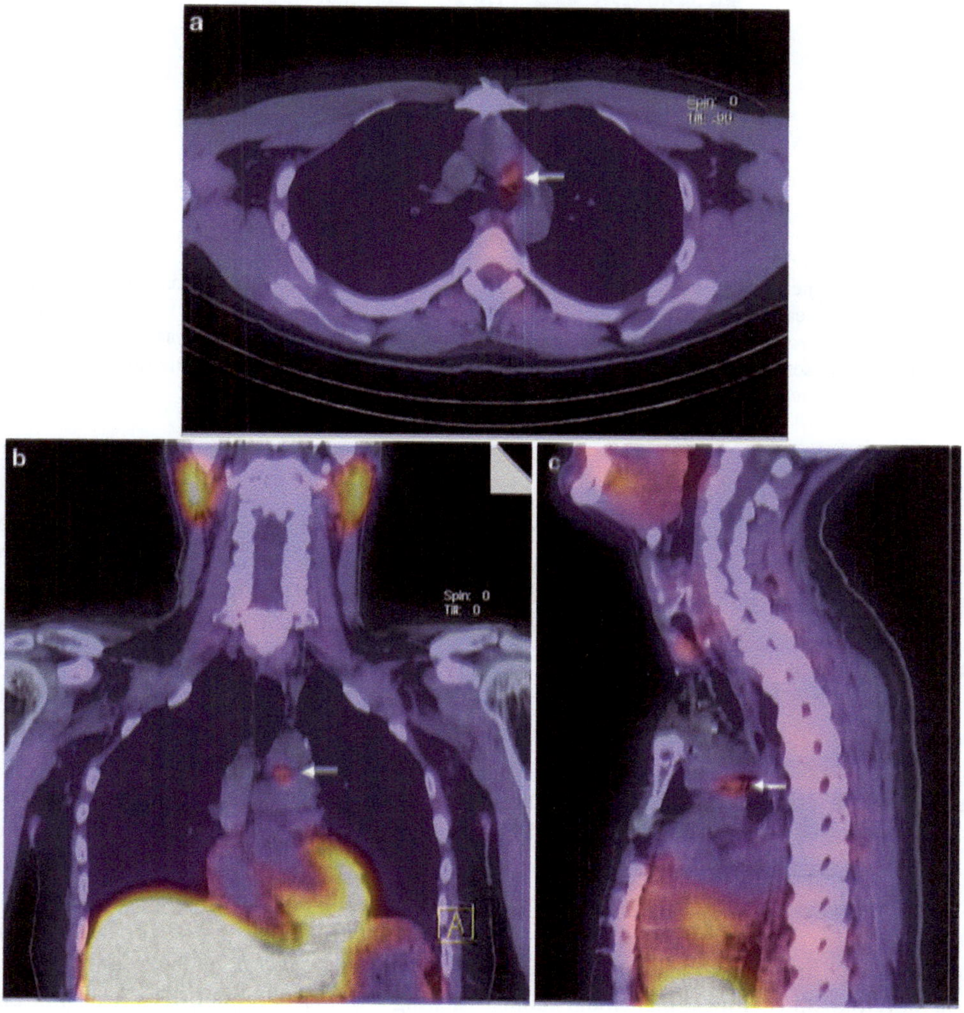

Fig. 19.13 Ectopic parathyroid adenoma (*arrow*) in the aortopulmonary window. Coregistered sestamibi SPECT/CT tomograms in the transverse (**a**), coronal (**b**), and sagittal (**c**) planes

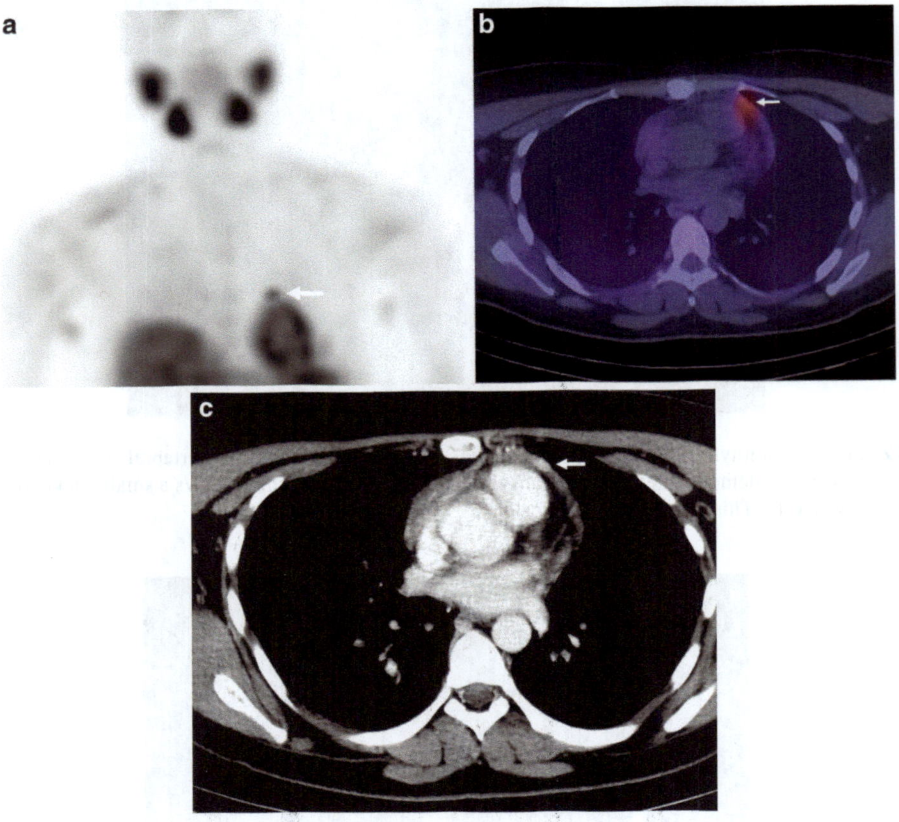

Fig. 19.14 Ectopic pericardial parathyroid adenoma. (**a**) Planar sestamibi scan shows a small focal site of radiotracer activity (*arrow*) just superior to the myocardium (**b**). Transverse sestamibi SPECT/CT shows focal sestamibi activity (*arrow*) associated with the pericardium anteriorly (**c**). Transverse contrast-enhanced CT shows a small enhancing lesion (*arrow*) in the anterior pericardium. A parathyroid adenoma was later resected from this site by minimally invasive robotic surgery

There are several identified limitations of CT for the detection of parathyroid lesions. Among them, CT has been found to have difficulty in identifying parathyroid lesions that are immediately adjacent to the thyroid due to similar enhancement patterns and occasional lack of tissue planes separating the two tissues (Fig. 19.17). In the reoperative patients, surgical clips from previous neck surgery may result in CT streak artifacts that can potentially obscure visualization of parathyroid lesions [68]. In addition, false-positive CT findings may result from contrast-enhancing vessels, lymph nodes, and thyroid nodules.

An emerging method in the evaluation of hyperparathyroidism is "four-dimensional" computed tomography (4D-CT), which provides both functional and detailed anatomic information about parathyroid lesions. In this technique, an initial unenhanced CT scan is obtained. This is followed by an IV contrast injection of 100 mL of nonionic iodinated radiographic contrast material. CT scanning is then repeated at 30, 60, and 90 s after the initiation of IV contrast administration. This results in a total of four 3-dimensional CT data sets. Parathyroid adenomas have been reported to show a characteristic pattern of early enhancement, allowing distinction from normal lymph nodes which show a slower, more progressive rate of enhancement [69]. The sensitivity of 4D-CT for parathyroid lesion localization has been reported as high as 88% in the reoperative setting [70, 71]. Although 4D-CT may be comparable to sestamibi imaging techniques for the

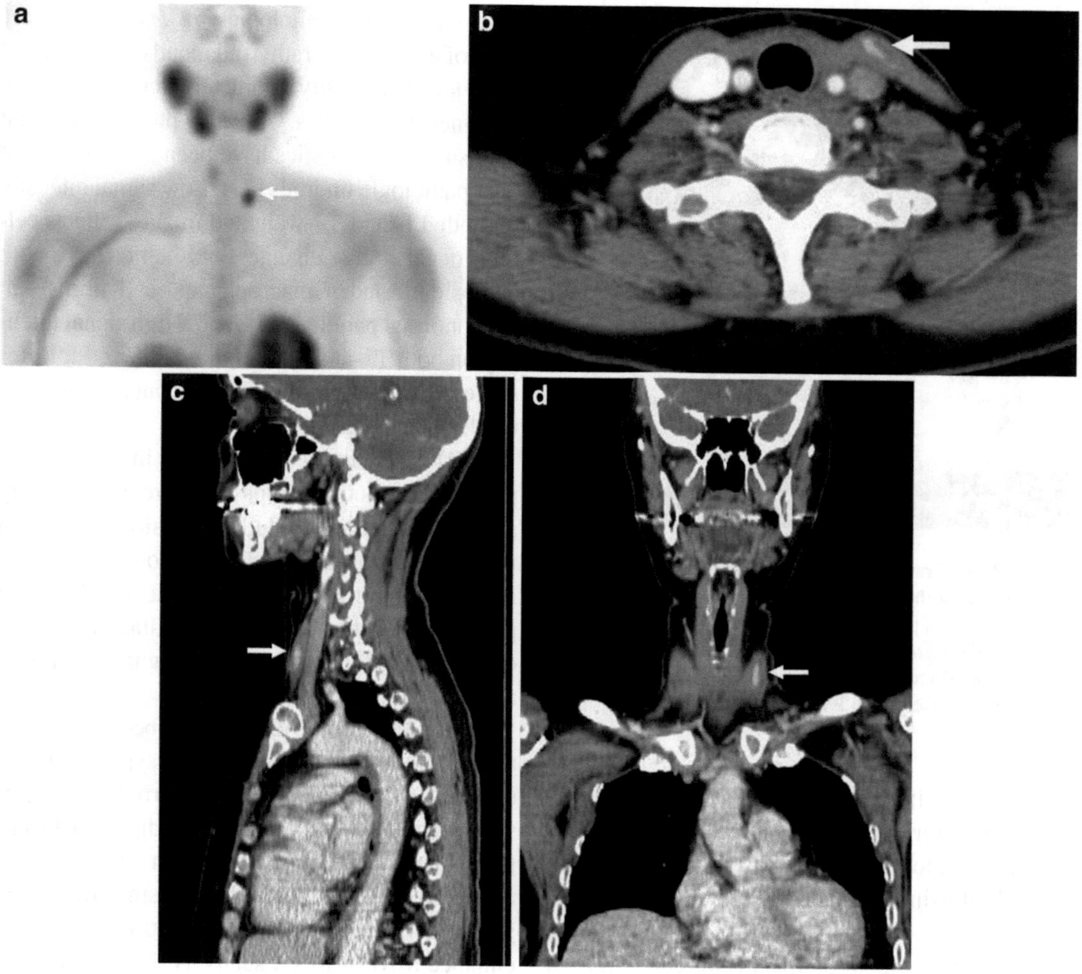

Fig. 19.15 Parathyroid autotransplant in the left sternocleidomastoid muscle. Planar sestamibi scan (**a**) shows focal radiotracer activity in the left neck laterally (*arrow*). Contrast-enhanced CT in the transverse (**b**), sagittal (**c**), and coronal (**d**) planes demonstrates an enhancing lesion (*arrow*) within the inferior portion of the left sternocleidomastoid muscle

detection of abnormal parathyroid tissue, further cost analyses, studies with larger sample sizes, and the resolution of radiation dosimetry concerns are needed before recommending 4D-CT as the imaging modality of choice in the setting of hyperparathyroidism.

Magnetic Resonance Imaging

The role of MRI is limited to parathyroid localization in the setting of persistent or recurrent postoperative hyperparathyroidism. MRI is not associated with ionizing radiation to the patient and can be used to examine both the neck and mediastinum. Multiplanar images are typically obtained from the hyoid bone to the thoracic inlet. In cases of suspected ectopic parathyroid disease, however, MR imaging can be extended further into the superior mediastinum. If needed, MR imaging of the inferior mediastinum can also be performed [72] .

Although normal parathyroid glands are not usually visualized on MRI, in general, parathyroid adenomas exhibit intermediate signal intensity on T1-weighted MR pulse sequences and

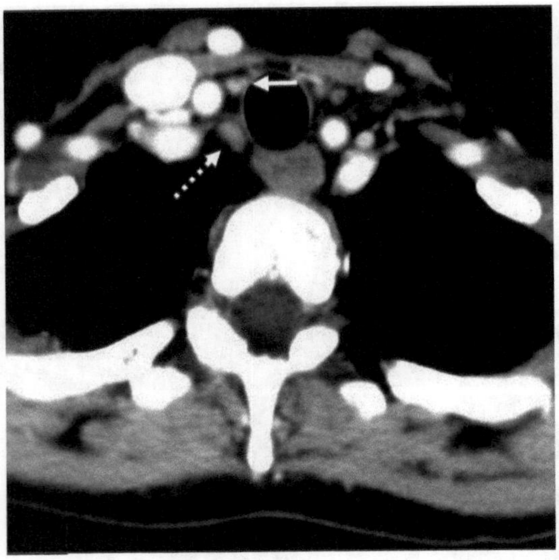

Fig. 19.16 Transverse contrast-enhanced CT image demonstrating the typical difference in contrast enhancement between a parathyroid adenoma (*solid arrow*) and a lymph node (*dashed arrow*), both in the right paratracheal region. Parathyroid adenomas typically enhance earlier and more intensely than lymph nodes

high signal intensity on T2-weighted images [73]. Superior and inferior presaturation pulses are also employed to suppress blood-flow artifact [74]. Following intravenous gadolinium-DTPA, parathyroid adenomas tend to demonstrate intense enhancement on the T1-weighted images compared with the adjacent thyroid gland and skeletal muscle [75] (Fig. 19.18).

Faster MR imaging can be performed using fast spin-echo techniques, which help reduce motion artifact that results from respiration and patient motion. The use of fat suppression pulse sequences has also been suggested as an aid to gadolinium-DTPA enhancement. CT and MRI in the neck show similar accuracy to ultrasonography, all three being modestly less accurate than Tc-99m-sestamibi scanning [73, 76, 77].

In most studies, MRI has not been as successful for parathyroid imaging compared to other imaging modalities. MRI suffers from a relatively high number of false-positive results, including coexistent thyroid pathology, particularly exophytic thyroid nodules, sarcoid nodules, neurofibromas, normal lymph nodes, follicular lymphadenitis, and other lymph node pathologies [78]. Approximately 30% of abnormal parathyroid glands have atypical MRI signal intensity characteristics, resulting in false-negative studies. These atypical MRI signal intensity characteristics have been correlated with histopathologic findings [79]. Low signal intensity on both T1- and T2-weighted images reflects cellular degenerative changes, old hemorrhage with hemosiderin-laden macrophages, and fibrosis in the abnormal parathyroid gland. High signal intensity on both T1-and T2-weighted images indicates acute hemorrhage without significant degenerative or fibrotic changes.

MRI is also limited by artifacts induced by the presence of metallic clips from previous surgery and patient motion, including physiologic motion from respiration and cardiac motion. In addition, MR imaging may be contraindicated in some patients, including those with cardiac pacemaker devices and those with paramagnetic cerebral aneurysm clips.

Also, gadolinium-DTPA has been linked to the development of nephrogenic systemic fibrosis (NSF). This disease has occurred in patients with moderate to end-stage renal disease (thus of particular concern in patients with either secondary or tertiary hyperpararthyroidism) after being given a gadolinium-based contrast agent to enhance MRI or MRA scans. NSF is a debilitating and sometimes fatal disease. Characteristics include red or dark patches on the skin; burning, itching, swelling, hardening, and tightening of the skin; yellow spots on the conjunctiva; joint stiffness; and muscle weakness [80].

Conclusion

A variety of imaging modalities and techniques are available for guiding accurate preoperative localization of parathyroid pathology in patients with hyperparathyroidism. The diagnostic imaging algorithms vary between institutions based on local availability and clinical expertise. Initial imaging usually includes ultrasonography and parathyroid scintigraphy. In the evaluation of hyperparathyroidism, tomographic SPECT imaging has been

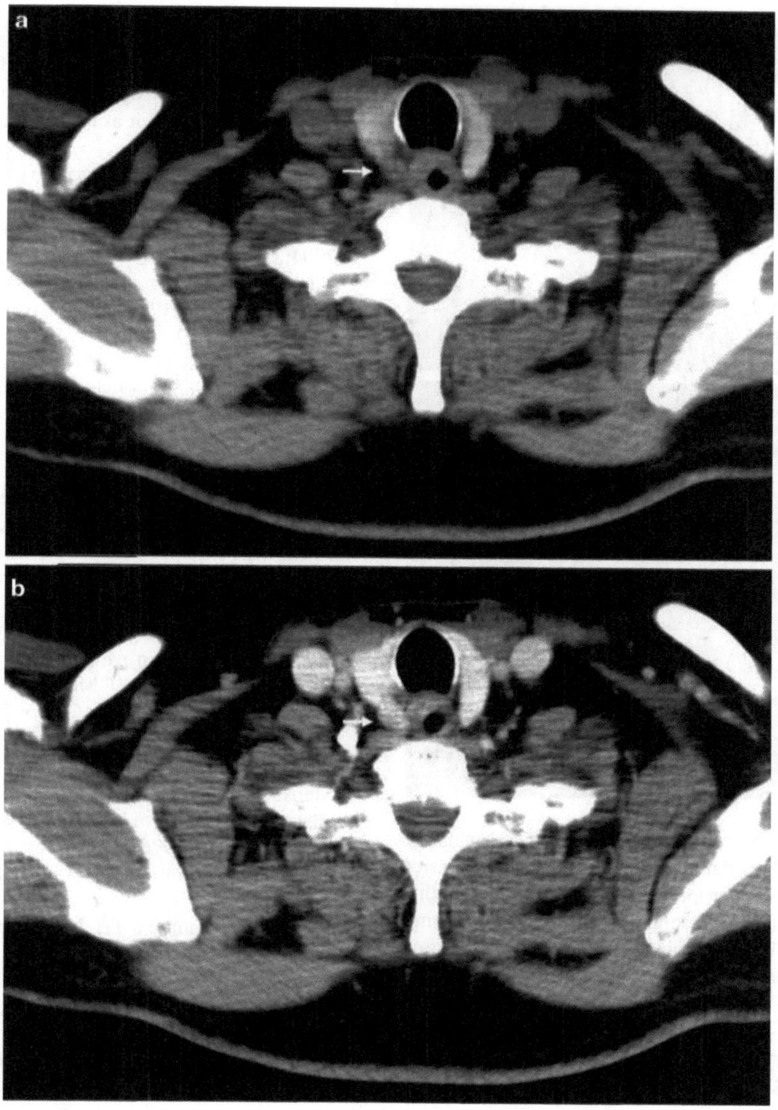

Fig. 19.17 Parathyroid adenoma in the right tracheoesophageal groove. (**a**) Transverse nonenhanced CT tomogram shows a soft tissue lesion (*arrow*) posterior to the right thyroid lobe. The thyroid is associated with higher CT attenuation characteristics due to its physiologic iodine concentration. (**b**) Contrast-enhanced CT shows enhancement of this nodule (*arrow*) similar to that of the adjacent thyroid lobe. Later, at surgery, a parathyroid adenoma was resected from this site

shown to have incremental value over planar scintigraphy for parathyroid lesion localization. Moreover, SPECT/CT has incremental value over SPECT for multiglandular parathyroid disease, detection of ectopic parathyroid lesions, and in those patients who have had previous neck surgery. MRI and contrast-enhanced CT are usually reserved for problem-solving when initial imaging studies are negative, equivocal or contradictory.

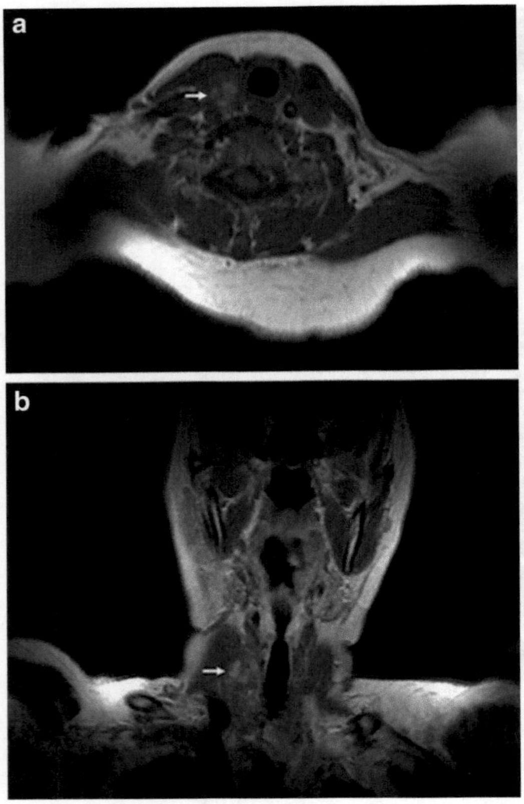

Fig. 19.18 Parathyroid adenoma. Gadolinium-enhanced T1-weighted MRI demonstrates an enhancing lesion (*arrow*) along the inferoposterior aspect of the right thyroid lobe on (**a**) transverse and (**b**) coronal tomograms. The left thyroid lobe is surgically absent. Later, a parathyroid adenoma was surgically resected from this site

References

1. Massaro A, Cittadin S, Rampin L, et al. Accurate planning of minimally invasive surgery of parathyroid adenomas by means of [(99m)Tc]MIBI SPECT. Minerva Endocrinol. 2007;32:9–16.
2. Pelizzo MR, Piotto A, Bergamasco A, Rubello D. Parathyroid carcinoma. Therapeutic strategies derived from 20 years of experience. Minerva Endocrinol. 2001;26:23–9.
3. Lumachi F, Zucchetta P, Marzola MC, et al. Advantages of combined technetium-99m-sestamibi scintigraphy and high-resolution ultrasonography in parathyroid localization. Eur J Endocrinol. 2000;26:755–60.
4. Udelsman R. Primary hyperparathyroidism. In: Cameron JL, editor. Current surgical therapy. St. Louis: Mosby; 2001. p. 662–7.
5. Marx SJ. Hyperparathyroid and hypoparathyroid disorders. N Engl J Med. 2000;343:1863–75.
6. Sackett WR, Barraclough B, Reeve TS, et al. Worldwide trends in the surgical treatment of primary hyperparathyroidism in the era of minimally invasive parathyroidectomy. Arch Surg. 2002;137:1055–9.
7. Gurnell EM, Thomas SK, McFarland I, et al. Focused parathyroid surgery with intraoperative parathyroid hormone measurement as a day-case procedure. Br J Surg. 2004;91:78–82.
8. Irvin GL, Caneiro DM, Solorzano CC. Progress in the operative management of sporadic primary hyperparathyroidism over 34 years. Ann Surg. 2004;239:704–8.
9. Udelsman R. Six hundred fifty-six consecutive explorations for primary hyperparathyroidism. Ann Surg. 2002;235:665–70.
10. Arora S, Balash PR, Yoo J, Smith GS, Prinz RA. Benefits of surgeon-performed ultrasound for primary hyperparathyroidism. Langenbecks Arch Surg. 2009;394:861–7.
11. Parel RJ, Bolton JS, Fuhrman GM. An analysis of sestamibi-positive versus -negative patients with primary hyperparathyroidism. Am Surg. 2001;67:1101–4.
12. Flynn MB, Bumpous JM, Schil K, McMasters KM. Minimally invasive radioguided parathyroidectomy. Am Surg. 2000;191:24–31.
13. Yao K, Singer FR, Roth SI, et al. Weight of normal parathyroid glands in patients with parathyroid adenomas. J Clin Endocrinol Metab. 2004;89:3208–13.
14. Bannister LH, Berry MM, Collins P, editors. Gray's anatomy. New York: Churchill Livingston; 1995. p. 17.
15. Mansberger Jr AR, Wei JP. Surgical embryology and anatomy of the thyroid and parathyroid glands. Surg Clin North Am. 1976;73:727–46.
16. Wang C. The anatomic basis of parathyroid surgery. Ann Surg. 1976;183:271–5.
17. Yadav R, Mohammed TL, Neumann DR, et al. Case of the season: ectopic parathyroid adenoma in the pericardium: a report of robotically assisted minimally invasive parathyroidectomy. Semin Roentgenol. 2010;45:53–6.
18. Roth SI, Belsley NA, Abu-Jawdeh GM. Parathyroid glands. In: Wells RJ, editor. Histology for pathologists. 3rd ed. Baltimore: Lippincott Williams and Wilkins; 2006. p. 1149–65.
19. Edis AJ, Evans Jr TC. High-resolution, real-time ultrasonography in the preoperative location of parathyroid tumors. Pilot study. N Engl J Med. 1979;301:532–4.
20. Purcell GP, Dirbas FM, Jeffrey RB, Lane MJ, Desser T, McDougall IR, et al. Parathyroid localization with high-resolution ultrasound and technetium Tc 99m sestamibi. Arch Surg. 1999;134:824–8. discussion 828–30.
21. Lane MJ, Desser TS, Weigel RJ, Jeffrey Jr RB. Use of color and power Doppler sonography to identify feeding arteries associated with parathyroid adenomas. AJR Am J Roentgenol. 1998;171:819–23.
22. Feingold DL, Alexander HR, Chen CC, Libutti SK, Shawker TH, Simonds WF, et al. Ultrasound and sestamibi scan as the only preoperative imaging tests in reoperation for parathyroid adenomas. Surgery. 2000;128:1103–9. discussion 1109–10.

23. Irvin 3rd GL, Carneiro DM, Solorzano CC. Progress in the operative management of sporadic primary hyperparathyroidism over 34 years. Ann Surg. 2004;239:704–8. discussion 708–11.
24. Haber RS, Kim CK, Inabnet WB. Ultrasonography for preoperative localization of enlarged parathyroid glands in primary hyperparathyroidism: comparison with (99m)technetium sestamibi scintigraphy. Clin Endocrinol (Oxf). 2002;57:241–9.
25. Solorzano CC, Carneiro-Pla DM, Irvin 3rd GL. Surgeon-performed ultrasonography as the initial and only localizing study in sporadic primary hyperparathyroidism. J Am Coll Surg. 2006;202:18–24.
26. Untch BR, Adam MA, Scheri RP, Bennett KM, Dixit D, Webb C, et al. Surgeon-performed ultrasound is superior to 99Tc-sestamibi scanning to localize parathyroid adenomas in patients with primary hyperparathyroidism: results in 516 patients over 10 years. J Am Coll Surg. 2011;212:522–9.
27. Abboud B, Sleilaty G, Rabaa L, Daher R, Abou Zeid H, Jabbour H, et al. Ultrasonography: highly accuracy technique for preoperative localization of parathyroid adenoma. Laryngoscope. 2008;118:1574–8.
28. Ulanovski D, Feinmesser R, Cohen M, Sulkes J, Dudkiewicz M, Shpitzer T. Preoperative evaluation of patients with parathyroid adenoma: role of high-resolution ultrasonography. Head Neck. 2002;24:1–5.
29. Lee L, Steward DL. Techniques for parathyroid localization with ultrasound. Otolaryngol Clin North Am. 2010;43:1229–39. vi.
30. Gritzmann N, Koischwitz D, Rettenbacher T. Sonography of the thyroid and parathyroid glands. Radiol Clin North Am. 2000;38:1131–45. xii.
31. Akerström G, Malmaeus J, Bergström R. Surgical anatomy of human parathyroid glands. Surgery. 1984;95:14–21.
32. Berber E, Parikh RT, Ballem N, Garner CN, Milas M, Siperstein AE. Factors contributing to negative parathyroid localization: an analysis of 1000 patients. Surgery. 2008;144:74–9.
33. Coakley AJ, Kettle AG, Wells CP, et al. ^{99m}Tc-sestamibi—a new agent for parathyroid imaging. Nucl Med Commun. 1989;10:791–4.
34. Arbab AS, Koizumi K, Toyama K, Araki T. Uptake of technetium-99m-tetrofosmin, technetium-99m-MIBI and thallium-201 in tumor cell lines. J Nucl Med. 1996;37:1551–6.
35. Chiu ML, Kronauge JF, Piwnica WD. Effect of mitochondrial and plasma membrane potential on accumulation of hexakis (2-Methoxyisobutylisonitrile) technetium in cultured mouse fibroblasts. J Nucl Med. 1990;31:1646–53.
36. Hetrakul N, Civelek AC, Stagg CA, et al. In vitro accumulation of technetium 99m sestamibi in human parathyroid mitochondria. Surgery. 2001;130:1011–8.
37. Taillefer R, Boucher Y, Polvin C, Lambert R. Detection and localization of parathyroid adenomas in patients with hyperparathyroidism using a single radionuclide imaging procedure with technetium-99m-sestamibi (double-phase study). J Nucl Med. 1992;33(180):1807–9.
38. Melloul M, Paz A, Koren R, et al. 99m Tc-MIBI scintigraphy of parathyroid adenomas and its relation to tumour size and oxyphil cell abundance. Eur J Nucl Med. 2001;28:209–13.
39. Ruda J, Hollenbeak CS, Stack BC. A systematic review of the diagnosis and treatment of primary hyperparathyroidism from 1995–2003. Otolaryngol Head Neck Surg. 2005;132:359–72.
40. Pinero A, Rodriguez JM, Ortiz S, et al. Relation of biochemical, cytologic, and morphologic parameters to the result of gammagraphy with technetium 99m sestamibi in primary hyperparathyroidism. Otolaryngol Head Neck Surg. 2000;122:851–5.
41. Mitchell BK, Cornelius EA, Zoghbi S, et al. Mechanism of technetium 99m sestamibi parathyroid imaging and the possible role of p-glycoprotein. Surgery. 1996;120:1039–45.
42. Rao VV, Chiu ML, Knonauge KF, Piwnica-Worms D. Expression of recombinant human multidrug resistance P-glycoprotein in insect cells confers decreased accumulation of technetium-99m-sestamibi. J Nucl Med. 1994;35:510–5.
43. Taki J, Sumiya H, Asada N, Ueda Y, Tsuchiya H, Tonami N. Assessment of P-glycoprotein in patients with malignant bone and soft tissue tumors using technetium-99m-MIBI scintigraphy. J Nucl Med. 1998;39:1179–84.
44. Gupta Y, Ahmed R, Happerfield L, Pinder SE, Balan KK, Wishart GC. P-glycoprotein expression is associated with sestamibi washout in primary hyperparathyroidism. Br J Surg. 2007;94:1491–5.
45. Palestro CJ, Tomas MB, Tronco GG. Radionuclide imaging of the parathyroid glands. Semin Nucl Med. 2005;35:266–76.
46. Neumann DR, Obuchowski NA, DiFilippo FP. Preoperative 123-I/99m-Tc-sestamibi subtraction SPECT and SPECT/CT in primary hyperparathyroidism. J Nucl Med. 2008;49:2012–7.
47. Ansquer C, Mirallie E, Carlier T, et al. Preoperative localization of parathyroid lesions. Value of 99mTc-MIBI tomography and factors influencing detection. Nuklearmedizin. 2008;47:158–62.
48. Carlier T, Oudoux A, Mirallie E, et al. 99mTc-MIBI pinhole SPECT in primary hyperparathyroidism: comparison with conventional SPECT, planar scintigraphy and ultrasonography. Eur J Nucl Med Mol Imaging. 2008;35:637–43.
49. Sharma J, Mazzaglia P, Milas M, et al. Radionuclide imaging for hyperparathyroidism (HPT): which is the best technetium-99m sestamibi modality? Surgery. 2006;140:856–63.
50. Loberboym ML, Minski I, Macadziob S, et al. Incremental diagnostic value of preoperative 99m Tc-MIBI SPECT in patients with a parathyroid adenoma. J Nucl Med. 2003;44:904–8.
51. Clark PB, Perrier ND, Morton KA. Detection of an intrathymic parathyroid adenoma using single-photon

emission CT, 99mTc sestamibi acintigraphy and CT. Am J Roentgenol. 2005;184:S16–8.
52. Sukan A, Reyhan M, Aydin M, Yapar AF, Sert Y, Canpolat T, et al. Preoperative evaluation of hyperparathyroidism: the role of dual-phase parathyroid scintigraphy and ultrasound imaging. Ann Nucl Med. 2008;22:123–31.
53. Hindie E, Melliere D, Jeanquillaume C, et al. Parathyroid imaging using simultaneous double-window recording of technetium-99m-sestamibi and iodine-123. J Nucl Med. 1998;39:1100–5.
54. Garvie NW. Imaging the parathyroids. In: Peters AM, editor. Nuclear medicine in radiologic diagnosis. London: Martin Dunitz; 2003. p. 681–94.
55. Erbil Y, Barbaros U, Yanik BT, et al. Impact of adenoma weight and ectopic location of parathyroid adenoma on localization study results. World J Surg. 2008;32:566–71.
56. Mehta NY, Ruda JM, Kapadia S, et al. Relationship of technetium Tc 99m sestamibi scans to histopathological features of hyperfunctioning parathyroid tissue. Arch Otolaryngol Head Neck Surg. 2005;131:493–8.
57. Stephen AE, Roth SI, Fardo DW, et al. Predictors of an accurate preoperative sestamibi scan for single-gland parathyroid adenomas. Arch Surg. 2007;142: 381–6.
58. Katz SC, Wang GJ, Kramer EL, et al. Limitations of technetium 99m sestamibi scintigraphic localization for primary hyperparathyroidism associated with multiglandular disease. Am Surg. 2003;69:170–5.
59. Bergson EJ, Snyter LA, Dubner S, et al. Sestamibi scans and intraoperative PTH measurement in the treatment of primary hyperparathyroidism due to multiple gland disease. Arch Otolaryngol Head Neck Surg. 2004;130:87–91.
60. Alexander HR, Chen CC, Shawker T, et al. Role of preoperative localization and intraoperative localization maneuvers including intraoperative PTH assay determination for patients with persistent or recurrent hyperparathyroidism. J Bone Miner Res. 2002;17 Suppl 2:N133–40.
61. Arici C, Cheah WK, Ituarte PH, et al. Can localization studies be used to direct focused parathyroid operations? Surgery. 2001;129:720–9.
62. Miura D, Wada N, Arici C, et al. Does intraoperative quick parathyroid hormone assay improve the results of parathyroidectomy? World J Surg. 2002;26:926–30.
63. Serra A, Bolasco P, Satta L, et al. Role of SPECT/CT in the preoperative assessment of hyperparathyroid patients. Radiol Med. 2006;111:999–1008.
64. Lavely WC, Goetze S, Friedman KP, et al. Comparison of SPECT/CT, SPECT, and planar imaging with single- and dual-phase (99m) Tc-sestamibi parathyroid scintigraphy. J Nucl Med. 2007;48:1084–9.
65. Reading CC, Gorman CA. Thyroid imaging techniques. Clin Lab Med. 1993;13:711–24.
66. Ernst O. Hyperparathyroidism: CT and MR findings. J Radiol. 2009;90:409–12.
67. Gotway MB, Higgins CB. MR imaging of the thyroid and parathyroid glands. Magn Reson Imaging Clin N Am. 2000;8:163–82.
68. Randall GJ, Zald PB, Cohen JI, Hamilton BE. Contrast-enhanced MDCT characteristics of parathyroid adenomas. AJR Am J Roentgenol. 2009;193:W139–43.
69. Beland MD, Mayo-Smith WW, Grand DJ, et al. Dynamic MDCT for localization of occult parathyroid adenomas in 26 patients with primary hyperparathyroidism. AJR Am J Roentgenol. 2011;196:61–5.
70. Mortenson MM, Evans DB, Lee JE, et al. Parathyroid explorationin the reoperative neck: improved preoperative localization with 4D-computed tomography. J Am Coll Surg. 2008;206:888–95.
71. Rodgers SE, Hunter GJ, Hamberg LM, et al. Improved preoperative planning for directed parthyroidectomy with 4-dimensional computed tomography. Surgery. 2006;140:932–40.
72. Jang YS, Rosen K, Clark OH, et al. Localization of abnormal parathyroid glands in the mediastinum with MR imaging. Radiology. 1993;189:137–41.
73. Kabala JE. Computed tomography and magnetic resonance imaging in diseases of the thyroid and parathyroid. Eur J Radiol. 2008;66:480–92.
74. Spritzer CE. Progress in MR imaging of the venous system. Perspect Vasc Surg Endovasc Ther. 2009; 21:105–16.
75. Seelos KC, DeMarco R, Clark OH, et al. Persistent and recurrent hyperparathyroidism: assessment with gadopentetate dimeglumine-enhanced MR imaging. Radiology. 1990;177:373–8.
76. Sekiyama K, Akakura K, Mikami K, et al. Usefulness of diagnostic imaging in primary hyperparathyroidism. Int J Urol. 2003;10:7–11.
77. Wakamatsu H, Noquchi S, Yamashita H, et al. Parathyroid scintigraphy with 99mTc-MIBI and 123-I subtraction: a comparison with magnetic resonance imaging and ultrasonography. Nucl Med Commun. 2003;24:755–62.
78. Gotway MB, Reddy GP, Webb WR, et al. Comparison between MR imaging and 99m-Tc MIBI scintigraphy in the evaluation of recurrent or persistent hyperparathyroidism. Radiology. 2001;218:783–90.
79. Auffermann W, Guis M, Taveras NJ, et al. MR signal intensity of parathyroid adenomas: correlation with histopathology. AJR Am J Roentgenol. 1989;153: 873–6.
80. Chen AY, Zirwas MJ, Hefferman MP. Nephrogenic systemic fibrosis: a review. J Drugs Dermatol. 2010;9: 829–34.

Parathyroid Surgery

20

Zvonimir L. Milas and Mira Milas

Abstract

Parathyroid surgery for hyperparathyroidism is a safe and effective strategy for durably reducing PTH hypersecretion and improving and/or reversing systemic consequences such as bone density loss and nephrocalcinosis. This overview provides a summary of currently available operative approaches for primary, secondary, and tertiary forms of hyperparathyroidism. Multidisciplinary communication is valuable at all phases of management. Surgeons should clearly communicate key details such as the method of parathyroid surgery and the extent of exploration (how many parathyroid glands were examined). The expertise of a surgeon, or specialized care for patients with parathyroid disease, is associated with improved outcomes. Parathyroid surgery remains the most effective method of treating hyperparathyroidism and can be accomplished with minimal morbidity. Long-term follow-up of patients who have been treated with parathyroidectomy is important to monitor for successful maintenance of normal calcium balance and resolution of sequelae of hyperparathyroidism.

Keywords

Parathyroidectomy • Cryopreservation • Autotransplantation • Intraoperative measurement of parathyroid hormone • Neck exploration

The Evolution of Parathyroid Surgery

Surgical management of parathyroid disease has evolved in response to several fundamentally new and important developments. Instead of being a rare endocrine disorder, primary hyperparathyroidism (PHPT) now accounts for the most common cause of hypercalcemia in the outpatient population, with estimated prevalence of 1 in 500 women and 1 in 2,000 men [1]. More patients are being diagnosed in earlier phases of PHPT in part

Z.L. Milas, MD (✉)
Head and Neck Surgical Oncology, MD Anderson Cancer Center, 1400 S. Orange Ave., MP 760, Orlando, FL 82806, USA
e-mail: zvonimir.milas@orlandohealth.com

M. Milas, MD
The Thyroid Center, Department of Endocrine Surgery, Cleveland Clinic, 9500 Euclid Ave F20, Cleveland, OH 44195, USA

A.A. Licata and E.V. Lerma (eds.), *Diseases of the Parathyroid Glands*,
DOI 10.1007/978-1-4419-5550-0_20, © Springer Science+Business Media, LLC 2012

incidentally because calcium has become a routine component of automated chemistry panels, and in part because practitioners are also recognizing the need to screen patients with osteoporosis, osteopenia, and kidney stones more comprehensively for underlying PHPT with panels that include calcium, intact parathyroid hormone (PHPT), and 25-hydroxyvitamin D levels. Technological innovations have also expanded the options available for parathyroid surgery. Once conducted predominantly via bilateral neck exploration, parathyroidectomy is now approached via a focused exploration to a radiologically identified abnormality [2]. Multiple methods of performing parathyroidectomy are available, and expertise in this surgery requires not only knowledge in evaluating parathyroid glands but also selection of operation appropriate for a specific patient's parathyroid diagnosis [3–5]. Several multidisciplinary publications have offered guidelines for the indications and timing of parathyroid surgery, in response to these epidemiologic and technologic shifts and to the challenge of what constitutes best treatment for apparently asymptomatic PHPT [6–8]. Despite these guidelines, patients with PHPT remain, as a group, under-referred and under-treated surgically [9]. This chapter catalogues the parathyroid operations in current surgical practice, while emphasizing those constant principles of management which are essential to surgical success.

The Goals of Parathyroid Surgery

The operative goals for the treatment of proven PHPT include achievement of a durable normocalcemic state and normal PTH, avoidance of injury to the laryngeal nerves, completion of surgery with minimal postoperative morbidity and negligible mortality, and consideration of cosmetic scar appearance that is acceptable to the patient. The operative goals for the treatment of secondary or tertiary hyperparathyroidism (SHPT/THPT) are identical, although the long-term durability of normal PTH levels can be more challenging to achieve. Operating on a patient without a clear diagnosis of PHPT undermines the ability to achieve these goals, thus proper patient selection and confirmation of the diagnosis before surgery cannot be overemphasized.

Indications for Parathyroid Surgery

In 2005, national professional associations of endocrine surgeons and endocrinologists jointly issued guidelines that operative management is clearly indicated for all patients with classic symptoms or complications of PHPT [7]. Less widespread has been the recognition that parathyroidectomy offers significant benefits to those with SHPT and THPT [10, 11]. Another challenge has been decision-making for those with apparently asymptomatic PHPT, not only in defining the timing of surgery (when to refer) but also, with some controversy, whether these patients require surgery. Experts organized by the National Institutes of Health in 2002 proposed parathyroidectomy for the following patients with PHPT: (1) those <50 years of age, (2) who cannot participate in appropriate follow-up, (3) with a serum calcium level >1.0 mg/dl above the normal range, (4) with urinary calcium >400 mg/24 h, (5) with a 30% decrease in renal function, or (6) with systemic complications of PHPT including nephrocalcinosis, osteoporosis (*T*-score lower than –2.5 SD at the lumbar spine, hip, or wrist), or a severe psychoneurologic disorder [12]. The development, timing, and progression of disease in patients with asymptomatic PHPT are difficult to predict. Long-term nonoperative management can be costly [13]. For these reasons, other experts have advised a more liberal approach to recommendations of parathyroidectomy beyond the NIH criteria, provided that surgery can be performed safely and with minimal risks for a disease that, in some patients, may be minimally problematic at the time of presentation [6, 8]. Thus, for example, parathyroidectomy may be appropriate to consider for patients with osteopenia (*T*-scores –1 to –2.5 SD) and mild neurocognitive symptoms. A recent multidisciplinary review advised, indeed, that surgery offers the best option for preventing or reversing complications of hyperparathyroidism and should be considered in discussions about management options upon diagnosis [6].

Some patients with indications for parathyroidectomy may not be medically fit for surgery or have other reasons to forego parathyroidectomy. Percutaneous ethanol ablation, bisphosphonates, and calcimimetic agents are available nonoperative treatment options. The calcimimetic agents reduce calcium and PTH levels while administered, are more frequently administered to patients with SHPT, but their long-term impact on improving systemic consequences of hyperparathyroidism is unclear [14]. Frequently monitoring laboratory values, avoiding dehydration and excess calcium intake, and periodic re-assessment for surgery are important components of nonoperative management.

Fundamental Concepts of Parathyroid Exploration

Parathyroid surgery relies on the knowledge of normal anatomical distribution of parathyroid glands, supranumerary and ectopic variations, and embryologic details that might affect the interpretation of parathyroid findings. It is also important to recognize variations of normal morphology and the spectrum of diseased parathyroid morphology. Proficiency with delicate surgery around the head and neck, upper mediastinum, and occasionally deeper intrathoracic mediastinal territory is necessary [15].

Although most patients receive some kind of parathyroid imaging studies, these are principally meant for localization of suspected site or sites of parathyroid disease, and not for diagnosis. A "positive" imaging study does not confirm the diagnosis of hyperparathyroidism (thyroid nodules can be a source of false positives, for example). A "negative" imaging study does not exclude the diagnosis of hyperparathyroidism. Because the risk of ectopic mediastinal or ectopic cervical parathyroid abnormalities is quite rare, conducting comprehensive bilateral neck exploration is possible without imaging studies and is advisable when imaging studies are negative. Indeed, this strategy has had a decades-long successful track-record [15–19]. Preoperative imaging is valuable, however, as it facilitates focal explorations and expedient surgery, and can alert to more challenging scenarios of ectopic or multigland disease.

Treatment of single adenomas is simple excision of the abnormal gland. Multigland hyperplasia is ideally treated with subtotal parathyroidectomy and parathyroid cryopreservation. While abnormal parathyroid glands need to be removed to ensure cure of hyperparathyroidism, it is likewise important to safeguard the viability of normal parathyroids and avoid hypoparathyroidism. Normal parathyroid glands are approximately 5–6 mm in greatest dimension, weigh 15–35 mg, and can be inconspicuous with their orange-tan color embedded or flattened within a surrounding yellow fatty tissue envelope (Fig. 20.1). The appearance of parathyroids can be variable even when they are biochemically functioning normally. When diseased, parathyroid glands may display variable morphological changes in size, shape, texture, and firmness (Fig. 20.2). For example, the median size (and range) of an individual abnormal parathyroid gland size varies with disease type: 700 mg (200–10,000 mg) for single adenomas, 150 mg (75–200 mg) in primary hyperplasia, and 1,000 mg (200–10,000 mg) for secondary hyperplasia [15]. Abnormal parathyroids are generally fuller in all dimensions, have a darker brown or reddish-brown color, and do not compress easily or are significantly firm when gently probed. They may have an irregular and knobby shape, more prominent vascular pedicles, or a plexus of vasculature. Glands of patients with secondary and THPT may be sclerotic and light in color from this fibrosis. There is ongoing interest and some controversy in defining what truly constitutes an abnormal parathyroid, and whether this is a matter of purely morphological form, biochemical function, or a combination of both.

In general, the search for parathyroid glands along the usual anatomical distribution of superior ("upper") and inferior ("lower") parathyroids can be viewed as a "primary parathyroid survey" [15]. It takes into consideration exploring all the regions shown in Fig. 20.3 until the remaining

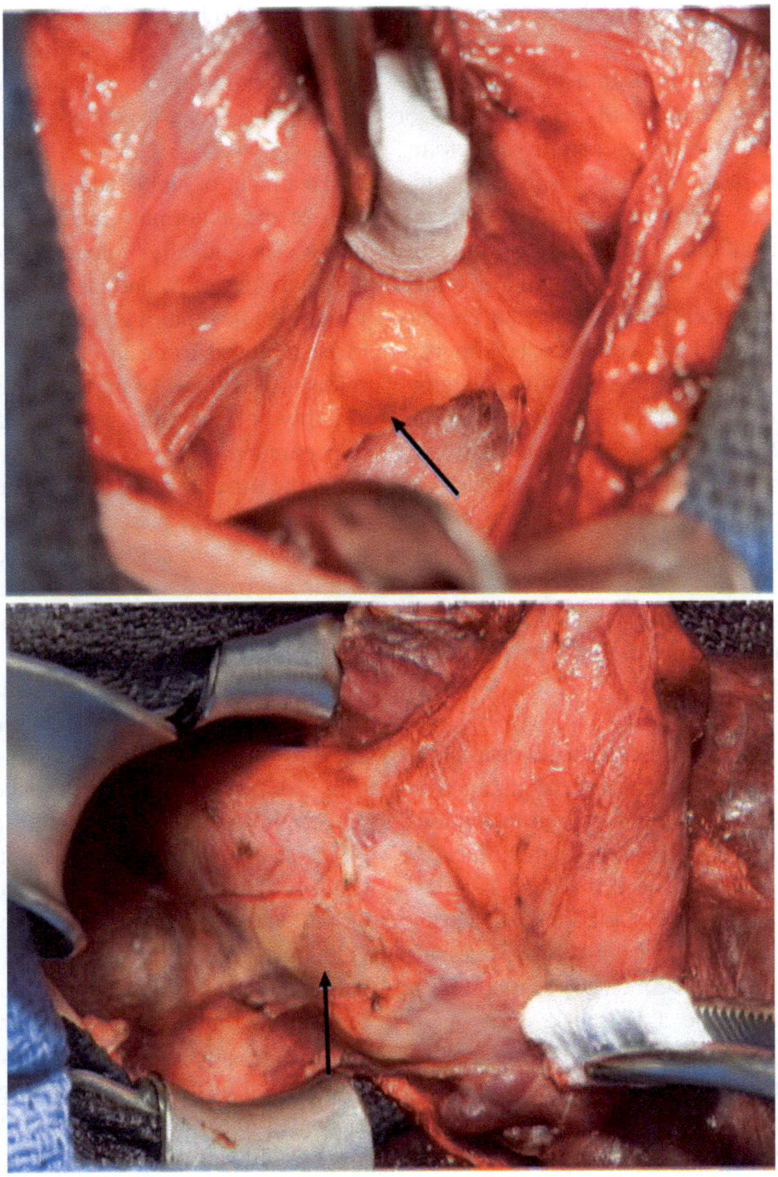

Fig. 20.1 Examples of normal parathyroid glands (*arrows*)

three parathyroids have been identified. It is useful to develop a systematic order of exploration and practice it routinely. A convenient strategy is to target exposure of the most abnormal parathyroid first, then the ipsilateral parathyroid, and finally explore the contralateral side. When all parathyroids have been identified, assessment about the disease process (single adenoma, double adenoma, or hyperplasia) can be made and a decision about which parathyroids to remove and in what order can be determined. A "secondary parathyroid survey" refers to exploration of cervical regions when parathyroid position is more unusual or ectopic, and when the above primary survey has not led to conclusive findings (Fig. 20.4) [15]. Important areas to examine are retroesophageal spaces, where parathyroid glands are most commonly missed because they have

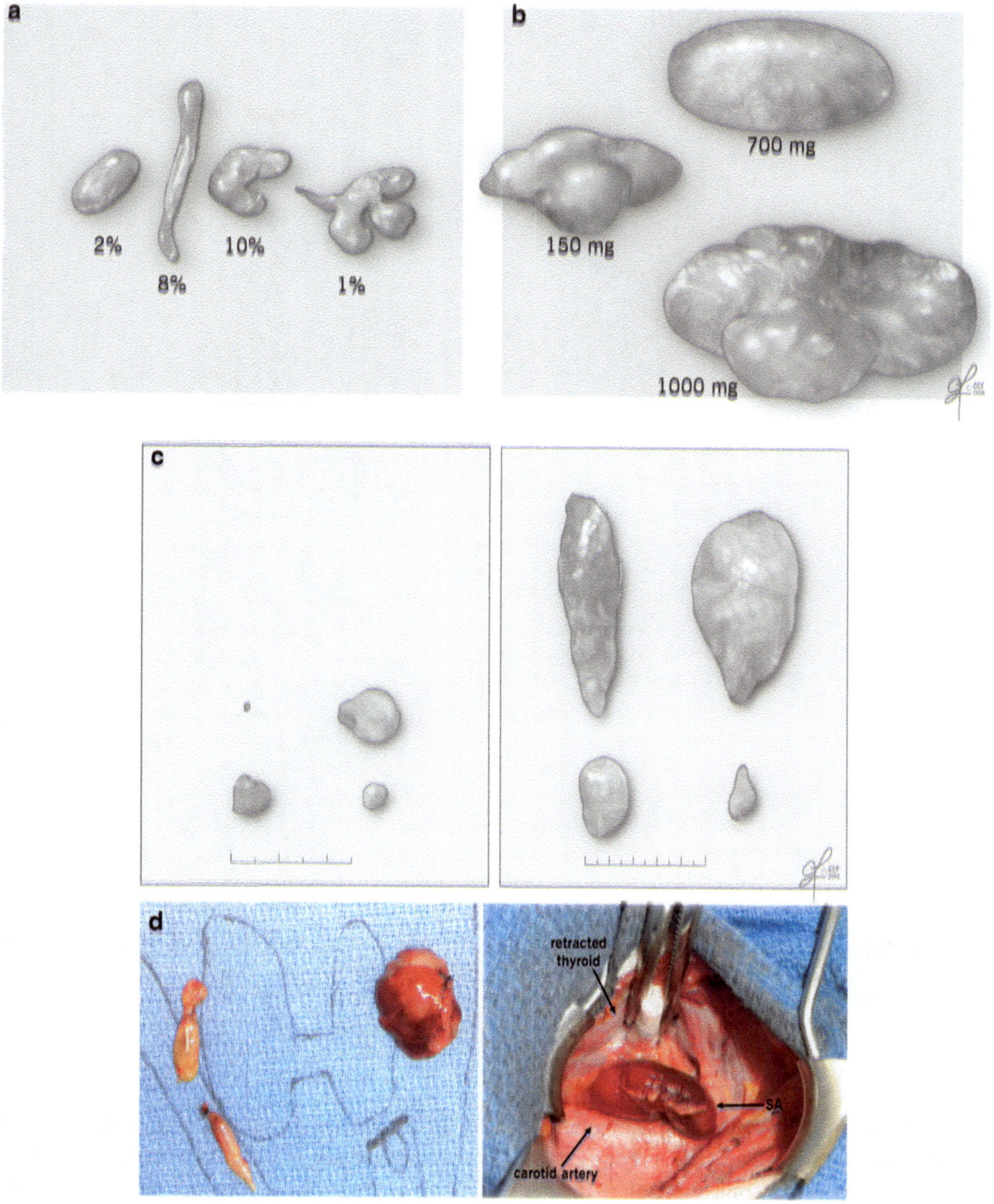

Fig. 20.2 Variable morphology of normal parathyroid glands (**a**), abnormal parathyroid glands (**b**), and parathyroid hyperplasia by illustrations (**c**) and in a surgical examples (**d**) of multigland disease (*left*) and single adenoma (SA) (*right*). (**a–c**) Reprinted with permission, Cleveland Clinic Center for Medical Art & Photography © 2008–2011. All Rights Reserved

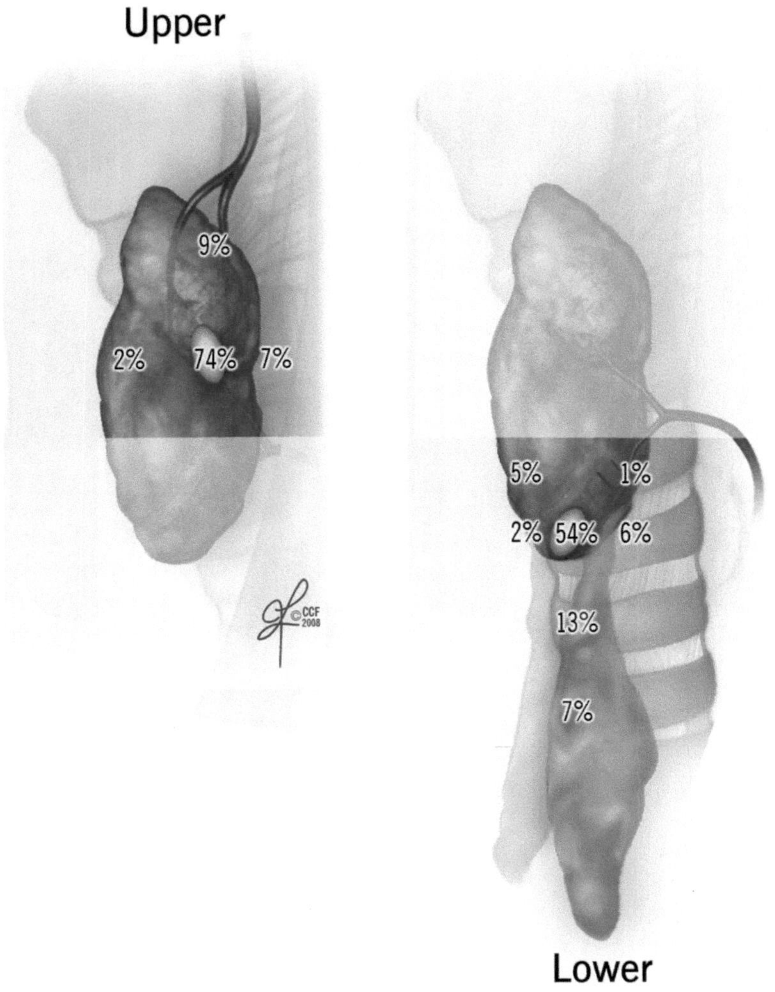

Fig. 20.3 Expected distribution of superior (*upper*) and inferior (*lower*) parathyroid glands where abnormalities develop. Reprinted with permission, Cleveland Clinic Center for Medical Art & Photography © 2008–2011. All Rights Reserved

sunken into the deep posterior space behind the tracheoesophageal groove, often lying on the anterior surface of the spine and below the main trunk of the inferior thyroid artery (Fig. 20.5) [20]. Other regions include the thymus, carotid and jugular sheath, and consideration of intrathyroidal parathyroid glands (which can be suspected from preoperative ultrasound). The secondary survey should *not* be performed just to locate a normal parathyroid, but a missing pathologic gland. In these cases, the thymus should be retracted out of the mediastinum as far as possible without avulsion, carefully examined, palpated, and removed (Fig. 20.6). For clearly mediastinal parathyroid glands, surgery often entails collaboration with thoracic surgeons, as operative approaches are tailored to the anatomical location within the chest and can include thoracotomy, median sternotomy, and various thoracoscopic surgeries [21].

The detailed description of operative findings is more important than the actual technology or method involved with parathyroid surgery. Thus, the operative report should specify what

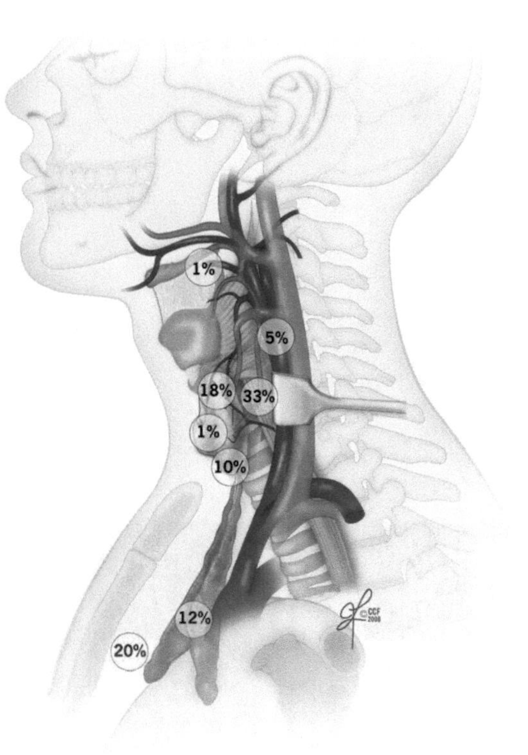

Fig. 20.4 Distribution of parathyroid glands found at re-exploration for persistent and recurrent disease, providing the basis for a "secondary survey" at the time of parathyroidectomy. Reprinted with permission, Cleveland Clinic Center for Medical Art & Photography © 2008–2011. All Rights Reserved

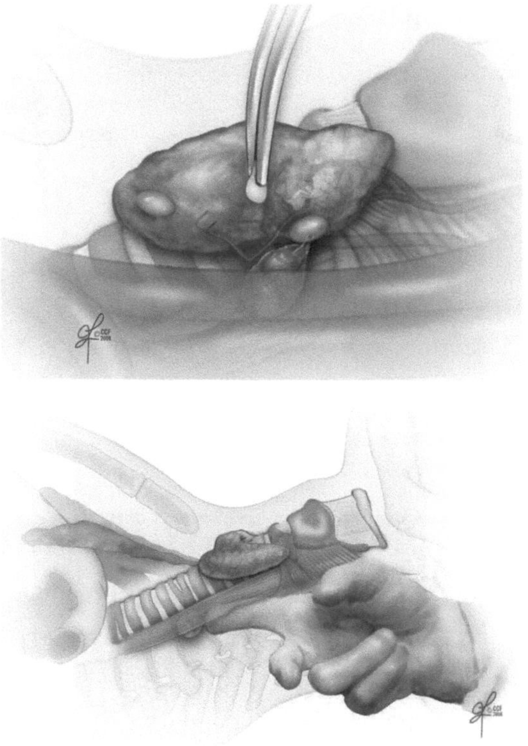

Fig. 20.5 The retroesophageal area is the most common source of missed parathyroid abnormalities. Reprinted with permission, Cleveland Clinic Center for Medical Art & Photography © 2008–2011. All Rights Reserved

parathyroid site or sites were explored (the intent and the extent of surgery), whether any ectopic regions needed evaluation, and the diagnosis based on the findings. The incisional length, the anesthetic or perioperative care, or the use of qualifiers such as "minimally invasive surgery" do not sufficiently describe what pathology was investigated and ultimately found. Instructive, for example, would be procedure titles such as "one-gland parathyroid exploration endoscopically via midline incision," "two-gland parathyroid exploration via robotic trans-axillary approach," "four-gland parathyroid exploration via 3 cm midline incision," "one-gland parathyroid exploration via 5 cm lateral neck approach," and "with or without radioguidance or IOPTH" added as qualifiers.

Surgical Options in Performing Parathyroidectomy

Bilateral Exploration

This approach involves directed and systematic examination of all four parathyroid glands in their expected anatomical distributions. It can be considered comprehensive parathyroid examination, in contrast to the majority of other operations which are focused on identifying just one suspected abnormality [17–19]. Bilateral exploration can be performed in a minimally invasive way, with small incisions and gentle dissection. The relevance of bilateral or comprehensive parathyroid exploration is that some patients have

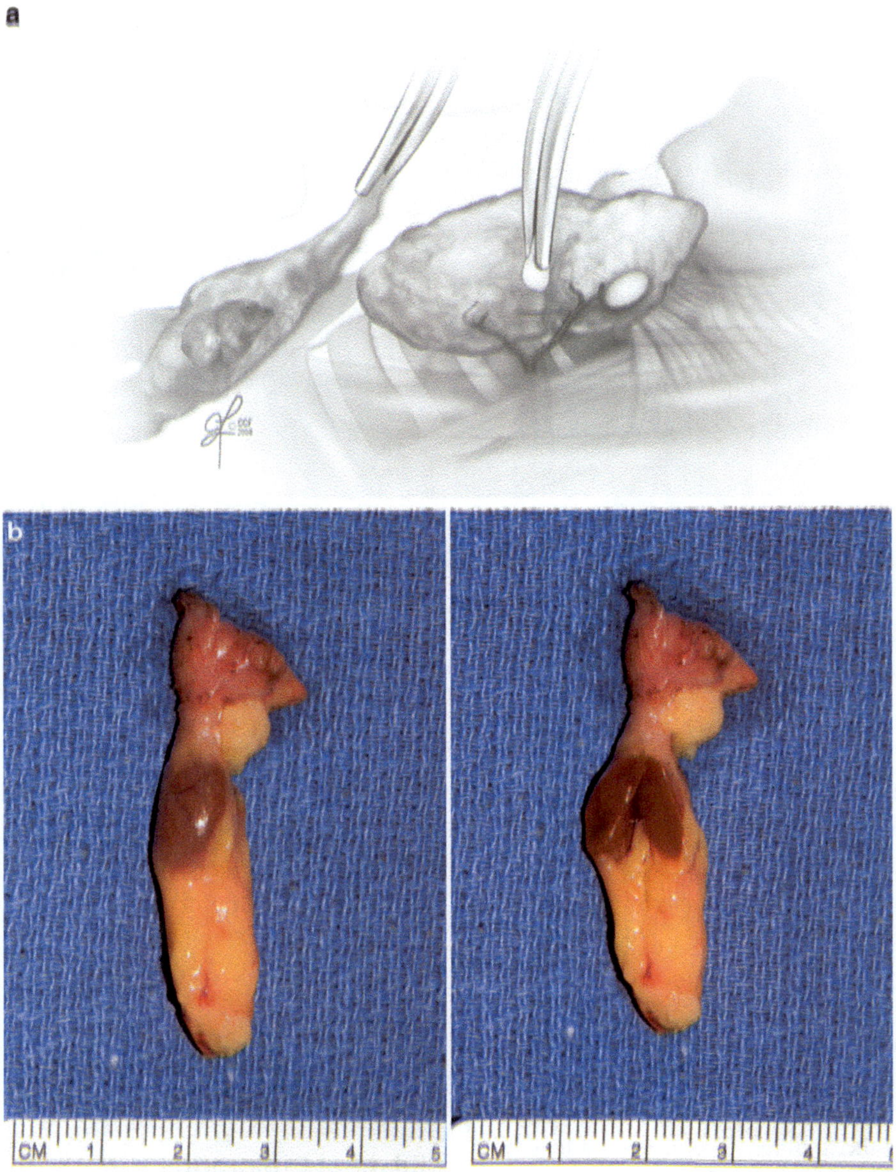

Fig. 20.6 Cervical thymectomy (**a**) removes abnormal ectopic parathyroid glands, as shown in operative specimen of single adenoma (**b**) with typical brown appearance surrounded by yellow thymic fat. (**a**) Reprinted with permission, Cleveland Clinic Center for Medical Art & Photography © 2008–2011. All Rights Reserved

significantly higher risk for multigland parathyroid disease (Table 20.1) and achieving normocalcemia is contingent on the evaluation of all parathyroid glands and the appropriate resection of those that are functionally and/or morphologically abnormal. Awareness of patterns of multigland disease, such as the asymmetric distribution of double adenomas to favor superior parathyroid glands is helpful. A recent survey of parathyroid surgeons, as well as published reports on large patient case series, have indicated that bilateral parathyroid exploration may be required in up to 30% of patients who are referred for surgery, and that a decision to convert from focal to bilateral exploration occurs intraoperatively in an additional 10% of patients [2].

Table 20.1 Indications for bilateral exploration of parathyroid glands as the initial surgery for primary hyperparathyroidism

Absolute indications
Known or suspected multiple endocrine neoplasia syndromes
Intraoperative PTH fails to drop after resection of suspected single adenoma
Failure to find diseased gland at location indicated by imaging studies
Finding more than one abnormal parathyroid during intended focal or unilateral neck exploration
Negative imaging studies
Imaging studies suggesting multiple sites of disease
Co-existing thyroid cancer or bilateral goiter requiring total thyroidectomy
Advisable indications
Discordant parathyroid imaging studies
Unavailability of intraoperative PTH measurement
Inability to obtain preoperative imaging
Lithium-induced PHPT
Non-MEN familial hyperparathyroidism
Co-existing thyroid pathology that may require operative intervention
Surgeon preference or experience

Focal Exploration

Focal exploration of one parathyroid site, guided by radiologic identification of suspected disease at that location, is the prevailing approach to modern parathyroid surgery [2, 22–25]. It is most often accompanied by intraoperative measurement of parathyroid hormone (IOPTH), although more recent reports are raising the possibility of conducting focal exploration without IOPTH [26]. The radiologic modalities useful for localization include Tc99-sestamibi scan, neck ultrasonography, four-dimensional computed tomography, and magnetic resonance imaging, while other types are reserved for use in challenging or re-operative parathyroid cases [27–32]. There are numerous methods of Tc99-sestamibi imaging and some can be more effective at localization of parathyroid disease [30]. It is important for a surgeon especially, and even nonsurgical specialists caring for patients with hyperparathyroidism, to know which method is used in their patients and become familiar with viewing and critically scrutinizing the images.

The sequence of operation is simple: a small incision is placed for optimal exposure of the underlying parathyroid gland, the abnormal gland is identified, IOPTH is measured before removing the gland and also 10 min afterwards, expecting that a drop of at least 50% in IOPTH value becomes the metric of disease cure and signals end of the operation.

Limited

Limited parathyroid exploration refers to the examination of both parathyroids on one side of the neck, or some contralateral combination that evaluates more than one, but less than the full complement of glands. It is often an incidental rather than planned approach, although some surgeons prefer to assess both unilateral parathyroid glands, even when only one is expected to be diseased [2].

Radioguided

The concept of radioguidance during surgery has been applied in two ways: the use of Tc-99 sestamibi injected before surgery to aid detection of an abnormal parathyroid in situ and the use, after similar injection, to judge the nature of parathyroid disease ex vivo after excising abnormal and biopsying normal parathyroid glands [33–38]. The radioactivity counts are obtained with a small hand-held, pencil-like probe and quantitatively displayed on a monitor. This approach has probably had most success in the latter, ex vivo application. The radioguided approach can also be helpful during surgery for ectopic mediastinal disease that requires sternotomy, here again performing better to confirm an abnormal parathyroid contained within the excised tissue. The strong background signals from adjacent thyroid tissue in the neck, or large vasculature and cardiac structures in the mediastinum, which both take up the radioisotope, limit its usefulness to pinpoint small areas of signal unique to the parathyroid in vivo.

Technical Innovations in Surgical Approach

A number of surgical approaches have been developed that can accomplish bilateral, focal, or limited parathyroid operations with innovative means, whether technical or cosmetic in nature. These include operating via smaller neck incisions (2–3 cm) using endoscopic tools and high-definition monitors that provide excellent visual display while allowing minimal dissection [23, 24]. The endoscopic and videoscopic equipment can function via incisions that are placed outside the neck region, such as in axillary folds and periareolar breast lines. Recently, robotic technology has emerged via a transaxillary approach, demonstrating feasibility but cautioning that its ultimate benefits and indications require further study [39].

Special Circumstances in Parathyroid Surgery

The descriptions of the basic surgical techniques above are most applicable to first-time parathyroid operations, where the epidemiology of PHPT particularly is expected to reveal a single adenoma. Nuances in surgical care are present for patients who undergo re-operative parathyroid surgery or have confirmed multigland disease from a number of etiologies—sporadic PHPT, hereditary syndromes such as the multiple endocrine neoplasias (MEN) and familial hyperparathyroidism, and SHPT or THPT. An individualized treatment plan is critical for these patients, taking into account all of the relevant details of their medical histories, including prior operations, imaging findings, and possible risks of higher long-term recurrence rates, such as seen with MEN patients and SHPT.

Subtotal Parathyroid Resections

When multiple abnormal parathyroid glands exist, surgical treatment has to balance the need to excise abnormal tissue with the need to have an adequate residual amount that maintains normal calcium and PTH balance. When two or three parathyroid glands are abnormal, the residual one or two normal glands are more than sufficient for this task. However, when all four parathyroid glands are abnormal, then the residual portion has to be crafted from one of the abnormal glands. This can be accomplished by leaving a small quantity of one parathyroid in situ, supplied by its own vascular pedicle, or by removing the entirety of parathyroids from their deep cervical location and autografting a small portion into another superficial site, where new vascular supply must be recruited [15]. A number of superficial locations have been used for this purpose, including the sternocleidomastoid muscle, the brachioradialis muscle of the nondominant forearm, and subcutaneous tissue pockets of the anterior chest wall. The definition of "small" is best judged by the operating surgeon. If there is availability to cryopreserve parathyroid tissue, more generous resection can be undertaken, leaving remnants that may be only 5×3×2 mm or about 25 mg in aggregate. If there is concern about viability or adequacy of parathyroid volume, or lack of cryopreservation, then the surgeon must estimate what "subtotal" degree of resection is best. In general, the aim is to leave remnants that might be equivalent to one normal parathyroid gland, significantly reducing the volume of abnormal glands which can be three- to tenfold hypertrophied.

The need for subtotal resections affects those patients with sporadic HPT, familial hyperparathyroidism and MEN, SHPT, and most patients with THPT. Cervical thymectomy is recommended for these patient groups, in order to remove small foci of ectopic parathyroid tissue in the thymus which are expected to be hyperplastic as well. The preferred surgery for those patients with primary sporadic hyperplasia or familial disease is subtotal parathyroidectomy that leaves a neck remnant in situ [40]. By contrast, patients with SHPT have benefited from total parathyroidectomy, leaving no residual parathyroid tissue, and near-total parathyroidectomy with extremely minimal amounts of tissue left in the neck or autotransplant sites [10, 11]. When there is concern to avoid any future re-operations in the neck, then autotransplantation into the brachioradialis muscle, especially in SHPT patients still undergoing dialysis, is convenient. Ideally, any of these operative interventions are accompanied by parathyroid cryopreservation.

Parathyroid Autotransplantation

This process of autotransplantation or autografting involves mincing parathyroid tissue into 2–3 mm fragments that are then inserted between muscle fibers or subcutaneous tissue pockets. They eventually become vascularized and function equally well to sense and regulate calcium balance from these new locations. This process is feasible using normal parathyroid tissue or benign hyperplastic tissue derived from multigland disease or single adenomas. Obviously, autografting too much tissue derived from a hyperplastic source is prone to regrowth and recurrent hyperparathyroidism that may require re-excision. Parathyroid autotransplantation is also the process by which patients who become severely hypocalcemic after parathyroid surgery can be rescued, provided they had autologous parathyroid tissue cryostored from the original surgery.

Parathyroid Cryopreservation

This process involves mincing excess parathyroid tissue obtained at the time of parathyroidectomy (Fig. 20.7) into 2–3 mm fragments which are then processed with serum and other protective substances for long-term storage at −80°F [15, 41]. They can be unthawed, prepared in a sterile fashion, and re-implanted into muscle or subcutaneous tissue. Viability tapers off with longer time in cryostorage, with decreasing chance of succesful grafting when using tissue stored for more than 2–3 years [42].

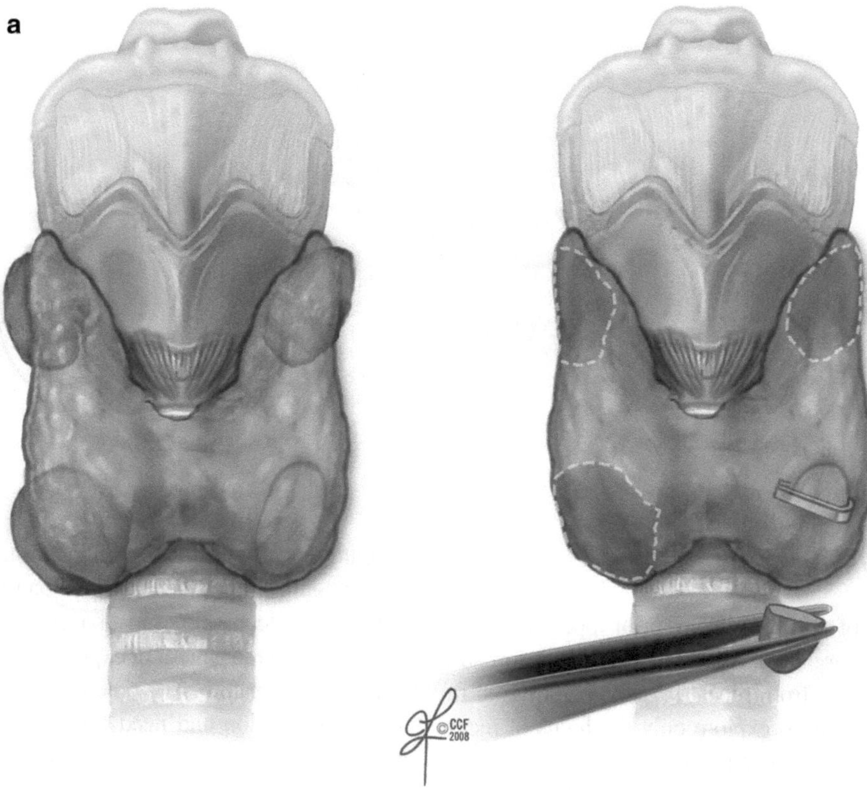

Fig. 20.7 Patients undergoing subtotal parathyroidectomy (**a**) benefit from parathyroid cryopreservation preparation (**b**) which may be needed for concomitant or later autotranplantation (**c**). (**a**) Reprinted with permission, Cleveland Clinic Center for Medical Art & Photography © 2008–2011. All Rights Reserved

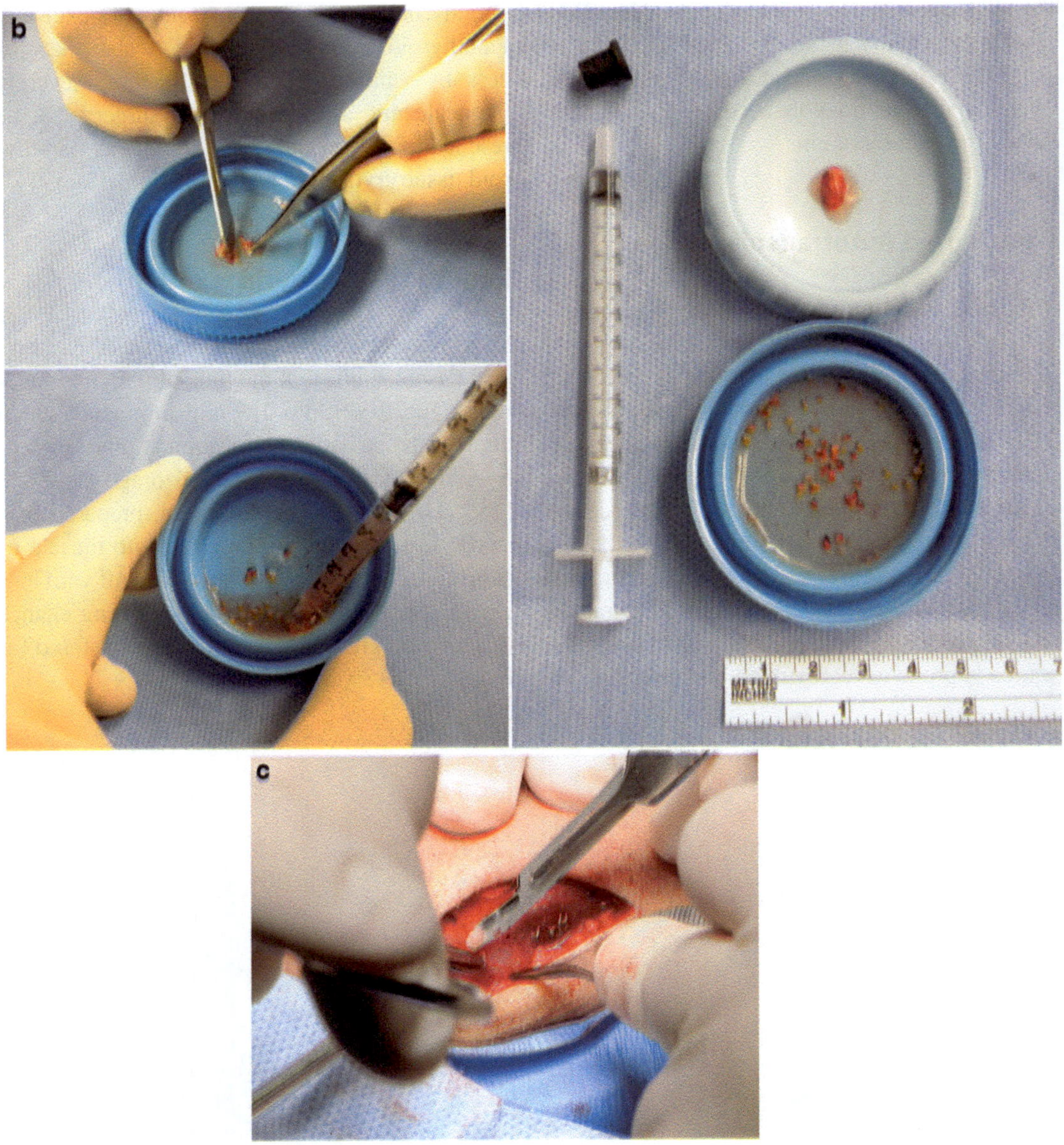

Fig. 20.7 (continued)

Parathyroid Re-operation

Because of scarring from prior operations that increases surgical risks and the potential to cause hypocalcemia from repeat surgery, parathyroid re-operations aim to explore only the focus of recurrent or missed parathyroid disease, rather than comprehensive bilateral dissection. Re-operations should not be embarked on without radiologic localization, and even the criteria for relying on imaging are stricter than at initial surgery: at least two imaging studies have to agree on the same site when a single parathyroid abnormality is anticipated or the same pattern of expected disease, if it is multigland in nature. The potential for parathyroid autotranplantation and need for parathyroid cryo-preservation is higher with re-operative surgery. A thoughtful, methodical, and detailed strategy is essential for treatment of patients with recurrent or persistent hyperparathyroidism [43–45].

Parathyroid Carcinoma

This has an incidence of less than 1% of all parathyroid operations and is not a multigland phenomenon. The surgery requires not just excision of the malignant parathyroid but also ipsilateral thyroid lobectomy and central neck dissection. It is not unusual for parathyroid cancer to invade the recurrent laryngeal nerve and have higher potential for postoperative hoarseness. In these cases, the decision to explore the contralateral parathyroids may be tempered by the need to avoid additional complications.

Concomitant Thyroid Surgery for Thyroid Disease

As many as 40% of patients with hyperparathyroidism may have co-existing thyroid disease, ranging from nonoperative conditions such as hypothyroidism and thyroiditis to nodular goiters (Fig. 20.8). This may become apparent preoperatively during examination or imaging, or intraoperatively. Use of neck ultrasound during parathyroid diagnostic evaluation allows identification of thyroid disease ahead of surgery and can identify more precisely those patients who may require partial or total thyroidectomy during the course of parathyroid surgery. A 4% incidence of previously undiagnosed thyroid cancer can be expected among patients undergoing parathyroid surgery [46–48].

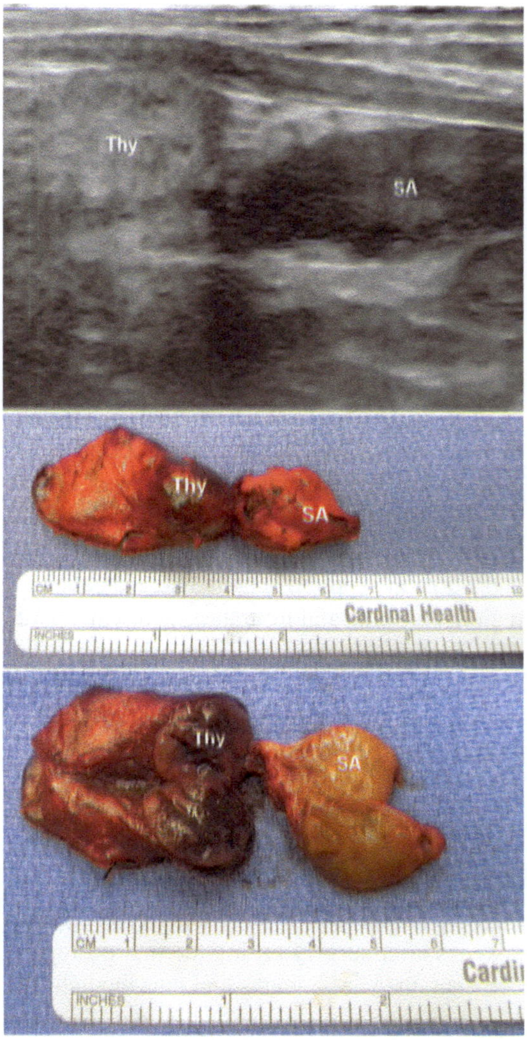

Fig. 20.8 Example of concomitant thyroid pathology in the form of a hyperplastic nodule (Thy) requiring thyroid lobectomy at the time of excision of large single parathyroid adenoma (SA). Both were evident on thyroid ultrasound

Perioperative Care

A thorough discussion of realistic benefits from parathyroid surgery and potential risks should precede any parathyroid operation. The overall risks associated with parathyroid surgery are small, and the aggregate of transient and permanent complications ought to be less than 5% [49, 50]. Infections occur exceptionally rarely with parathyroidectomy. Neck hematomas requiring operative evacuation and permanent hoarseness from recurrent laryngeal nerve injury should likewise be minimal (0.5–1%). There must be delicate tissue handling to avoid damage to normal parathyroids or disruption of abnormal glands. The actual tissue of these structures should never be grasped itself; rather, forceps and instruments should handle the surrounding fatty tissue, filmy adventitia, or vessels. Transient hypocalcemia can readily be treated with calcium and vitamin D supplements when there is a known sufficient quantity of residual parathyroid tissue. Long-term hypocalcemia becomes a greater risk (thought still rare at <1%) with subtotal or near-total excision of multigland parathyroid hyperplasia. The need to re-implant cryopreserved parathyroid tissue usually becomes evident within 6 months of surgery if the cervical remnants become nonfunctional. The potential for missed ectopic or supranumerary parathyroids and persistent or recurrent hyperparathyroidism (1–2%) should be discussed with patients before surgery to properly inform expectations of surgery.

Parathyroid surgery can be performed with local/regional anesthesia or a general anesthetic [2, 51]. Postoperative management as an inpatient hospitalization, outpatient visit or overnight observation is contingent on many factors, including the patient's type of parathyroid disease and overall health, the operation that was performed and surgeon's preference in management, and regional hospital and insurance requirements [2]. The incisional discomfort from parathyroid surgery is usually minimal and treated by over-the-counter analgesics. Recuperation with full return to normal activities and work occurs typically in a week. Long-term management relies on diligent monitoring of calcium and PTH levels to observe durable cure of hyperparathyroidism. A full biochemical panel that includes calcium, PTH, and vitamin D levels should be checked at 2 weeks after surgery during the first postoperative visit, then at 6 months and then annually for the remainder of the patient's lifetime. Transient SHPT from vitamin D deficiency in an otherwise cured patient can be seen in up to 20–30% of patients in the first year after surgery and requires reassurance (of both patient and referring physicians), treatment, and monitoring [52]. It is important to ensure that the patient receives adequate calcium and vitamin D supplementation after surgery. Minimal daily calcium carbonate or citrate supplementation is 500–600 mg taken 2–3 times daily. Depending on the degree of vitamin D deficiency, some patients may require over-the-counter supplements of 800–2,000 IU daily of vitamin D3 cholecalciferol, while others need a prescription-level strength such as 50,000 IU ergocalciferol weekly (for 25-hydroxyvitamin D <20 ng/ml) and very rarely 0.25 or 0.5 μg daily of calcitriol (for 1,25-dihydroxyvitamin D deficiency or significant hypocalcemic symptoms). These patients should be re-evaluated with blood tests at 3 months after surgery to determine the need for ongoing vitamin D supplementation. Durable cure after comprehensive parathyroidectomy means 95–98% success rate, with 2–5% of patients at risk to develop recurrent hyperparathyroidism.

Conclusion

Parathyroid surgery for hyperparathyroidism is a safe and effective strategy for durably reducing PTH hypersecretion and improving and/or reversing systemic consequences such as bone density loss and nephrocalcinosis. This overview provided a summary of currently available operative approaches for primary, secondary, and tertiary forms of hyperparathyroidism. Multidisciplinary communication is important at all phases of management, and is valuable postoperatively to know what type and extent of parathyroid surgery was performed. The expertise of a surgeon or specialized care for patients with parathyroid disease is associated with improved outcomes [50]. Parathyroid surgery remains the most effective method of treating hyperparathyroidism and can be accomplished with minimal morbidity. Long-term follow-up of patients who have been treated with parathyroidectomy is essential to monitor for successful maintenance of normal calcium balance and resolution of sequelae of hyperparathyroidism.

References

1. Mazzaglia PJ, Berber E, Kovach A, Milas M, Siperstein A. The changing presentation of hyperparathyroidism over three decades. Arch Surg. 2008;143: 260–6.
2. Greene A, Mitchell J, Davis R, Barbosa G, Tsinberg M, Berber E, et al. National trends in parathyroid surgery from 1997–2007: a decade of change. J Am Coll Surg. 2009;209:332–43.
3. Phitayakorn R, McHenry CR. Parathyroidectomy: overview of the anatomic basis and surgical strategies for parathyroid operations. Clin Rev Bone Miner Metabol. 2007;5(2):89–102.

4. Terris DJ, Stack Jr BC, Gourin CG. Contemporary parathyroidectomy: exploiting technology. Am J Otolaryngol. 2007;28(6):408–14.
5. Lew JI, Solorzano CC. Surgical management of primary hyperparathyroidism: state of the art. Surg Clin North Am. 2009;89(5):1205–25. Review.
6. Udelsman R, Pasieka JL, Sturgeon C, et al. Surgery for asymptomatic primary hyperparathyroidism: proceedings of the third international workshop. J Clin Endocrinol Metab. 2009;94(2):366–72.
7. AACE/AAES Task Force on Primary Hyperparathyroidism. The American Association of Clinical Endocrinologists and the American Association of Endocrine surgeons position statement on the diagnosis and management of primary hyperparathyroidism. Endocr Pract. 2005;11(1):49–54.
8. Bilezikian JP, Khan AA, Potts Jr JT. Guidelines for the management of asymptomatic primary hyperparathyroidism: summary statement from the third international workshop. third international workshop on the management of asymptomatic primary hyperthyroidism. J Clin Endocrinol Metab. 2009;94(2):335–9.
9. Wu B, Haigh PI, Hwang R, et al. Underutilization of parathyroidectomy in elderly patients with primary hyperparathyroidism. J Clin Endocrinol Metab. 2010;95(9):4324–30.
10. Pitt SC, Sippel RS, Chen H. Secondary and tertiary hyperparathyroidism, state of the art surgical management. Surg Clin North Am. 2009;89(5):1227–39.
11. Milas M, Weber CJ. Near-total parathyroidectomy is beneficial for patients with secondary and tertiary hyperparathyroidism. Surgery. 2004;136(6):1252–60.
12. Bilezikian JP, Potts Jr JT, Fuleihan G-H, et al. Summary statement from a workshop on asymptomatic primary hyperparathyroidism: a perspective for the 21st century. J Bone Miner Res. 2002;17 Suppl 2: N2–11.
13. Zanocco K, Angelos P, Sturgeon C. Cost-Effectiveness analysis of parathyroidectomy for asymptomatic primary hyperparathyroidism. Surgery. 2006;140(6): 874–81. discussion 881–2.
14. Wüthrich RP, Martin D, Bilezikian JP. The role of calcimimetics in the treatment of hyperparathyroidism. Eur J Clin Invest. 2007;37(12):915–22.
15. Ritter H, Milas M. Parathyroidectomy: bilateral neck exploration. In: Terris D, editor. Operative techniques in otolaryngology. St. Louis, MO: Elsevier; 2009. p. 44–53.
16. Ruda JM, Hollenbeak CS, Stack Jr BC. A systematic review of the diagnosis and treatment of primary hyperparathyroidism from 1995 to 2003. Otolaryngol Head Neck Surg. 2005;132(3):359–72.
17. Siperstein A, Berber E, Wagner K, Alghoul M, Stephen A, Milas M. Prospective evaluation of sestamibi, ultrasound, and rapid PTH to predict the success of limited exploration for sporadic primary hyperparathyroidism. Surgery. 2004;136:872–80.
18. Siperstein A, Berber E, Barbosa G, Tsinberg M, Greene A, Mitchell J, et al. Predicting success of limited exploration for 1o hyperparathyroidism using ultrasound, sestamibi scan, and intraoperative PTH: analysis of 1,055 cases. Ann Surg. 2008;248(3):420–8.
19. Moalem J, Guerrero M, Kebebew E. Bilateral neck exploration in primary hyperparathyroidism—when is it selected and how is it performed? World J Surg. 2009;33(11):2282–91.
20. Perrier ND, Edeiken B, Nunez R, Gayed I, Jimenez C, Busaidy N, et al. A novel nomenclature to classify parathyroid adenomas. World J Surg. 2009;33(3): 412–6.
21. Iacobone M, Mondi I, Viel G, Citton M, Tropea S, Frego M, et al. The results of surgery for mediastinal parathyroid tumors: a comparative study of 63 patients. Langenbecks Arch Surg. 2010;395(7):947–53.
22. Miccoli P. Parathyroid surgery: we only need a minimal surgical approach. J Endocrinol Invest. 2005; 28(6):570–3.
23. Seybt MW, Terris DJ. Minimally invasive thyroid and parathyroid surgery: where are we now and where are we going? Otolaryngol Clin North Am. 2010; 43(2):375–80.
24. Miccoli P, Berti P, Materazzi G, Ambrosini CE, Fregoli L, Donatini G. Endoscopic bilateral neck exploration versus quick intraoperative parathormone assay (qPTHa) during endoscopic parathyroidectomy: a prospective randomized trial. Surg Endosc. 2008; 22(2):398–400.
25. Lew JI, Irvin 3rd GL. Focused parathyroidectomy guided by intra-operative parathormone monitoring does not miss multiglandular disease in patients with sporadic primary hyperparathyroidism: a 10-year outcome. Surgery. 2009;146(6):1021–7.
26. Sugino K, Ito K, Nagahama M, Kitagawa W, Shibuya H, Ohkuwa K, et al. Minimally invasive surgery for primary hyperparathyroidism with or without intraoperative parathyroid hormone monitoring. Endocr J. 2010;57(11):953–8.
27. Milas M, Stephen A, Berber E, Wagner K, Miskulin J, Siperstein A. Ultrasound for the endocrine surgeon: a valuable clinical tool to enhance diagnostic and therapeutic outcomes. Surgery. 2005;138:1193–201.
28. Solorzano CC, Lee TM, Ramirez MC, Carneiro DM, Irvin GL. Surgeon-performed ultrasound improves localization of abnormal parathyroid glands. Am Surg. 2005;71(7):557–62. discussion 562–3.
29. Gurney TA, Orloff LA. Otolaryngologist—head and neck surgeon—performed ultrasonography for parathyroid adenoma localization. Laryngoscope. 2008; 118(2):243–6.
30. Sharma J, Mazzaglia P, Milas M, Berber E, Schuster D, Halkar R, et al. Radionuclide Imaging for hyperparathyrodism: which is the best ^{99}Tc-sestamibi modality? Surgery. 2006;140:856–65.
31. Rodgers SE, Hunter GJ, Hamberg LM, Schellingerhout D, Doherty DB, Ayers GD, et al. Improved preoperative planning for directed parathyroidectomy with 4-dimensional computed tomography. Surgery. 2006; 140(6):932–40. discussion 940–1.
32. Yen TW, Wang TS, Doffek KM, Krzywda EA, Wilson SD. Reoperative parathyroidectomy: an algorithm for

imaging and monitoring of intraoperative parathyroid hormone levels that results in a successful focused approach. Surgery. 2008;144(4):611–9. discussion 619–21.
33. Norman J, Politz D. 5,000 parathyroid operations without frozen section or PTH assays: measuring individual parathyroid gland hormone production in real time. Ann Surg Oncol. 2009;16(3):656–66.
34. Norman J, Politz D. Measuring individual parathyroid gland hormone production in real-time during radioguided parathyroidectomy. Experience in over 8,000 operations. Minerva Endocrinol. 2008;33(3):147–57.
35. Wineland A, Siegel E, Stack Jr BC. Reexamining normative radiation data for radioguided parathyroid surgery. Arch Otolaryngol Head Neck Surg. 2008; 134(11):1209–13.
36. Chen H. Radioguided parathyroid surgery. Adv Surg. 2004;38:377–92.
37. Olson J, Repplinger D, Bianco J, Chen H. Ex vivo radioactive counts and decay rates of tissues resected during radioguided parathyroidectomy. J Surg Res. 2006;136(2):187–91.
38. Chen H, Sippel RS, Schaefer S. The effectiveness of radioguided parathyroidectomy in patients with negative technetium tc 99 m-sestamibi scans. Arch Surg. 2009;144(7):643–8.
39. Landry CS, Grubbs EG, Morris GS, Turner NS, Holsinger FC, Lee JE, et al. Robot assisted transaxillary surgery (RATS) for the removal of thyroid and parathyroid glands. Surgery. 2011;149(4):549–55.
40. Melck AL, Carty SE, Seethala RR, Armstrong MJ, Stang MT, Ogilvie JB, et al. Recurrent hyperparathyroidism and forearm parathyromatosis after total parathyroidectomy. Surgery. 2010;148(4):867–73. discussion 873–5.
41. Cohen MS, Dilley WG, Wells Jr SA, Moley JF, Doherty GM, Sicard GA, et al. Long-term functionality of cryopreserved parathyroid autografts: a 13-year prospective analysis. Surgery. 2005;138(6):1033–40. discussion 1040–1.
42. Guerrero MA, Evans DB, Lee JE, Bao R, Bereket A, Gantela S, et al. Viability of cryopreserved parathyroid tissue: when is continued storage versus disposal indicated? World J Surg. 2008;32(5):836–9.
43. Richards ML, Thompson GB, Farley DR, Grant CS. Reoperative parathyroidectomy in 228 patients during the era of minimal-access surgery and intraoperative parathyroid hormone monitoring. Am J Surg. 2008; 196(6):937–42. discussion 942–3.
44. Henry JF. Reoperation for primary hyperparathyroidism: tips and tricks. Langenbecks Arch Surg. 2010;395(2):103–9.
45. Bonjer HJ, Bruining HA. Technique of parathyroidectomy. In: Clerk O, Duh Q, Kebebew E, editors. Textbook of endocrine surgery. 2nd ed. Philadelphia: W.B. Saunders; 2005. p. 439–48.
46. Gul K, Ozdemir D, Korukluoglu B, Ersoy PE, Aydin R, Ugras SN, et al. Evaluation of preoperative and postoperative thyroid pathologies in patients operated for primary hyperparathyroidism. Endocr Pract. 2009;24:1–18.
47. Morita SY, Somervell H, Umbricht CB, Dackiw AP, Zeiger MA. Evaluation for concomitant thyroid nodules and primary hyperparathyroidism in patients undergoing parathyroidectomy or thyroidectomy. Surgery. 2008;144(6):862–6. discussion 866–8.
48. Milas M, Alghoul M, Berber E, Stephen A, Mensah A, Siperstein A, et al. Impact of office neck ultrasonography on reducing unnecessary thyroid surgery in patients undergoing parathyroidectomy. Thyroid. 2005;15:1055–9.
49. Lew JI, Rivera M, Irvin 3rd GL, Solorzano CC. Operative failure in the era of focused parathyroidectomy: a contemporary series of 845 patients. Arch Surg. 2010;145(7):628–33.
50. Mitchell J, Milas M, Barbosa G, Sutton J, Berber E, Siperstein A. Avoidable reoperations for thyroid and parathyroid surgery: effect of hospital volume. Surgery. 2008;144(6):899–906. discussion 906–7.
51. Miccoli P, Barellini L, Monchik JM, Rago R, Berti PF. Randomized clinical trial comparing regional and general anesthesia in minimally invasive video-assisted parathyroidectomy. Br J Surg. 2005;92(7):814–8.
52. Carty SE, Roberts MM, Virji MA, Haywood L, Yim JH. Elevated serum parathormone level after "concise parathyroidectomy" for primary sporadic hyperparathyroidism. Surgery. 2002;132(6):1086–92. discussion 1092–3.

Index

A

Abnormal calcium
  hypercalcemia
    bisphosphonate therapy, 62
    bone radiographs, 58
    calcitonin, 62
    cinacalcet, 63
    DEXA, 58
    diagnostic approach, 56
    electrocardiography, 58
    FHH, 59
    gallium nitrate, 62
    glucocorticoid therapy, 63
    hypercalciuria, 60
    laboratory studies, 57–58
    MEN syndromes, 56
    parathyroid carcinoma, 63
    physical examination, 57
    plicamycin, 62
    primary hyperparathyroidism, 58–59
    PTH-independent hypercalcemia, 60–61
    saline hydration, 62
    symptoms, 55
    tertiary hyperparathyroidism, 59–60
    treatment, 61–62
  hypocalcemia
    differential diagnosis, 64–65
    laboratory studies, 64
    physical findings, 64
    symptoms, 63
    treatment of, 65–66
  serum calcium
    blood calcium, 55
    bone remodeling, 54
    CaSR signaling, 55
    intracellular signal, 54
    plasma proteins, 54
    PTH secretion, 55
Acidic serine and aspartate-rich motif (ASARM), 21
Acute hypocalcaemia, 275, 277
Adenomatous polyposis coli (APC), 168
α2-Heremans-Schmid glycoprotein (AHSG), 120
Akerstrom, G., 204, 205, 207
Albright, F., 315, 317
Alfacalcidol, 277, 307
Amifostine, 172
Amyloidosis, 279
Apolipoprotein E (ApoE), 120
Arch-Ferrer, J.E., 138
AREDIA®, 294
Argatroban, 134
Arteriolopathy, 122
Attie, M.F., 242
Atypical parathyroid adenomas, 254
AU-rich elements (AREs), 5
Autoimmune hypocalciuric hypercalcemia (AHH), 81, 241
Autoimmune polyendocrinopathy candidiasis ectodermal dystrophy (APECED) syndrome, 306
Autosomal disorder, 279
Autosomal dominant hypocalcemia (ADH), 304–305
Autosomal recessive hypophosphatemic rickets (ARHR), 39
Autotransplantation, 215

B

Barakat syndrome, 282, 304
Bartter syndrome, 31
Bastepe, M., 319
Beige, J., 91
Bergstrom, R., 204, 205
Bisphosphonate therapy, 62
Blomstrand lethal osteochondrodysplasia (BOCD), 185
Blomstrand's disease, 282–283
Bone dysplasia, 315
Bone morphogenic proteins (BMPs), 119, 120
Brachytelephalangy, 282
Bradley, K.J., 266
Breast cancer
  bone metastasis, 188, 189
  CaSR, 188
  connective tissue growth factor, 189

A.A. Licata and E.V. Lerma (eds.), *Diseases of the Parathyroid Glands*,
DOI 10.1007/978-1-4419-5550-0, © Springer Science+Business Media, LLC 2012

Breast cancer (*cont.*)
 immunohistochemistry PTHrP, 187
 osteolytic lesions, 187
 PTHrP secretion, 188
 TGFβ, 188
Breast carcinoma susceptibility (BRCA2), 161
Brennan, M.F., 93, 103
Broome, J.T., 219
Brown, E.M., 237, 242
Brown tumors, 257
Bryant, 114

C
Calabria, A.C., 253
Calcific uremic arteriolopathy (CUA)
 clinical manifestations
  calciphylactic lesions, 122–125
  comorbidities, 129–130
  demographic factors, 126–127
  diagnosis, 131–132
  laboratory abnormalities, 127–129
  medications, 130–131
  overview, 122
  prevention, 132–133
  treatment, 133–139
  uremic calciphylaxis, 125–126
 etiology and pathogenesis
  BMPs, 120
  Cbfa-1, 121
  extraskeletal calcium deposition, 116
  Fetuin-A, 120
  HPT, role of, 116–117
  hyperphosphatemia, role of, 117
  inorganic phosphorus, 121
  MGP, 119
  molecular factors, 118
  OPG, 119
  OPN, 121
  oxidative stress and inflammation, role of, 117–118
  proinflammatory cytokines, 121
  uremia, role of, 116
  vascular calcification, 115–116
 historical perspective, 114
 prevalence and mortality, 114–115
Calcilytics, 82, 84
Calcimimetics
 agents, 136
 NSHPT and FHH, 84
 primary and secondary hyperparathyroidism, 104
Calciphylactic lesions
 description, 122–123
 location and distribution, 122
 tissue ischemia and secondary infection, 123–125
Calciphylaxis
 comorbidities
  diabetes, 129
  HPT, 129
  hypercoaguable states, 129
  hypoalbuminemia, 129
  inflammatory diseases, 129–130
  liver disease, 130
  obesity, 129
  POEMS syndrome, 130
 demographic factors
  Caucasian race, 126
  female gender, 126–127
  younger age, 127
 diagnosis
  clinical diagnosis *vs.* biopsy, 131
  diagnostic imaging, 132
  histopathology, 131–132
 laboratory abnormalities
  elevated calcium-phosphorus product, 128
  elevated serum alkaline phosphatase, 128
  elevated serum aluminum, 128–129
  elevated serum PTH, 128
  hypercalcemia and vitamin D therapy, 127
  hyperphosphatemia, 127–128
 medications
  corticosteroid therapy, 130–131
  warfarin, 130
 prevention, 132–133
 prognosis, 138–139
 treatment
  anticoagulation, 137
  bisphosphonates, 137
  calcimimetic agents, 136
  corticosteroids, 137
  dialysis therapy, 134
  discontinuation, 134
  hyperbaric oxygen therapy, 138
  multidisciplinary approach, 133–134
  pain management, 138
  parathyroidectomy, 135–136
  phosphorus binders, 134–135
  sodium thiosulfate, 136–137
  wound management, 137–138
 uremia, 125–126
Calcitonin
 bone resorption, 37
 hydrocortisone, 172
 PHP-Ia, 317
Calcitriol
 bone remodeling, 36–37
 calcium absorption, 26
 FGF-23 expression, 21
 25-hydroxyvitamin D, 18–20, 277
 hypophosphatemia, 35
Calcium and phosphate metabolism
 adult humans, 15
 Bartter syndrome, 31
 β-glucuronidase activity, 31
 bone and cartilage, roles of, 34
 bone mineral hydroxyapatite, 14
 bone mineralization, 37–38
 bone resorption and regulation
  β-adrenergic signaling, 37
  calcitonin, 37

calcitriol, 36–37
estrogens, 37
osteocytes, 37
PTH-induced remodeling, 36
calcitriol and 25-hydroxyvitamin D
1α-hydroxylase expression, 18
CYP27B1, 19
D binding protein, 20
macronutrient digestion and absorption, 19
VDR, 20
calcitriol-dependent activation, 26
calcium-sensing mechanism, 22–23
calcium transport mechanisms
paracellular Ca^{2+} transport mechanisms, 23–25
transcellular Ca^{2+} transport mechanisms, 23
CaSR, 31
DCT and connecting tubules, 29
estrogens, 27
FGF-23 and Klotho, 20–22
hormonal regulation
claudins, 30
cTAL, 30
parathyroid hormone, 29–30
hydroxyapatite
calcium deficiency, 34–35
mineral metabolism, 34
phosphate deficiency, 35
inorganic phosphate transporters, 25
intestinal calcium absorption, 25–26
intestinal phosphate absorption, 27
intracellular and extracellular roles, 16
α-Klotho, 22
macronutrient-dependent stimulation
carbohydrates, 26–27
protein, 27
mineral-regulating hormones, 17
Npt2b expression, 27
osteoclast-specific ablation, 31
parathyroid hormone
bone formation and mineralization, 18
calcitriol, 17
chronic kidney disease, 17, 18
distal nephron, 17
hypocalcemia, 17
phosphatonin FGF-23, 18
serum phosphate levels, 18
phosphate-sensing mechanism, 23
proximal tubular phosphate transport
CaSR, 33
FGF-23 and α-Klotho, 32–33
PTH, 32
proximal tubule, 28
renal tubular calcium transport, 28
renal tubular phosphate transport, 31–32
rickets and osteomalacia, 38–39
secondary hyperparathyroidism, 30
small intestinal phosphate sensing, 33–34
thick ascending limb, 28
TRPV5, 30
Calcium-sensing receptor (CaSR)
autoimmune hypocalciuric hypercalcemia, 80–81
bone, 73
calcium homeostasis, 70–71
clinical features, 79
differential diagnosis, 80
etiology, 78–79
FHH, 78
genetics, 78–79
hypercalcemic disorders
activating mutations, 77–78
autoimmune hypocalciuric hypercalcemia, 81
clinical features, 79
differential diagnosis, 80
etiology, 78–79
FHH, 78
genetics, 78–79
inactivating mutations, 74–77
laboratory findings, 80
NSHPT, 80–81
pathogenesis, 78–79
treatment, 80
hypocalcemic disorders
autoimmune acquired hypoparathyroidism, 83
autosomal dominant hypocalcemia, 81
Bartter syndrome type V, 82–83
clinical features, 82
differential diagnosis, 82
etiology, 81–82
genetics, 81–82
laboratory findings, 82
pathogenesis, 81–82
pharmacological target, 83–84
polymorphic variants, 83
treatment, 82
inherited disorders, 73–78
kidney, 73
laboratory findings, 80
NSHPT, 80–81
parathyroid and C-cells, 73
pathogenesis, 78–79
structure and function of, 71–73
treatment, 80
cAMP response element (CRE), 182
Carcinoid tumors, 220
Cardiac arrhythmias, 64
Cardiomyopathy, 282
Carling, T., 254
Carpten, J.D., 262
Castanet, M., 289
Castleman, B., 165
Caudal pharyngeal complex, 204
Celiac disease, 290
Cellular hyperplasia, 290
Cervical thymectomy, 368, 370
Chakravarti, B., 179
Chattopadhyay, N., 179
Chloramphenicol acetyltransferase (CAT), 3
Cholecalciferol, 66, 277
Cholecystokinin secretion, 23
Chromosome 11p15, 279

Chronic kidney disease (CKD)
functional hyperplasia and hypertrophy, 92
late-stage, 127, 128
MBD, 94–95
phosphorus control, 104–105
ROD, 99
vitamin D deficiency, 101
Chvostek sign, 300
CINACALCET ®, 294
Coakley, A.J., 346
Computed tomography (CT)
4D-CT, 356–357
hounsfield unit, 353
parathyroid adenoma, 356, 359
parathyroid autotransplant, 353, 357
thin-slice contrast-enhanced imaging, 353
transverse contrast-enhanced CT image, 353, 358
Concomitant thyroid surgery, 375
Congenital ectopias
abnormal embryological migration, 205
ectopic mediastinal location, 207, 208
inferior parathyroid glands, 206
intrathyroid localization, 205, 206
reoperative parathyroid surgery, 206
ultimobranchial bodies fusion, 205–206
undescended parathyroid adenomas, 207
undescended PIII, 206, 207
Conigrave, A.D., 13
Core-binding factor α-1 (Cbfa-1), 121
Corticosteroids, 171
Crohn's disease, 280
Cryopreservation, 215
CUA. *See* Calcific uremic arteriolopathy (CUA)
Cystic parathyroid lesions (CPLs)
functional parathyroid cysts
clinical presentation, 152
diagnosis, 152–153
etiopathogeny, 151–152
management, 153–154
nonfunctional parathyroid cysts
clinical presentation, 148
diagnosis, 148–150
etiopathogeny, 151
management, 150–151

D
Demay, M., 3
Dendritic cell immunotherapy, 172
De Quervain, F., 158
Diabetes mellitus, 282, 283
DiGeorge syndrome, 64, 280, 302–303
1,25 Dihydroxy vitamin D, 278
Distal convoluted tubule (DCT), 22
Dual energy X-ray absorptiometry (DEXA), 58
Dwivedi, S.K.D., 179
Dysimmunity, 303

E
Ectopic parathyroid glands
congenital ectopias
abnormal embryological migration, 205
ectopic mediastinal location, 207, 208
inferior parathyroid glands, 206
intrathyroid localization, 205, 206
reoperative parathyroid surgery, 206
ultimobranchial bodies fusion, 205–206
undescended parathyroid adenomas, 207
undescended PIII, 206, 207
hyperfunctional parathyroid gland
diagnosis, 211
initial surgery, 214–215
localization, 211–213
reoperation, 214–215
surgery indications, 213–214
normal location, 204–205
supernumerary parathyroid glands, 205
acquired ectopias, 209–211
aorto-pulmonary window, 207–208
HPT syndrome, 207
intravagal parathyroid tissue, 209
parathyroid fragments, 207
paravagus complex, 209
vagus nerve, 208, 209
Egbuna, O.I., 237, 242
Eiken syndrome, 185
Ellsworth-Howard test, 317
Endocrinopathy, 274
End-stage renal disease (ESRD), 115
Epidermal growth factor receptors (EGFRs), 117
Ergocalciferol, 277
Ericsoussi, B., 123, 133
Estradiol, 194
Etiopathogeny
FPCs, 151–152
NFPCs, 151

F
Facial dysmorphia, 303
Familial hypocalciuric hypercalcemia (FHH)
CaSR, 238
clinical presentation
encephalitis, 244
family screening, 242
genetic screening, 243
heterozygous mutations, 244
homozygous/compound heterozygous mutations, 244
mutations screening, 243
parathyroid surgery, 243
presumably coincidental parathyroid adenoma, 243
Pro39Ala mutation, 244
Q459R mutation, 244
SPINK1 gene, 243
differential diagnoses, 246–247
epidemiology, 239

gene encoding mutation, 238
imaging studies, 245–246
laboratory evaluation, 244–245
mineral metabolism, 238
NSHPT, 238, 241
pathogenetic basis
AHH, 241
dimeric CaSR, 240
extracellular domains, 240
FBHOk, 239
gain-of-function mutations, 240
glucocorticoid therapy, 242
hypocalcemia, 241
linkage analysis, 239
missense mutations, 240
SNP, 241
pathophysiology, 242
prognosis, 248
treatment, 247–248
Familial isolated hyperparathyroidism (FIHP), 259
Farr syndrome, 301
Fetuin-A, 120
Fibroblast growth factor-23 (FGF-23), 16
Fine, A., 138
Fine needle aspiration (FNA), 148
Fluorode-oxyglucose positron emission tomography (FDG-PET), 165
Foley, T.P. Jr., 238
Four-dimensional computed tomography (4D-CT), 356–357
Frazer, J.E., 208
Functional parathyroid cysts (FPCs)
clinical presentation, 152
diagnosis, 152–153
etiopathogeny, 151–152
management, 153–154

G
Gaffney-Stomberg, E., 27
Galactorrhea, 222
Gallium nitrate, 172
Genomic hybridization technique, 294
GHRHoma, 220, 221
Gilmour, J.R., 208
Gipstein, R.M., 114
Glial Cell Missing B (GCMB) gene, 279, 303
Glucagonoma, 221
Glucocorticoid therapy, 242
Goris, D., 147
G-protein-coupled receptor (GPCR), 312
Guanine nucleotide binding protein (GNAS), 312–313

H
Haag, C., 69
Haemochromatosis, 279
Haploinsufficiency, 281
HaraldJueppner, 319
Hematuria, 290
Henry, J.-F., 147, 157, 203
Heparin-induced thrombocytopenia (HIT), 134
Heterotopic ossification, 316–317
Huang, 240
Human embryonic kidney (HEK), 6
Human T-cell leukemia virus type 1 (HTLV-1), 191
Humoral hypercalcemia of malignancy (HHM), 181
Hungry bone syndrome, 64, 170, 297
Hürthle cell thyroid adenoma, 259
Hydroxyl-tamoxifen, 194
Hypercalcemia
causes of
FHH, 59
primary hyperparathyroidism, 58–59
tertiary hyperparathyroidism, 59–60
diagnostic evaluation
bone radiographs, 58
DEXA, 58
electrocardiography, 58
laboratory studies, 57–58
history and physical examination
diagnostic approach, 56
MEN syndromes, 56
physical examination, 57
symptoms, 55
treatment
bisphosphonate therapy, 62
glucocorticoid therapy, 63
saline hydration, 62
vitamin D deficiency, 63
Hypercalciuria
primary hyperparathyroidism, 80, 256
PTH resistance, 320
renal complications, 256
serum calcium level, 66
Hyperfunctional parathyroid gland
diagnosis, 211
initial surgery, 214–215
localization, 211–213
reoperation, 214–215
surgery indications, 213–214
Hyperparathyroidism (HPT)
blood test, 59
calciphylaxis, 116–17
FHH, 59
jaw tumor syndrome (*see* Jaw tumor syndrome)
kidney transplantation, 102, 192, 203
MEN syndromes, 56
primary and secondary (*see* Primary and secondary hyperparathyroidism)
PTH-mediated hypercalcemia, 58
supernumerary parathyroids, 207
tertiary, 59–60
Hyperphosphatemia, 317
Hypertelorism, 303, 304
Hypocalcemia
diagnostic evaluation
differential diagnosis, 64–65
laboratory studies, 64
treatment, 65–66

Hypocalcemia (*cont.*)
history and physical examination
physical findings, 64
symptoms, 63
Hypogonadism, 222
Hypoparathyroidism
acute hypocalcaemia, 275, 277
autoimmune acquired hypoparathyroidism, 284
autosomal hypoparathyroidism, 279
Barakat syndrome, 282
Blomstrand's disease, 282–283
calcium homeostasis, 274, 276
calcium-sensing receptor abnormalities, 283–284
causes, 274
children
ADH, 304–305
anti-CaSR antibodies, 306
APECED syndrome, 306
biochemistry, 300–301
differential diagnosis, 307
DiGeorge syndrome, 302–303
etiologies, 302, 305–307
GCMB, 303
gene mutation, 305
HDR syndrome, 304
HRD syndrome, 304
maternal hyperparathyroidism, 306
mitochondrial diseases, 305–306
parathyroid glands, impaired embryonic development, 302
radiological findings, 301
surgery, 306
symptoms, 300
treatment, 307–308
X-linked recessive transmission, 304
clinical features, 274–275, 277
complex syndromes, 280
deafness, 281
DiGeorge syndrome, 280
hypocalcaemic symptoms, 280
hypomagnesaemia, 280
inherited forms and chromosomal locations, 274, 275
isolated hypoparathyroidism, 279
Kenney–Caffey syndromes, 282
Kirk-Richardson syndromes, 282
mitochondrial disorders, 281–282
neonatal hypoparathyroidism, 280
persistent hypocalcaemia, 277–279
pluriglandular autoimmune, 283
renal anomalies syndrome, 281
Sanjad–Sakati syndromes, 282
X-linked recessive hypoparathyroidism, 279
Hypoparathyroidism retardation dysmorphism (HRD) syndrome, 304
Hypophosphatemia, 16
Hypotonia, 290

I

Iacobone, M., 147, 157, 203
Ibandronate, 137
Imaging, parathyroid diseases
anatomic and functional imaging techniques, 344
computed tomography
4D-CT, 356–357
hounsfield unit, 353
parathyroid adenoma, 356, 359
parathyroid autotransplant, 353, 357
thin-slice contrast-enhanced imaging, 353
transverse contrast-enhanced CT image, 353, 358
magnetic resonance imaging, 357–358, 360
minimally invasive parathyroid surgery, 344–345
parathyroid anatomy, embryology, and histology, 345
parathyroid scintigraphy
false-negative dual-phase sestamibi scan, 348, 349
lesion size, 351
oxyphil cells, 348, 350
P-glycoprotein, 350
selenium-75-methionine, 348
single-isotope double-phase technique, 348
SPECT, 350
subtraction imaging, 350
Tc-99m sestamibi, 348
thallium-201, 348
true-positive double-phase sestamibi scan, 348, 349
SPECT/CT
anterior superior mediastinum, parathyroid adenoma, 352, 354
aortopulmonary window, parathyroid adenoma, 352, 355
ectopic pericardial parathyroid adenoma, 352, 356
posterior mediastinum, parathyroid adenoma, 352, 355
retroesophageal parathyroid adenoma, 352, 353
sestamibi-avid soft tissue nodule, parathyroid adenoma, 351, 352
Tc-99m sestamibi scanning, 351–352
tissue attenuation correction, 351
tracheoesophageal groove , parathyroid adenoma, 352, 353
undescended parathyroid adenoma, 352
ultrasonography
advantages, 345
color Doppler sonography, 346
ectopic locations, 347
homogeneous hypoechoic texture, 346, 347
hyperechoic rim of adventitia, 346, 347
microcalcifications, 346
preoperative localization, parathyroid adenomas, 345
transverse and longitudinal ultrasonographic views, 346
ultrasound-guided fine-needle aspiration biopsy, 347
Immunochemiluminometric assay (ICMA), 58
Inabnet, W.B., 338
Indian hedgehog (Ihh), 185
Infiltrating metastase, 279
Insulinoma, 221, 222
Intracystic tetracycline injection, 150
In vitro degradation assay (IVDA), 5
Isolated albright osteodystrophy, 318

J

Jackson, C.E., 257
Jaw tumor syndrome
  axial and coronal, 257, 258
  brown tumors, 257
  calcium homeostasis, 259, 260
  CASR gene, 260, 261
  cemento-ossifying fibroma, 257, 258
  clinical genetic testing, 254
  clinical presentation, 256
  diagnostic evaluation
    additional baseline testing, 266
    gene sequencing and screening, 266
    preoperative imaging, 264–265
    primary hyperparathyroidism, 264, 265
    screening recommendations, 266–277
  fibro-osseous lesions, 257
  FIHP, 259
  history, 256–257
  kidney involvement, 258–259
  maxillary and mandibular tumors, 257
  parafibromin and HRPT2 gene
    apoptosis, 263
    cell division cycle 7 mutation, 261
    chromosomal map location, 261
    C-terminal domain, 263
    DNA sequence analysis, 261
    gene silencing, 262
    immunohistochemical analysis, 262
    Knudson's two-hit model, 262
    parathyroid tumorigenesis, 262
    PCR-based analysis, 262
    PGP9.5, diffuse positive staining, 262
    polymerase-associated factor 1, 263
    somatic and germ line mutations, 263
    sporadic parathyroid carcinomas, 263
    tumor suppressor, 262
    Wnt signaling pathway, 263
  pathophysiology, 255–256
  primary hyperparathyroidism, familial forms, 254
  RET proto-oncogene, 261
  sporadic disorder, 254
  treatment, 267–269

K

Kaplan, F.S., 318
Kato, S., 3
Kearns–Sayre syndrome (KSS), 281, 305
Kenney–Caffey syndromes, 282
Ketoconazole, 307
Keutel syndrome, 119
Kirk-Richardson syndromes, 282
Knudson's two-hit model, 262
Kocher's incision, 102

L

Lactic acidosis, 282
Lakhani, V.T., 219
Lamesch, P., 91
Laryngospasm, 300
Lehmann, G., 99, 100
Leptin, 127
Lerma, E.V., 113
Levine, M.A., 253
Lienhardt-Roussie, A., 299
Linglart, A., 299, 311
Lithiasis, 307
Lithium therapy, 59
Liu, S.M., 3
Lorenz, K., 102
Low-density lipoprotein (LDL), 120
Lung cancer, 191
Lymphoedema, 276, 280

M

Magnetic resonance imaging (MRI), 164, 357–358, 360
Malabsorption syndromes, 290
Mallet, E., 289, 311
Mallette, L.E., 256
Malmaeus, J., 204, 205
Mantovani, G., 319
Marx, S.J., 238
Masi, G., 263
Maternal hyperparathyroidism, 306
Matrix extracellular phosphoglycoprotein (MEPE), 28
Matrix Gla protein (MGP), 119
Matrix metalloproteinase (MMP), 190
Mayer, A., 306
MELAS syndrome, 281, 282
MEN 2
  clinical presentation, 229
  diagnosis, 230–231
  epidemiology, 228
  imaging studies, 231
  laboratory evaluation, 229–230
  MEN 2A, 228–229
  MEN 2B, 229
  prognosis, 231–232
  treatment, 231
Menin, 222
Menorrhagia, 259
Mibi scans, 338
MIBI scintigraphy, 294
Microcephaly, 303
Microcyst theory, 151
Micrognathia, 303, 304
Mihai, R., 97
Milas, M., 323, 363
Milas, Z.L., 323, 363
Milk-alkali syndrome, 61
Millot, J., 158
Minimal invasive parathyroidectomy (MIP), 295
Mithal, A., 179
Mitochondrial trifunctional protein deficiency syndrome, 281–282
Mouallem, M., 317
99mTectnetium-methylene diphosphonate (99mTe-MDP), 132
Multigland parathyroid hyperplasia, 330, 336

Multiple endocrine neoplasia (MEN)
definition, 220
MEN 1 (*see* Wermer syndrome)
MEN 2 (*see* MEN 2)MEN 4, 232

N
National Cancer Data Base, 158
Naveh-Many, T., 1
Nechama, M., 1
Necrolytic migratory erythema, 221
Neonatal hypoparathyroidism, 280
Neonatal severe hyperparathyroidism (NSHPT), 238
Nephrocalcinosis, 307
Nephrolithiasis, 279, 291
Nephrotic syndrome, 64
Neumann, D.R., 343
Neuroendocrinopathies, 293
Neuromuscular irritability, 300
Nonfunctional neuroendocrine tumors, 221
Nonfunctional parathyroid cysts (NFPCs)
clinical presentation, 148
diagnosis, 148–150
etiopathogeny, 151
management, 150–151
Nuclear localization sequence (NLS), 181

O
Octreotide, 172
Oklahoma variant (FBHOk), 239
Ophthalmoplegia, 282
Opossum kidney (OK), 3
Orthopantomographic X-ray, 159
Osteoma cutis, 316–317
Osteomalacia, 38–39, 100
Osteopontin (OPN), 121
Osteoprotegerin (OPG), 36, 119
Osteosclerosis, 282
Osteostatin, 181
Osterix (OSX), 39
Oxygen therapy, 124

P
Pancreatic islets, 187
Papillary thyroid cancer (PTC), 331, 337
Papilloedema, 275
Parafibromin, 159
Parathormone resistance, children
GNAS, 312–313
PHP (*see* pseudohypoparathyroidism)
PTHR1 signaling, 312
treatment, 320
Parathyroid carcinoma
clinical features, 163
clinical presentation, 161–162
diagnosis, 162
epidemiology, 158
etiopathogenesis
BRCA2 gene, 161
CT scan, 160
cyclin D1, 161
end-stage renal disease, 158
hemodialysis, 158
heterozygosity, 161
HRPT2 mutations, 160
hyperparathyroidism, 158
jaw tumor syndrome, 159
menin, 160
neck irradiation, 158
orthopantomographic X-ray, 159
parafibromin, 159
p53 expression, 161
retinoblastoma, 161
sporadic parathyroid carcinomas, 160
imaging techniques, 164–165
intraoperative diagnosis, 165
laboratory studies, 163–164
medical and adjuvant treatments, 171–172
postoperative diagnosis
APC expression, 168
atypical parathyroid adenoma, 167
degenerative changes, 166
electron microscopy, 168
histopathological findings, 165
immunohistochemical staining, 168
mitotic activity, 165
parathyromatosis, 167
vascular invasion, 167
preoperative diagnosis, 162–163
prognosis, 168–169
surgical treatment, 169–171
Parathyroidectomy, 238, 241
Parathyroid hormone (PTH)
AUF1, 6
FGF23, 9–10
IVDA, 5
KSRP, 7
lanthanum carbonate (La), 4
$1,25(OH)_2$ vitamin D (1,25D)
bovine parathyroid cells, 2
calreticulin, 3
chloramphenicol acetyltransferase, 3
CKD, 4
opossum kidney, 3
serum calcium, 2
VDRE, 3
oral Pi binders, 4
secondary hyperparathyroidism, 7–8
serum phosphate (Pi), 2
untranslated regions (UTRs), 5
up-stream of N-ras (Unr), 6
Parathyroid hormone-related peptide (PTHrP)
biochemical features, 181
breast cancer, 187–189
cardiovascular system, 186–187
cartilage development, 185–186
ectopic sources, 191–192
hematological malignancies, 190–191

lung cancer, 191
mammary gland development, 184
pancreatic islets, 187
pathophysiological role, 187
physiological roles, 183
pregnancy and lactation, 184
prostate cancer, 189–190
regulation of
androgens, 194
calcium homeostasis, 193
cAMP responsive element, 192
CpG islands, 194
DNA methylation, 194
Ets binding site, 192
glucocorticoids, 194
hypercalcemia, 192
Ras-MAPK pathway, 192
retinoid-X-receptor, 193
schematic representations, 193
testosterone, 194
TGFβ, 192
VDRE, 193
renal carcinoma, 191
signaling aspects, 181–183
Parathyroid scintigraphy
false-negative dual-phase sestamibi scan, 348, 349
lesion size, 351
oxyphil cells, 348, 350
P-glycoprotein, 350
selenium-75-methionine, 348
single-isotope double-phase technique, 348
SPECT, 350
subtraction imaging, 350
Tc-99m sestamibi, 348
thallium-201, 348
true-positive double-phase sestamibi scan, 348, 349
Parathyroid surgery, 243
abnormal parathyroid glands, 365, 367
autotransplantation, 373
carcinoma, 375
cervical thymectomy, 368, 370
concomitant thyroid surgery, 375
cryopreservation, 373–374
durable normocalcemic state, 364
ectopic mediastinal/cervical parathyroid abnormalities, 365
evolution, 363–364
hereditary syndromes, 372
indications, 364–365
injury avoidance, laryngeal nerves, 364
minimally invasive surgery, 369
mortality, 364
multigland hyperplasia, 365
"negative" imaging, 365
normal parathyroid glands, 365, 366
operative finding, 368
parathyroid hyperplasia, 365, 367
perioperative care, 375–376
postoperative morbidity, 364
preoperative imaging, 365
primary parathyroid survey, 365
re-operation, 374
retroesophageal area, parathyroid abnormalities, 368, 369
secondary parathyroid survey, 366, 369
single adenoma, 365, 367
subtotal parathyroid resections, 372–373
surgical options
bilateral exploration, 369–371
endoscopic and videoscopic equipment, 372
endoscopic tools, 372
focal exploration, 371
limited parathyroid exploration, 371
radioguidance, 371
robotic technology, 372
Parathyroid ultrasound
abnormal parathyroid disease entities
ectopic parathyroid adenoma, 330, 337
intrathyroidal cysts, 331, 337
Mibi scan, 338
multigland parathyroid hyperplasia, 330, 336
parathyroid cancer, 330, 336
PTC, 331, 337
abnormal parathyroid sonographic features
"fingertip" curvilinear prob, 328, 331
hypoechoic density, 329, 335
sclerotic changes and calcification, 328, 331–332
teardrop shape, 328, 330
triangularization, central neck, 329, 335
triple circle sign, 329, 333, 334
vascular pedicle, 328–329, 333
advantages, 324
clinical management
advantages, 336, 338
ethanol injection, 335
focal parathyroid exploration, 332
Mibi scan, 338
minimally invasive parathyroid surgery, 332
negative ultrasound, 332
radiation risks, 334
recurrent hyperparathyroidism, 334
re-operative setting, 338
secondary and tertiary hyperparathyroidism, 338
surgical management plan, 332
equipment and technique, 325–326
parathyroid anatomy, 327–328
Parental imprinting, 312–313
Peripheral vascular disease (PVD), 131
Persistent hypocalcaemia, 277–279
P-glycoprotein, 350
Pheochromocytoma, 228–230
Philtrum, 303
Phospholipase C (PLC), 182
Pigmentary retinopathy, 282
Plöthner, J., 95
Plötner, A., 92, 107
POEMS syndrome, 130
Polyuropolydipsic syndrome, 290
Porter, S.E., 183
pPHP. *See* Pseudopseudohypoparathyroidism (pPHP)

Primary and secondary hyperparathyroidism
biochemical fine needle aspiration, 100
bone disorder, CKD-MBD, 94–95
calciphylaxis, 95–96
clinical course, 96
diagnostic techniques
bone disease assessment, 98–100
imaging, 96–98
laboratory techniques, 98
history, 96
jugular venous sampling, 100
pathophysiology and epidemiology
dead bone disease, 94
endocrinological disorders, 92
glomerular fiiltration rate, 93
healthy kidneys, 92
hypercalcemia, 92
mineral metabolism, 94
phosphaturia, 93
serum phosphorus elevation, 93
vitamin D receptor, 94
physical findings, 96
treatment
bone metabolism, 105–106
calcimimetics, 104
CKD, 104–105
dialysis techniques, 101
integrative CKD-MBD therapy, 106–107
operative technique, 102–103
parathyroidectomy, 101–102
parathyroid tissue, 103
vitamin D analogues, 101
Primary parathyroid (HP1) disorder
adolescents, 290–291
biological data, 291–292
children, 290–291
medical treatment, 294
preoperative investigations, 294–295
surgical treatment, 295–297
etiologies
familial hypocalciuric hypercalcemia, 292–293
hereditary forms, 292
HPT-JT syndrome, 293
neuroendocrinopathies, 293
primary parathyroid adenoma, 294
neonatal, 290, 291
Prolactinoma, 220, 222
Prostate cancer, 189–190
Protein kinase C (PKC), 182
Pseudo-Bartter syndrome, 305
Pseudohypoparathyroidism (PHP), 284–285, 312
isolated albright osteodystrophy, 318
PHP-Ib, 318–320
type I, 313, 314
type Ia
ACTH resistance, 317
antiadipogeneic effect, 316
A366S mutation, 317
bone dysplasia, 315
brachydactyly, 315
brachymetacarpy, 315
Ellsworth-Howard test, 317
epinephrine resistance, 316
gonadotropin signal, 317
Gsa, mono-or biallelic transcription, 313
heterotopic ossification, 316
isoleucine deletion, 318
PTHLH, 315
rheumatologic complications, 315
symptomatic hypocalcemia, 317
Pseudopseudohypoparathyroidism (pPHP), 318–320
PTH gene mutation, 279

Q
Quick parathyroid hormone (QPTH), 153

R
Raue, F., 69
Receptor activator of nuclear factor-kB (RANK), 118
Recklinghausen's disease, 158
Renal anomalies syndrome, 281
Renal carcinoma, 191
Renal dysplasia, 281
Renal osteodystrophy (ROD), 94, 117
Reoperative parathyroid surgery, 226–227
RET codon 634 mutations, 228–229
Retinoblastoma (Rb), 161
Rickets, 38–39, 290
Rudolph, E.H., 113
Russell, J., 3

S
Sainton, P., 158
Sandstrom, I., 147
Sanjad–Sakati syndrome, 282, 304
Sarcoidosis, 279
Schantz, A., 165
Sela-Brown, A., 3
Selective estrogen receptor modulators (SERMs), 37
Selective venous sampling (SVS), 211, 213
Selenium-75-methionine, 348
Selye, H., 114, 116, 125, 128
Sensorineural deafness, 281, 282
Serine 193 (S193), 8
Sestamibi scintigraphy, 164
Shin, J.J., 343
Single nucleotide polymorphisms (SNP), 241
Single photon emission computerized tomography/Computed tomography (SPECT/CT)
anterior superior mediastinum, parathyroid adenoma, 352, 354
aortopulmonary window, parathyroid adenoma, 352, 355
ectopic pericardial parathyroid adenoma, 352, 356
posterior mediastinum, parathyroid adenoma, 352, 355
retroesophageal parathyroid adenoma, 352, 353
sestamibi-avid soft tissue nodule, parathyroid adenoma, 351, 352
Tc-99m sestamibi scanning, 351–352

tissue attenuation correction, 351
tracheoesophageal groove, parathyroid adenoma, 352, 353
undescended parathyroid adenoma, 352
Sipple syndrome, 228–229, 293
Small integrin-binding ligand N-linked glycoproteins (SIBLInGs), 21
Somatostatinoma, 221
Sporadic parathyroid carcinomas, 160
Strewler, G.J., 245
Subcapsular cataract, 275
Subtotal parathyroid resections, 372–373
Supernumerary parathyroid glands, 205
acquired ectopias, 209–211
aorto-pulmonary window, 207–208
HPT syndrome, 207
intravagal parathyroid tissue, 209
parathyroid fragments, 207
paravagus complex, 209
vagus nerve, 208, 209

T
Tachyphylaxis, 62
Taillefer, R., 348
Tamoxifen, 194
Technetium-99 m sestamibi, 164
Tetany, 277
Thakker, R.V., 273, 277
Thallium-201, 348
Thallium/Tc scintigraphy, 294
Thiazide diuretics, 82
Thick ascending limb (TAL), 28
Threonine residue 692 (T692), 8
Thymic parathyroids, 204
Tissue nonspecific alkaline phosphatase (TNAP), 38
Tonelli, M., 105
Transforming growth factor-alpha (TGF-α), 117
Trousseau sign, 300
Tsukazaki, 183
Tubulin specific Chaperone E (TBCE) gene, 304
Tumor lysis syndrome, 65

U
Udelsman, R., 254
Ultrasonography
advantages, 345
color Doppler sonography, 346
ectopic locations, 347
homogeneous hypoechoic texture, 346, 347
hyperechoic rim of adventitia, 346, 347
microcalcifications, 346
preoperative localization, parathyroid adenomas, 345
transverse and longitudinal ultrasonographic views, 346
ultrasound-guided fine-needle aspiration biopsy, 347
Undescended parathyroid adenomas, 207
Uremia, 116
Urinary calcium, 301, 304, 305, 307
US National Library of Medicine, 324
Uterine tumors, 259

V
Various congenital cardiac malformations, 303
Vascular calcification
active mechanisms, 115–116
BMPs, 120
Cbfa-1, 121
ESRD, 115
extraskeletal calcium deposition, 115–116
Fetuin-A, 120
HPT, 116–117
hyperphosphatemia, 117
inorganic phosphorus, 121
MGP, 119
molecular factors, 118
OPG, 119
OPN, 121
oxidative stress and inflammation, 117–118
proinflammatory cytokines, 121
uremia, 116
Vascular endothelial growth factor (VEGF), 130
Vascular smooth muscle cells (VSMCs), 186
Vasoactive intestinal peptide, 221–222
VIPoma, 220–222
Vitamin D-responsive element (VDRE), 193

W
Wells, S.A. Jr., 103
Wermer syndrome
clinical presentation, 221–222
diagnosis, 222–223
differential diagnosis, 223
epidemiology, 220
hyperparathyroidism, 220–221
imaging studies, 223–224
laboratory evaluation, 222
prognosis, 228
treatment
complications, 224
hypo and hyperparathyroidism, 226
initial surgery, 224–225
medical management, 227
reoperative parathyroid surgery, 226–227
surgical intervention, 224
total and subtotal parathyroidectomy, 225–226
White, 114
Wilson's disease, 280

X
X-linked hypophosphatemia (XLH), 20

Y
Yamashita, Y., 258

Z
Zaidi, S.S., 219
Zolendronate, 171
Zollinger-Ellison syndrome, 220, 221